Essentials for Aesthetic Dermatology in Ethnic Skin

This book focuses on creating awareness and detailing the nuances of aesthetic dermatology practice in skin of color. It highlights practical considerations in pre-/intra-/post-procedure care with an emphasis on patient selection for aesthetic procedures and the associated challenges involved in real-time practice. It aims to cater to audiences of countries with both high and low populations of dark-skinned patients, as clinicians often have limited experience in treating this group. Numerous topics are explored through case-based discussions and practical tips. This is a practical ready reference manual for a cosmetic dermatologist dealing with darker skin.

Key Features

- Covers the geo-ethnic skin types of Asians, Southeast Asians, Africans, and Hispanics
- Explores the topics through case-based discussions
- Provides comprehensive details about the use of machines on skin of color

Essentials for Aesthetic Dermatology in Ethnic Skin
Practice and Procedure

Edited by

Mukta Sachdev, MD
Head of Department and Consultant Dermatologist
Manipal Hospitals, Bangalore, India
Director, MS Skin Centre, Bangalore, India

Niti Khunger, MD, DDV, DNB
Professor and Consultant Dermatologist
VM Medical College
Safdarjung Hospital
New Delhi, India

Junior Editor
Ninon Patrao
Department of Dermatology
Manipal Hospitals
Bangalore, India

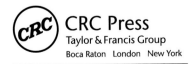

CRC Press
Taylor & Francis Group
Boca Raton   London   New York

CRC Press is an imprint of the
Taylor & Francis Group, an **informa** business

First edition published 2023
by CRC Press
6000 Broken Sound Parkway NW, Suite 300, Boca Raton, FL 33487–2742

and by CRC Press
4 Park Square, Milton Park, Abingdon, Oxon, OX14 4RN

CRC Press is an imprint of Taylor & Francis Group, LLC

© 2023 Taylor & Francis Group, LLC

ISBN: 978-0-367-19857-2 (hbk)
ISBN: 978-1-032-46015-4 (pbk)
ISBN: 978-0-429-24376-9 (ebk)

DOI: 10.1201/9780429243769

Typeset in Warnock Pro
by Apex CoVantage, LLC

I wish to dedicate this book to Dev and Dr. Rani Bhardwaj, my wonderful parents who left us during the pandemic—my source of love, support, and constant inspiration.

My big thank you always to my husband, Rohit, and my lovely boy, Aahan, who support my choices and endeavors with the greatest of enthusiasm, which allows me to constantly grow and aspire to new heights. Thank you always.

Mukta Sachdev

CONTENTS

PART III: COSMECEUTICALS

Contents

ACKNOWLEDGMENTS

We sincerely thank all the contributing authors for their efforts and patience in submitting chapters during the past challenging COVID-19 pandemic period.

Dr. Niti and I would both like to acknowledge Dr. Ninon Patrao, the junior editor, whose tireless efforts and persistence have culminated in this wonderful manual, which we hope will be a valuable tool for all readers.

I would like to dedicate this to my late parents, both of whom I lost during the pandemic and whose support and encouragement have been my inspiration to achieve and continue to learn.

EDITORS

Mukta Sachdev, MD, is Head of the Department and Consultant Dermatologist at Manipal Hospitals, Bangalore, and Director of the MS Skin Centre, Bangalore. She has numerous academic and professional achievements to her credit and has been an invited speaker and training faculty at various national and international conferences. She has also authored textbooks and publications and has been an investigator and consultant with several clinical trials.

Niti Khunger, MD, DDV, DNB, is presently Professor and Consultant Dermatologist at VM Medical College, Safdarjang Hospital, New Delhi, India. She completed her graduation and postgraduation at Grant Medical College, Mumbai. She was Editor in Chief of the *Journal of Cutaneous & Aesthetic Surgery* (2014–2017) and President of the Association of Cutaneous Surgeons of India (2007–2008). She has edited books on chemical peels, acne scars, cosmeceuticals, and cosmetic dermatology and dermatosurgery. She is the recipient of the Dr. PN Behl Oration Award in Dermatosurgery (2014) and the Prof. K. C. Kandhari Award for Best Dermatologist (2015).

Ninon Patrao, MD, completed her graduate and postgraduate training at Father Muller Medical College, Mangalore, and is currently working in the Department of Dermatology at Manipal Hospitals, Bangalore. She has actively participated in various conferences and workshops and has been involved academically with many publications to her credit.

CONTRIBUTORS

Pooja Agarwal, MD
Associate Professor
Department of Dermatology
SVPIMSR Hospital
NHL Municipal Medical College
Ahmedabad, India

Sandip Agrawal, MD
Department of Dermatology
LTMMC and GH
Mumbai, India

Awa Bakayoko
Lewis Katz School of Medicine at Temple University
Philadelphia, PA

Eliot Battle MD
Department of Dermatology
Howard University College of Medicine
and
Cultura Dermatology and Laser Center
Washington, DC

Valerie D. Callender
Howard University College of Medicine
Washington, DC
and
Callender Dermatology & Cosmetic Center
Glenn Dale, MD

Charvi Chanana, MD
VM Medical College & Safdarjang Hospital
New Delhi, India

Vandana Chatrath, MD
Vanila Dermologie
New Delhi, India

Banani Choudhury, MD, DNB, MNAMS
Sir HN Reliance Foundation Hospital and Research Centre
Jaslok Hospital and Research Centre
Mumbai, India

Sandeep Cliff, FRCP
East Surrey Hospital
Surrey, UK

Abirami Pararajasingam
East Surrey Hospital
Surrey, UK

Libin Mathew
East Surrey Hospital
Surrey, UK

Jennifer David, DO, MBA
Skin & Scripts Virtual Dermatology
Philadelphia, PA

Seemal R. Desai, MD, FAAD
Innovative Dermatology
Havertown, PA
and
Department of Dermatology
University of Texas Southwestern Medical
    Center
Dallas, TX

Rachita Dhurat, MD
Department of Dermatology
LTMMC and GH
Mumbai, India

Christine Dierickx
Skinperium
Luxembourg

Zoe Diana Draelos, MD
Dermatology Consulting Services, PLLC
High Point, NC

Sahar Ghannam, MD, PhD
Sahar Polyclinic
Salmiya, Kuwait
and
Department of Dermatology and
    Venereology
University of Alexandria
Alexandria, Egypt

Michael H. Gold, MD
Gold Skin Care
Tennessee Clinical Research Center
Nashville, TN

Kimberly A. Huerth, MD, MEd
Gateway Aesthetic Institute and Laser Center
Salt Lake City, UT

Natthachat Jurairattanaporn, MD, MSc
Ramathibodi University Hospital
Mahidol University
Bangkok, Thailand

**Bhavjit Kaur, MS, DNB, DRCOG,
DFSRH**
Health & Aesthetic Clinic
London, UK

Kaleem Khan, MD
Wockhardt Hospital and
Skin Indulgence Clinic
Andheri, Mumbai, India

Ayushi Khandelwal, MD
M. S. Skin Centre
Bangalore, India

Contributors

Meenaz Khoja, MD
Joshi Hospital and Ruby Hall Clinic
Pune, India

Niti Khunger, MD, DDV, DNB
VM Medical College & Safdarjang
   Hospital
New Delhi, India

Malavika Kohli, MD, DVD, DNB
Skin Secrets
and
Jaslok Hospital and Research Centre
Breach Candy Hospital
Mumbai, India

C. R. Satish Kumar, MSc, MPhil, PhD
Manipal Hospitals
Bangalore, India

Shirin Lakhani, MBBS, MRCA, DRCOG, MRCGP
ELITE Aesthetics
Kent, UK

Wendy Lewis
Wendy Lewis & Co. Ltd.
New York, NY

Nina Madnani, MD
PD Hinduja National Hospital & Sir HN Reliance Foundation
   Hospital
Mumbai, India

Kavita Mariwalla, MD, FAAD
Mariwalla Dermatology
West Islip, NY

Vivek Mehta, MD
Pulastya Skin Clinic
New Delhi, India

Milind Naik, MD
Ophthalmic Plastic Surgery Service
LV Prasad Eye Institute
Hyderabad, India
and
University of Rochester
Rochester, NY
and
Stein Eye Institute
UCLA
Los Angeles, CA

Paula Celeste Rubiano Mojica, MD
Universidad del Rosario
Bogota, Colombia

O. Nefertiti Nwaobasi (Umeh), MD
St. George's University School of Medicine
Grenada, British West Indies

Sanjeev Nelogi, MD
SNATI, AMI Faculty
Mumbai, India

Nordeep Panesar, MS
Department of Dermatology
Howard University College of Medicine
Washington, DC

Ginette Okoye, MD
Department of Dermatology
Howard University College of Medicine
Washington, DC

Ninon Patrao, MD
Manipal Hospitals
Bangalore, India

Sahana P. Raju, MD, DNB, FRGUHS
Department of Dermatology
Bowring and Lady Curzon
   Hospital
Bangalore, India.

Mukta Sachdev, MD
Manipal Hospitals
and
MS Skin Centre
and
MS Clinical Research Private
   Limited
Bangalore, India

Suraj Sachidanand, MD
Department of Dermatology
Manipal Hospitals
Bangalore, India

Rashmi Sarkar, MD, FAMS
Department of Dermatology
Lady Hardinge Medical College
New Delhi, India

Jaishree Sharad, MD
Skinfiniti Aesthetic & Laser Clinic
Mumbai, India

Franklin Sujith Kumar, MD
Department of Dermatology
Manipal Hospitals
Bangalore, India

Atchima Suwanchinda, MD, MSc
Ramathibodi University Hospital
Mahidol University
Bangkok, Thailand

Sumayah Taliaferro
Atlanta Dermatology and Aesthetics
Atlanta, GA

Susan C. Taylor, MD
Department of Dermatology
Perelman School of
    Medicine
University of Pennsylvania
Philadelphia, PA

Godfrey Town, PhD
Department of Dermatology
Aalborg University
    Hospital
Aalborg, Denmark

Amanda A. Onalaja-Underwood, MD
Department of Dermatology
Perelman Center for Advanced Medicine
Philadelphia, PA

Maya Vedamurthy
RSV Skin and Laser Centre
Apollo Hospitals
Chennai, India

Keerthi Velugotla, MD
Femiint Health Hospital
Whitefield, Bangalore, India

Part I
Fundamentals in Understanding Ethnic Skin/Skin of Color

CHAPTER 1: INTRODUCTION

Mukta Sachdev and Niti Khunger

The diversity that we see in the skin landscape today is immense. More than 75% of the global population is people with skin of color. The varying racial, cultural, and ethnic skin backgrounds and the amalgamation and intermixing of individuals across borders have given rise to a diverse milieu of skin types. The field of cosmetic and aesthetic dermatology has expanded considerably over the past decade with the advent of numerous invasive and noninvasive cosmetic procedures. All this has contributed to certain challenges when treating this subset of patients. The aim of our book is to understand pigmented skin and treat it effectively and correctly. Although there is an overlap in the approach for any dermatology patient, irrespective of skin type, emphasis is laid on treating a patient with skin of color. Global experts have shared their valuable clinical expertise, with pearls and pointers to achieve a desirable outcome for both patient and physician.

We hope you enjoy reading!

DOI: 10.1201/9780429243769-1

CHAPTER 2: ANATOMY
Skin, Hair, Nails

Ninon Patrao

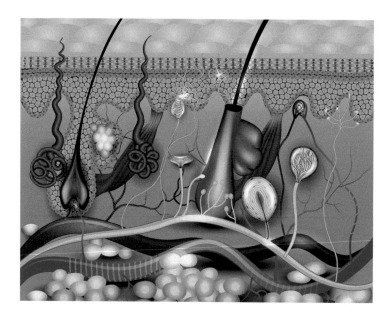

FIGURE 2.1   Human skin.

THE SKIN

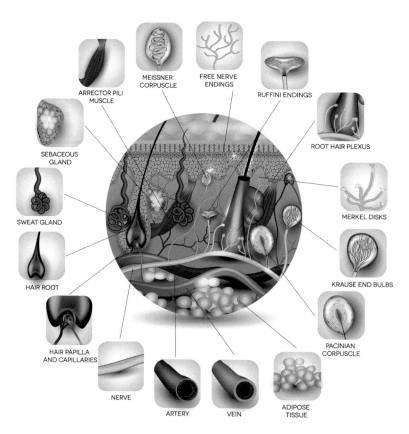

FIGURE 2.2   Structure of the skin.

DOI: 10.1201/9780429243769-2

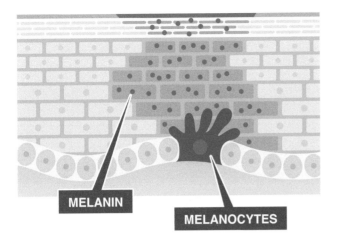

FIGURE 2.3 Melanin and melanocyte.

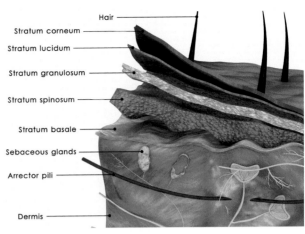

FIGURE 2.4 Layers of the skin.

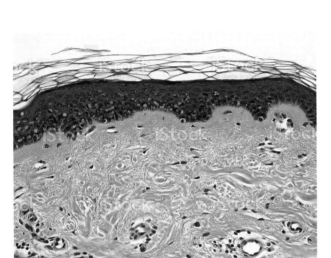

FIGURE 2.5 Histology of the skin.

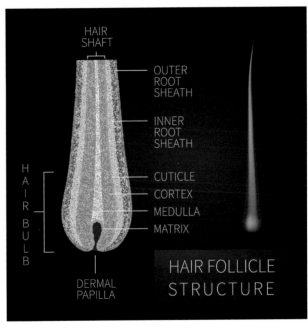

FIGURE 2.6 Structure of the hair follicle.

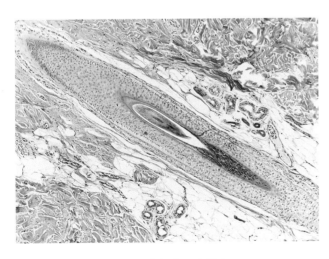

FIGURE 2.7 Histology of the hair follicle.

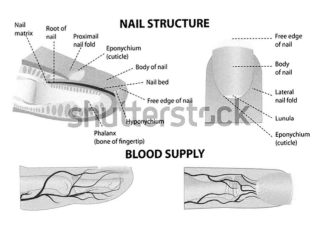

FIGURE 2.8 Structure of the nail.

CHAPTER 3: FACTORS AFFECTING SKIN INTEGRITY

Ninon Patrao

3.1 Introduction

Our skin, as we know, is the largest organ of the body, weighing approximately 8 pounds and comprising a huge surface area of approximately 2 m^2.

It forms an integral interface between the body and its environment, and thus, factors, both internal and external, play a very important role in skin health. Apart from being an organ that has various important functions, its sensitivity and visibility are two crucial aspects that play a significant role in the mind of a patient seeking treatment.

Although there is an interplay of many factors that affect the skin, we have touched upon a few relevant aspects as part of this chapter.

3.2 Microbiome

The skin ecosystem is intricate and complex, and essentially, the biodiversity of the skin microbiome depends both on the local topographic environment, as well that of the macrobiome—that is, one's surroundings and one's interaction with them.[1]

Various skin microorganisms exist as commensals on the skin, but they can sometimes turn pathogenic, depending on an individual's immune status, microbial imbalance, and genetic susceptibility. Certain microenvironments have their distinct microbial communities.

Some of those include sebaceous areas where *Propionibacterium* and *Staphylococcus* species predominate and moist areas where *Corynebacterium* and *Malassezia* species are present.[2]

Apart from these site-specific interactions, one must also recognize the importance of age-related differences, nutrition, medications, household and cosmetic products, ambient temperature, air quality, ventilation, occupation, co-occupancy, domestic pets, and device surfaces, all of which and many more factors have an influence on the colonizing microbiota, and thus the microbial-immune interactions in the skin, which are vital to maintaining healthy tissue homeostasis.

3.3 Endocrine

The human skin has been a target for several hormones, the effects of which have been meticulously described over the years as also their production in the skin and their role in the development and physiological function of skin tissues. Hair follicles and sebaceous glands, for example, are the targets for androgen steroids secreted by the gonads and the adrenal cortex. The circulating androgens dehydroepiandrosterone (DHEA) and androstenedione are converted in the skin through different pathways to testosterone or androstenedione and further into more potent androgen 5α-dihydrotestosterone (5α-DHT).[3]

The ability of the skin to produce hormones and similar substances, along with their ability to metabolize them and synthesize derivatives with systemic activity, have paved the way for the understanding of dermato-endocrinological homeostasis and their pharmacological and therapeutic function. Vitamin D analogs, retinoids, and corticosteroids are a few noteworthy examples of having been used to that effect.

3.4 Climate

3.4.1 Sunlight and Humidity

Exposure to ultraviolet radiation (UV) is associated with both health benefits and risks. On the one hand, it aids in the natural synthesis of vitamin D and endorphins in the skin, and on the other, it is termed as a mutagen with both tumor initiator and promoter properties, in addition to its being a risk factor for other skin disorders such as pigmentary changes. The genetic predisposition of an individual also mediates the sensitivity, color, and malignancy risk, and hence, the effects are multifold and complex.[4]

Extremes in humidity similarly present their own set of troubles, with high humidity being associated with heat rashes and acne eruptions and low humidity leading to a decreased barrier function and thereby making the skin increasingly susceptible to irritants and allergens.[5]

3.4.2 Cold and Dry

The stratum corneum (SC), with its functioning of corneocytes, lipids, natural moisturizing factor, and desquamation, provides important physical blockade against external factors, and its integrity remains very crucial to overall skin health.

The water from the deeper epidermal layers ascends to hydrate the SC and eventually evaporates. It is this loss of epidermal water content that contributes to skin dryness.[6]

The winter weather and dry climatic conditions, along with frequent bathing, add to its severity by sapping moisture.

It is important to keep in mind that the physiological properties of skin vary between races, and even if exposed to a similar external environment, dry skin can be distressing.

Although few studies are being carried out lately to assess the variations in quantifiable parameters across different skin types, such as trans epidermal water loss, water content, ceramide levels, and skin reactivity, an interesting observation among them has been a higher value of these parameters in the Asian skin as opposed to the others.[7] However, more large-scale studies are needed to delve deeper, and efforts are being made to understand these structural and functional nuances.

3.5 Allergens and Irritants

3.5.1 Skin

Although there a variety of allergic skin disorders that one may come across, a basis of understanding the concepts of allergy lies within the realm of atopic dermatitis, mainly because the pathogenesis involves a complex interaction between skin barrier dysfunction and environmental factors, such as allergens and microbes.

An important observation was that the mutation of the skin barrier protein filaggrin is associated with an allergen sensitization and that an altered skin barrier function, caused by several factors, results in the passage of allergens through the skin and to systemic responses. A key factor in such a response is exerted by Langerhans cells, which, via their immunoglobulin E (IgE) receptor, capture the allergens and present them to T cells. When T helper type 2 (Th2) cells are activated, the production of proinflammatory cytokines and chemokines pattern sustains the persistence of inflammation.[8]

DOI: 10.1201/9780429243769-3

Contact skin lesions involving allergens and irritants are other common inflammatory skin disorders. While allergic contact dermatitis (CD) is a delayed hypersensitivity reaction (type IV) to allergens, irritant CD is a nonspecific skin response to direct chemical skin damage with the release of inflammatory mediators.[9]

3.5.2 Hair

Although the chemical composition of hair remains the same, there are differences in morphological shapes and structural properties across ethnicities. For instance, the cuticular layers, the scalp density, and hair diameter and growth rate are relatively lesser in African ethnicities as compared to those of others.

Moreover, the daily habits and hair care practices owing to societal and cultural norms increase the susceptibility of hair to damage over a period of time as measured intensile properties.

Chemicals used in hair coloring and straightening treatments create breaks in hair shafts resulting in their damage as well those closer to the root. Constant combing and brushing along may cause frictional harm. Thermal styling treatments, such as ironing and blow-drying, can cause hair protein denaturation, dehydration, and cuticular destruction, thus making it very sensitive and highly prone to damage.[10]

As hair ages, there is also a loss of pigment and protein with resultant oxidative damage, and as such, the resilience of an individual's hair to damage is also reduced; consequently, both surface and internal weathering ensue.

3.5.3 Genetic

While there have been different schools of thought on the origin of the human species, genetic variation has been a gradual process. Interbreeding in archaic populations may have hardly existed but with migration over time, this has changed, and today an individual may have attributes from different continental groups.

Thus, we see patterns of variation, and with regard to skin color, there is roughly a 10%variance that occurs within racial and genetic groups and 90%between groups. This poses a challenge to a dermatologist at times because of varied presentation of a skin disorder and how to fine-tune different aspects of treatment to provide the best possible outcome and avoid complications.[11]

Another fascinating concept is that of convergent adaptation, which contributes toward similar skin colors owing to selective pressure. For instance, equatorial populations exhibit a darker skin color so as to prevent skin cancers and photodermatoses.

3.5.4 Cultural Practices

Ethnic differences exist not only with appearances but also with respect to what is viewed by an individual as an acceptable social norm. This can range from the desire to look fair by some ethnicities to preferring a tanned look by others.

Certain cultural practices such as coining, cupping, and moxibustion maybe harmful to the skin, as is the use of traditional hairstyling practices such as hair dyeing and using straightening appliances and products, creams, rollers, and extensions, which can damage the hair, along with the use of hennas and bindis for social occasions, which can cause dyspigmentation over a period of time.[12]

3.5.5 Aging

The aging process involves a myriad of factors that involve photodamage, fat redistribution, bone shifting, and the loss of connective tissue, with also genetic and environmental influences affecting the process. Individuals with darker skin are overall thought to have firmer and smoother skin than individuals with lighter skin of the same age. However, with the intermixing of races, ethnicities, and cultures, the cutaneous effects are varied and dynamic as is the growing desire for a youthful appearance.[13]

3.6 Conclusion

Skin vitality is of the essence in today's world, and with advances in the field of dermatology, factors affecting skin integrity are being studied in greater depth to understand the different facets of micro and macro environments affecting it, which ultimately facilitates skin health, healing, and care.

References

1. Findley K, Grice EA. The skin microbiome: A focus on pathogens and their association with skin disease. PLoS Pathog. 2014;10(11):e1004436.
2. Prescott SL, Larcombe DL, Logan AC, et al. The skin microbiome: Impact of modern environments on skin ecology, barrier integrity, and systemic immune programming. World Allergy Organ J. 2017;10(1):29.
3. Zouboulis CC. The skin as an endocrine organ. Dermatoendocrinol. 2009;1(5):250–252.
4. D'Orazio J, Jarrett S, Amaro-Ortiz A, Scott T. UV radiation and the skin. Int J Mol Sci. 2013;14(6):12222–12248.
5. Engebretsen KA, Johansen JD, Kezic S, Linneberg A, Thyssen JP. The effect of environmental humidity and temperature on skin barrier function and dermatitis. J Eur Acad Dermatol Venereol. 2016 Feb;30(2):223–249.
6. Purnamawati S, Indrastuti N, Danarti R, Saefudin T. The role of moisturizers in addressing various kinds of dermatitis: A review. Clin Med Res. 2017;15(3–4):75–87.
7. Wan DC, Wong VW, Longaker MT, Yang GP, Wei FC. Moisturizing different racial skin types. J Clin Aesthet Dermatol. 2014;7(6):25–32.
8. Incorvaia C, Frati F, Verna N, D'Alò S, Motolese A, Pucci S. Allergy and the skin. Clin Exp Immunol. 2008;153(Suppl 1):27–29. doi:10.1111/j.1365-2249.2008.03718.x
9. Novak-Bilić G, Vučić M, Japundžić I, Meštrović-Štefekov J, Stanić-Duktaj S, Lugović-Mihić L. Irritant and allergic contact dermatitis—skin lesion characteristics. Acta Clin Croat. 2018 Dec;57(4):713–720
10. Maymone MBC, Laughter M, Pollock S, et al. Hair aging in different races and ethnicities. J Clin Aesthet Dermatol. 2021;14(1):38–44
11. Torres V, Herane MI, Costa A, Martin JP, Troielli P. Refining the ideas of "ethnic" skin. An Bras Dermatol. 2017;92(2):221–225.
12. Albares MP, Belinchón I. Cultural practices in immigrant populations and their relevance to dermatology. Actas Dermosifiliogr. 2012 Dec;103(10):849–852.
13. Vashi NA, de Castro Maymone MB, Kundu RV. Aging differences in ethnic skin. J Clin Aesthet Dermatol. 2016 Jan;9(1):31–38.

CHAPTER 4: GEO-ETHNIC VARIATIONS IN SKIN

Ayushi Khandelwal

4.1 Introduction

The majority of the world's population has skin of color, and Asians comprise more than half of the total population of the earth.[1] Skin conditions occur globally, affecting people of all ethnicities. These conditions may have a genetic factor and may present differently in specific population groups. If population-based differences exist, it is practical to assume that understanding these differences may optimize treatment outcomes. The idea that racial or genetic differences between groups have a relation with health or disease has been supported by sequencing of the human genome and the ongoing international effort to catalog common haplotypes in various populations.[2] With this active research, it is time to examine the complex relation between genetic research and the concepts of race, ethnicity, and ancestry and disease in dermatology.

4.2 The Origin of Humans

Modern humans ventured out of Africa ~100,000 years ago, and they spread across continents into a variety of habitats, from tropical zones to the arctic, and from lowlands to highlands. During migration, selective pressures in local environments (e.g., the cold climate, hypoxia, and endemic pathogens), together with random drift, have resulted in population-specific genetic variants, which further influenced variable phenotypes, such as lactose tolerance, height, immune system, and metabolic efficiency. Skin color variation is one of the most striking examples of human phenotypic diversity. It is dominated by melanin, a pigment located in the base of the epidermis and produced by melanocytes. Melanin has two forms, pheomelanin (yellow-reddish) and eumelanin (black-brown). The former is mainly accumulated in light-complexioned people, while the latter is mostly produced in dark-complexioned people. In addition, the number and size of melanin particles differ among individuals and are even more important than the proportions of the two forms of melanin in the determination of human skin color. Other skin-related factors, such as keratin, also contribute to skin color variation. In global populations, skin color is highly correlated with latitude and, fundamentally, the distribution of ultraviolet (UV) radiation. Populations closer to the equator tend to have dark skin for protection against UV since overexposure to UV may decrease folic acid levels and cause skin cancer. The lighter skin in populations at higher latitudes is the underlying selection to maintain vitamin D photosynthesis, which is a UV-dependent process.

4.3 Differences in Skin Coloration

Pigmentation is the most obvious difference in skin characteristics between different racial groups.[3] This racial variation is dependent on the quantity of melanin, amount of UV exposure, genetics, melanosome content, and type of pigments found in the skin. Four chromophores are responsible for the varying colors found in human skin: hemoglobin, oxyhemoglobin, melanin, and carotenoids. Hemoglobin and oxyhemoglobin contribute to the pinkish color of Caucasian skin by absorbing specific wavelengths of light and allowing red

to be reflected back. The various brown shades seen in black and sun-tanned skin are a result of melanin. Carotenes are the source of yellow-orange pigmentation. Other hues are caused by a combination of all the pigments. Melanin is a natural skin pigment that protects the skin from UV damage. It is synthesized in melanocytes and packaged into melanosomes that are found dispersed throughout the epidermis. Melanosomes are found most prominently in the basal layer of the epidermis and serve to protect germinating nuclei of epidermal cells from UV radiation damage. The packaging and arrangement of skin pigments are responsible for the differences in skin pigmentation that serve to protect an individual.

4.4 Racial Differences in Stratum Corneum Structure

Differences in stratum corneum (SC) biology are apparent in different skin types. Black skin contains more corneocyte cell layers than that from Caucasian skin (mean 21.8 vs. mean 16.7 cell layers).[4] Since no significant difference in thickness of the stratum corneum between white people and black people was found, the cell layers in black skin were thought to be more compact, perhaps reflecting greater intercellular cohesion.[5] The desquamation rate was higher in the black subjects. The lipid content of the stratum corneum of black skin was higher than that of white skin. Asians, in general, have the lowest transepidermal water loss (TEWL), highest water content, and highest SC lipid levels. The findings are the opposite for black skin. Black subjects have been reported to have a greater density of *Propionibacterium acnes* compared to white subjects, but the values were not statistically significant.[6] Rebora et al. have also shown increased aerobic bacteria (650% greater) and *Candida albicans* (150% greater) on black skin compared with white skin.[7]

4.5 Racial Differences in Epidermal-Dermal Function

Racial differences in epidermal-dermal structure become especially pronounced during photoaging. Naturally, the darker the skin phenotype, the greater the skin protection against UV irradiation. White subjects exhibit numerous focal areas of atrophy and necrosis.[3] Equally, there is greater dermal damage in the lighter ethnic groups. Skin thickness was increased on the sun-exposed site in all racial groups. However, skin extensibility was the same on both sites for black subjects, whereas both dorsal sites on Hispanic subjects and white subjects showed reduced extensibility.[5] However, the elastic modulus was only increased on the dorsal skin of the Caucasians. Black subjects showed the same elastic recovery on both sites, whereas both Hispanic and white subjects showed reduced recovery and viscoelasticity on the dorsal forearm.[3] These differences are probably due to the greater sun protection capability of black skin. Warrier et al. found that the elastic recovery was 1.5 times greater in black subjects compared with white subjects on the cheeks, with no differences in the legs.[6] Overall, one would expect fewer signs of aging—that is, the maintenance of skin elasticity in darker-skinned individuals. Black

DOI: 10.1201/9780429243769-4

people are reported to have an intrinsic sun protection factor (SPF) value of approximately.[3]

4.6 Racial Differences in Cutaneous Appendages: Eccrine, Apocrine, and Apoeccrine Sweat Glands

Several papers suggest that there are differences in the number of sweat glands between different racial groups.[3] However, when measuring sweat gland functionality, acclimatization needs to be taken into consideration as this will influence the onset and type of sweating process. Thus, there is probably a greater density of actively sweating glands in the tropics rather than real differences in gland numbers. Differences in electrolyte content may occur where black people do not resorb as much sodium chloride as Caucasians.[8] Apart from this, no other compositional differences are reported, but they are highly likely to occur. There are some very early studies in this area that indicate that black subjects have larger apocrine glands and in greater numbers than Caucasian and Chinese subjects. They can be as much as three times greater in black subjects. There is also a greater proportion of secretion of apocrine fluid by black subjects; secretions were more turbid and had a different odor. The apoeccrine gland is a somewhat forgotten gland that develops at puberty from the eccrine gland. It is present in the axilla, in the perianal regions, and on the face, particularly in the nasal skin. Its fluid does contain some lipids, but it is mainly water and electrolyte. However, it is a much bigger gland and is reported to secrete at ten times the rate of the eccrine gland. Again, these are found in greater numbers in black facial skin compared to white facial skin. In the axilla, these glands are reported to represent up to 45% of the glands present, and they secrete fluid directly on the skin surface, unlike apocrine glands.

4.7 Sebaceous Glands

The sebaceous gland is attached to the hair follicle by a duct, and it produces sebum; a mixture of squalene, cholesterol, and cholesterol esters; wax esters; and triglycerides that are secreted on to the skin surface. On route, the triglycerides can be hydrolyzed to free fatty acids by bacterial lipases. Sebum should not be considered a liquid but a semisolid. Various crystalline lipid domains are present, and these will vary according to composition, which may be due to racial or seasonal variations. For the latter, there is less oleate in sebum in summer compared with winter, for instance. Comparing lipid in hair samples, it has been shown that black subjects have 60–70% more lipid in their hair compared with white subjects. Black subjects also have bigger sebaceous glands, which contribute to the increased sebum secretion. Consistent with these reports, studies by Hillebrand et al. recently reported a greater pore count fraction in African Americans, but the number of pores increases with age in all racial groups.[9] The level of sebum secretion on the forehead was reported to increase during the early decades, peaking in the 30–40s, and then declining. African Americans showed significantly more sebum excretion than East Asians, whereas Hispanics had the lowest. There are few studies on sebum composition and the effect of race. One study examining Caucasians and the Japanese found that, like Caucasians, Japanese subjects have a greater predominance of straight-chain fatty acids in their sebum wax esters than branched-chain fatty acids, but the Japanese had a greater quantity of C16 isobranched-chain fatty acids.[10] Japanese men

also appear to have greater sebaceous gland activity compared with Caucasians. Nevertheless, sebum levels decline with age. The incidence of acne is similar across different racial groups, but acne responses appear to show differences between the different racial groups. In response to coal tar, Caucasians develop inflammatory lesions, whereas subjects with Black skin open comedones develop.[9] Thus, in subjects with white skin, the rupture of the follicles occurs, but in black subjects, hyperproliferation and retention of horny cells occur.

4.8 Cutaneous Irritation in Different Racial Groups

As mentioned earlier, differences in SC biology are apparent in different skin types with Asians in general having the lowest TEWL, highest water content, and highest SC lipid levels with the reverse being true for black skin. Due to its enhanced spontaneous desquamation (and probably increased sebum levels), tape stripping revealed a weaker barrier when only using a few strips.[3] However, on further tape stripping, black skin has a stronger barrier presumably due to its increased cohesiveness. This increased cohesivity may also explain the reduced potential to irritate black skin using a variety of chemical stimuli. Asian skin, on the contrary, is reported to be more sensitive to chemical stimuli presumably due to the higher sweat gland density or possibly due to a thinner SC where the number of tape strippings to break the barrier is reported to be less.

4.9 Clinically Relevant Structural and Functional Differences

Structural and functional differences observed among darkly pigmented populations compared with lightly pigmented populations have been reported. Key biological characteristics to consider when performing laser or light-based aesthetic procedures in dark skin types include the following:

1. Increased epidermal melanin
2. Larger melanosomes that are more singly dispersed and widely distributed within epidermal keratinocytes
3. Labile melanocyte responses
4. Reactive fibroblasts

These features, in turn, contribute to differences in the frequency of specific dermatological disorders and the safety of laser or light-based procedures. Increased melanin content, packaging, and epidermal distribution confer greater protection against the deleterious effects of ultraviolet radiation, and therefore, signs of photoaging tend to be less marked and delayed in higher SPT.[11] Labile melanocyte responses contribute to an increased prevalence of pigmentary disorders in nonwhite populations, and as such, the treatment of dyschromia is among the most frequent reasons for which individuals with skin of color visit dermatologists. Of particular relevance to laser or light procedures, the tendency for injury or inflammation to incite alterations in pigment production is associated with a greater risk for post-procedure hyper- or hypopigmentation in individuals with SPT IV–VI. Racial differences exist in the frequency of keloids, with the highest prevalence being observed in populations of African ancestry.[12] This is probably due to genetic factors that contribute to increased fibroblast reactivity among individuals at risk. Therefore, a greater overall risk of keloids and hypertrophic scars associated with iatrogenic dermal injury is observed in ethnic populations. With these characteristics in mind, minimization of epidermal and dermal injury through careful selection of treatment modality and settings, as well as the use of pre- and post-treatment precautions, are paramount when performing laser or light-based procedures in dark-skinned patients.

4.10 Complications

It is very important to be cautious in laser skin-resurfacing procedures in patients with Fitzpatrick skin types III to VI because of the well-known and well-documented side effects that may occur in this group, including the following:

1. Hyperpigmentation
2. Hypopigmentation
3. Scarring

Hyperpigmentation occurs from six weeks to six months after laser ablation in almost 100% of dark-skinned patients. Although transient in most patients, it can persist from nine months to a year.[13] Treatment for this condition is bleaching with hydroquinone. Hypopigmentation may occur six months after laser abrasion. Although the incidence of hypopigmentation is much less than that of hyperpigmentation, hypopigmentation may result in permanent hypopigmented scars. In dark-skinned people, these scars are much more obvious and difficult to conceal. A careful pre-treatment history, including the patient's previous exposure to trauma, dermabrasion, or chemical peels, must be taken. These factors carry an increased risk for hypopigmentation. Scarring is a consideration with laser resurfacing. Darker skin types are more predisposed to the formation of hypertrophic and keloid scars.

References

1. Taylor, S. Understanding skin of colour. Suppl. Am. Acad. Dermatol. 46, S41–S42 (2002).
2. Taylor, S.C. Epidemiology of skin diseases in ethnic populations. Dermatol Clin. 21, 601–607 (2003).
3. Deng, L. and Xu, S. Adaptation of human skin color in various populations. Hereditas 155 (2018)
4. Weigand, D.A., Haygood, C. and Gaylor, J.R. Cell layers and density of Negro and Caucasian stratum corneum. J. Invest. Dermatol. 62, 563–568 (1974).
5. Johnson, L.C. and Corah, N.L. Racial differences in skin resistance. Science 139, 766–769 (1963).
6. Warrier, A.G., Kligmn, A.M., Harper, R.A., Bowman, J. and Wickett, R.R. A comparison of black and white skin using non-invasive methods. J. Soc. Cosmet. Chem. 47, 229–240 (1996).
7. Rebora, A. and Guarrera, M. Racial differences in experimental skin infection with Candida albicans. Acta Derm. Venereol. (Stockh) 68, 165–168 (1988).
8. Quinton, P.M., Elder, H.Y., McEwan Jenkinson, D. and Bovell, D.L. Structure and function of human sweat glands. In: Antiperspirants & deodorants, Chapter 2 (Laden, K., ed.), Taylor and Francis, pp. 17–58 (1999).
9. Hillebrand, G.G., Levine, M.J. and Miyamoto, K. The age dependent changes in skin condition in African-Americans, Asian Indians, Caucasians, East Asians & Latino's. IFSCC Mag. 4, 259–266 (2001).
10. Yamamoto, A., Serizawa, S. and Ito, M. Effect of aging on sebaceous gland activity and on the fatty acid composition of wax eaters. Invest. Dermatol. 89, 507 (1987).
11. Taylor, S.C. Chemical peels. In: Cosmetic procedures. Treatments of skin of color, 1st edn. Saunders, Chapter 17 (2011).
12. Sachdeva, S. Fitzpatrick skin typing: Applications in dermatology. Indian J Dermatol Venereol Leprol. 75, 93–96 (2009).
13. Anthony, C. Griffin. Laser resurfacing procedures in dark-skinned patients. Aesthet Surg J. 25 (6), 625–627 (November 2005), https://doi.org/10.1016/j.asj.2005.09.019

Part II
Cases Encountered in Cosmetic Dermatology Practice

CHAPTER 5: SENSITIVE SKIN

Seemal R. Desai and O. Nefertiti Nwaobasi (Umeh)

5.1 Definition

Sensitive skin is a sensory reaction triggered by various phenomena and characterized by a plethora of symptoms, such as erythema, itching, tingling, pricking, or burning.

It is an emerging phenomenon owing to a host of factors contributing to the condition, and both patient perception and clinician evaluation are of utmost importance in the care of these individuals.

5.2 Introduction

Approaching aesthetic procedures, especially from a safety perspective, in patients of different ethnic backgrounds, including those with Fitzpatrick skin types IV–VI, may be related to the differences observed in structure and composition as well as sociocultural influences in comparison to the Caucasian counterpart (1). A detailed history and physical examination are crucial to evaluate subjective symptoms of cosmetic intolerance, such as post-inflammatory hyperpigmentation, dermatitis, and keloid formation, to name a few (1). Methodologies, such as reactivity tests, followed up by dermoscopy, can also be used to demonstrate irritation reactions locally. Psychiatric evaluations could be considered to rule out underlying negative mental perceptions that make patients seek out certain cosmetic treatments outside the scope of normal anti-aging techniques, blemish correcting, and even disease-modifying treatments.

One must be aware of the effects of age, gender, race/ethnicity, cultural influences, and environmental factors that contribute to the physical and psychological makeup of skin sensitivities in this population (2) (Table 5.1). Beauty is perceived via means of cultural, environmental, and historical influences. Skin of color comprises a phenotypically heterogeneous group of patients. Understanding the difference within this group, both genetically and physiologically, will aid in good cosmetic management outcomes.

Ethnocentric beauty is one that should be celebrated. More ethnic patients are requesting aesthetic procedures than ever before; however, they do not all necessarily desire "Westernized" appearances (3). They often wish to enhance their culture-specific beauty. The understanding of these culture and ethnic-specific features is the first step in taking care of ethnic patients and using specialized aesthetic approaches to their care (3).

TABLE 5.1: Cutaneous Factors Contributing to Sensitive Skin

Stratum corneum	Decrease in hydration and thickness, thus increase in permeability and release of mediators that stimulate nerve endings
Transepidermal water loss (TEWL)	Decrease in TEWL, thus causing intolerance to ingredients in products
Lipids	Decrease in ceramides, thus compromising integrity
Cutaneous nerves	Certain thermal receptors are stimulated, causing neurogenic inflammation and thus the unpleasant sensation

5.2.1 Key Considerations before Moving Forward with Cosmetic Procedures

5.2.1.1 Aging

Skin of color has many characteristics that make its aging process unique. A thicker dermis provides a reduced appearance of fine lines and preserved skin elasticity for longer. Melanin concentration is markedly higher in darker skin types, which provides for greater photoprotection and lower incidence of skin cancer. On the other hand, epidermal melanin also makes darkly pigmented persons more vulnerable to dyspigmentation.

As skin ages, it becomes more sensitive. Clinical features of wrinkles, sunspots, uneven skin color, dryness and itchiness, skin tags, easy bruising, and sagging skin are all descriptors used when discussing the topic of skin aging. These characteristics are all influenced by both intrinsic and extrinsic factors and often are varied based on structural and functional differences from one ethnicity to another (4).

Some considerations when dealing with aged skin are sensitivity reactivity testing, irritation tests, epidermal function tests, dermoscopy, and contact tests before any cosmetic procedure takes place.

5.2.1.2 Xerosis (Dry Skin)

It has been shown that the changes to the stratum corneum (SC) and its lipid composition vary over time, giving way to dry, less elastic, and in some instances, itchy skin. However, these manifestations are present in individuals of all ages that concurrently seek out cosmetic services. Dry skin is predisposed to irritation and fragility and is more prone to develop skin shears, ulcers, inflammation, and infections (5). In addition, it

DOI: 10.1201/9780429243769-5

recovers more slowly after insult (1). Exacerbations are associated with environmental and personal habits. Alternatively, xerosis can be acquired and associated with other pathologies, such as malignancy, infectious disease, nutritional deficiencies, and endocrine diseases (2).

The goal in xerosis should be to maintain the skin surface in its physiological acidic state, which is in turn crucial for the permeability barrier function, stratum corneum integrity/cohesion, and antimicrobial defense (6, 7). With xerosis, the natural acidity of the SC is hard to maintain. Therefore, advising patients to use skin care products formulated with an effective buffer system at a more acidic pH may be the best option to ensure skin durability for any future cosmetic procedures and for maintenance (8).

In addition, emollients are well recognized as essential in the management of all dry skin disorders as they reduce TEWL while helping to restore the intercorneocyte lipid structure and thus strengthening the cutaneous barrier. The enhanced hydration of the skin, after emollient application, also strengthens the stratum corneum's extensibility and flexibility, providing an ideal base upon which to conduct cosmetic procedures.

5.2.1.3 Atopy: Cosmetic Dermatology in Atopic Dermatitis Patients

Atopic dermatitis is an itchy inflammatory skin condition associated with epidermal barrier dysfunction, the root of sensitive skin. The interplay between genetics, immune response, impairments in the stratum corneum, and hypersensitivities to the environment all come together and make the skin's potential to withstand the assault of a cosmetic procedure much less than patients who do not have AD. As a result, managing these patients adequately before starting any cosmetic treatment may be beneficial in reducing the incidence of post-treatment flares. It would also be advisable to omit any cosmetic manipulation in the midst of an active flare to avoid further irritation.

5.2.1.4 Post-Inflammatory Hyperpigmentation (PIH)

A ubiquitous issue to be mindful of when designing a treatment regimen for skin-of-color patients is the importance of addressing PIH. One simple example is acne, one of the most common cutaneous conditions, regardless of race or ethnicity, which has the same pathogenesis across borders. However, despite these similarities, there are unique characteristics in the expression of acne in skin of color, such as the presence of inflammation in a seemingly noninflammatory lesion and the tendency for post-treatment and post-resolution hyperpigmentation. These clinical features and a patient's irritation potential should influence the choice of anti-acne agents used when designing a treatment regimen.

TABLE 5.2: Key Considerations before Cosmetic Procedures

1. Aging
2. Xerosis
3. Atopy
4. Post-inflammatory hyperpigmentation

5.3 Aesthetic Procedures and Considerations in Skin of Color

5.3.1 Chemical Peels

Indications for peeling in darker-skinned patients include treatment of dyschromia, PIH, acne, melasma, scarring, and pseudofolliculitis barbae. Clinicians must keep in mind that different ethnicities may respond unpredictably despite similarities in complexions. For example, Latin Americans and Hispanics have a wide range of skin phenotypes and are more prone to PIH, so inquiring about a patient's history of PIH is very useful. In addition, studies have shown that Asians will develop more pigmentary changes from UV radiation than Caucasians.

With proper technique, chemical peels can be beneficial in the treatment of photoaging and dyschromia. Mild superficial peels should be used and gradually titrated to minimize irritation and worsening dyspigmentation (9). Peels are often paired with topical regimens to minimize any potential dyspigmentation side effects. Deep peels are not recommended for skin types IV–VI due to the higher probability of peel-induced post-inflammatory hyperpigmentation.

Positive outcomes depend on various factors, such as peel agents, concentration, depth, skin type, and concomitant use of skin care products. It is important to highlight the risks of increased complications from poor sun protection practices after a peel. Patients should be monitored closely for SPF compliance. Pre-treatment with bleaching agents prior to therapy with peels possibly decreases the appearance of PIH. Post-treatment corticosteroids may be used for prolonged post-peel erythema to prevent PIH. Treatment options for post-peel PIH include topical hydroquinone, kojic acid, and other tyrosinase inhibitors combined with enhanced sun protection.

5.3.2 Lasers

Skin-of-color patients and dermatologists have historically been hesitant to use lasers in darker skin types, given the risk of scarring and dyspigmentation. However, nonablative fractional resurfacing has been shown to be a safe and efficacious treatment option for various dermatological disorders in skin of color (10). This type of laser is a mid-infrared laser and targets water instead of melanin, therefore reducing the dyspigmentation side effects, which were once of major concern using the modality. It has also been shown to be better than the chemical reconstruction of skin scars (CROSS) in treating rolling type acne scars. Available evidence supports that nonablative fractional lasers are comparable in efficacy to triple combination creams in the treatment of melasma.

Skin-of-color-specific indications for lasers include hair removal, pseudofolliculitis barbae, dermatosis papulosa nigra, photoaging, melasma, lentigines, nevus of Ota, Hori's nevus, and tattoo removal. Newer laser devices with better surface cooling, longer pulse durations, and longer wavelengths are now safer and more efficacious in darker complexions.

Other ways to reduce risk of adverse effects are modifying the number of passes per treatment session, increasing treatment intervals, and providing additional cooling between passes to reduce bulk heating. It is also advised to space out the duration between two treatment sessions, especially if PIH occurs between the last two laser treatment sessions.

5.3.3 Hair Removal

It has been noted that both epilation methods (plucking out the entire hair, for example, by electrical epilation and waxing) and depilation methods (dry shaving–physical skin/material interaction) cause a moderate decrease in skin barrier function, which is known to be one of the building blocks of sensitive skin (11). Baseline transepidermal water loss (TEWL) is fundamental for barrier function. Skin of color generally has a higher baseline TEWL value, making the skin more sensitive, with an increased susceptibility to irritants.

With the exception of pseudofolliculitis barbae, in which the benefit of hair removal outweighs the cost of potential scarring or dyspigmentation, judicious use must be employed.

5.3.4 Injectables

Understanding the unique aesthetic considerations in a population that is quickly growing and diversifying is important for patient satisfaction in the upcoming years. The Hispanic population reported the highest consideration rate for injectables (85%), followed by Asians (74%) and African Americans (64%) (12).

Awareness of treatment area preference based on ethnicity and culture is important. For example, darker-skinned patients develop significantly more volume loss in the lower face compared with deep furrows and rhytides of the lower face seen in Caucasian patients (2).

Soft tissue augmentation can be very effective in treating volume loss evident in skin-of-color patients. Excellent outcomes have been seen with the appropriate choice of tissue depth, injection technique, and choice of filler. In skin-of-color patients, it is advisable to avoid multiple puncture techniques or minimize injection pricks, keeping in mind the risk of PIH at the puncture site. In addition, an awareness of regional perceptions of beauty is extremely important in this population.

Understanding the variety in aging patterns, cultural considerations, and aesthetic goals for each patient population may help optimize treatment expectations and outcomes.

5.3.5 Microdermabrasion (MDA)

MDA should be used cautiously in individuals with a known history of hypertrophic scarring, keloids, rosacea, and telangiectasias. Any skin of color resurfacing procedures, such as dermabrasion, chemical peels, and laser therapy, can be effective but can also be associated with prolonged recovery and a higher risk of dyspigmentation, scarring, and unsatisfactory clinical outcomes (6, 13, 14).

5.3.6 Hair Transplantation

Caution must be exercised in darker skin tones to avoid the development of keloids or hypertrophic scars, particularly at the donor site.

5.3.7 Other Considerations: Keloids and Hypertrophic Scars

Prevention is of extremely importance in this patient population. Therefore, a complete history should be obtained before any cosmetic procedure to determine if there is a personal or family history of keloids or hypertrophic scarring. All surgical cosmetic procedures should be avoided in patients with any positive history. However, if a keloid or scar still develops despite precautionary efforts, intralesional corticosteroids are the mainstay of treatment. Complications that may arise from this treatment include hypopigmentation and atrophy at the injection site. Surgical removal of keloids is typically associated with a high recurrence rate and a more involved therapy regimen to prevent reoccurrence.

TABLE 5.3: Quick Assessment of Sensitive Skin

- Do you feel that you have sensitive skin, especially after the application of cosmetic or toiletry products?
- How would you characterize the sensation? Red, stinging, burning, itchy?
  How long does it last?
- Has the avoidance/change of the product made a difference and has reapplication triggered the same issue?
- If so, have you checked the ingredient list of the product?
- Does a change in climate affect your skin? warm or cold weather? increased sun exposure?
- Has a cosmetic sensitivity patch test been performed to determine an allergy?

TABLE 5.4: Practical Approach to Treatment of Sensitive Skin

- Assess the skin involving a detailed history.
- Examine for any noticeable color change, compromise of skin, and dermatitis.
- Discontinue the product use for three weeks.
- Reassess patient for any change/improvement.
- Consider cosmetic patch test, provocation tests, and dermoscopy.
- Counsel patient on potential cosmetic sensitizers.
- Reintroduce cosmetics gradually one by one after three weeks

---

TABLE 5.5: Strategies for the Management of Sensitive Skin

Skin Care	Cosmetics
Fragrance-free	Avoid old/stale products—check expiration dates
Paraben-free	Products with minimal ingredients
Non-comedogenic	Powder and mineral-based cosmetics preferable
Water-based products	Oil-free products
Physical sunscreens	Elimination of sensitizing vehicles, such as menthol
Product labels (e.g., "suitable for sensitive skin")	Low-sensitizing preservatives, as opposed to sensitizers, such as isothiazolinones and formaldehyde

5.4 Conclusion

Sensitive skin is becoming an increasingly recognized dermatological entity in all skin types, including skin of color. Management involves the recognition of the condition with proper detailed advice on avoidance of potentially sensitizing products and customization of a personalized skin care regimen.

Frequently Asked Questions

1. *Q: How can we be more focused on obtaining a history and physical in hopes of being more accurate in our evaluation of aesthetic skin-of-color sensitivities?*
   A: Consider administering a self-assessment questionnaire to identify not-so-obvious signs of sensitive skin. This will be helpful in constructing a plan prior to cosmetic management.

2. *Q: What are some red flags to pay attention to in a psychiatric evaluation for a skin-of-color patient seeking cosmetic procedures?*

A: Including but not limited to a history of frequent bleaching with minimal satisfaction or a history of numerous cosmetic procedures.

3. *Q: How can we measure TEWL clinically to detect levels and predict sensitive skin before clinical disease presentation?*

A: The most popular non-invasive test is the TEWL measurement. It is based on the estimation of the water pressure gradient above the skin surface. It is done by two different techniques: open chamber method and ventilated chamber method. A detailed account of methods can be found in the article by Primavera and Berardesca. There are now simpler instruments available for in-clinic physician use.

4. *Q: How can we assess the safety and reduce risks of keloids after hair transplant surgery?*

A: It is suggested that test grafts are performed with a three-month wait before proceeding with the procedure.

5. *Q: What is the best way to evaluate a patient's history indicating a potential for skin irritation?*

A: Paying attention to skin care practices and particular cultural trends of beautifying skin is essential to formulating a culturally competent treatment strategy.

Citations

1) Davis EC, Callender VD. Aesthetic dermatology for aging ethnic skin. Dermatol Surg. 2011;37:901–917. doi:10.1111/j.1524-4725.2011.02007.x

2) Duarte IAG, Silveira JEPS, Hafner MFS, Toyota R, Pedroso DMM. Sensitive skin: Review of an ascending concept. An Bras Dermatol. 2017;92(4):521–525.

3) Inamadar AC, Palit A. Sensitive skin: An overview. Indian J Dermatol Venereol Leprol. 2013;79:9–16.

4) Vashi NA, de Castro Maymone MB, Kundu RV. Aging differences in ethnic skin. J Clin Aesthet Dermatol. 2016;9(1):31–38.

5) Pons-Guiraud, A. Dry skin in dermatology: A complex physiopathology. J Eur Acad Dermatol Venereol. 2007;21:1–4.

6) Shah M, Crane JS. Microdermabrasion. [Updated 2019 Mar 3]. In: StatPearls [Internet]. Treasure Island (FL): StatPearls Publishing; 2019 Jan. Available from: www.ncbi.nlm.nih.gov/books/NBK535383/

7) Tončić RJ, et al. Skin barrier and dry skin in the mature patient. Clin Dermatol. 2018;36(2):109–115.

8) Abels C, Angelova-Fischer, I. Skin care products: Age-appropriate cosmetics. pH of the Skin: Issues and Challenges. Vol. 54. Karger Publishers, 2018.173–182.

9) Talakoub L, Wesley NO. Differences in perceptions of beauty and cosmetic procedures performed in ethnic. Semin Cutan Med Surg. 2009;28:115–129.

10) Kaushik SB, Alexis AF. Nonablative fractional laser resurfacing in skin of color: Evidence-based review. J Clin Aesthet Dermatol. 2017;10(6):51–67.

11) Pany A, Klang V, Brunner M, Ruthofer J, Schwarz E, Valenta C: Effect of physical and chemical hair removal methods on skin barrier function in vitro: Consequences for a hydrophilic model permeant. Skin Pharmacol Physiol. 2019;32:8–21.

12) Boyd C, et al. Differential facial aesthetic treatment considerations for skin of color populations: African American, Asian, and Hispanic. SKIN: The J Cutaneous Med. 2017;1(3.1):s66.

13) Cohen BE, Elbuluk N. Microneedling in skin of color: A review of uses and efficacy. J Am Acad Dermatol. 2016 Feb;74(2):348–355.

14) Rendon MI, Berson DS, Cohen JL, Roberts WE, Starker I, Wang B. Evidence and considerations in the application of chemical peels in skin disorders and aesthetic resurfacing. J Clin Aesthet Dermatol. 2010;3(7):32–43

CHAPTER 6: ACNE VULGARIS

Suraj Sachidanand

6.1 Introduction

Acne vulgaris is a chronic, self-limiting, inflammatory disorder of the pilosebaceous unit resulting in increased sebum production and altered keratinization and colonization of the hair follicle by *Cutibacterium acnes*. It is one of the most common dermatological disorders encountered in clinical practice, with a prevalence rate of around 91% in adolescent males and 79% in adolescent females (1). It is typically characterized by chronic or recurrent development of papules, pustules, or nodules on the face, trunk, and sometimes proximal upper limbs. The pathogenesis of acne vulgaris involves the interaction of multiple factors that result in the formation of comedones and the development of inflammation. Hyperpigmentation and scarring are some of the common complications (2).

6.2 Classification

Acne can be classified into mild, moderate, or severe, based on its clinical appearance (2):

6.2.1 Mild Acne Vulgaris

* Scattered, small (<5 mm), comedones, papules or pustules without associated scarring
* Involvement of one body area or relatively few lesions in more than one body area
* Absence of nodules
* Absence of near-confluent skin involvement

6.2.2 Moderate to Severe Acne Vulgaris

* Visually prominent acne consisting of comedones/papules/pustules
* Presence of nodules
* Involvement of multiple body areas with more than a few scattered lesions
* Associated scarring

6.3 Epidemiological and Etiological Aspects

Acne vulgaris is quite common and usually occurs in adolescents and young adults. Acne often begins in preadolescents (7 to 12 years) and resolves in the third decade but may persist into adulthood or sometimes start only in adulthood. Adolescent acne exhibits a male predominance, whereas post-adolescent acne predominantly affects women (2).

The pathogenesis of acne involves a complex interplay of host factors, such as androgen-mediated stimulation of sebaceous glands, dysbiosis within the microbiome of the pilosebaceous follicle, and innate and cellular immune responses, and may be influenced by factors such as genetics and diet (3).

The microcomedo (a small, hyperkeratotic plug) is considered the precursor for acne vulgaris, which includes closed comedones (whiteheads), open comedones (blackheads), and inflammatory papules, pustules, and nodules. A complex interaction of these four factors results in these lesions (2):

* Follicular hyperkeratinization
* Increased sebum production by sebaceous glands
* *Cutibacterium acnes* (*C. acnes*, formerly *Propionibacterium acnes*), an anaerobic diphtheroid that is a normal component of skin flora
* Inflammation

Role of androgens on sebaceous glands—Androgens are directly responsible for increased sebum production by stimulating sebaceous glands. Sebum acts as a growth medium for *C. acnes* (2).

Androgens are mostly produced by the adrenal gland, gonads, and sebaceous glands, which convert dehydroepiandrosterone sulfate (DHEAS) to testosterone. Testosterone is subsequently converted to 5-alpha-dihydrotestosterone (DHT) via the action of type I 5-alpha reductase in the sebaceous gland (2).

The effects of androgens are mediated through androgen receptors. Androgen receptors that bind DHT and testosterone are present in the sebaceous glands and the outer root sheath keratinocytes of the follicular epithelium. DHT has a greater affinity for androgen receptors than testosterone (2).

Although the majority of patients with acne have normal androgen levels, androgen excess due to conditions such as polycystic ovarian syndrome, congenital adrenal hyperplasia, or adrenal or ovarian tumors can cause acne. In addition, acne typically does not develop prior to adrenarche (the prepubertal period in which levels of DHEAS rise), with the exception of infantile acne, a condition seen in infants that results from excess androgen production by immature adrenal glands or gonads. Moreover, men with androgen insensitivity do not produce sebum and do not develop acne (4).

Cutibacterium acnes **and inflammation**—The ability of *C. acnes*, the prominent commensal bacteria within the microbiome of pilosebaceous follicles (5–7) to activate innate and adaptive immune responses contributes to the inflammation observed in acne (2). *C. acnes* activates the innate immune response to produce proinflammatory IL-1 via activation of the nod-like receptor P3 (NLRP3) inflammasome in human sebocytes and monocytes (8, 9). It also binds and activates toll-like receptor 2, located on perifollicular macrophages, and triggers the release of proinflammatory cytokines (including IL-8 and IL-12) (10, 11). These cytokines contribute to the attraction of neutrophils and the release of neutrophil lysosomal enzymes that promote follicular rupture. Differences in the host inflammatory response to *C. acnes* or the pathogenicity of specific strains of *C. acnes* that colonize skin may contribute to the variation in the prevalence and severity of acne (12, 13). *C. acnes* may also form biofilms within follicles that could contribute to resistance to therapy (14).

Gene expression studies have been performed on the skin of patients with acne to further elucidate the inflammatory response. Upregulation of matrix metalloproteinases 1 and 3, inflammatory cytokines (IL-8), and antimicrobial peptides (human beta-defensin 4 and granzyme B) have been detected in inflammatory acne lesions (15). In addition, human beta-defensin 1 and 2 immunoreactivity is also upregulated in acne patients (16). Individuals having close relatives with acne are

DOI: 10.1201/9780429243769-6

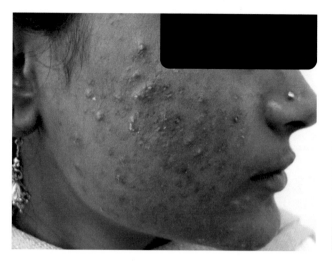

FIGURE 6.1   Papulopustular acne.

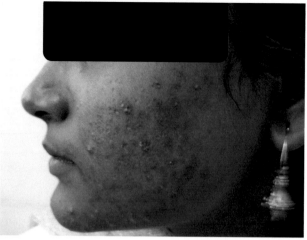

FIGURE 6.2   Nodular acne.

at an increased risk of developing the lesions, thus proving a genetic link to the disease. Aggravating factors of acne include skin trauma, dairy-rich and high glycemic diet, stress, insulin resistance, and high body mass index (2).

6.3.1 Acne Grading System

Acne vulgaris can be classified into four grades as follows (17):

- Grade 1: Comedones, occasional papules
- Grade 2: Papules, comedones, few pustules
- Grade 3: Predominant pustules, nodules, abscesses
- Grade 4: Mainly cysts, abscesses, widespread scarring

Classic features—The typical distribution of acne vulgaris correlates with areas of the body with large, hormonally responsive sebaceous glands, including the face, neck, chest, upper back, and upper arms. One or more types of active lesions may be present, including the following (2):

- *Closed comedones*: Noninflammatory; <5 mm; dome-shaped; smooth; skin-colored, gray-white papule
- *Open comedones*: Noninflammatory, <5 mm papules with a central, dilated, follicular orifice containing gray or black keratotic material
- *Papulopustular acne*: Inflamed superficial papules and pustules, typically <5 mm in diameter (Figure 6.1)
- *Nodular acne*: Deep-seated, inflamed, tender, large papules (≥0.5 mm) or nodules (≥1 cm) (Figure 6.2)

The active acne lesions in ethnic patients can clinically appear similar to those seen in Caucasian patients (18). Dark-skinned patients can develop inflammatory papules, pustules, nodules, and cysts, and it is these inflammatory lesions that promote the development of post-inflammatory hyperpigmentation (PIH), scarring, and keloids (18). Inflammatory papules inlighter-skinned patients typically have associated erythema; however, in darker skin phototypes, these lesions can also develop overlying hyperpigmentation, mimicking PIH, but the distinction is made upon palpation (18). Nodulocystic acne is thought to be less common in African Americans than Caucasians based on a study published in 1970 by Wilkins et al. (19) of 4,654 incarcerated men. However, Hispanics and Asians are thought to have

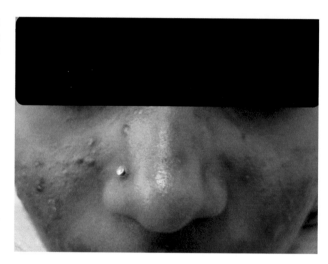

FIGURE 6.3   Hyperpigmentation and scarring.

similar prevalence rates of nodulocystic acne as Caucasians, although supporting evidence is lacking (20, 21). A study of acnein skin of color by Taylor et al. (20) showed cystic lesions to be present in 18% of African American (n = 239), 25.5% of Hispanic (n = 55), and 10.5% of Asian (n = 19) patients. However, larger studies are needed to confirm these findings.

However, an interesting study by Halder et al. (22) of 30 African American female patients with acne showed marked inflammation in all types of lesions. The histology from biopsy specimens showed some degree of inflammation, even around simple comedones that showed no evidence of inflammation on clinical exam. In addition, there was also extensive inflammation surrounding papules and pustules, inflamed tissue far away from the lesion, foreign body granulomas with giant cells, and epidermalmelanin granules and melanophages extending into the reticular dermis in areas of hyperpigmentation, which was not consistent to what was seen clinically. This could be a major reason why African Americans with even mild-to-moderate acne develop hyperpigmented macules (18).

Common sequelae—Resolution of individual acne lesions may leave transient or permanent changes on the skin. Post-inflammatory hyperpigmentation (Figures 6.3 and 6.4) and

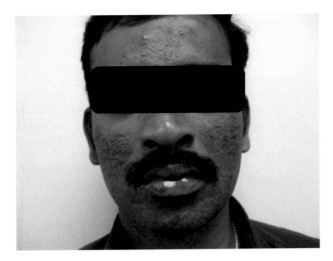

FIGURE 6.4 Post-inflammatory hyperpigmentation.

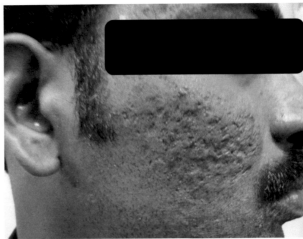

FIGURE 6.5 Atrophic scars.

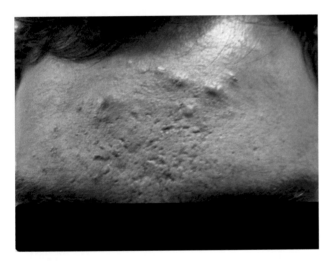

FIGURE 6.6 Atrophic scars.

scarring are common sequelae that can be highly distressing for patients (2).

Post-inflammatory hyperpigmentation—As with other inflammatory skin conditions, acne vulgaris may lead to the development of hyperpigmentation at the site of an active or resolving lesion. The risk of hyperpigmentation increases with increasing baseline skin pigmentation and is particularly common in individuals with skin phototypes IV to VI (Figures 6.3 and 6.4) (2).

Post-inflammatory hyperpigmentation typically resolves spontaneously, but an individual hyperpigmented macule may persist for several months or longer without treatment. As a result, even patients with relatively mild, active acne can exhibit post-inflammatory hyperpigmentation as a prominent disfiguring feature (2).

Scarring—Acne scarring is a common consequence of acne vulgaris that occurs in some patients. Inflammatory acne is considered more likely to result in scarring than noninflammatory acne (2). Various types of scars can result from acne vulgaris, including atrophic scars (ice pick scars, rolling scars, and boxcar scars), hypertrophic scars, and keloids (Figures 6.5 and 6.6). Some variants of acne vulgaris include acne conglobata and acne excoriée (2).

Acne conglobata—Acne conglobata is a severe form of nodular acne that mostly occurs in young males. Skin involvement tends to be more on the back, chest, and buttocks but can also appear on the face or other sites. Large draining lesions, sinus tracts, and severe scarring may occur. Sinus tracts manifest as fluctuant, linear lesions and are formed when nodules merge. Systemic symptoms are absent. Acne conglobata is distinct from acne fulminans, an acute condition characterized by nodules, friable plaques, erosions, and ulcers (2).

Acne excoriée—Acne excoriée typically presents with relatively mild acne comedones or inflammatory papules that are chronically and obsessively picked and excoriated, leading to erosions and scarring. This condition is often, but not always, seen in young women. An underlying psychiatric disorder can be associated, and treatment may involve antidepressants and psychotherapy (2).

6.4 Investigations

The diagnosis of acne vulgaris is usually made on physical examination. Laboratory or radiologic tests are generally limited to patients with signs of hyperandrogenism, seen in polycystic ovarian syndrome, congenital adrenal hyperplasia, and adrenal or ovarian tumors (2).

History—Patient history is particularly helpful for identifying patients with acne caused or exacerbated by an exposure (e.g., drug-induced acne) or who may need further evaluation for associated disease (e.g., hyperandrogenism, SAPHO [synovitis, acne, pustulosis, hyperostosis, and osteitis] syndrome, acne fulminans) (2).

Some of the clues include the following (2):

* Age of onset and current age
* Drug history (corticosteroids, lithium, phenytoin, androgens)
* Menstrual history in females (frequency, association with acne flares)
* Medical history
* Family history of acne
* Signs of virilization in young children or females (hirsutism, male pattern hair loss, deepening of voice)
* Joint, bone, or systemic symptoms in patients with severe acne
* Skin care regimen (using comedogenic products)
* Prior treatments and response

Physical examination—Diagnosis is based upon identifying typical lesions (closed comedones, open comedones, inflammatory papules, inflammatory pustules, inflamed nodules) in a characteristic distribution (e.g., face, chest, back, or upper arms) during skin examination (2).

Helpful factors to assess include the following:

- Lesion type and distribution
- Lesion stages (monomorphous to polymorphous)
- Signs of hyperandrogenism in children and females (hirsutism, male pattern hair loss)
- Extent of post-inflammatory hyperpigmentation/scarring

The identification of comedones with or without other lesion types strongly supports the diagnosis. In addition, acne lesions are generally in various stages of development and resolution, in contrast to some presentations of drug-induced acne, which exhibit the acute development of monomorphous lesions. Pityrosporum folliculitis, one of the differentials of acne vulgaris, often presents with monomorphous inflammatory lesions (2).

Tests are usually not necessary in a routine case of acne vulgaris. But inorder to rule out folliculitis by *Staphylococcus aureus* or *Malassezia furfur*, aswab can be obtained from the pustule and sent for microbial culture and sensitivity (2).

Women with signs of hyperandrogenism can be tested for certain markers of polycystic ovaries by taking a blood sample during the first half of the menstrual cycle (2). These include the following:

- Luteinizing hormone (LH) and follicular-stimulating hormone (FSH)
- Prolactin
- Sex hormone-binding globulin (SHBG)
- Dehydroepiandrosterone sulfate (DHEAS)
- 17-hydroxyprogesterone
- Free testosterone

USG abdomen and pelvis can be done to rule out cysts and tumors of the ovaries and adrenal gland (2).

6.5 Management/Approach to Ethnic Skin

Skin of color—Patients with moderately to highly pigmented skin (skin phototypes IV–VI) are more likely to develop post-inflammatory hyperpigmentation than patients with lower skin phototypes. Post-inflammatory hyperpigmentation may result from both active acne vulgaris and skin irritation related to topical acne treatments (2).

With topical retinoid therapy, slow titration of the frequency of application along with a lower concentration of the retinoid may help in alleviating the potential to irritate the skin (23).

Post-inflammatory hyperpigmentation—Post-inflammatory hyperpigmentation can be a distressing problem for patients with acne vulgaris, particularly patients with skin of color (skin phototypes IV to VI). It can have a significant psychological impact, at times more than the acne itself (2).

6.6 Clinical Pearls in Treating Skin of Color

- *Photoprotection*—Sun (UV) protection is of significant importance in the treatment of post-inflammatory hyperpigmentation. Daily use of sunscreen, wide-rimmed hats, and shade-seeking behaviour are encouraged (2).

- *Topical retinoids and azelaic acid* (Table 6.1)—Topical retinoids can be used for patients with acne-induced, post-inflammatory hyperpigmentation (24). Azelaic acid is an alternative to a topical retinoid in patients who experience side effects with retinoids. Both these agents hasten the resolution of post-inflammatory hyperpigmentation (4, 25). In one randomized trial, African American patients who applied tretinoin 0.1% cream exhibited significantly greater lightening of facial post-inflammatory hyperpigmentation than those treated with a vehicle (4).
  - For topical therapies, it is ideal to start at lower concentrations and titrate up based on patient response (17). Given the lower starting doses for skin of color, treatment failures should prompt an increase in dosage or addition of another product rather than switching to another agent (18).
- *Oral antibiotics and retinoids* (Table 6.1)—These should be started in patients with inflammatory lesions, then can be discontinued once the inflammatory lesions resolve (26). If stopping oral antibiotics is not an option and a longer course of treatment is needed, patients should use either BPO alone or BPO/antibiotic combinations to combat any risk of bacterial resistance. Topical retinoids can be used as maintenance therapy once antimicrobials are stopped (26).
- *Topical hydroquinone*—Topical hydroquinone can be applied once or twice daily on hyperpigmented lesions to lighten the marks. Topical hydroquinone is a depigmenting agent that inhibits melanin production and is considered the "gold standard" for the treatment of hyperpigmentation (25–27).
- *Superficial chemical peels* (Table 6.1)—Peels with glycolic acid or salicylic acid can significantly help patients with acne vulgaris, although care must be taken to avoid chemical peel-induced post-inflammatory hyperpigmentation (2).

TABLE 6.1: Managing Acne in Skin of Color (18)

Mild Acne

- Topical retinoids
- Clindamycin + tretinoin or benzoyl peroxide gel
- Adapalene + benzoyl peroxide gel
- Topical benzoyl peroxide
- Topical dapsone
- Azelaic acid for acne with post-inflammatory hyperpigmentation
- Salicylic acid
- Oral contraceptive pills for women

Moderate Acne

- Oral antibiotics like doxycycline, minocycline, and tetracycline
- Clindamycin + tretinoin or benzoyl peroxide gel
- Adapalene + benzoyl peroxide gel
- Comedo extraction
- Oral contraceptive pills for women
- Chemical peels
- Laser and light-based interventions

Nodulocystic Acne

- Oral isotretinoin
- Oral antibiotics with topical retinoids +/– benzoyl peroxide
- Oral contraceptives for women

- *Chemical peeling* (Table 6.1) is another modality that can address both acne and PIH simultaneously in skin-of-color patients (18). Patients with FST IV to VI typically undergo superficial or medium-depth chemical peels. Their response to chemical peeling may vary, and thus, the selection of the peelingagent must be made with caution. Glycolic acid (GA) is a naturally occurringalpha-hydroxy acid that works by inducing epidermolysis, dispersing basal layer melanin, and increasing dermal collagen synthesis (28, 29). GA peel concentrations range from 20% to 70% and require neutralization to terminatethe peel. Salicylic acid (SA) causes keratolysis by disrupting intercellular lipid linkages between epithelioid cells (28, 30). Superficial SA peels range from 20% to 30%, without the need for neutralization. Jessner's solution is acombination of 14 g of resorcinol, 14 g of salicylic acid, and 14 g of lactic acid in 95%ethanol, which causes keratolysis by decreasing corneocyte cohesion (31). It's used as a combination peel to decrease the concentration of anyone agent used in the solution, thereby decreasing not only the risk for side effects but also producing a synergistic effect (28, 31).

6.7 Conclusion

Post-inflammatory hyperpigmentation and scarring appear to be much more common and severe in ethnic skin types, and hence, medical therapy should be started early in these patients (18). Sun protection is paramount in the prevention and treatment of PIH and using effective depigmentingagents (17). Initiating treatment strategies early for both acne and it's sequelae work best in managing skin-of-color patients.

Frequently Asked Questions

1. Q: *Is acne due to poor personal hygiene?*
   A: No, acne is due to the overactivity of sebaceous glands due to high circulating androgens leading to seborrhea (increased sebum production).
2. Q: *Nobody in my family has acne. Why did I get it?*
   A: Although there is a small genetic component to it, the majority of acne patients do not have other family members affected by it. It occurs due to increased sebum production precipitated by increased androgens.
3. Q: *Is my acne due to junk/oily food?*
   A: Acne is not caused by a poor diet but may be aggravated by it. It is a hormonal problem caused by high androgens.
4. Q: *Will my acne improve if I wash my face multiple times a day?*
   A: Acne is not due to poor hygiene and will not improve with repeated cleansing. In fact, excess washing may dry up and irritate the skin.
5. Q: *Does acne worsen with exercise?*
   A: There is no correlation between acne and physical activity. It is due to the overactivity of sebaceous glands and the colonization of hair follicles by *Cutibacterium acnes*.

References

1. Kaushik M, Gupta S, Mahendra A. Living with acne: Belief and perception in a sample of Indian youths. Indian J Dermatol 2017;62:491–497.
2. Thiboutot D, Zaenglein A. Pathogenesis, clinical manifestations, and diagnosis of acne vulgaris, 2021, accessed May 28, 2021. <www.uptodate.com>
3. O'Neill AM, Gallo RL. Host-microbiome interactions and recent progress into understanding the biology of acne vulgaris. Microbiome 2018;6:177.
4. Grice EA, Kong HH, Conlan S, et al. Topographical and temporal diversity of the human skin microbiome. Science 2009;324:1190.
5. Fitz-Gibbon S, Tomida S, Chiu BH, et al. Propionibacterium acnes strain populations in the human skin microbiome associated with acne. J Invest Dermatol 2013;133:2152.
6. Hall JB, Cong Z, Imamura-Kawasawa Y, et al. Isolation and identification of the follicular microbiome: Implications for acne research. J Invest Dermatol 2018;138:2033.
7. Brüggemann H, Henne A, Hoster F, et al. The complete genome sequence of Propionibacterium acnes, a commensal of human skin. Science 2004;305:671.
8. Qin M, Pirouz A, Kim MH, et al. Propionibacterium acnes Induces IL-1β secretion via the NLRP3 inflammasome in human monocytes. J Invest Dermatol 2014;134:381.
9. Alexis AF, Harper JC, Stein Gold LF, Tan JKL. Treating acne in patients with skin of color. Semin Cutan Med Surg 2018;37:S71.
10. Leachman SA, Reed BR. The use of dermatologic drugs in pregnancy and lactation. Dermatol Clin 2006;24:167.
11. Leyden JJ, Del Rosso JQ, Webster GF. Clinical considerations in the treatment of acne vulgaris and other inflammatory skin disorders: A status report. Dermatol Clin 2009;27:1.
12. Agak GW, Qin M, Nobe J, et al. Propionibacterium acnes induces an IL-17 response in acne vulgaris that is regulated by vitamin A and vitamin D. J Invest Dermatol 2014;134:366.
13. Webster GF, Graber EM. Antibiotic treatment for acne vulgaris. Semin Cutan Med Surg 2008;27:183.
14. Cunliffe WJ, Holland KT, Bojar R, Levy SF. A randomized, double-blind comparison of a clindamycin phosphate/benzoyl peroxide gel formulation and a matching clindamycin gel with respect to microbiologic activity and clinical efficacy in the topical treatment of acne vulgaris. Clin Ther 2002;24:1117.
15. Eady EA, Farmery MR, Ross JI, et al. Effects of benzoyl peroxide and erythromycin alone and in combination against antibiotic-sensitive and -resistant skin bacteria from acne patients. Br J Dermatol 1994;131:331.
16. Thiboutot D, Zaenglein A, Weiss J, et al. An aqueous gel fixed combination of clindamycin phosphate 1.2% and benzoyl peroxide 2.5% for the once-daily treatment of moderate to severe acne vulgaris: Assessment of efficacy and safety in 2813 patients. J Am Acad Dermatol 2008;59:792.
17. Tutakne MA, Chari KVR. Acne, rosacea and perioral dermatitis. In: Valia RG, Valia AR, editors. IADVL Textbook and atlas of dermatology, 2nd ed., Mumbai: Bhalani Publishing House; 2003. pp. 689–710.
18. Davis EC, Callender VD. A review of acne in ethnic skin pathogenesis, clinical manifestations, and management strategies. J Clin Aesthet Dermatol 2010 Apr;3(4):24–38.
19. Taylor SC, Cook-Bolden F, Rahman Z, Strachan D. Acne vulgaris in skin of color. J Am Acad Dermatol 2002;46:S98.
20. Callender VD. Considerations for treating acne in ethnic skin. Cutis 2005;76:19.
21. Draelos ZD. Skin lightening preparations and the hydroquinone controversy. Dermatol Ther 2007;20:308.
22. Palumbo A, d'Ischia M, Misuraca G, Prota G. Mechanism of inhibition of melanogenesis by hydroquinone. Biochim Biophys Acta 1991;1073:85.
23. Li ZJ, Choi DK, Sohn KC, et al. Propionibacterium acnes activates the NLRP3 inflammasome in human sebocytes. J Invest Dermatol 2014;134:2747.
24. Callender VD. Considerations for treating acne in ethnic skin. Cutis 2005;76:19.
25. Draelos ZD. Skin lightening preparations and the hydroquinone controversy. Dermatol Ther 2007;20:308.
26. Taylor SC, Cook-Bolden F, Rahman Z, Strachan D. Acne vulgaris in skin of color. J Am Acad Dermatol 2002;46:S98.
27. Palumbo A, d'Ischia M, Misuraca G, Prota G. Mechanism of inhibition of melanogenesis by hydroquinone. Biochim Biophys Acta 1991;1073:85.
28. Roberts WE. Chemical peeling in ethnic/dark skin. Dermatol Ther 2004;17:196–205.
29. Song JY, Kang HA, Kim MY, et al. Damage and recovery of skin barrier function after glycolic acid chemical peeling and crystal microdermabrasion. Dermatol Surg 2004;30:390–394.
30. Grimes PE. Management of hyperpigmentation in darker racial ethnic groups. Semin Cutan Med Surg 2009;28:77–85.
31. Grimes PE, Rendon MI, Pellerano J. Superficial chemical peels. In: Grimes PE, editor. Aesthetics and cosmetic surgery for darker skin types, Philadelphia, PA: Lippincott Williams & Wilkins; 2008. pp. 154–169.

CHAPTER 7: ROSACEA

Suraj Sachidanand

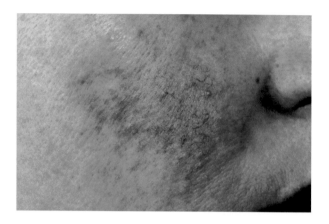

FIGURE 7.1 Rosacea.

7.1 Introduction

Rosacea is an inflammatory facial dermatosis with varied clinical presentations, facial erythema being the most common, mostly affecting the facial convexities along with some vascular changes, inflammatory lesions, hypertrophic changes, or ocular involvement (Figure 7.1). The diagnosis is harder to ascertain in people with colored skin (Fitzpatrick skin types IV, V, or VI), as the hallmark erythema is difficult to discern. As a result, this condition remains undiagnosed in ethnic races, although its incidence is increasing in this group (1).

7.2 Epidemiology

The exact prevalence of rosacea remains unknown; lighter-skinned individuals usually being affected more commonly. A review of population studies has revealed a widely varying prevalence: 0.1% in the Faroe Islands, 5% in Russia, 12.3% in Germany, 10% in Sweden, and 22% in Estonia. These studies mainly included patients with phototypes 1–3 (2). Although rosacea is not uncommon in colored skin, typical clinical features are hard to detect, thus leading to underdiagnosis and underestimation of the prevalence of rosacea among people with colored skin (3). Delayed diagnosis could lead to advanced disease, inadequate treatment, greater morbidity, loss of sight in ocular rosacea, and facial disfigurement with disease progression (e.g., rhinophyma and otophyma) (4, 5–14).

In India, rosacea (especially steroid-induced) is being increasingly reported (15). One Indian study showed that rosacea accounted for almost 0.5% of all dermatology patients indicating that it is more prevalent than earlier thought (4). A study conducted among Saudi females with rosacea reported its highest prevalence in skin type 6 (42%), followed by skin type 4 (40%) and skin type 5 (18%) (16). In China, Taiwan, Korea, and Japan, rosacea is a common disease (17). In Tunisia, Khaled et al. (18) reported 224 cases of rosacea in a predominantly dark-skinned population, with a hospital prevalence of 0.2%. The

onset is usually in middle age (30–50 years), although children may also be affected. Although sexual predilection is absent, men appear to be worse affected, with a higher risk of developing rhinophyma (1).

7.3 Pathophysiology of Rosacea in Skin of Color

Reduced flushing seen in Fitzpatrick skin phototype VI (19, 20) could be explained by studies of skin circulation in various populations (21–23). In studies involving microvascular endothelial function, the skin blood flow response to reactive hyperemia under occlusion and local heating was examined; these studies showed differences in the microvascular structure and function between white patients and Afro-Caribbean, Korean, and Southeast Asian patients, who all displayed lower vascular endothelial function. Nevertheless, any physiological differences that exist for skin of color do not change the risk factors for rosacea, and people with skin of color show the same rosacea triggers (24).

7.4 Clinical Features and Subtypes of Rosacea (1)

Erythematotelangiectactic type—Here, patients present with erythema on the face with multiple telangiectases.

Papulopustular type—Patients present with a mixture of papules and pustules with a little less flushing.

Phymatous type—Papules and nodules can be seen on the nose, forehead, and ears, leading to altered contours of these sites.

Ocular type—Mild itching, dryness, or gritty sensation of the eyes. Conjunctival telangiectases can also be seen. In patients with skin phototype ≥4, erythema is often times hard to discern, which makes the diagnosis difficult (1). In a study done on Saudi women (skin phototypes 3, 4, and 5), sun exposure was seen to worsen rosacea in 72% of the patients. Pruritus was most significant in contrast to burning or stinging seen in Europeans or white Americans. Erythematotelengiectatic and papulopustular rosacea were the commonest varieties, and severity was not related to skin type. Extrafacial sites were also commonly involved (14%). Phymatous and granulomatous types were not seen. Post-inflammatory hyper-/hypopigmentation was not reported in any of the patients (16). Khaled et al. reported sun exposure to be a major triggering factor (64%) along with other thermal stimuli (25%) in Tunisian patients (18). The most common clinical subtype was papulopustular rosacea (69%), followed by erythematotelangiectatic type (12%) and rhinophyma (3.7%). Other types were rare, and the amount of sun exposure was noted to have a major effect on the occurrence and severity of the erythematotelangiectatic variant (25).

A study conducted in China among 586 patients evaluated the differences in epidemiological and clinical characteristics among rosacea patients according to different facial sites—full-face, cheeks, nose, or perioral involvement. There were 471 (80.4%), 49 (8.4%), 52 (8.9%), and

DOI: 10.1201/9780429243769-7

14 (2.4%) cases in the full-face, cheek, nasal, and perioral groups, respectively. Compared with the full-face group, the nasal group had more severe phymatous changes and less severe self-reported and dermatologist-evaluated grading of symptoms (26).

Rosacea is usually reported less commonly in skin of color, probably because darker skin types are less prone to photodamage and also because flushing and telangiectasia are harder to detect on examination (1).

Cutaneous presentations of rosacea in a patient with skin of color, outside of visible erythema or telangiectasia, might include dryness, edema, and hyperpigmentation (27). Another important indicator to consider is the presence of acneiform papules and pustules, which are often present with rosacea in skin of color. Papules and pustules without comedones help differentiate rosacea from acne. Ocular symptoms like itching, foreign body sensation, and irritation might be present. Thickening of the nasal and medial cheek skin may indicate early phymatous changes associated with rosacea (27).

7.5 Differential Diagnoses to Be Considered in Patients with Skin of Color (27)

- Acne vulgaris
- Steroid-induced acne
- Contact dermatitis
- Perioral dermatitis
- Seborrheic dermatitis
- Lupus erythematosus
- Sarcoidosis
- Dermatomyositis
- Keratosis pilaris rubra

7.6 Treatment of Rosacea (1)

Treatment of rosacea can be challenging due to the multitude of factors involved and can be categorized into general and specific measures: the latter including topical, systemic, and physical/light-based modalities (1).

For the erythematotelangiectatic type, topical brimonidine, oral beta blockers, intense pulsed light, and pulsed dye laser are some of the treatment modalities.

In patients presenting with inflamed papules and pustules, topical azelaic acid/metronidazole and oral doxycycline can be used for mild/moderate cases, whereas oral isotretinoin is the treatment of choice for severe cases. Patients with phymatous type are best managed with oral doxycycline or isotretinoin.

7.7 General Measures/Non-Pharmacologic Treatments

General measures are aimed at identifying the triggering factors and minimizing their effects to hasten improvement.

7.7a Patient Education
Educating patients regarding the benign nature of rosacea is important to allay any fears that they might have. They must be counseled to avoid all the common triggering factors like sun exposure, strong winds, temperature variations,

exercise, spicy foods, alcohol, and physical and/or emotional stress (2). History of drug intake should be noted to identify aggravating drugs, like niacin and topical corticosteroids (28).

7.7b Photoprotection/Sunscreens
Exposure to ultraviolet rays resulting in photodamaged skin is a well-known trigger for the occurrence and/or worsening of rosacea, and hence, photoprotection is an important component of its treatment (2). Apart from physical measures, such as covered clothing, shade-seeking behavior, and umbrella, broad-spectrum sunscreens (sun protection factor 30+) are recommended to achieve effective photoprotection against UVA and UVB radiation. Conventional sticky sunscreens may worsen the condition by increasing the warmth of the skin by converting ultraviolet radiation into heat. Inorganic sunscreens with zinc oxide and titanium oxide are preferred as they do not have this effect (5). Sunscreens should also be advocated in women staying indoors before they go near hot stoves or consume hot liquids.

7.7c Facial Cleansers
Facial cleansers are needed to remove excess sebum, exfoliated keratinocytes, environmental debris, and some microorganisms (*Demodex*, *Pityrosporum*, etc.) to maintain a healthy and clean biofilm (1). However, mild cleansers must be prescribed to preserve the epidermal barrier (1). Selection of appropriate cleansers is essential—such as soaps, syndets, and lipid-free cleansers for oily, normal, and dry skins, respectively—to achieve optimum results (5). Ideally, cleansers should be used twice daily, followed by rinsing with water to clean the biofilm maintaining the normal skin barrier. Nasolabial areas, eyebrows, and beard areas must be cleaned meticulously, as these sites have high sebum concentration (1).

7.7d Facial Moisturizers
Facial moisturizers may be helpful when patients have normal or dry skin. These substances act by helping in barrier repair and minimizing transepidermal water loss (28). However, they should not promote bacterial overgrowth (plant and animal oils like coconut, olive, argan, and sunflower oils) or occlude the sweat ducts to cause miliaria, acneiform eruptions, and facial irritation (1). Broadly, three classes of moisturizers are available—occlusive (oily substances that retard transepidermal water loss), humectants (substances that attract water to the epidermis from underlying dermis and environment), and hydrocolloids (large molecules that cover the epidermis and minimize transepidermal water loss). A mixture of occlusive and humectant properties provides the best results in these patients (5).

The treatment approach for rosacea in skin of color is similar to that in lighter skin types, involving the same topical, oral, laser, light-based, or surgical treatments targeted to the patient's individual signs of rosacea (6, 7)—although data on the treatment of rosacea in this patient population are limited (24). Patients with skin of color might have unique clinical features that need to be addressed during rosacea treatment, such as post-inflammatory pigment alteration and the risk of developing this complication on the administration of laser and light-based therapies. The treatment approach for rosacea might also need to include cultural and geographic variations in skin care that might affect the skin condition (8). For example, patients with skin of color might be accustomed to using skin lighteners or brighteners, astringent or abrasive skin care products, or occlusive moisturizers, such as shea butter or cocoa butter (27). In the authors' experience, exfoliation is common in East Asian populations (e.g., Korean), and patients of sub-Saharan African ancestry might use shea or cocoa butter products (27). There also are geographic factors that tend to trigger rosacea, such as variations in temperature, humidity, sun exposure, or local popularity of spicy food (27). Ultimately, managing patients with skin of color should consist of controlling the occurrence of papules and pustules, reducing the risk of post-inflammatory hyperpigmentation, and educating patients about the stubbornness of the condition and long-term treatment (27).

Skin-of-color patients should be properly counseled about their skin care routine. A critical component is the use of sunscreen or a physical sunblock. In addition, patients should be taught about identifying rosacea triggers (dietary, environmental, lifestyle) and measures to avoid them (27).

The use of topical medications to address vascular involvement might be warranted (9–11). Foams, creams, and aqueous gels might be less irritating to the skin. Oral medications can be added to reduce inflammation of papules and pustules. Laser and light-based therapies may be considered for reducing the capillary network of the skin or for resurfacing phymatous changes (27). Recent studies have also shown the effectiveness and safety of microsecond-pulsed 1,064 nm neodymium-doped yttrium-aluminum-garnet (Nd-YAG) laser treatment in patients with skin of color (12–14). With laser devices, the use of lower fluences is recommended to reduce the risk of pigmentation and scarring (27).

7.8 Conclusion

Rosacea is a multifactorial disease that is largely underdiagnosed in skin-of-color patients. Treatment strategies should be tailored differently and started early due to the risk of post-inflammatory hyperpigmentation and scarring in these patients. Identifying and avoiding rosacea triggers also plays an important role in the management of this difficult condition.

References

1. Sarkar R, Podder I, Jagadeesan S. Rosacea in skin of colour: A comprehensive review. Indian J Dermatol Venereol Leprol 2020;86:611–621.
2. Berth-Jones J. Rosacea, perioral dermatitis and similar dermatoses, flushing and flushing syndromes. In: Burns T, Breathnach S, Cox N, Griffiths C, editors. Rook's textbook of dermatology. 7th ed. UK: Wiley-Blackwell Publishing Ltd.; 2004. p. 2197–2216.
3. Al-Dabagh A, Davis SA, McMichael AJ, Feldman SR. Rosacea in skin of color: Not a rare diagnosis. Dermatol Online J 2014;20:13030.
4. Wollina U, Verma SB. Rosacea and rhinophyma: Not curse of the Celts but Indo Eurasians. J Cosmet Dermatol 2009;8:234–235.
5. Draelos ZD. Cosmeceuticals for rosacea. Clin Dermatol 2017;35:213–217.
6. Tan J, Almeida LM, Bewley A, et al. Updating the diagnosis, classification and assessment of rosacea: Recommendations from the global ROSacea COnsensus (ROSCO) panel. Br J Dermatol 2017;176:431–438.
7. Gallo RL, Granstein RD, Kang S, et al. Standard classification and pathophysiology of rosacea: The 2017 update by the National Rosacea Society Expert Committee. J Am Acad Dermatol 2018;78:148–155.
8. Cole PD, Hatef DA, Taylor S, Bullocks JM. Skin care in ethnic populations. Semin Plast Surg 2009;23:168–172.
9. Baumann L, Goldberg DJ, Stein-Gold L, et al. Efficacy and safety of topical oxymetazoline cream 1.0% for the treatment of facial erythema associated with rosacea: Findings from the second of 2 pivotal trials [abstract]. Presented at: Annual Meeting of the American Academy of Dermatology; March 3–7, 2017; Orlando, FL.
10. Kircik LH, DuBois J, Draelos ZD, et al. Efficacy and safety of topical oxymetazoline cream 1.0% for the treatment of facial erythema associated with rosacea: Findings from 1 of 2 pivotal trials [abstract]. Presented at: Annual Meeting of the American Academy of Dermatology; March 3–7, 2017; Orlando, FL.
11. Fowler Jr. J, Jackson M, Moore A, et al. Efficacy and safety of once-daily topical brimonidine tartrate gel 0.5% for the treatment of moderate to severe facial erythema of rosacea: Results of two randomized, double-blind, and vehicle-controlled pivotal studies. J Drugs Dermatol 2013;12:650–656.
12. Battle Jr. EF. Cosmetic laser treatments for skin of color: A focus on safety and efficacy. J Drugs Dermatol 2011;10:35–38.
13. Alexis AF. Lasers and light-based therapies in ethnic skin: Treatment options and recommendations for Fitzpatrick skin types V and VI. Br J Dermatol 2013;169:91–97.
14. Alexis AF, Webster G, Preston NJ, et al. Effectiveness and safety of once-daily doxycycline capsules as monotherapy in patients with rosacea: An analysis by Fitzpatrick skin type. J Drugs Dermatol 2012;11:1219–1222.
15. Bhat YJ, Manzoor S, Qayoom S. Steroid-induced rosacea: A clinical study of 200 patients. Indian J Dermatol 2011;56:30–32.
16. Al Balbeesi AO, Halawani MR. Unusual features of rosacea in Saudi females with dark skin. Ochsner J 2014;14:321–327.
17. Chang AL, Raber I, Xu J, et al. Assessment of the genetic basis of rosacea by genome-wide association study. J Invest Dermatol 2015;135:1548–1555.
18. Khaled A, Hammami H, Zeglaoui F, et al. Rosacea: 244 Tunisian cases. Tunis Med 2010;88:597–601.
19. Rosen T, Stone MS. Acne rosacea in blacks. J Am Acad Dermatol 1987;17:70–73.
20. Guy RH, Tur E, Bjerke S, Maibach HI. Are there age and racial differences to methyl nicotinate-induced vasodilatation in human skin? J Am Acad Dermatol 1985;12(6):1001–1006.
21. Strain WD, Chaturvedi N, Leggetter S, et al. Ethnic differences in skin microvascular function and their relation to cardiac target-organ damage. J Hypertens 2005;23(1):133–140.
22. Yim J, Petrofsky J, Berk L, et al. Differences in endothelial function between Korean-Asians and Caucasians. Med Sci Monit 2012;18(6):Cr337–Cr343.
23. Petrofsky JS, Alshahmmari F, Lee H, et al. Reduced endothelial function in the skin in Southeast Asians compared to Caucasians. Med Sci Monit 2012;18(1):Cr1–Cr8.
24. Shah S, Alexis AF. Acne and rosacea in skin of color. In: Alexis AF, Barbosa VH, editors. Skin color: A practical guide to dermatologic diagnosis and treatment. New York, NY: Springer; 2013. p. 21–36.
25. Bae YI, Yun SJ, Lee JB, Kim SJ, et al. Clinical evaluation of 168 Korean patients with rosacea: The sun exposure correlates with the erythematotelangiectatic subtype. Ann Dermatol 2009;21:243–249.
26. Xie HF, Huang YX, He L, et al. An observational descriptive survey of rosacea in the Chinese population: Clinical features based on the affected locations. PeerJ 2017;5:e3527.
27. Alexis AF, Callender VD, Baldwin HE, et al. Global epidemiology and clinical spectrum of rosacea, highlighting skin of color: Review and clinical practice experience. J Am Acad Dermatol. June 1, 2019;80(6):1722–1729. E7
28. Two AM, Wu W, Gallo RL, Hata TR. Rosacea: Part II. Topical and systemic therapies in the treatment of rosacea. J Am Acad Dermatol 2015;72:761–770.

CHAPTER 8: PIGMENTARY DISORDERS

Pooja Agarwal and Rashmi Sarkar

8.1 Introduction

The color of the skin imparts an important visible social and cultural characteristic to an individual, and any deviation from the assumed normal pattern of pigmentation for that culture results in significant concerns. The racial and ethnic differences in skin color arise from differences in number, shape, size, and distribution of the melanin-laden organelles called melanosomes. Two different types of melanin pigmentation can be seen: *constitutive* skin color (genetically determined in the absence of any external influence) and *facultative* skin color (inducible by sun exposure).

Pigmentation disorders pose a diagnostic and therapeutic challenge many a time, and some of the disorders are even difficult to classify.

Morphologically, disorders of pigmentation may be classified into two types: hypermelanosis and hypomelanosis. In hypermelanosis, there is an increased amount of melanin in the skin, which may be present in epidermis, dermis, or both. In hypomelanosis, there is a relative lack of pigment, which makes the skin appear lighter than the normal color. A third disorder of pigmentation can also be considered, which is amelanosis, where melanin is completely lacking from the skin.

8.2 Hyperpigmentation

Increased pigmentation of the skin can arise in a number of ways and can be due to a variety of genetic and environmental factors. It can be due to an increase in the number of melanocytes in the skin or an increase in melanogenesis in the normal melanocytes. Hyperpigmentation may be classified according to distribution as being diffuse or localized.

Diffuse hyperpigmentation may be congenital or acquired. The congenital variant is known as *melanosis diffusa congenita*, also known by a multitude of names, such as familial progressive hyperpigmentation or carbon baby. It is a diffuse dirty brown hyperpigmentation covering almost the whole body. No systemic involvement is seen. It presumably follows an autosomal dominant inheritance pattern. As the child grows, there is a tendency for the skin to become lighter.

8.2a Acquired Diffuse Hyperpigmentation

A diffuse brown pigmentation of the skin may be caused by various disorders, as outlined in Table 8.1. This type of pigmentation is especially typical for Addison disease (primary adrenal cortical insufficiency). Systemic symptoms in Addison disease arise from corticosteroid deficiency and present as easy fatigue, hypotension, weight loss, hypothermia, and a tendency toward hypoglycemia. However, hyperpigmentation usually precedes all the other symptoms of the disease and is most intensified at sites of pressure and frequent sun exposure, palmar creases, and areas of scarring (Figure 8.1). Lentiginous pigmentation may also be found in the oral mucosa, lips, and anogenital regions. Acromegaly and Cushing syndrome can also lead to diffuse hyperpigmentation, which is caused by excessive stimulation of melanocyte activity by melanocyte-stimulating hormone (MSH). During pregnancy, hyperpigmentation appears

TABLE 8.1: Acquired Hyperpigmentation

Etiology	Gray/Blue Color	Brown Color
Metabolic	Hemochromatosis	Liver diseases Porphyria
Endocrine		Addison disease Pregnancy MSH-producing tumors Chloasma Hormonal therapy
Chemicals	Minocycline Fixed drug eruptions	Psoralens Bleomycin Arsenic
Nutritional	Chronic deficiency	Pellagra Kwashiorkor Vitamin B12 deficiency
Post-inflammatory	Erythema dyschromicum perstans	Eczema/acne/psoriasis/pemphigus/insect bite reactions/lichen planus/etc.
Neoplastic	Metastatic melanoma	Malignant melanoma Acanthosis nigricans with underlying malignancy

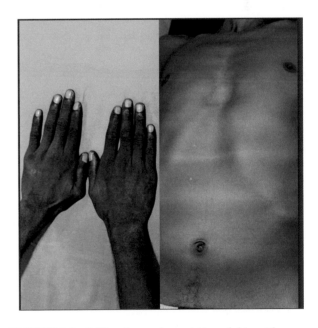

FIGURE 8.1 Diffuse hyperpigmentation of skin with accentuation of the pigment over the knuckles and relative sparing of body folds in Addison disease.

on the face (chloasma), nipples, linea alba, neck, and anogenital regions. Both estrogens and progesterone appear to play a role, as does perhaps MSH.

Diffuse grayish-brown discoloration of the skin develops, typically in hemochromatosis, which is also known as bronze diabetes. Hyperpigmentation mainly affects the face and hands and sometimes is associated with mucosal changes. It

DOI: 10.1201/9780429243769-8

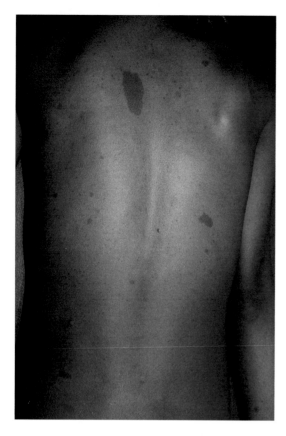

FIGURE 8.2 Multiple café-au-lait macules, freckles, and neurofibromas in neurofibromatosis

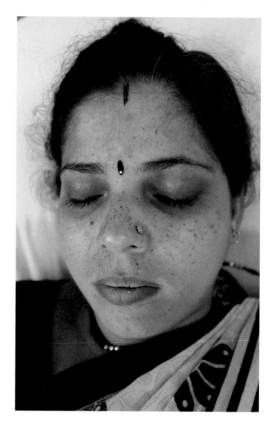

FIGURE 8.3 Diffusely distributed freckles in a fair-skinned female.

TABLE 8.2: Hyperpigmentation due to Genetic and Nevoid Factors

Gray/Blue Color	Brown Color
• Mongolian spot	• Freckles
• Nevus of Ota	• Lentigines
• Nevus of Ito	• Café au lait macules
• Becker's nevus	• Hypermelanotic macules in McCune-Albright syndrome
	• Peutz-Jeghers syndrome

TABLE 8.3: Syndromes Associated with Multiple Lentigines

• LEOPARD syndrome (*l*entiginosis, *e*lectrocardiographic changes, *o*cular hypertelorism, *p*ulmonary stenosis, *a*bnormalities of the genitalia, *r*etarded growth, *d*eafness)
• Centrofacial lentiginosis
• Peutz-Jeghers syndrome
• Cronkhite-Canada syndrome
• Carney complex
• LAMB syndrome (*l*entigines, *a*trial myxomas, *m*ucocutaneous myxomas, *b*lue nevi)
• NAME syndrome (*n*evi, *a*trial myxomas, *m*yxoid neurofibromas, *e*phelides)
• Laugier-Hunziker syndrome

is a result of both increased melanogenesis and iron deposits in the deeper dermis. Other systems may also be affected by the excess iron. Diffuse hyperpigmentation is also seen in other forms of chronic liver disorders, porphyrias, chronic renal insufficiency, and systemic sclerosis.

Another way to classify hyperpigmentation disorders can be according to the factors implicated in pathogenesis. (Table 8.2)

8.2b Hyperpigmentation of Genetic/ Nevoid Origin

Café-au-lait spots usually develop during the first years of life and may sometimes be present at the time of birth also. In 2% of the Caucasian population, they can be present without any other genodermatoses. Café-au-lait spots have a uniform brown pigmentation and a sharp border (Figure 8.2). The brown color results from increased melanin content of the

melanocytes and the basal keratinocytes. They are also considered markers for various genodermatoses, like neurofibromatosis, Albright syndrome, and Cowden syndrome.

Lentigines are dark 2–20 mm benign pigmented macules that can appear anywhere on the skin. There is an increased number of melanocytes in the epidermis. When lentigines are present in an exceptionally large number or a typical distribution, it is referred to as *lentiginosis*. Various syndromes associated with multiple lentigines are enumerated in Table 8.3.

Freckles or *ephelides* are small hyperpigmented macules (2–4 mm) appearing predominantly on sun-exposed skin (Figures 8.3 and 8.4). They increase during summers and have a tendency to lighten during the winters. They result from

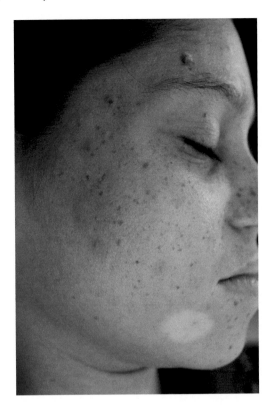

FIGURE 8.4 Light brown-colored freckles along with a single depigmented macule.

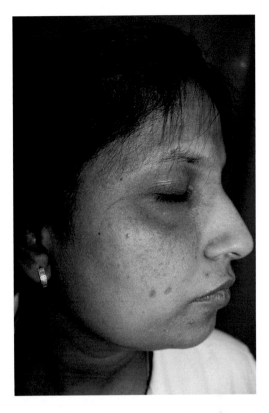

FIGURE 8.5 Nevus of Ota involving the right side of the forehead and zygoma region.

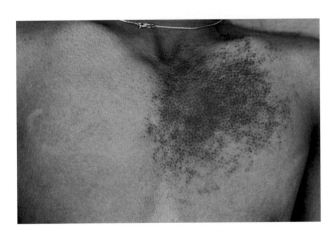

FIGURE 8.6 Becker's nevus over the left side of the chest.

an increase in melanogenesis on sun exposure in normal melanocytes.

Mongolian spots are bluish-colored macules seen commonly in Oriental babies. They are poorly circumscribed and are usually present over the lumbosacral area. They fade in early childhood, though extrasacral aberrant spots may persist.

Nevus of Ota is usually congenital but may also appear later in life. It is a unilateral bluish-gray macule sometimes involving the sclera and nasal mucosa also (Figure 8.5). Hyperpigmentation affects the area supplied by the ophthalmic and mandibular divisions of the trigeminal nerve.[1] A bilateral, acquired dermal melanosis of the face, which resembles the nevus of Ota, has been described as *Hori's nevus*.[2]

Becker nevus presents with a unilateral hyperpigmented macule, which has ill-defined margins. It commonly affects the shoulder region or upper chest (Figure 8.6). It usually manifests during puberty, and there is a growth of darker and thicker hair on the lesion. Many other cutaneous lesions, like acneiform eruptions, can appear over the nevus. The rare Becker nevus syndrome features ipsilateral hypoplasia of the breast tissue and pectoral muscle, often associated with scoliosis and urogenital malformations.

8.2c Acquired Localized Hyperpigmentation

Disorders with acquired localized pigmentation are seen more commonly in routine practice as compared to the diffuse pigmentation. In this section, common causes of acquired localized pigmentation are discussed.

Melasma Melasma is a commonly acquired localized pigmentary disorder that presents as mostly symmetric hyperpigmented macules, most commonly over the face (Figures 8.7, 8.8, and 8.9). They can also be seen over the neck and hands in case of extrafacial melasma.[3] Etiology of melasma is elusive and multifactorial. These include genetic predisposition, ultraviolet radiation, thyroid autoimmunity, pregnancy, and drugs, such as oral contraceptive pills and phenytoin.[4-6] Both melanocytosis and increased melanogenesis are responsible for the pigmentation in melasma. Vascular endothelial growth factor (VEGF) levels have been found to be increased in the lesional skin of melasma, signifying increased vascularization.[7]

Traditionally melasma has been classified on the basis of the depth of the melanin pigment in the skin and is helpful in predicting the therapeutic outcome.[8] Hydroqinone (HQ) is the gold standard in the treatment of melasma and can be

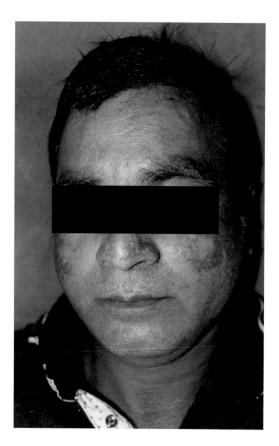

FIGURE 8.7   Centrofacial melasma in a male.

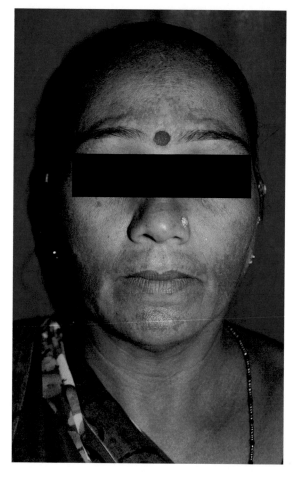

FIGURE 8.8   Melasma over centrofacial and mandibular area.

TABLE 8.4: Botanical Extracts Used in the Treatment of Melasma

- Grape seed extract
- Orchid extract
- Aloe vera extract
- Pycnogenol
- Marine algae extract
- Green tea extracts
- Mulberry extract
- Soy
- Licorice extract

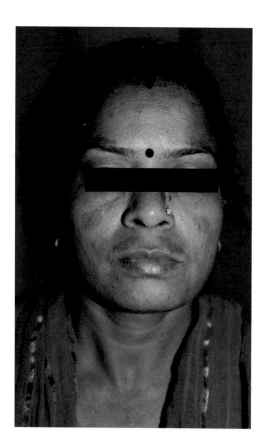

FIGURE 8.9   Centrofacial melasma in a female.

used alone (2–4%) or in combination with other agents. These combinations include the Kligman formula (5% HQ, 0.1% tretinoin, and 0.1% dexamethasone), modified Kligman's formula (4% HQ, 0.05% tretinoin, and 1% hydrocortisone acetate), Pathak's (2% HQ and 0.05–0.1% tretinoin) and Westerhof's formula (4.7% N-acetylcysteine, 2% HQ, and 0.1% triamcinolone acetonide).[9]

Various chemical peels like glycolic acid, tretinoin peel, mandelic acid, and Jessner's solution have shown efficacy in the treatment of melasma. Various botanical extracts are also being used for the treatment of melasma (Table 8.4).

Pigmented Contact Dermatitis (Riehl Melanosis) Riehl melanosis is now almost synonymous with pigmented contact dermatitis. The most common causes are sensitizing chemicals in cosmetics. It is characterized by a brownish-gray pigmentation that is more marked on the forehead and temples (Figure 8.10). The patches usually have a reticular pattern and a black to brown-violet hue.[10] Avoidance of the implicated chemicals and cosmetics results in a slow improvement in pigmentation.

Case—A 42-year-old male presents with blackish-brown hyperpigmentation over the forehead for two to three months (Figure 8.10). He denies a history of excessive sun exposure; however, on probing, he gave a history of rubbing balms over his forehead for colds and headaches for almost one year. A diagnosis of pigmented contact dermatitis is suspected. Management of Riehl's melanosis involves promptly stopping the offending agent. A broad-spectrum sunscreen is advised to be used regularly along with Kligman's formula for nighttime application. The improvement is slow, and exposure to any similar chemical will result in delayed results.

Erythema Dyschromicum Perstans Erythema dyschromicum perstans, or ashy dermatosis, is an idiopathic and chronic skin disorder. It is characterized by round or oval-shaped blue-gray patches over the face, trunk, and extremities. The trunk and proximal extremities are more commonly affected, followed by the face and neck. There appears to be no predilection for exposed areas. There is considerable evidence that an immunologic mechanism may be involved in the pathogenesis of the disease.[11] NB-UVB and topical tacrolimus have shown promising results in the treatment of erythema dyschromicum perstans.

Phototoxic Dermatitis As the name suggests, phototoxic dermatitis is initiated by a photochemical reaction between a phototoxic substance and UV radiation. Exposure to these phototoxic substances could be topical application (psoralens), systemic, or contacted accidentally (photo-toxic plants). After exposure to the sun, initially erythema and blisters develop, followed by prominent post-inflammatory hyperpigmentation.

Berloque dermatitis is a type of phototoxic dermatitis resulting from the application of a phototoxic oil found in several perfumes. The hyperpigmentation usually develops in a streaked pattern following the lines of the flow of the perfume.

8.2d Drug-Induced Hyperpigmentation

Drugs can cause hyperpigmentation of skin and mucosa by stimulating melanogenesis through nonspecific cutaneous inflammation. Drug-induced hyperpigmentation may range from the usual brownish hyperpigmentation to a blue-gray hue. Commonly implicated drugs are enumerated in Table 8.5.

8.2e Reticulate Pigmentary Disorders

Reticulate pigmentary disorders encompass a group of disorders that present with hyperpigmented macules similar to freckles.[12] They can be inherited or acquired; in the latter, a reticular or net-like pigmentation is seen more commonly, varying in pigment and size. Another set of disorders that have both hypo- and hyperpigmented lesions over the body is termed *dyschromatosis*. *Poikilodermatous* conditions are characterized by atrophy, macular or reticulate pigmentation, and telengietasias. Various genetic disorders with reticulate pigmentation, dyschromatosis, and poikiloderma are summarized in Table 8.6.

Case—A 15-year-old male presented with chief complains of recurrent episodes of diarrhea on and off since four years of age, dark-colored pigmentation over the whole body since six years of age, and nail changes since seven years of age. There was a history of mild mental retardation. On examination, fine, reticulate, gray-brown pigmentation was seen over the neck, both thighs, the back, and both arms (Figures 8.15 and 8.16). The skin over the dorsum of the hands and feet was diffusely atrophic. Palms were thickened and hyperhydrotic. Nail dystrophy was present in the nails of both hands and feet. Oral leucoplakia was seen. Investigations revealed leucopenia, and colonoscopy was suggestive of celiac disease. No active management for dermatological findings is described, and the patient was referred to a gastroenterologist for the management of celiac disease. A final diagnosis of dyskeratosis congenita with coeliac disease was made. These patients require multidisciplinary management and regular screening for bone marrow suppression and malignancy.

Many acquired cutaneous disorders may also have the classic reticular pattern. These include Riehl's melanosis, erythema ab igne, cutis marmorata, livedo reticularis, and

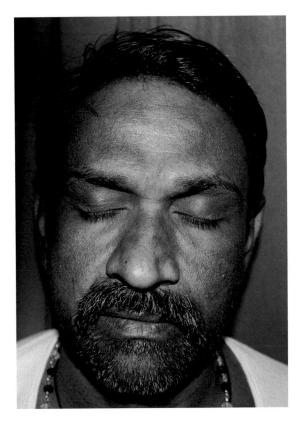

FIGURE 8.10 Pigmented contact dermatitis over areas or repeated rubbing of a balm.

TABLE 8.5: Drugs That Cause Pigmentation of Skin and Mucosa

• Antimalarials	• Heavy metals (e.g., gold, silver, mercury)
• Amiodarone	• Clofazimine
• Bleomycin	• Antiretrovirals (e.g., zidovudine)
• 5 fluoro uracil	• Oral contraceptives
• Cyclophosphamide	• Psoralens
• Minocycline	• Tricyclic antidepressants
• Phenothiazines	• Bimatoprost/latanoprost

TABLE 8.6: Genetic Disorders with Reticulate Pigmentation, Dyschromatosis, and Poikiloderma

Disorder	Distribution of Pigmentation	Clinical Features
Dowling-Degos disease (Figure 8.11)	Flexural	Pigmented reticulate macules Comedone-like papules on the back and neck (seborrheic distribution) Worsens in hot weather Perioral acneform pits; keratoses; epidermal cysts
Acropigmentation of Kitamura	Acral	Hyperpigmented mildly atrophic macules primarily localized to the dorsum of hands and feet Rarely may involve the flexures and the palms and soles Palmar pits characteristic
Acropigmentation of Dohi (dyschromatosis symmetrica hereditaria) (Figures 8.12 and 13)	Acral	Hypopigmented and hyperpigmented macules without atrophy over both the dorsal and ventral surface of hands and legs Freckle-like macules on the face
Naegeli-Franceschetti-Jadassohn syndrome	Generalized	Onset in childhood, fading in adolescence Palmoplantar keratoderma Dental defects
Dyschromatosis universalis hereditaria (Figure 8.14)	Generalized	Hypo- and hyperpigmented macules involving the whole body Can also involve palms, soles, and oral mucosa Extracutaneous features may be associated
Dermatopathia pigmentosa reticularis	Generalized	Diagnostic triad of reticulate hyperpigmentation, non-cicatricial alopecia, and onychodystrophy Associated hypo- or hyperhidrosis, absent dermatoglyphics; acral blisters Palmarpolantar hyperkeratoses
Kindler syndrome	Acral	Spontaneous blistering Photosensitivity and palmoplantar hyperkeratosis Widespread poikiloderma Marked skin atrophy
Rothmund-Thomson syndrome	Generalized	Poikiloderma in photodistributed pattern Bullae over photoexposed areas Photosensitivity Cataracts Alopecia
Dyskeratosis congenita (Figures 8.15 and 8.16)	Generalized	Poikiloderma seen on the face, neck, trunk, and upper thighs Hyperhidrosis of palms and soles may be present Leukokeratosis in oral, anorectal, or urogenital mucosae Dystrophic nails with pterygium formation Thin, lusterless hair May be associated with dental defects, aplastic anemia, growth retardation, hypogonadism, and mental retardation

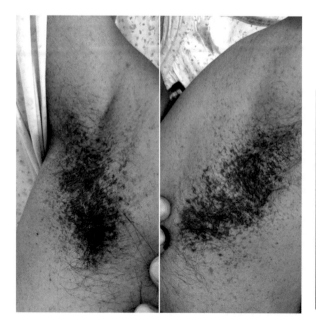

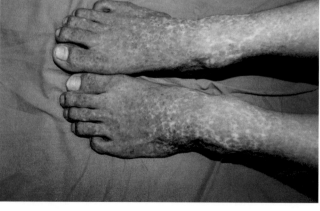

FIGURE 8.11 Pigmented reticulate macules in axillae in Dowling-Degos disease.

FIGURE 8.12 Hypo- and hyperpigmented macules over legs in dyschromatosis symmetrica hereditaria.

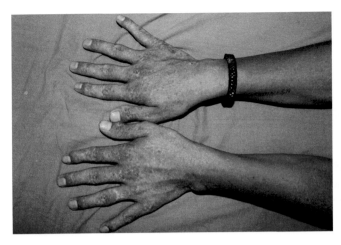

FIGURE 8.13 Hypo- and hyperpigmented macules over hands in dyschromatosis symmetrica hereditaria.

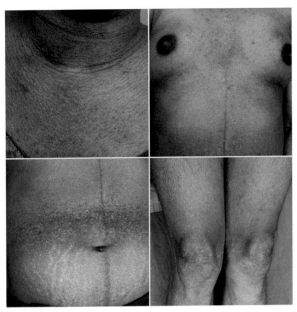

FIGURE 8.14 Hypo- and hyperpigmented macules involving the whole body in dyschromatosis universalis hereditaria.

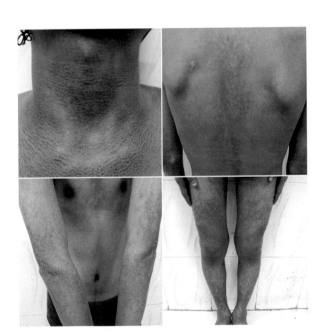

FIGURE 8.15 Poikiloderma seen on the neck, trunk, and extremities in dyskeratosis congenita.

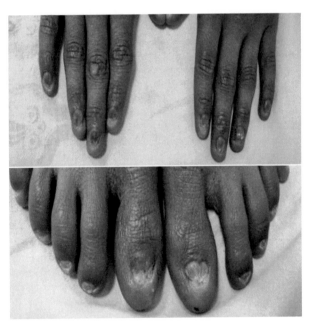

FIGURE 8.16 Dystrophic nails with pterygium formation in dyskeratosis congenita.

post-inflammatory hyperpigmentation. Infections like oncocerchiasis, pityriasis versicolor, and pediculosis corporis may also give rise to mottled pigmentation in a few cases.

8.2f Hyperpigmentation Affecting Flexures

Hyperpigmentation limited to flexures is most commonly seen in acanthosis nigricans and Dowling-Degos disease. *Acanthosis nigricans* is characterized by hyperpigmented velvety skin lesions that are symmetrically distributed over the neck (Figure 8.17) and axillae, less commonly over antecubital and popliteal fossae, and groin folds. It may be benign, obesity-associated, syndromic, or malignancy-associated.

Due to a common association with underlying insulin resistance, a proper workup for metabolic syndrome is needed. Malignancies most commonly associated with acanthosis nigricans include gastric adenocarcinoma and lung carcinomas. The therapeutic approach aims at the treatment of underlying insulin resistance/malignancy, removal of inciting drugs, and various oral/topical medications. Topical retinoids form the first line of therapy and may be supplemented with peels like 15% trichloroacetic acid peel or topical calcipotriol. Oral metformin is also found to be useful in increasing peripheral insulin responsiveness.

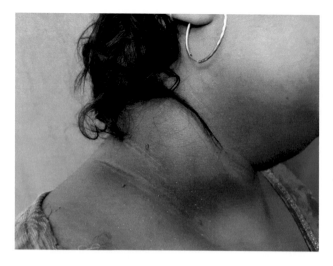

FIGURE 8.17   Hyperpigmented velvety plaque with skin tags over the neck in acanthosis nigricans.

8.2g Pigmented Lesions in Oral Mucosa

The most common cause of oral mucosal pigmentation is racial and is an incidental finding on examination in dark-skinned individuals. It is completely asymptomatic and is usually symmetrical and most prominent on labial gingivae and the palatal mucosa. The dorsal surface of the tongue may also be commonly affected. No treatment other than reassurance is warranted. Other causes of asymptomatic hyperpigmented lesions in oral mucosa include melanotic macules and amalgam tattoos. Melanotic macules are flat brown or black lesions similar to the ephelides. They can normally be found in up to 3% of individuals as a normal finding and are seen most commonly over the lips, gingiva, and buccal mucosa. Oral mucosal pigmentation may also be seen in many systemic diseases that cause diffuse pigmentation over the body. These include Addison disease, Laugier-Hunziker syndrome, and Peutz-Jeghers syndrome. Less commonly seen pigmented lesions in oral mucosae are the pigmented nevi. They are seen more commonly over the skin as compared to mucosae. Intradermal (intramucosal) type is the most common, followed by blue nevi and junctional nevus. Rarely, malignancies like malignant melanoma and Kaposi sarcoma can also present as well-defined hyperpigmented lesions in the oral cavity. Other causes of mucosal pigmentation are enumerated in Table 8.7.

8.2h Pigmented Lesions of the Vulva

Increased pigmentation in the vulva is usually caused by increased melanin. Rarely, hemosiderin deposition can also cause bluish-brown macules in the genital mucosa. Vulval melanosis may be seen as an isolated finding, or it can be associated with oral mucosal pigmentation, as seen in Laugier-Hunziker syndrome. There is intense macular pigmentation, and a biopsy is warranted, sometimes to exclude malignant melanoma. They are otherwise asymptomatic, and hence, a regular follow-up with photographic documentation is advisable. Pregnancy can cause diffuse pigmentation over the vulva and mons and extend upward toward the umbilicus as linea nigra. These are due to hormonal changes and slowly improve by themselves during postpartum period without any intervention. Post-inflammatory hyperpigmentation is also a very common cause of localized hyperpigmentation over the vulva. It can arise after various infectious disorders like folliculitis,

TABLE 8.7: Pigmented Lesions in Oral Mucosa

Localized	Generalized
• Post-inflammatory (lichen planus)	• Race
• Melanotic macules	• Smoking
• Nevus	• Drug-induced (minocycline,
• Amalgam tattoo	antimalarials, heavy metals)
• Malignant melanoma	• Addison disease
• Kaposi sarcoma	• Nelson syndrome
• Peutz-Jeghers syndrome	• Malignant acanthosis
• Laughier-Hunziker syndrome	nigricans
• Centrofacial lentiginosis	

TABLE 8.8: Causes of Pigmented Lesions in the Vulva

Localized	Generalized
• Post-inflammatory (folliculitis, furuncle, tinea, lichen planus, fixed drug eruption)	• Racial
	• Pregnancy
• Nevus	• Drug-induced (minocycline, antimalarials, heavy metals)
• Malignant melanoma	• Malignant acanthosis nigricans
• Dowling-Degos disease	
• Laughier-Hunziker syndrome	

furuncles, tinea cruris, and genital ulcers, as well as inflammatory disorders like lichen planus and fixed drug eruption. Increased vulval pigmentation as a result of hemosiderin deposition is seen in conditions with extravasation of red blood cells like plasma cell vulvitis (Zoon's vulvitis) and lichen sclerosus et atrophicus. Other causes of pigmented lesions in the vulva are mentioned in Table 8.8.

With an increasing trend toward gynecological cosmetology, there is an increase in demands for the treatment of these lesions with no well-defined consensus.

8.3 Hypopigmentation Disorders

Hypopigmentation disorders may be classified by the age of onset, as shown in Table 8.9.

Congenital causes of hypopigmentation can further be classified according to the pathogenesis, as mentioned in Table 8.10.

8.3a Piebaldism

This is a rare genetic disorder with a specific form of pigmentary abnormality. Multiple sharply demarcated and symmetric depigmented macules that generally affect the frontal scalp, forehead, chest, abdomen, and extremities are present since birth. The hands, feet, and back remain normally pigmented. Another characteristic feature is the localized lock of white hair of the frontal scalp and/or eyebrows.

8.3b Waardenburg Syndrome

It is characterized by a white forelock, congenital depigmented macules, heterochromia irides, typical facies, congenital sensorineural deafness, and aganglionic megacolon. It is considered to be a more severe version of neural crest development disorder and has four subtypes.

8.3c Albinism

Albinism results from a genetic defect in the enzyme tyrosinase, which is important in melanin formation.[12] The term

TABLE 8.9: Hypopigmentation Disorders According to Age of Onset

Congenital/Early Childhood	Adult
Diffuse hypopigmentation	*Diffuse hypopigmentation*
• Piebaldism	• Vitiligo universalis
• Waardenburg syndrome	• Pan hypopituitarism
• Menkes syndrome	
• Griscelli syndrome	*Localized hypopigmentation*
• Elejalde syndrome	• Focal/acral vitiligo
• Malnutrition	• Chemical leukoderma
• Ectodermal dysplasia	• Scleroderma
• Phenylketonuria	• Post-inflammatory (lichen
• Histidinemia, homocystinuria	striatus, lichen sclerosus et
• Chédiak-Higashi syndrome	atrophicus, pityriasis lichenoides
• Oculocutaneous albinism	chronica, progressive macular
	hypomelanosis, syphilis,
Localized hypopigmentation	pityriasis rosea, leprosy)
• Ash leaf macules	• Idiopathic guttate hypomelanosis
• Nevus depigmentosus	
• Nevus anemicus	
• Hypomelanosis of Ito	
• Phylloid hypomelanosis	
• Incontinentia pigmenti	
• Segmental vitiligo	
• Post-inflammatory	
• Pityriasis alba	

TABLE 8.10: Congenital Hypopigmentation Disorders According to Pathogenesis

Abnormal Migration of Melanoblasts from the Neuroectoderm	Abnormal Melanogenesis	Abnormal Melanosome Formation	Abnormal Melanosome Transfer
Piebaldism Waardenburg syndrome	Albinism Menkes syndrome Phenylketonuria Histidinemia, homocystinuria	Hermansky-Pudlak (HPS) disease Chediak-Higashi syndrome	Griscelli syndrome Elejalde syndrome

refers to a mixed group of diseases that may have the following features: poor vision, nystagmus, very light hair, and skin. A distinction can be made between the oculocutaneous and purely ocular forms of albinism. In the ocular form, instead of diffuse depigmentation, there is discrete depigmentation of the skin and hair.

8.3d Griscelli Syndrome

Along with systemic manifestations, there is hypopigmentation of skin and hair in Griscelli syndrome. Systemic associations include neurological involvement (type 1) and immunodeficiency (type 2).

8.3e Ash Leaf Macules

They are single or multiple, lanceolate-shaped, sharply demarcated hypopigmented macules present over the trunk and extremities. They are usually present at birth and are nonprogressive. Ash leaf macules are considered the earliest cutaneous manifestation of tuberous sclerosis complex and sometimes may be the only cutaneous feature of the complex. However, they may also be found in approximately 4.7% of normal individuals.

8.3f Nevus Anemicus

It appears as a congenital hypopigmented patch anywhere over the body but most commonly over the chest. There is no true pigmentary abnormality, as the apparent hypopigmentation is a result of persistent vasoconstriction due to the enhanced reactivity of catechols.

8.3g Nevus Depigmentosus

It usually manifests early in life but may develop later in childhood.[13] The lesion is completely hypopigmented with irregular margins and is mostly single, but segmental or extensive lesions with a sharp midline cut-off can also be seen (Figure 8.18). The trunk is the most common site. It is sometimes divided into two types—type 1 (<10 cm) or type 2 (>10 cm).

8.3h Hypomelanosis of Ito

This is characterized by the presence of various patterns of hypopigmentation (whorls/linear streaks) in a Blaschkoid distribution. In up to 70% of cases, it manifests in infancy. It has a strong association with the involvement of other systems, like the nervous system, eyes, hair, teeth, and musculoskeletal system. Psychomotor retardation and cognitive deficit are the most significant associated features. Cerebral hypoplasia, cortical atrophy, kyphoscoliosis, genital anomalies, and congenital heart defects may also be seen.

8.3i Idiopathic Guttate Hypomelanosis

It is a very common disorder with confetti-like depigmentation affecting predominantly the legs (Figure 8.19) and sometimes the trunk and arms in patients with actinic skin damage.

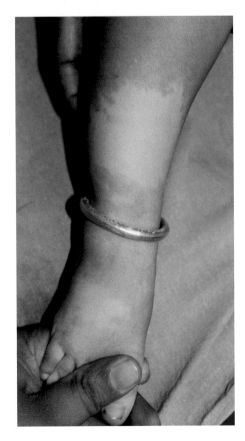

FIGURE 8.18   Nevus depigmentosus over the left leg.

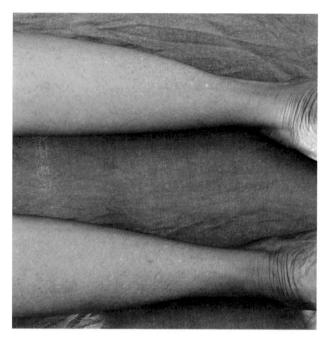

FIGURE 8.19 Idiopathic guttate hypomelanosis over legs.

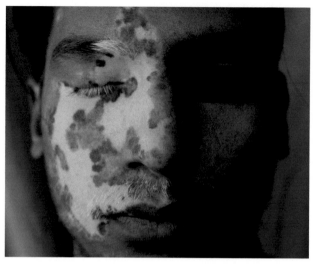

FIGURE 8.20 Segmental vitiligo with leucotrichia of eyebrows, eyelashes, and mustache.

8.3j Vitiligo

It is an acquired skin condition occurring in approximately 1% of the population worldwide. Clinically vitiligo is classified into two major forms:[14]

1. Segmental vitiligo (SV) (Figure 8.20)
2. Non-segmental vitiligo (NSV), which includes several variants (generalized vitiligo, acrofacial vitiligo, universal vitiligo)

Vitiligo is characterized by multiple asymptomatic, milky-white, well-circumscribed macules over the body, usually in a symmetrical pattern (Figures 8.21 and 8.22). The most common sites of initial involvement are the fingers, hands, and face.

In *acrofacial vitiligo*, as the name suggests, the involved sites are usually limited to the face, hands, and feet. The involvement of distal fingers and facial orifices is a distinctive feature.

Vitiligo universalis is the most extensive form of vitiligo, and the term is used when depigmentation is virtually universal (80–90% of the body). *Mucosal vitiligo* refers to the involvement of the oral and/or genital mucosae. *Mixed vitiligo* refers to the concomitant occurrence of segmental and nonsegmental vitiligo.

Focal vitiligo deserves special mention as it refers to a small isolated depigmented patch that is not in a segmental distribution and has not yet evolved into vitiligo after a period of at least two years.

Segmental vitiligo has a distinct natural history and unique clinical features. It is characterized by early onset, rapid progression, and then stable persistence. The clinical pattern of the lesions in a specific dermatome is the most defining characteristic of segmental vitiligo. Various treatment modalities are summarized in Table 8.11.

Case—A 17-year-old male presented with a depigmented lesion over the right side of his face for ten years. There was

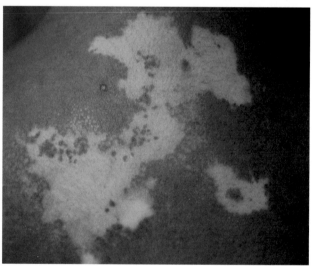

FIGURE 8.21 Milky-white macule with scalloped margins in vitiligo.

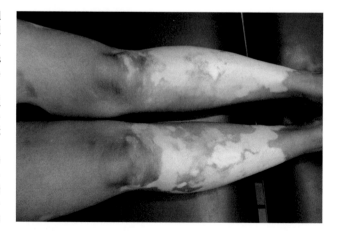

FIGURE 8.22 Symmetrical distribution of the depigmented macules in vitiligo.

TABLE 8.11: Therapeutic Modalities for Vitiligo

Medical management
- Topical potent corticosteroids
- Calcineurin inhibitors
- Phototherapy—photochemotherapy/NBUVB/targeted phototherapy
- Combination treatments—oral antioxidant + UVB
- Psoralen + UVA
- Low-dose azathioprine + PUVA
- Oral steroids and other immunosuppressants
- Oral steroid mini pulse therapy
- Biologics
- 308 nm excimer laser + tacrolimus
- Topical pseudocatalase + UVR
- NBUVB + laser dermabrasion
- Punch grafting + topical flucinolone

Surgical management
- Punch grafting
- Epidermal suction blister grafting
- Split-skin grafting
- Cellular grafts
- Transplant of pure cultured melanocytes
- Transplant of noncultured melanocytes

Excimer LASER
Camouflage
Depigmentation
Psychological interventions

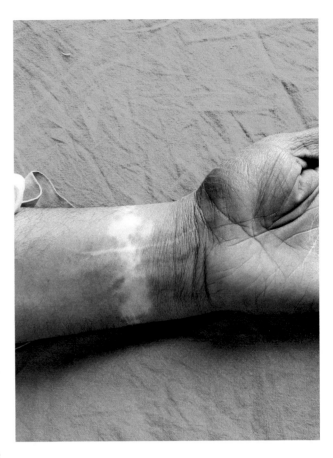

FIGURE 8.23 Chemical leukoderma due to a band of a wristwatch.

a history of multiple oral and topical treatments with little response over the last seven years. On examination, a well-defined depigmented macule with intervening areas of normal and hyperpigmentation was seen involving the right side of the cheek, eyelid, and forehead with sharp demarcation at midline and overlying leucotrichosis. The patient was diagnosed with segmental vitiligo, and since medical management has a limited role, the patient was taken up for suction blister grafting. Surgical management forms the main therapeutic stay for segmental vitiligo, and with the advent of cultured and noncultured melanocyte transplantation, the results obtained are satisfactory.

8.3k Other Hypopigmentation Disorders

Chemical leucoderma denotes the development of vitiligo-like depigmentation over sites of repeated exposure to specific chemical compounds (Figure 8.23).[15] Due to the sensitization in susceptible indivuduals, depigmented macules may appear at remote sites also.[13]

Common contributory chemical agents in the development of chemical leukoderma are monobenzyl, monomethyl, and monoethyl ethers of hydroquinone; para-tertiary butylphenol in bindi adhesives; paraphenylenediamine in hair dyes and tattoo; mercapto and thiuram in rubber sandals; and cinnamic acid in toothpaste.[16, 17]

Progressive macular hypomelanosis is a common asymptomatic skin condition characterized by the presence of multiple variable-sized, discrete, and coalescing hypopigmented macules over the body (Figure 8.24). The most common sites of involvement are the posterior trunk and abdomen, suggesting a possible etiological role of *Propionibacterium acnes*. The lesions are ill-defined and can range from 0.5 cm to more than 20 cm in size. In the case of larger lesions, it may become difficult at times to differentiate between normal and hypopigmented areas. The natural course of the disease is appearance in young adult life, slow progression over many years with a slow natural improvement.

Case—A 42-year-old male, resident of Bihar, presented with light-colored lesions over the back for six months. There was no history to suggest leprosy in the patient or his close family. Examination revealed multiple well-defined 10–15 cm hypopigmented patches only over the back. There was no overlying sensory loss. No peripheral nerves were enlarged. Slit-skin smear was negative, and the skin biopsy was unremarkable. The final diagnosis of progressive macular hypomelanosis was made, and the patient was counseled regarding the course. Exclusion of leprosy in these patients is essential. There is no standard response to therapy with slow improvement over the years.

Pityriasis alba is a very common cause of ill-defined hypopigmented macules seen in children and sometimes in young adults also (Figure 8.25). It is more commonly seen in patients with atopic dermatitis. The etiology has not yet been fully explained.

In infectious causes of hypopigmentation, the most common cause is leprosy, where well-defined hypopigmented hypoesthetic lesions are seen over the body (Figure 8.26). Indeterminate type of leprosy is a common cause of single well-defined hypopigmented macule over the face in young children from endemic areas. Other causes of post-infectious pigment lightening include secondary syphilis, post-kala-azar dermal lesihmaniasis, and oncocerchiasis.

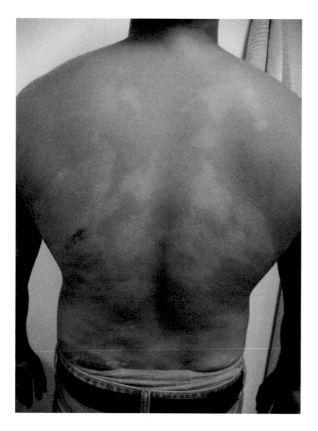

FIGURE 8.24 Large hypopigmented macules in progressive macular hypomelanosis.

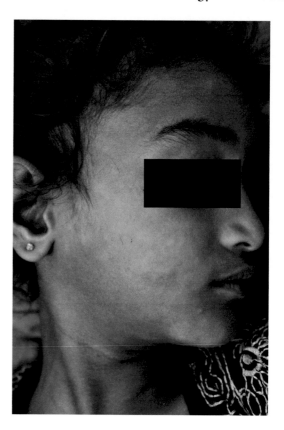

FIGURE 8.25 Ill-defined hypopigmented macules of pityriasis alba.

8.4 Conclusion

Disorders of pigmentation are an integral part of dermatology, but the varied presentations often make the diagnosis challenging. Once a proper understanding of the disease is developed, the learning becomes easier, and the cases become less daunting. Multiple therapeutic options are developing at a decent pace, so even the diseases that were earlier difficult to treat are now becoming manageable with proper compliance and counseling.

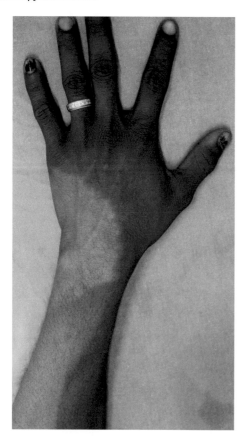

FIGURE 8.26 Well-defined hypopigmented hypoesthetic macule of borderline leprosy.

Frequently Asked Questions

1. *Q: What is the reason for the pigmentation change in pityriasis versicolor?*

   A: The causative organism of pityriasis versicolor, *Malassezia* sp., secretes enzymes in its pathogenic hyphal form. These enzymes inhibit the melanocyte tyrosinase enzyme, thus leading to hypopigmentation.

2. *Q: What causes tanning, and how can it be prevented?*

   A: Exposure to sunlight causes stimulation of epidermal melanocytes, which increases melanin production and increases the transfer of melanosomes to keratinocytes. This response is visible as the darkening of the skin, known as tanning. Avoidance of sun exposure during peak hours and proper application of broad-spectrum sunscreen helps in reducing tanning.

3. *Q: What is the familial incidence and possibility of transmission of vitiligo?*

   A: Around 15–30% of patients have a positive family history of vitiligo in first-degree relatives; however, the risk of transmission to further generations cannot be predicted.

4. *Q: Can some pigmentary disorders act as markers for systemic diseases?*

A: Yes, for example, generalized hyperpigmentation (Addison disease), ash leaf macules and confetti lesions (tuberous sclerosis), multiple lentigines (various multiple lentigine syndromes), hypomelanosis of Ito (disorders of the central nervous system and the musculoskeletal system), rain drop pigmentation (arsenic poisoning), and so on.

5. *Q: Can nutritional deficiency lead to pigmentation changes?*

A: Yes. Protein loss or vitamin deficiencies can lead to facial and extremity hypopigmentation in patients with kwashiorkor, marasmus, malabsorption, nephrotic syndrome, worm infestation, and pellagra.

References

1. Hidano A, Kajima H, Ikeda S, Mizutani H, Miyasato H, Niimura M. Natural history of nevus of Ota. Arch Dermatol. 1967 Feb;95(2):187–195.
2. Hori Y, Kawashima M, Oohara K, Kukita A. Acquired bilateral nevus of Ota like macules. J Am Acad Dermatol. 1984;10:961–964.
3. Sarkar R, Arora P, Garg VK, Sonthalia S, Gokhale N. Melasma update. Indian J Dermatol. Oct–Dec 2014;5(4).
4. Resnik S. Melasma induced by oral contraceptive drugs. JAMA. 1967;199:601–5.10.
5. Lutfi RJ, Fridmanis M, Misiunas AL, Pafume O, Gonzalez EA, Villemur JA. Association of melasma with thyroid autoimmunity and other thyroidal abnormalities and their relationship to the origin of the melasma. J Clin Endocrinol Metab. 1985;61:28–31.
6. Moin A, Jabery Z, Fallah N. Prevalence and awareness of melasma during pregnancy. Int J Dermatol. 2006;45:285–288.
7. Grimes PE. Melasma. Etiologic and therapeutic considerations. Arch Dermatol. 1995;131:1453–1457.
8. Kim EH, Kim YC, Lee ES, Kang HY. The vascular characteristics of melasma. J Dermatol Sci. 2007;46:111–116.
9. Victor FC, Gelber J, Rao B. Melasma: A review. J Cutan Med Surg. 2004;8:97–102.
10. Cestari TF, Hexsel D, Viegas ML, Azulay L, Hassun K, Almeida AR, et al. Validation of a melasma quality of life questionnaire for Brazilian Portuguese language: The MelasQoL-BP study and improvement of QoL of melasma patients after triple combination therapy. Br J Dermatol. 2006;156 Suppl 1:13–20.
11. Riehl G. Uber eine eigenartige melanose. Wien Klin Wochensschr. 1917;30:280–281.
12. Schwartz RA. Erythema dyschromicum perstans: The continuing enigma of Cinderella or ashy dermatosis. Int J Dermatol. 2004;43:230–232.
13. Ezzedine K, Lim HW, Suzuki T, Katayama I, Hamzavi I, Lan CC, et al. Revised classification/nomenclature of vitiligo and related issues: The Vitiligo Global Issues Consensus Conference. Pigment Cell Melanoma Res. 2012;25:E1–13.
14. Ramrath K, Stolz W. Disorders of melanin pigmentation. In: Burgdorf P, Wolff L, editors. Braun Falco's dermatology. 3rd ed. New York: Springer; 2009. p. 772–774.
15. Rees JL. The genetics of sun sensitivity in humans. Am J Hum Genet. 2004;75:739–751.
16. Jimbow K, Jimbow M. Chemical and pharmacologic agents. In: Norlund JJ, Boissy RE, Hearing VJ, editors. The pigmentary system: Physiology and pathophysiology. New York: Oxford University Press; 1998. p. 618–624.
17. Ghosh S. Chemical leukoderma: What's new on etiopathological and clinical aspects? Indian J Dermatol. 2010;55:255–258.

CHAPTER 9: CONTACT DERMATITIS

Keerthi Velugotla

9.1 Introduction

The human skin, being a barrier, encounters a variety of environmental and exogenous agents. Thankfully, not all these agents incite an immunological reaction and disease. Contact dermatitis is an eczematous inflammation of the skin, secondary to exposure to environmental irritants or allergens. The inflammatory reaction can be classified as acute, subacute, or chronic based on the duration of onset and clinical features. Contact dermatitis is divided into two distinct entities, allergic contact dermatitis (ACD) and irritant contact dermatitis (ICD), based on etiologic and causative factors. The irritant contact dermatitis accounts for 80% of total contact dermatitis cases.[1] The current chapter focuses on the discussion of allergic contact dermatitis.

9.2 Allergic Contact Dermatitis

Also known as contact allergy or contact eczema, it is an immunologically mediated eczematous reaction, which occurs on exposure to a chemical agent to which the individual has been previously sensitized. ACD is a delayed type of hypersensitivity reaction, antigen-specific and predominantly T-cell mediated.

9.2.1 Epidemiology

There is a gradually progressing trend in the prevalence of contact eczema.[2–4] Multiple studies have been done and published to determine the prevalence of ACD worldwide.[5] Fifteen to twenty percent of the German population are affected by some form of contact dermatitis.[6] Nearly 20% of the European population is reported to be suffering from contact allergy to one or more allergens.[7] Fragrances, preservatives, nickel, and para-phenylenediamine are found to be the most common culprits in the majority of studies.[8, 9]

Allergic contact dermatitis can affect both sexes equally. However, few studies suggest a higher incidence in women.[10] This observation is proposed to be due to higher exposure of women to nickel or due to hormonal factors.[11–13] It can affect an individual at any age. Studies show an increasing incidence of allergic contact dermatitis, with nickel being the most common sensitizer in childhood ACD.[14–16] Frequency of exposure to the allergens, presence of pre-existing dermatoses and medical ailments, and decreased epidermal barrier integrity are few of the factors responsible for the frequency of ACD in older age group.[16]

9.3 Risk Factors[7]

Certain inherent and acquired conditions are identified as risk factors for ACD. Various steps in the ACD pathogenesis, such as antigen uptake or antigen metabolism by enzymes, such as N-acetyltransferases (NATs), glutathione S-transferases (GSTs), and angiotensin-converting enzyme, are genetically influenced. Polymorphism in genes controlling these enzymes is associated with an increased incidence of ACD to allergens, such as PPD, thiomersal, and chromate.[17–19] Occupational exposure is the single largest risk factor for ACD in adults.

9.4 Ethnicity

Individuals with skin of color are supposed to be resistant to sensitization by allergens, as the stratum corneum has higher lipid compaction and provides better barrier function.[16, 20, 21]

9.5 Pathogenesis

ACD is delayed-type, or type IV, hypersensitivity reaction and is an allergen-specific reaction. ACD is seen in individuals who are sensitized to an allergen previously. Pathogenesis of ACD comprises two distinct phases: (1) sensitization phase and (2) elicitation phase.

9.6 Sensitization Phase

Sensitization is an essential step in the pathogenesis of ACD. Low-molecular-weight hydrophilic or electrophilic chemical molecules known as haptens initiate the cascade. Haptens bind with epidermal carrier proteins covalently to form a complete allergen. These hapten-protein complexes bind to the MHC complex II, initiating a sensitization reaction.[22] Cytokines, such as IL-1β, TNF-α, and GM-CSF, produced by the injured keratinocytes enable Langerhans cell activation and maturation.[23, 24] These allergens bound to Langerhans cells migrate to the regional lymph nodes and present to T-lymphocytes. Upon recognition of the allergen, numerous cytokines, such as interleukins, are released, which induce CD8+ and CD4+ T-lymphocytes that are allergen-specific. This phase usually lasts for 10–15 days.

9.7 Elicitation Phase

Once an individual is adequately sensitized to the allergen, upon re-exposure sensitized T-lymphocytes in the epidermis produce cytokines, which are responsible for further T-lymphocyte proliferation and release of inflammatory mediators. These inflammatory mediators are responsible for the clinical manifestations of ACD, which appear within 12–48 hours of allergen re-exposure.

9.8 Clinical Presentation

Patterns of clinical presentation of ACD are (1) localized dermatitis, (2) systemic or generalized dermatitis, (3) non-eczematous variant, and (4) allergic contact urticaria (ACU).

9.8.1 Localized ACD

This is the most common clinical form of ACD. It typically presents with well-demarcated eczematous patches, which may be acute or chronic. Papules and vesicles with erythema are characteristic of acute ACD, whereas lichenified patches and excoriation are seen in chronic ACD.[25] The eruption is usually pruritic and limited to the area of contact with the allergen. The shape and location of the dermatitis point toward the possible allergen. However, generalized rashes may be seen, especially in cases where the allergen is airborne (Figures 9.1 and 9.2).[26]

DOI: 10.1201/9780429243769-9

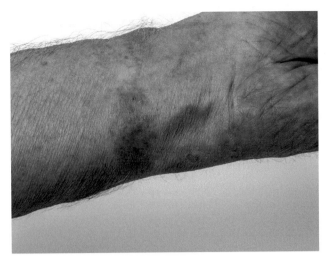

FIGURE 9.1   Leather watch strap allergy.

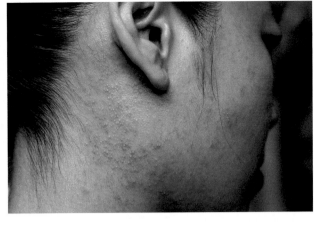

FIGURE 9.2   Allergic contact dermatitis over the neck.

TABLE 9.1: Possible Allergens and Sources of Allergens to Consider Depending on the Anatomical Areas Involved

Location	Allergen/Source of Allergen
Scalp	Hair dyes, shampoos, surfactants, topical medications
Face and eyelids	Skin care products, cosmetics, hair dyes, preservatives, nail varnish, nail varnish remover, topical ophthalmological preparations, metal spectacle frames, contact lens solutions, eye makeup, eye makeup remover, mascaras, airborne allergens
Lips	Lip cosmetics, toothpaste, colophonium in chewing gum, foods, food additives, dentures
Ears	Earplugs, external otitis, jewelry, hearing aids, eyeglasses
Neck	Jewelry (especially nickel-based), fragrances, airborne allergens
Trunk	Fragrances, textile allergens, detergents, body washes
Axillae	Deodorants, antiperspirants
Hands	Soaps, detergents, occupational allergens (such as hair dyes, industrial solvents, and rubber gloves), nail varnish, acrylates, food, poison ivy, chromates in cement, disinfectants, watch straps, moisturizers
Legs and feet	Rubber footwear, airborne allergens, topical medications, fragrances, chromates in cement,
Anogenital	Topical medicaments (such as antihemorrhoid creams and vaginal pessaries), allergens in food, textile allergens, poison ivy, rubber/latex condoms, sanitary napkins
Mucous membrane (oral)	Dentures, dental fillings, spices, food additives, toothpaste

9.8.2 Systemic/Generalized CD

It is a relatively uncommon form of ACD presenting as diffuse areas of dermatitis or generalized erythroderma. It is seen in individuals who had a history of localized ACD and sensitized to an allergen. These individuals develop generalized reactions when exposed to the same or related allergen in systemic routes, such as percutaneous penetration, ingestion, and inhalation. Balsam of Peru, metals (such as nickel, chromium, and cobalt), and poison ivy dermatitis are the most common allergens causing systemic CD.[27] Airborne contact dermatitis and photo contact dermatitis commonly present as generalized ACD.

9.8.3 Non-Eczematous ACD

Lichenoid dermatitis is the most common form of non-eczematous ACD. Other less common forms are contact purpura, contact leukoderma, and erythema multiforme.[28–31] Dental amalgams, PPD derivatives, tattoo pigments, and plant derivatives commonly present as lichenoid dermatitis.[32–34]

9.8.4 Allergic Contact Urticaria (ACU)[27]

It is an atypical form of contact dermatitis. It is an IgE-mediated immunological reaction manifesting as urticaria when a sensitized individual meets an offending allergen. Mostly seen in atopic individuals. A skin prick test must be performed to establish the diagnosis. Latex is the most common allergen to cause ACU.

9.8.5 Diagnosis

Mostly the diagnosis of ACD is not difficult to make when the presentation is typical and localized. However, it can be difficult to differentiate from other eczematous disorders, such as stasis dermatitis, atopic dermatitis, and irritant contact dermatitis. Generalized ACD must be differentiated from erythroderma. A thorough history and examination are necessary to ascertain the possible allergen. Occupational exposure must be looked into in every case of ACD. Patch testing with suspected allergens helps in establishing the culprit allergen and in further management.

9.9 Patch Test

A patch test is the most reliable method to diagnose ACD. It is indicated in patients with a history of dermatitis in whom a contact allergy is suspected. It is also indicated in patients with a flare-up of existing dermatoses (like stasis dermatitis or atopic or seborrheic dermatitis), in patients with atypical forms of ACD, and so on[35, 36] to rule out the role of contact allergens. Patch testing can be done in cases where there is no improvement despite avoidance of a suspected allergen. Patch testing to establish the allergen as a cause of contact allergy was first done by Jadassohn.

9.9.1 Types
9.9.1.1 Standard Patch Test

An appropriate concentration of allergen is loaded in aluminum chambers known as Finn chambers. These chambers are

TABLE 9.2: ICDRG Grading System

+/−, ?	Doubtful reaction
−	Negative reaction
+	Weak positive, faint erythema, infiltration
++	Strong positive, erythema, infiltration, papules, vesicles
+++	Highly positive, infiltration, coalescing vesicles, bullous, ulcers
IR	Irritant reaction
NT	Not tested

applied to the skin and fixed with the help of tapes to create occlusion. A patch test is read after 48 hours, and a second reading is taken on the fourth day. Studies suggest that a delayed reading is important to get accurate results.[37, 38] Positive reactions are graded using the International Contact Dermatitis Research Group (ICDRG) grading system (Table 9.2). The upper back is the most preferred site for a patch test. In cases where patch testing is not possible on the upper back, the lateral aspect of the thigh, and the volar aspect of the forearms can be preferred to lay patches.

Individuals can be patch tested with suspected allergens alone in appropriate concentrations or can be tested with a standard series of allergens if multiple allergens are suspected. The standard series and the allergen in the series vary among countries, and they vary according to the statistical trends in that country. European Standard Series, TRUE Test Series, North American Contact Dermatitis Group (NACDG) Standard Series, and International Standard Series are a few of the standard series of patch tests used.

9.9.1.2 False Positive and False Negative Reactions

Using a high concentration of allergens or using the wrong allergens, in cases with multiple positive reactions (angry back syndrome or status eczematicus), can give false positive reactions. A low concentration of allergens, faulty technique, early removal of patches, patients on oral corticosteroids, and a high dose antihistamines may result in false negative reactions.

9.9.1.3 Complications

Anaphylaxis, sensitization, persistent positive reaction, plaster reaction, post-inflammatory hyperpigmentation/depigmentation, and scars are a few of the complications. In patients with skin of color a positive reaction may lead to a post-inflammatory reaction, scars, and keloids in rare cases.

9.9.1.4 Open and Semi-Open Test[39, 40]

Usually performed for substances that are highly acidic or highly alkaline.[41] In an open test, the suspected allergen is applied directly on the upper arm or upper back twice a day for two days. The test material is left uncovered until the reading is taken.

In a semi-open test, the test material is applied with a Q-tip in an area of 1 cm² and allowed to dry. The area is covered with acrylic tape. The reading is taken on two and four days of application. Topical medicaments; cosmeceutical products containing propylene glycol and sodium lauryl sulfate; cosmetics like mascara, nail lacquers, shampoos, and hair dyes; and industrial products such as paints and resins are a few of the products that can be tested using semi-open tests.

9.9.1.5 Repeat Open Application Test (ROAT)[39]

The test material is applied to an area of 5 cm² area, preferably to the area close to the cubital fossa. About 0.1 ml of material is applied twice daily for a period ranging from 7 days to 21 days until a positive reaction is observed. ROAT is performed in cases with doubtful patch test results to preparations in which the suspected allergen is present in very low concentrations.

9.9.1.6 Prick Test

This test is used in conditions such as contact urticaria syndrome and protein contact dermatitis in which the suspected allergens are low-molecular-weight or high-molecular-weight proteins.[42, 43] Prick tests determine the ability of the allergens to induce an immediate hypersensitivity reaction. Test material is applied to the upper back or volar aspect of the forearm and pricked with a lancet. Positive (histamine) and negative (saline) controls are tested at the same time. The test is read in 15–20 minutes. A wheal and flare of greater than 3 mm diameter at the test site is considered a positive reaction.

9.9.1.7 Photo Patch Test

In cases of suspected photo allergy, the patches are applied as duplicates on the upper back and removed on the second day. One site is irradiated with UV light while the other site serves as a control. A positive reaction on the irradiated site indicates the role of photo allergy.

9.9.1.8 Management

Identification of the causative allergen forms the cornerstone in the management of ACD. Detailed history, examination, and patch testing for the suspected antigens enable the physician to identify the causative allergens. Occupational exposure must be strongly considered in doubtful cases. Once the allergens are identified, the patients are to be adequately educated on the sources of the allergen and avoidance of the same.

Topical steroids are the gold standard in treating ACD and alleviating symptoms, though their long-term side effects forbid their prolonged use. Topical calcineurin inhibitors (tacrolimus, pimecrolimus) may be considered for maintenance. Acute weeping eczematous lesions benefit from wet compresses, whereas emollients are helpful in chronic lichenified lesions. Antihistamines to control pruritus may also be given. Oral corticosteroids may be required in cases of generalized ACD and acute exacerbation of eczema.

9.10 Conclusion

Allergic contact dermatitis causes a significant lowering of quality of life, especially if the dermatitis is chronic. Identification of the culprit allergen is possible by a thorough history taking, examination, and patch testing. Occupational exposure is to be considered and excluded in all doubtful cases and in cases non-responsive to treatment. Topical steroids are the drug of choice in the treatment of acute cases. However, educating the patient in appropriately avoiding the allergen is the cornerstone in the treatment and prevention of ACD.

References

1. Marks JG Jr, Elsner P, DeLeo VA. Allergy and ICD. In: Contact and Occupational Dermatology, 3rd edn. Philadelphia: Mosby, 2002. p. 3–15.
2. Nguyen SH, Dang TP, MacPherson C, Maibach H, Maibach HI. Prevalence of patch test results from 1970 to 2002 in a multi-centre population in North America (NACDG). Contact Dermat. 2008;58(2):101–106.
3. Kohl L, Blondeel A, Song M. Allergic contact dermatitis from cosmetics. Retrospective analysis of 819 patch-tested patients. Dermatology. 2002;204(4):334–337.

4. Lunder T, Kansky A. Increase in contact allergy to fragrances: Patch-test results 1989–1998. Contact Dermat. 2000;43(2):107–109.

5. Brasch J, Becker D, Aberer W, Bircher A, Kränke B, Jung K, et al. Guideline contact dermatitis: S1-Guidelines of the German Contact Allergy Group (DKG) of the German Dermatology Society (DDG), the Information Network of Dermatological Clinics (IVDK), the German Society for Allergology and Clinical Immunology (DGAKI), the Working Group for Occupational and Environmental Dermatology (ABD) of the DDG, the Medical Association of German Allergologists (AeDA), the Professional Association of German Dermatologists (BVDD) and the DDG. Allergo J Int. 2014;23:126–138

6. Peiser M, Tralau T, Heidler J, Api AM, Arts JH, Basketter DA, et al. Allergic contact dermatitis: Epidemiology, molecular mechanisms, in vitro methods and regulatory aspects. Current knowledge assembled at an international workshop at BfR, Germany. Cell Mol Life Sci. 2012;69:763–781.

7. Dhingra N, Shemer A, Correa da Rosa J, et al. Molecular profiling of contact dermatitis skin identifies allergen-dependent differences in immune response. J Allergy Clin Immunol. 2014;134(2):362–372.

8. Wilkinson M, Orton D. Allergic contact dermatitis. In: Griffiths CEM, Barker J, Bleiker T, Chalmers R, Creamer D. Rook's Textbook of Dermatology. 9th edn. 2016, Chapter 128.

9. Milam EC, Jacob SE, Cohen DE. Contact dermatitis in the patient with atopic dermatitis. J Allergy Clin Immunol Pract. 2019 Jan;7(1):18–26.

10. Hermann-Kunz E. Allergische Krankheiten in Deutschland Ergebnisse einer repräsentativen Studie. Bundesgesundheitsbl Gesundheitsforsch Gesundheitssch. 2000;43(6):400–406. doi: 10.1007/s001030070045.

11. Jensen CS, Lisby S, Baadsgaard O, Vølund A, Menné T. Decrease in nickel sensitization in a Danish schoolgirl population with ears pierced after implementation of a nickel-exposure regulation. Br J Dermatol. 2002;146(4):636–642.

12. Uter W, Pfahlberg A, Gefeller O, Geier J, Schnuch A. Risk factors for contact allergy to nickel—results of a multifactorial analysis. Contact Dermat. 2003;48(1):33–38.

13. Rees JL, Friedmann PS, Matthews JN. Sex differences in susceptibility to development of contact hypersensitivity to dinitrochlorobenzene (DNCB). Br J Dermatol. 1989;120(3):371–374.

14. Pigatto P, Martelli A, Marsili C, Fiocchi A. Contact dermatitis in children. Ital J Pediatr. 2010;36:2.

15. Simonsen AB, Deleuran M, Johansen JD, Sommerlund M. Contact allergy and allergic contact dermatitis in children – a review of current data. Contact Dermatitis. 2011 Nov;65(5):254–265.

16. Jurado-Palomo J, Moreno-Ancillo A, Bobolea ID, et al. Epidemiology of contact dermatitis. www.intechopen.com.

17. Blömeke B, Brans R, Coenraads PJ, Dickel H, Bruckner T, Hein DW, et al. para-Phenylenediamine and allergic sensitization: Risk modification by N-acetyltransferase 1 and 2 genotypes. Br J Dermatol. 2009;161(5):1130–1135.

18. Westphal GA, Schnuch A, Schulz TG, Reich K, Aberer W, Brasch J, et al. Homozygous gene deletions of the glutathione S-transferases M1 and T1 are associated with thimerosal sensitization. Int Arch Occup Environ Health. 2000;73(6):384–388.

19. Wang BJ, Shiao JS, Chen CJ, Lee YC, Guo YL. Tumour necrotizing factor-α promoter and GST-T1 genotype predict skin allergy to chromate in cement workers in Taiwan. Contact Dermat. 2007;57(5):309–315.

20. Robinson MK. Population differences in skin structure and physiology and the susceptibility to irritant and allergic contact dermatitis: Implications for skin safety testing and risk assessment (1999). Contact Dermatitis. August 1999;41(2):65–79, ISSN 0105-1873

21. Astner S, Burnett N, Rius-Díaz F, Doukas AG, González S, González E. Irritant contact dermatitis induced by a common household irritant: A noninvasive evaluation of ethnic variability in skin response. J Am Acad Dermatol. March 2006;54(3):458–465, ISSN 0190-9622

22. Rajagopalan R, Anderson RT, Sarma S, et al. A n economic evaluation of patch testing in the diagnosis and management of allergic contact dermatitis. Am J Contact Dermatis. 1998;9:149–154.

23. McFadden JP, White IR, Frosch PJ, Sosted H, Johansen JD, Menne T. Allergy to hair dye. BMJ. 2007;334:220.

24. Griffiths C, Barker J, Bleiker T, Chalmers R, Creamer D. Rook's Textbook of Dermatology. 9th edn. Wiley Blackwell, 2016, Chapter 41.

25. Mowad CM, Marks Jr, JG. Allergic contact dermatitis. In: Bolognia JL, Jorizzo JL, Rapini RP. Dermatology. Vol. 1. 2nd edn. Mosby Elsevier. 2008, Chapter 15. p. 209–222.

26. Habif T. Clinical Dermatology Acolour Guide to Diagnosis and Therapy, 5th edn. Mosby Elsevier. 2010, Chapter 4. p. 130–153.

27. Wolff K, Goldsmith L, Katz S, Gilchrest B, Paller A, Leffell D. Allergic contact dermatitis. In Fitzpatrick's Dermatology in General Medicine, 7th edn. Chapter 13. p. 135–146.

28. Belsito DV. The diagnostic evaluation, treatment, and prevention of allergic contact dermatitis in the new millennium. J Allergy Clin Immunol. 2000;105:409.

29. Mizoguchi S, Setoyama M, Kanzaki, T. Linear lichen planus in the region of the mandibular nerve caused by an allergy to palladium in dental metals. Dermatology. 1998;196:268–270

30. Oliver EA, Schwartz L, Warren L. Occupational leukoderma: Preliminary report. JAMA. 1939;113:927.

31. Fisher, AA. Allergic petechial and purpuric rubber dermatitis: The PPPP syndrome. Cutis. 1974;14:25–27.

32. Sharma VK, Mandal SK, Sethuraman G, Bakshi NA. Para-phenylenediaminehb induced lichenoid eruptions. Contact Dermatitis. 1999;41:40–41.

33. Ancona A, Monroy F, Fernandez-Diez J. Occupational dermatitis from IPPD in tyres. Contact Dermatitis. 1982;8:91–94.

34. Yasuda H, Kumakiri M, Miura Y, Tsuchiya K, Shiratori, A. Primula dermatitis. Hokkaido Igaku Zasshi. 1983;58:617–621.

35. Johansen JD, Aalto-Korte K, Agner T, et al. European Society of Contact Dermatitis guideline for diagnostic patch testing—recommendations on best practice. Contact Dermatitis. 2015;73:195–221.

36. Goncalo M, Bruynzeel D. Patch testing in adverse drug reactions. In: Johansen JD, Frosch PJ, Lepoittevin J-P, editors. Contact Dermatitis, 5th edn. Heidelberg, Dordrecht, London, New York: Springer, 2011. p. 475–491.

37. Geier J, Gefeller O, Weichmann K, et al. Patch test reactions at D4, D5, D6. Contact Dermatitis. 1999;40:119–126.

38. Jonker MJ, Bruynzeel DP. The outcome of an additional patch test reading on days 6 or 7. Contact Dermatitis. 2000;42:330–335.

39. Goosens A. Recognizing and testing allergens. Dermatol Clin. 2009;27:219–226.

40. Frosch PJ, Geier J, Uter W, et al. Patch testing with the patient's own products. In: Frosch PJ, Menne T, Lepoittevin JP, editors. Textbook of Contact Dermatitis, 4th edn. Berlin: Springer—Verlag, 2006. p. 929–941.

41. Bruze M. Use of buffer solutions for patch testing. Contact Dermatitis. 1984;10:267–269.

42. Amaro C, Goosens A. Immunological occupational contact urticaria and contact dermatitis from proteins: A review. Contact Dermatitis. 2008;58:757–767.

43. Levin C, Warshaw E. Protein contact dermatitis: Allergens, pathogenesis and management. Dermatitis. 2008;19:241–251.

CHAPTER 10: KELOIDS AND HYPERTROPHIC SCARS

Franklin Sujith Kumar

10.1 Introduction

Hypertrophic scars and keloids may follow local skin trauma or inflammatory skin disorders like laceration, tattoos, burns, injections, ear-piercing, vaccination, bites, acne, abscess, or surgery. They are the consequences of uncontrolled synthesis and deposition of dermal collagen.

A keloid extends beyond the borders of the original wound, does not regress spontaneously, grows in a pseudo-tumor fashion with distortion of the lesion, and tends to recur after excision. On the other hand, hypertrophic scars remain confined to the borders of the original wound and, most of the time, retain their shape.

In hypertrophic scars, collagen fibers are oriented somewhat parallel to the long axis of the scar. On the other hand, in keloid, collagen is arranged in a complete haphazard manner with the presence of keloidal collagen bundles.

Anatomically predisposed sites for keloids are the shoulders, sternum, mandible, and arms [1]. They are more commonly observed in Asians and dark-skinned races [1]. The basic cause of this abnormal wound healing still remains unknown. Medical advice is sought for relief of pruritus, pain, and restricted movement and mainly for cosmetic disfigurement.

10.1.1 Etiology

Studies have demonstrated that keloid development is driven by three dysfunctional pathways.

Though the pathophysiology of keloid and hypertrophic scars is not completely known, various cytokines have been implicated, including interleukins, such as IL-6, IL-8, and IL-10, as well as various growth factors, including transforming growth factor beta and platelet-derived growth factor [2].

1. Altered apoptosis
2. Altered transcription of growth factors, such as transforming growth factor beta (TGF-β) and vascular endothelial growth factor (VEGF)
3. Deregulation of the immune system

10.1.2 Psychological Impact

Despite their common occurrence, keloid remains one of the most challenging dermatologic conditions to successfully treat and may have a significant psychosocial impact on the patient. Keloid and hypertrophic scars have affected patients and frustrated physicians for centuries. More than a cosmetic nuisance, they are often symptomatic and can have a significant psychosocial burden for the patient. They might turn out as an aesthetically unacceptable complication of wound healing, and some scars might even cause anatomic dysfunction[3]. Worse still is the fact that the swellings may be multiple, located in a site that cannot be masked, and constitute an embarrassment to the patients from friends and other people. While typically only impinging on cosmesis, large or recurrent keloids may require therapeutic intervention. In such instances, treatment may be impossible or difficult. Patients may therefore be psychologically affected. Scars can have many significant functional, cosmetic, and psychological sequelae [4].

10.1.3 Case

A 35-year-old female patient presented with a history of two nodular lesions on the left pinna. There is no family history of keloids or similar lesions and no history of metabolic disorders. The lesions had developed at the site of an ear piercing.

On examination, two flesh-colored, firm, and rubbery fibrous nodules were seen and diagnosed as keloids. After taking consent for excision from the patient, under strict aseptic measures, we excised the lesions with CO_2 laser, injected the base with 10% triamcinolone injection, and asked the patient to review for dressing and further intralesional injections.

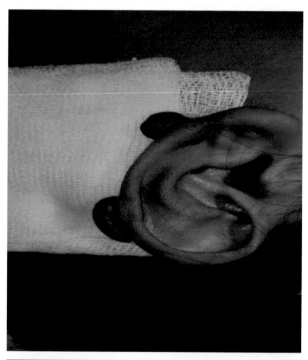

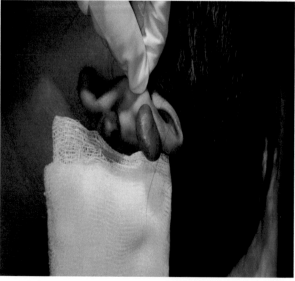

FIGURE 10.1 Earlobe keloids before excision.

DOI: 10.1201/9780429243769-10

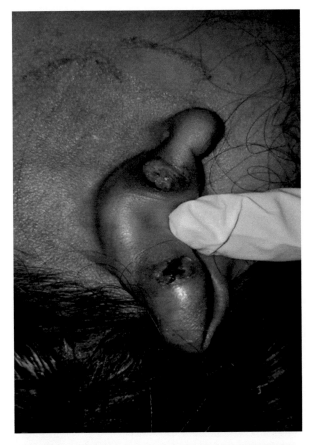

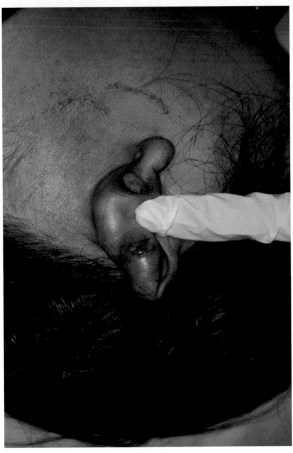

FIGURE 10.2 Earlobe keloids after excision.

10.1.4 Standard Guidelines of Care for Keloids and Hypertrophic Scars

10.1.4.1 Rationale and Scope

No single treatment is uniformly effective in all patients, and multiple treatment options may be needed in a patient with keloids or hypertrophic scars. These guidelines review current evidence for the efficacy of each treatment modality and provide basic recommendations based on them so that the physician can choose the treatment modality appropriate for an individual patient while taking efficacy, therapeutic effects, adverse effects, and cosmetic outcome, feasibility, patient's preference, and cost into consideration [5].

10.1.4.2 Physician's Qualification and Facility

Physicians involved in the management of keloids and hypertrophic scars should have a postgraduate qualification in dermatology or super-specialization in plastic surgery. Radiotherapy needs to be delivered by a specialist [5].

Some of the procedures, such as intralesional injections or surface cryosurgery, can be done in the physician's treatment room. Invasive modalities, such as ablative procedures with CO_2 lasers and surgical excision, may require minor OT with a trained nurse as an assistant. An anesthetist should be ready on call [5].

10.1.4.3 Counseling

Patients should be informed about the nature and course of the disease, available treatment options, their efficacy and adverse effects, and cost. They should be informed about the possibility of recurrences after treatment. The final decision to undertake treatment should lie with the patients. Informed consent should be obtained in all cases. Pre-treatment photography is recommended [5].

10.1.4.4 Different Modalities and Their Current Status in the Management of Keloids

While planning a treatment protocol for a patient with keloids and hypertrophic scars, the treating doctor should primarily consider a low recurrence rate, significant cosmetic outcome, and symptomatic improvement with minimal adverse effects.

10.1.4a Intralesional Corticosteroids

This is the most frequently used modality and the steroid most commonly used is depot preparation of triamcinolone acetonide. The concentration of triamcinolone acetonide depends upon the size and site of the lesion and the age of the individual. Generally, it is used in a concentration of 10–20 mg/ml, though it can be given at a dose of 40 mg/ml for a tough bulky lesion. It is important to inject the steroid at a correct depth in mid-dermis; otherwise, it may lead to irreversible atrophy of the epidermis.

Injections are repeated once in three to four weeks, depending on the bulk of the keloid and therapeutic response. The total number of injections depends on the response and possible side effects. Pain during injection is an important limiting factor.

Triamcinolone injection alone is effective in reducing the volume of lesions in a majority of patients [6]. Ardehali et al. [7] reported that mean scar volume reduced significantly after monthly intralesional injections of triamcinolone acetate. The combination of 5-fluorouracil (5-FU) and triamcinolone seems to be superior to intralesional steroid therapy alone in the treatment of keloids (92% average reduction in lesion size with a combination compared with 73% with steroid alone) [8].

Postoperative intralesional triamcinolone injections, after surgical excision, seem to prevent recurrence. With these pieces of evidence available, intralesional steroids should be considered as the first-line treatment for keloids and hypertrophic scars [9].

10.1.4b 5-Fluorouracil (5-FU) Intralesional Injections

This treatment is increasingly becoming popular. 5-FU alone is effective in the treatment of keloids [10, 11]. The combination of 5-FU injections with surgical excision of keloids showed significant results, especially in cases that failed to respond to intralesional triamcinolone injections alone, and the recurrence rate of the keloid was seen in a very small percentage of patients [12].

There is also evidence that a combination of triamcinolone and 5-FU results in less skin atrophy and telangiectasia than triamcinolone alone [13].

10.1.4c Bleomycin

Intralesional injection of bleomycin appears to be an effective therapy in the treatment of keloids, with almost three-fourths of the patients showing good to excellent results. It is administered either by intralesional injections or by multiple punctures using a 22-G needle [14–17].

Hyperpigmentation is one of the reported adverse effects of intralesional injection of bleomycin [18].

10.1.4d Interferon α-2b

Intralesional injection of a combination of interferon α-2b with triamcinolone has been reported to be superior to triamcinolone alone in reducing the depth and volume of keloids [19]. Due to contradictory results reported, interferon α-2b is not recommend for routine use [20].

10.1.4e Verapamil

Verapamil has been known to stimulate the synthesis of procollagenase, thus increasing collagenase activity, thereby leading to a reduction in fibrous tissue production. However, there has been limited clinical data showing its efficacy in keloids. Therefore, more studies are needed before it is recommended as a routine treatment for keloids [21, 22].

10.1.4f Imiquimod

Imiquimod 5% cream, an immune modulator with localized therapeutic effects at the site of application, is capable of enhancing the local production of immune-stimulating cytokines. In a few studies, imiquimod cream has been used in combination with surgical excision, with the objective of preventing recurrence after surgical excision. However, the antifibrotic effect seems to be short-lived, and the lesions reappeared. The evidence is thus not adequate to establish the efficacy and the role of imiquimod in the prevention of the recurrence of keloids after surgical excision [23–25].

10.1.4g Radiotherapy

Radiotherapy has been used as a monotherapy or as an adjuvant to surgical excision. A combination of surgery followed 24 hours later by radiotherapy is thought to be the most effective approach for the management of extensive hypertrophic scars and keloids. The recurrence rate varies from 9% to 72%, which generally depends on the total dose of radiation and duration of follow-up. Keloids and intractable hypertrophic scars should be treated with dose protocols customized by site [26–28].

Radiation is associated with the risk of carcinogenesis in the long run, and there is hesitation and apprehension about its use for a benign condition, such as keloids. However, there are only a few reports in the literature of malignancies arising from the treatment of keloid scars with radiotherapy.

Some studies have shown that patients with keloids treated with orthovoltage-based radiotherapy post-surgical excision have tolerated the treatment well with less toxicity and high patient satisfaction level [29–31].

10.1.4h Pressure Therapy

Though it is a popular treatment modality for keloids and hypertrophic scars, there is no proven mechanism of action in keloid treatment. The expert recommendation is to apply 20–40 mmHg of pressure for 24 hours a day [32].

Some of the limitations and problems of pressure therapy are pressure loss, discomfort from heat and sweating, swelling of limbs, rashes, eczema, friction, and poor compliance [33].

10.1.4i Lasers

Pulsed dye laser (PDL) has been reported to decrease transforming growth factor-beta 1 (TGF-β 1) induction and upregulation of matrix metalloproteinase (MMP) expression in keloid tissue. This may be responsible for the keloid regression with PDL treatment [34, 35].

Carbon dioxide laser monotherapy has a recurrence rate as high as 90% and is therefore not recommended [36, 37].

10.1.4j Surgical Excision

Surgical excision alone is associated with recurrence in 50–100% of patients; however, an exception is earlobe keloid which recurs much less frequently [38]. Thus, after the excision of a keloid, adjuvant therapy is recommended. Radiation, intralesional steroid, and 5-FU prevent recurrence more efficiently than topical imiquimod and interferons. Postoperative pressure therapy designed to suit the individual patient is important and can be tried to prevent recurrence, but the problems and limitations of pressure therapy must be considered by the treating doctor.

10.1.4k Cryosurgery

Cryosurgery with liquid nitrogen leads to total or partial success in almost two-thirds to three-fourths of patients with keloids after at least three sessions [39–41]. Hypopigmentation, blistering, delayed healing, and infection are the major side effects [42]. A combination of liquid nitrogen cryosurgery and intralesional steroids seems to have a synergistic effect over liquid nitrogen cryosurgery alone [43]. Cryotherapy induces edema and cellular breakdown, causing a decrease in the density of fibrous tissue so that the injection can be given easily, and also, it softens the keloid and leads to uniform dispersal of the drug into the pathological tissues.

10.1.4l Botulinum Toxin

Botulinum toxin type A is an exotoxin of the anaerobic spore-forming bacterium, *Clostridium botulinum*. It has become a useful tool for treating the hyperactive muscles of facial expression. It acts by inhibiting the exocytosis of acetylcholine, which indirectly blocks neuromuscular transmission resulting in muscle flaccidity or relaxation [44].

Several papers have reported that botulinum toxin type A can minimize facial scarring by reducing the muscle tension that acts on the healing wound. It may produce changes in the muscle spindles that could lead to altered sensory input and changes in the cell cycle distribution of fibroblasts derived from the hypertrophic scar [45, 46].

The action of botulinum toxin type A on hypertrophic scars is believed to be a temporary denervation of smooth muscle fibers decreasing the tension in the scar tissue. This is one of the main factors that determine the degree of scar formation [47]. Hypertrophic scars result from fibroblast proliferation, which is responsible for enhanced collagen production that leads to excessive scarring [48]. By decreasing the tension in the scar, botulinum toxin causes local fibroblasts to gradually change their functional status to proliferate slower, secrete less biologically active mediators, and synthesize less extracellular matrix and collagen, resulting in an improvement of hypertrophic scars [49].

Monthly injections of intralesional botulinum toxin type A for a period of three months are associated with an improvement of erythema, pliability, and itching in hypertrophic scars. It is a novel and promising therapeutic agent with no side effects noted so far [50].

10.2 Conclusion

The evidence available for many therapeutic modalities for keloids is poor- and high-quality randomized studies are not available. This may be due to a lack of support in research on keloids and various treatment options for the same.

Good evidence of efficacy in the treatment of keloids is available for intralesional steroids, 5-FU, bleomycin, cryosurgery, and surgical excision combined with radiotherapy. Surgical excision and carbon dioxide laser should never be used alone in the management of keloids.

Overall, in spite of several limitations, significant improvement is achievable with the available treatments.

References

1) Mutalik S. Treatment of keloids and hypertrophic scars. Indian J Dermatol Venereol Leprol. 2005 Jan–Feb;71(1):3–8

2) Berman B, Maderal A, Raphael B. Keloids and hypertrophic scars: Pathophysiology, classification, and treatment. Dermatol Surg. 2017 Jan;43 Suppl 1:S3–S18. doi: 10.1097/DSS.0000000000000819. PMID: 27347634.

3) Olaitan PB. Keloids: Assessment of effects and psychosocial- impacts on subjects in a black African population. Indian J Dermatol Venereol Leprol. 2009;75:368–372

4) Jalali M, Bayat A. Current use of steroids in management of abnormal raised skin scars. The Surgeon. 2007;5(3):175–180.

5) Gupta S, Sharma VK. Standard guidelines of care: Keloids and hypertrophic scars. Indian J Dermatol Venereol Leprol. 2011;77:94–100

6) Muneuchi G, Suzuki S, Onodera M, Ito O, Hata Y, Igawa HH. Long-term outcome of intralesional injection of triamcinolone acetonide for the treatment of keloid scars in Asian patients. Scand J Plast Reconstr Surg Hand Surg. 2006;40:111–116 (LEVEL B).

7) Ardehali B, Nouraei SA, van Dam H, Dex E, Wood S, Nduka C. Objective assessment of keloid scars with three-dimensional imaging: Quantifying response to intralesional steroid therapy. Plast Reconstr Surg. 2007;119:556–561 (LEVEL A).

8) Davison SP, Dayan JH, Clemens MW, Sonni S, Wang A, Crane A. Efficacy of intralesional 5-fluorouracil and triamcinolone in the treatment of keloids. Aesthet Surg J. 2009;29:40–46 (LEVEL C).

9) Chowdri NA, Masarat M, Mattoo A, Darzi MA. Keloids and hypertrophic scars: Results with intraoperative and serial postoperative corticosteroid injection therapy. Aust N Z J Surg. 1999;69:655–659 (LEVEL B).

10) Gupta S, Kalra A. Efficacy and safety of intralesional 5-fluorouracil in the treatment of keloids. Dermatology. 2002;204(2):130–132. doi: 10.1159/000051830. PMID: 11937738.

11) Nanda S, Reddy BS. Intralesional 5-fluorouracil as a treatment modality of keloids. Dermatol Surg. 2004;30:54–56 (LEVEL B).

12) Haurani MJ, Foreman K, Yang JJ, Siddiqui A. 5-Fluorouracil treatment of problematic scars. Plast Reconstr Surg. 2009;123:139–148 (LEVEL B)

13) Manuskiatti W, Fitzpatrick RE. Treatment response of keloidal and hypertrophic sternotomy scars: Comparison among intralesional corticosteroid, 5-fluorouracil, and 585-nm flashlamp-pumped pulsed-dye laser treatments. Arch Dermatol. 2002;138:1149–1155 (LEVEL C).

14) Bodokh I, Brun P. Treatment of keloid with intralesional bleomycin. Ann Dermatol Venereol. 1996;123:791–794 (LEVEL B).

15) España A, Solano T, Quintanilla E. Bleomycin in the treatment of keloids and hypertrophic scars by multiple needle punctures. Dermatol Surg. 2001;27:23–27 (LEVEL B).

16) Naeini FF, Najafian J, Ahmadpour K. Bleomycin tattooing as a promising therapeutic modality in large keloids and hypertrophic scars. Dermatol Surg. 2006;32:1023–1029 (LEVEL B).

17) Aggarwal H, Saxena A, Lubana PS, Mathur RK, Jain DK. Treatment of keloids and hypertrophic scars using bleom. J Cosmet Dermatol. 2008;7:43–49 (LEVEL B).

18) Saray Y, Güleп AT. Treatment of keloids and hypertrophic scars with dermojet injections of bleomycin: A preliminary study. Int J Dermatol. 2005;44:777–784 (LEVEL B).

19) Lee JH, Kim SE, Lee AY. Effects of interferon-alpha2b on keloid treatment with triamcinolone acetonide intralesional injection. Int J Dermatol. 2008;47:183–186 (LEVEL C).

20) Davison SP, Mess S, Kauffman LC, Al-Attar A. Ineffective treatment of keloids with interferon alpha-2b. Plast Reconstr Surg. 2006;117:247–252 (LEVEL C)

21) D'Andrea F, Brongo S, Ferraro G, Baroni A. Prevention and treatment of keloids with intralesional verapamil. Dermatology. 2002;204:60–62 (LEVEL C).

22) Xu SJ, Teng JY, Xie J, Shen MQ, Chen DM. Comparison of the mechanisms of intralesional steroid, interferon or verapamil injection in the treatment of proliferative scars. Zhonghua Zheng Xing Wai Ke Za Zhi. 2009;25:37–40 (LEVEL C).

23) Malhotra AK, Gupta S, Khaitan BK, Sharma VK. Imiquimod 5% cream for the prevention of recurrence after excision of presternal keloids. Dermatology. 2007;215:63–65 (LEVEL B).

24) Martin-Garcva RF, Busquets AC. Postsurgical use of imiquimod 5% cream in the prevention of earlobe keloid recurrences: Results of an open-label, pilot study. Dermatol Surg. 2005;31:1394–1398 (LEVEL B).

25) Caпγo FM, Tanaka V, Messina MC. Failure of imiquimod 5% cream to prevent recurrence of surgically excised trunk keloids. Dermatol Surg. 2009;35:629–633 (LEVEL B).

26) Ragoowansi R, Cornes PG, Moss AL, Glees JP. Treatment of keloids by surgical excision and immediate post-operative single-fraction radiotherapy. Plast Reconstr Surg. 2003;111:1853–1859 (LEVEL B).

27) Ogawa R, Miyashita T, Hyakusoku H, Akaishi S, Kuribayashi S, Tateno A. Postoperative radiation protocol for keloids and hypertrophic scars: Statistical analysis of 370 sites followed for over 18 months. Ann Plast Surg. 2007;59:688–691 (LEVEL B).

28) Veen RE, Kal HB. Postoperative high-dose-rate brachytherapy in the prevention of keloids. Int J Radiat Oncol Biol Phys. 2007;69:1205–1208 (LEVEL B)

29) Botwood N, Lewinski C, Lowdell C. The risks of treating keloids with radiotherapy. Br J Radiol. 1999;72:1222–1224 (LEVEL B).

30) Bilbey JH, Muller NL, Miller RR, Nelems B. Localised fibrous mesothelioma of pleura following external ionizing radiation therapy. Chest. 1988;94:1291–1292 (LEVEL B).

31) Speranza G, Sultanem K, Muanza T. Descriptive study of patients receiving excision and radiotherapy for keloids. Int J Radiat Oncol Biol Phys. 2008 Aug 1;71(5):1465–1469. doi: 10.1016/j.ijrobp.2007.12.015. Epub 2008 Feb 4. PMID: 18249504.

32) Leung P, Ng M. Pressure treatment for hypertrophic scars resulting from burns. Burns. 1980;6:244 (LEVEL C).

33) Cheng JC, Evans JH, Leung KS, Clark JA, Choy TT, Leung PC. Pressure therapy in the treatment of postburn hypertrophic scars: A critical look into its usefulness and fallacies by pressure monitoring. Burns Incl Therm Inj. 1984;10:154–163 (LEVEL B).

34) Kuo YR, Wu WS, Jeng SF, Wang FS, Huang HC, Lin CZ, et al. Suppressed TGF-beta1 expression is correlated with up-regulation of matrix metalloproteinase-13 in keloid regression after flashlamp pulsed-dye laser treatment. Lasers Surg Med. 2005;36:38–42 (LEVEL C).

35) Kuo YR, Wu WS, Jeng SF, Nicolini J, Zubillaga M. Activation of ERK and p38 kinase mediated keloid fibroblast apoptosis after flashlamp pulsed-dye laser treatment. Lasers Surg Med. 2005;36:31–37 (LEVEL C).

36) Norris JE. The effect of carbon dioxide laser surgery on the recurrence of keloids. Plast Reconstr Surg. 1991;87:44–49(LEVEL B).

37) Apfelberg DB, Maser MR, White DN, Lash H. Failure of carbon dioxide laser excision of keloids. Lasers Surg Med. 1989;9:382–388 (LEVEL B)

38) Kim DY, Kim ES, Eo SR, Kim KS, Lee SY, Cho BH. A surgical approach for earlobe keloid: Keloid fillet flap. Arch Facial Plast Surg. 2005;7:172–175 (LEVEL B).

39) Zouboulis CC, Blume U, Büttner P, Orfanos CE. Outcomes of cryosurgery in keloids and hypertrophic scars. A prospective consecutive trial of case series. Arch Dermatol. 1993;129:1146–1151 (LEVEL B).

40) Ernst K, Hundeiker M. Results of cryosurgery in 394 patients with hypertrophic scars and keloids. Hautarzt. 1995;46:462–466 (LEVEL B).

41) Rusciani L, Rossi G, Bono R. Use of cryotherapy in the treatment of keloids. J Dermatol Surg Oncol. 1993;19:529–534 (LEVEL B).

42) Zouboulis CC, Orfanos CE. Cryosurgical treatment of hypertrophic scars and keloids. Hautarzt. 1990;41:683–688 (LEVEL B)

43) Sharma S, Bhanot A, Kaur A, Dewan SP. Role of liquid nitrogen alone compared with combination of liquid nitrogen and intralesional triamcinolone acetonide in treatment of small keloids. J Cosmet Dermatol. 2007;6:258–261 (LEVEL B.

44) Naumann M, So Y, Argoff CE, Childers MK, Dykstra DD, Gronseth GS, et al. Assessment: Botulinum neurotoxin in the treatment of autonomic disorders and pain (an evidence-based review): Report of the Therapeutics and Technology Assessment Subcommittee of the American Academy of Neurology. Neurology. 2008;70:1707–1714.

45) Aoki KR. Botulinum toxin: A successful therapeutic protein. Curr Med Chem. 2004;11:3085–3092.

46) Zhibo X, Miaobo Z. Botulinum toxin type A affects cell cycle distribution of fibroblasts derived from hypertrophic scar. J Plast Reconstr Aesthet Surg. 2008;61:1128–1129.

47) Scheffer AR, Erasmus C, van Hulst K, van Limbeek J, Jongerius PH, van den Hoogen FJ. Efficacy and duration of botulinum toxin treatment for drooling in 131 children. Arch Otolaryngol Head Neck Surg. 2010;136:873–877

48) Nordlund JJ. Keloids and hypertrophic scars. Arch Dermatol. 2000;137:77.

49) Xiao Z, Qu G. Effects of botulinum toxin type a on collagen deposition in hypertrophic scars. Molecules. 2012;17:2169–2177.

50) Elhefnawy AM. Assessment of intralesional injection of botulinum toxin type A injection for hypertrophic scars. Indian J Dermatol Venereol Leprol. 2016;82:279–283.

CHAPTER 11: HIRSUTISM

Sahana P. Raju and Mukta Sachdev

11.1 Introduction

Hirsutism is defined as the occurrence of excessive terminal hair in a male pattern distribution in females. The etiology of hirsutism is widely varied. It most commonly occurs as part of an underlying syndrome due to androgen excess. Hirsutism must be differentiated from hypertrichosis, which is increased growth of hair in a non-sexual generalized manner and is usually androgen-independent. Hirsutism is one of the most established health problems in women of childbearing age and is a major cause of psychological stress in them. The successful treatment of hirsutism, in addition to the various modalities of treatment available, also requires a great deal of patience from both the treating physician and the patient.

11.2 Epidemiology

Hirsutism is said to affect 5–10% of the women in the reproductive age group.[1] It can also occur in post-menopausal women due to the relative hyperandrogenism caused by the cessation of ovarian function. Cultural, genetic, ethnic, and racial factors must also be taken into account while quantifying the amount and distribution of terminal hair in women. Women of American and Asian descent have very little body hair, while Mediterranean women have moderate to large amounts of body hair. Similarly, the cut-off value for the diagnosis of hirsutism and its severity varies according to race and ethnicity.

11.3 Pathophysiology

There are many factors contributing to the development of hirsutism. However, none of them are definite as there is a dearth of molecular techniques required to prove the hypothesis.

11.3.1 Types of Hair

Lanugo hair, vellus hair, and terminal hair are the three distinguished hair types. Lanugo hair is the soft, dense hair covering the fetus, which is shed post-partum. Vellus hair is the non-pigmented, non-medullated, fine short hair, whereas terminal hair is the pigmented, coarse, thick hair found on androgen-sensitive areas like the scalp, beard, axilla, and pubis. The transformation of vellus hair into terminal hair, which usually occurs at puberty, is an androgen-sensitive process.[2]

11.3.2 Normal Enzymatic Activity of the Skin

The enzyme 5α-reductase (5α-RA), which plays a major role in the conversion of sex hormones like testosterone, androstenedione, and dehydroepiandrosterone, to their active form, dihydrotestosterone (DHT), is in fact the function of two separate iso-enzymes, type 1 and type 2 5α-RA. The distribution of the two iso-enzymes varies, as shown in Table 11.1. DHT is essentially formed by the peripheral conversion of testosterone in males and androstenedione in females by the enzyme 5α-reductase. The activity of 5α-RA is increased by local growth factors, circulating growth factors, and androgens, which could explain the increased presence of terminal hair in conditions with hyperandrogenism, leading to hirsutism.

TABLE 11.1: Distribution of Iso-Enzymes of 5α-Reductase

Type 1	Type 2
Skin–hair follicles and distal lobules of sebaceous glands	Skin–hair follicles and duct of sebaceous glands
Liver	Liver
Adrenal glands	Prostate
Kidney	Epididymis, seminal vesicles, and testes

It has been proposed that idiopathic hirsutism, a type of non-androgenic form of hirsutism, results from androgen receptor polymorphisms or increased peripheral 5α-reductase activity.[3]

11.3.3 Androgens and Hair Growth

Androgens are the predominant hormones involved in the modulation of hair growth. They bring about the differentiation of pilosebaceous unit into either a terminal hair follicle or sebaceous gland. They also cause an increase in hair follicle size and hair fiber diameter. Increased levels of DHT result in thicker and longer hair due to the prolongation of the anagen phase.[4]

The action of androgens on hair growth is area-specific due to variations in the androgen receptor and 5α-RA levels. These areas can be divided into three types—namely, non-sexual skin, which is independent of effects of androgens (eyebrows and eyelashes); ambisexual skin, which is sensitive to even low levels of androgens (pubic and axillary hair); and sexual skin, which are sensitive to only high levels of androgens (chest, abdomen, back, thighs, upper arms, and face). While the presence of terminal hair in ambisexual areas is considered to be normal even in females, their presence in the sexual areas is considered pathological and termed hirsutism.

11.3.4 Insulin Resistance and Hirsutism

The pathways of insulin resistance and hyper-androgenemia are interlinked, which may explain the occurrence of hirsutism and other features of hyperandrogenism in patients with PCOS, diabetes mellitus, and metabolic syndrome. In addition to androgens, hair growth regulation and the anagen phase are influenced by multiple growth factors, including insulin-like growth factor 1 (IGF-1). Hyperinsulinemia increases the circulating IGF-1 levels, which in turn results in an increased cell turnover of the pilosebaceous unit, resulting in hirsutism and acne vulgaris.[5]

11.4 Etiology

Understanding the various causes of hirsutism is essential as it could be the only presenting sign of an underlying disorder of androgen excess. Hirsutism can be broadly classified into androgenic type and non-androgenic type (Figure 11.1).[6] Polycystic ovarian syndrome (PCOS) is the commonest cause of androgenic hirsutism, whereas idiopathic hirsutism (IH) is the most common form of non-androgen-induced hirsutism. Together, they account for more than 95% of all cases of hirsutism. Drugs causing hirsutism are listed in Table 11.2.[7]

DOI: 10.1201/9780429243769-11

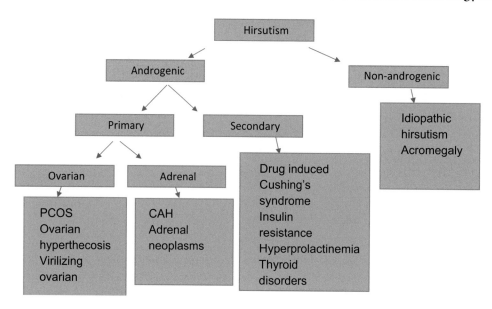

FIGURE 11.1: Classification of hirsutism.

TABLE 11.2: Drugs Leading to Hirsutism

- Androgens
- Glucocorticoids
- Progestins
- Minoxidil
- Cyclosporine
- Danazol
- Phenytoin
- D-penicillamine
- Interferon-α
- Clomiphene and tamoxifen

11.5 Clinical Features

Some of the common endocrinological conditions associated with hirsutism are outlined in Table 11.3. Although there is considerable overlap in clinical features of these conditions, they still serve as important diagnostic clues.[8, 9]

Benign causes of hirsutism usually have a pubertal onset, slow progression, positive family history, and rarely signs of virilization, whereas late-onset hirsutism with rapid development, treatment-resistant hirsutism, and signs of virilization indicate a malignant pathology, which could be an androgen-secreting tumor either of adrenal or ovarian origin.

The two most common causes accounting for 95% of cases of hirsutism are explained as follows:

1. *Polycystic ovarian syndrome (PCOS)*
   PCOS affects 4–6% of reproductive-age women and is the most common cause of androgen-induced hirsutism. The etiology of PCOS remains ambiguous, with hyperandrogenism, insulin resistance, HPA axis dysfunction, oxidative stress, and genetic and prenatal factors playing a role in its pathogenesis. The diagnosis of PCOS is made based on the Rotterdam criteria, in which two of the following three criteria are required:[10]

TABLE 11.3: Diagnostic Clues to Common Causes of Hirsutism

Underlying Condition	Clinical Clues
PCOS	• Oligo-/amenorrhea • Hirsutism • Acne • Acanthosis nigricans • Alopecia • Obesity • Infertility
HAIR-AN syndrome	• Acne, hirsutism • Acanthosis nigricans • Features of insulin resistance
SAHA syndrome	• Seborrhea • Acne • Hirsutism • Male-pattern alopecia
CAH	• High-risk ethnic groups (Hispanics, Azhkenazi Jews) • Hirsutism • Amenorrhea • Infertility
Cushing's syndrome	• Central obesity • Purple skin striae • Moon facies, buffalo hump • Acne, hirsutism • Proximal muscle weakness
Thyroid dysfunction	• Menstrual irregularities • Features of hyper- or hypothyroidism
Pituitary tumor	• Headaches and visual disturbances • Galactorrhea
Adrenal or ovarian tumor	• Palpable abdominal or pelvis mass • Rapid-onset hirsutism • Treatment-resistant hirsutism • Signs of virilization like clitoromegaly, deep voice, increased muscle mass, and atrophy of breast tissue

a. Menstrual irregularity
   • Clinical—oligomenorrhea or amenorrhea
   • Biochemical—high levels of luteinizing hormone (LH)
b. Features of hyperandrogenism
   • Clinical—hirsutism, acne, male pattern alopecia, acanthosis nigricans
   • Biochemical—raised free androgen index or free testosterone
c. Pelvis ultrasound showing polycystic ovaries (ovary with ≥12 follicles measuring 2–9 mm in diameter or ovarian volume of >10 cc)

More recently, a serum called anti-Mullerian hormone (AMH) assay is said to be a more sensitive and specific biomarker for detecting PCOS.[11] Patients diagnosed with PCOS should be regularly screened for hypertension, dyslipidemia, atherosclerosis, and endometrial carcinoma.

2. *Idiopathic hirsutism (IH)*
   Although hirsutism is associated with the discussed endocrinological disorders, certain patients show regular ovulation and an absence of hyperandrogenemia. This is termed as idiopathic hirsutism.[3] It is also known as simple or peripheral hirsutism. IH is a diagnosis of exclusion and accounts for 5–15% of the total cases.

The following categories of patients are included in IH:
a. Hirsutism of unknown causes
b. Hirsutism with regular menstrual cycles and a normal ovulatory function
c. Hirsutism with normal circulating androgen levels

11.6 Classification of Severity

In 1961, Ferriman and Gallwey proposed a scoring system to quantify hirsutism in 11 androgen-dependent areas.[12, 13] This was modified later on to include only nine of the androgen-dependent sites and is known as the modified Ferriman Gallwey scoring system (mFG), which is extensively used till date to assess the severity of hirsutism.[14] (Figure 11.2)

Although an mFG score of more than or equal to 8 is considered hirsutism, the cut-off scores differ by race and ethnicity. A cut-off score of 2 or greater is considered hirsutism in Asian women, 6 or greater in South American women, 8 or greater in British and American women, and 9 or greater in Mediterranean, Hispanic, and Middle Eastern women.[15]

11.7 Approach to a Hirsute Patient

After establishing the distribution of the terminal hair and assessing the severity, the following steps can be initiated to determine the cause of hirsutism:[16]

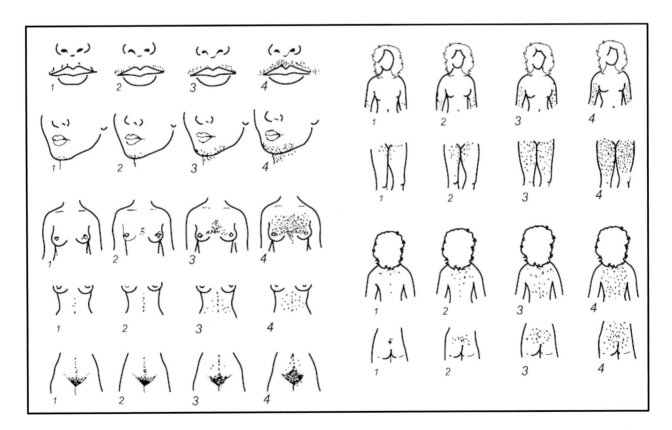

FIGURE 11.2 The modified Ferriman-Gallwey scoring system involving nine sites. The sum of scores in each site is considered to be the final score.

(From Yildiz BO, Bolour S, Woods K, Moore A, Azziz R. Visually scoring hirsutism, Hum Reprod Update, 2010, vol. 16 (pg. 51–64)10.1093/humupd/dmp024.)

- A detailed history of the age of onset and progression of hirsutism, menstrual and reproductive history, family history of hirsutism, infertility or obesity, history of medication use, and history of acne and hair loss.
- A thorough examination including a routine physical with a complete systemic examination (breast, thyroid, and pelvis), BMI calculation, examination for any signs of virilization like deepening of the voice, male pattern hair loss, clitoromegaly, increase in muscle mass, measuring the content and distribution of body fat, and presence of any Cushingoid features or signs of insulin resistance like acanthosis nigricans, obesity, and acrochordons.
- Biochemical evaluation: When must it be done?—It has been suggested that routine evaluation of androgen levels must be done only in sudden-onset hirsutism, rapidly progressive hirsutism, moderate to severe hirsutism, and hirsutism associated with infertility and irregular menstrual cycles. It is not indicated in mild hirsutism.[17, 18] The various serum markers used and the conditions tested for are enumerated in Table 11.4.
- Imaging studies: A pelvic ultrasonography can be done to confirm PCOS or an ovarian neoplasm. Computed tomography (CT) or magnetic resonance imaging (MRI) of the adrenals can be done in suspected adrenal gland pathology.

11.8 Management

Patients should be counseled about the need for long-term treatment and the adverse effects of the drugs or procedures involved.

Lifestyle modification measures: Numerous studies have reported reductions in total or free testosterone, adrenal androgens, and hirsutism with dietary modifications, exercise, and behavioral treatment with the aim of weight reduction in women with PCOS and insulin resistance. Menstrual function and ovulation also improved in these women. In women with hirsutism associated with obesity and PCOS, lifestyle modification measures must be advocated along with pharmacologic therapy for a fruitful outcome.[19]

TABLE 11.4: Biochemical Markers for Diagnosis of Hirsutism

Serum Marker	Value	Underlying Condition
Serum total testosterone	>200 ng/mL	Malignant adrenal or ovarian tumor
DHEA-S	>700 ng/mL	Benign or malignant adrenal cause
17-Hydroxy progesterone	300–1000 ng/mL and >1,000 mg/mL post-ACTH stimulation test	Congenital adrenal hyperplasia
24-hour urinary-free cortisol		Cushing's syndrome
LH/FSH	>3	PCOS
Lipid profile, fasting blood sugar, and insulin levels		Metabolic syndrome
Prolactin levels		Hypothalamic or pituitary disease
Thyroid function tests (T3, T4, serum TSH)		Could be a co-factor in hirsutism

Physical methods of hair removal: Plucking, tweezing, waxing, and shaving are common methods of hair removal used by women. These methods, though safe and effective, are only temporary means and have no effect on hair growth. They can also cause irritation of the skin, folliculitis, and pseudofolliculitis.

Electrolysis: It involves the passage of a small needle or probe into the hair follicle, through which an electric current is passed. This results in the permanent destruction of the hair follicle. Multiple treatment sessions are necessary to minimize thermal cutaneous injury. Even though electrolysis is the only modality that can produce permanent hair removal, it must be done cautiously due to a high propensity for adverse effects like the risk of transmission of infectious agents, pain, and cutaneous pigmentation.[20]

Topical eflornithine: Eflornithine, initially synthesized as a chemotherapeutic agent, is the first US FDA-approved topical preparation for treating facial hirsutism in women. Eflornithine inhibits the enzyme ornithine decarboxylase, which is involved in the conversion of ornithine to polyamines. Polyamines play a regulatory role in hair growth and differentiation. A 13.5% cream used twice daily for four to eight weeks is proven to be effective.[21] Some of the adverse effects related to its use are headache, dryness, pruritis, acne, and folliculitis. Once treatment with eflornithine is stopped, hair growth reverts in eight to ten weeks' time. The use of eflornithine only as an adjunct along with laser hair removal and not as monotherapy is advocated.

Oral therapy:[22] The aim of systemic oral therapy in hirsutism is to correct the hormonal imbalance and reduce the level of androgens responsible for hirsutism. The various agents used are as follows:

1. **Oral contraceptive pills (OCPs)**
   OCPs are used as the first line drugs in treatment of hirsutism, in combination with anti-androgens. OCPs act by increasing the production of sex-hormone-binding globulin (SHBG) from the liver, which ultimately suppresses androgen secretion. A combination of ethinylestradiol in a low dose (0.03 to 0.035 mg) and a progestin with anti-androgenic properties, like cyproterone acetate (CPA) and drospirenone, can be started. Therapy must be continued for a minimum period of six months for optimum results. Adverse effects, including but not limited to the risk of thromboembolism, myocardial infarction, stroke, and breast cancer, have to be diligently monitored.
2. **Anti-androgen therapy**
   - *Spironolactone*: It is an androgen receptor blocker and an aldosterone antagonist which competes with DHT for binding with androgen receptors. It also has additional mechanisms useful in the treatment of hirsutism, like inhibiting 5-alpha reductase and decreasing the circulating LH/FSH ratio. Therefore, it can be used in the treatment of both androgenic and idiopathic hirsutism. A dose of 100 mg/day is generally used in the treatment of hirsutism. Higher doses of 250–300 mg/day can be used in severe hirsutism in morbidly obese women. Some of the adverse effects associated with its use are gastritis, xerosis, headaches, fatigue, and syncope. Absolute contraindications for its use include hyperkalemia, chronic renal impairment, pregnancy, and abnormal uterine bleeding. Monitoring of electrolyte levels and renal function tests must be done periodically.

- *Flutamide*: It is an androgen receptor blocker whose active metabolite, 2-hydroxyflutamide, inhibits the binding of DHT to its androgen receptor. Doses ranging from 62.5 mg to 250 mg/day are used for the treatment of hirsutism. The regular monitoring of liver function tests, including enzyme markers, is recommended as flutamide can cause hepatotoxicity. Other minor side effects include xerosis and discoloration of urine.
- *Cyproterone acetate (CPA)*: CPA is a derivative of 17-hydroxyprogesterone acetate, which is an anti-androgen with strong progestogenic properties. It has contraceptive properties and is also used as an effective treatment for hirsutism. CPA in doses of 50–100 mg/day in combination with 30–35 mg of ethinylestradiol was found to be effective in the management of hirsutism.
- *Finasteride*: It selectively inhibits the type 2 isoform of 5α-reductase and hence the peripheral conversion of testosterone to DHT. It can be used in doses of 1–7.5 mg.

3. **Insulin sensitizing agents**

This group of drugs includes metformin and thiazolidinediones like pioglitazone. They act by depleting insulin levels and thereby reduce hyperandrogenemia. They are primarily used in the management of hirsutism associated with PCOS, in combination with OCPs and anti-androgens, in order to reduce androgen levels, help in weight reduction and normalize menstrual cycles. The use of insulin-sensitizing drugs in the treatment of hirsutism without hyperinsulinemia is inconsistent and not recommended.[23]

4. **Glucocorticoids**

A low dose of dexamethasone can be used to treat hirsutism associated with congenital adrenal hyperplasia (CAH).

5. **Gonadotropic-releasing hormone (GnRH) agonists**

Long-acting GnRH agonists act by suppressing the hypothalamic-pituitary-ovarian axis in androgenized or hyper-insulinemic patients. It is only indicated when OCPs, anti-androgens, and corticosteroid therapy fails. GnRH analogs must be for two to three months before their effects manifest, during which long-term adverse effects like atrophic vaginitis, hot flushes, demineralization of bones, and so on must be carefully monitored.[24]

Some of the important considerations to be made while using systemic oral therapy for hirsutism are as follows:[25]

- Mild hirsutism, without any evidence of an underlying condition, does not require treatment other than for cosmetic purposes.
- OCPs are the first-line therapy for moderate to severe hirsutism.
- Monotherapy with anti-androgens is contraindicated in women of childbearing group as they are teratogenic.

Lasers: The successful treatment of hirsutism requires a combination of therapies. While the further progression of the disease is prevented by hormonal therapy, strategies to permanently remove unwanted hair also have to be employed. The age-old method of hair destruction, electrolysis, or epilation is now applied to laser therapy, also known as photo-epilation. The use of lasers for hair removal works on the principle of selective photo-thermolysis, wherein energy delivered at a particular wavelength to a targeted site can cause selective destruction of the hair follicle, sparing the surrounding structures. The target for laser hair removal can be a hair bulb and bulge melanin or an exogenous chromophore. Lasers have the advantages of causing fewer adverse effects, providing a longer hair-free interval, and are more convenient.

Various parameters and patient factors have to be taken into consideration to ensure a predictable and favorable outcome.

Laser parameters

1. Spot size—Larger spot sizes are preferred to prevent scattering of energy.
2. Pulse duration is selected based on the thermal relaxation time (TRT). The concept of thermal damage time (TDT), which is significantly longer than the TRT, in order to achieve permanent damage to the hair bulb and also disperse an amount of energy to the surrounding non-pigmented stem cells, comes into play here.[26] The TDT and hence the pulse duration for terminal hair is calculated to be around 100 milliseconds.
3. Fluence has to be determined by the upper limit of the energy that produces perifollicular erythema and edema. In general, higher fluences achieve greater hair reduction but also come with a higher side effect profile. Lower fluences in the range of 20–24 J/cm^2 are preferred for darker skin types.

Patient factors[27]

1. Skin type—The chances of effective hair removal are increased with light skin (Fitzpatrick I–IV skin types) and dark hair.
2. Site of hair removal—Axillae and belt areas have better response rates than arms, legs, and chest due to anatomic variations in anagen-telogen ratios.
3. Stage of hair cycle—Terminal anagen hair have the best response rates due to the presence of higher levels of melanin in these types of hair.
4. Any underlying condition—Evaluation for the cause of hirsutism must be carried out in all patients. Untreated hormonal and endocrinological conditions can result in poor laser hair removal outcomes. Collateral hormonal therapy and increased laser hair removal sessions are required for such patients. The occurrence of paradoxical hypertrichosis after laser hair removal and PCOS has been reported in darker skin types.

Different lasers used: An ideal laser for hair removal should have the following properties:

- Wavelength absorbed preferentially only by melanin
- Sufficient penetration to reach hair follicles
- Effective fluence to prevent scattering
  1. Continuous mode ruby laser delivers a wavelength of 694 nm, which is especially useful in individuals with light skin and dark hair due to higher melanin absorption at 694 nm.
  2. Alexandrite laser has a greater wavelength of 755 nm, with an increased depth of penetration.
  3. Diode laser, with a wavelength of 800–980 nm, can be used to treat darker skin types (Fitzpatrick IV–VI) safely.
  4. The long-pulsed 1,064 nm Nd:YAG laser can be safely used in darker skin types due to its deeper penetration and poor melanin absorption capacity. However, the pain associated with the use of this laser and its overall reduced efficacy are some of the drawbacks of the Nd:YAG laser. It also requires the use of an epidermal cooling device to reduce epidermal injury.

5. Intense pulse light therapy (IPL) is the laser-equivalent device that delivers non-coherent wavelengths of 550–1,200 nm, which are useful for light-colored hair.

6. Newer methods like vacuum-assisted low-fluence laser hair removal use a low fluence and large spot size under vacuum, which has the advantages of specifically targeting the chromophore, treating large body surface areas, and is comparatively less painful.

Pre-treatment preparation

Application of broad-spectrum sunscreens must be advised three to four weeks prior to laser hair removal to avoid post-inflammatory hyperpigmentation and tanning. Patients should be advised not to undergo waxing, plucking, threading, or electrolysis prior to laser therapy as this removes the target chromophore. Shaving or depilation, however, is acceptable. Topical anesthesia can be used prior to the procedure to minimize discomfort.

After a thorough evaluation, the starting pulse duration and fluence is predetermined according to the skin type. The treatment sessions are performed at four-week intervals, with the fluence increased by 10% at each session. Most studies report a 25–75% clearance rate achieved after six months of therapy, depending on the anatomic location and skin phototype.

Side effects of laser hair removal therapy include epidermal injury with blistering, pigmentary changes, thrombophlebitis, and rarely scarring. All adverse effects are more common in darker skin types (Fitzpatrick IV–VI) due to the absorption of energy by epidermal melanin.[28]

To summarize, the 755 alexandrite laser or the 800 nm diode laser can be used in lighter skin types (Fitzpatrick I–III). Although long-pulsed Nd:YAG laser is found to be the safest device for darker skin types (Fitzpatrick IV–VI), the 800 nm diode laser is found to be more efficacious and is considered the gold standard.[29]

Newer modalities[30]

- *Statins*: Statins are HMG-CoA reductase inhibitors that have been shown to reduce hyperandrogenism by inhibiting ovarian theca cell proliferation and testosterone production. Further studies are required to decide their role in the treatment of hirsutism.

- *Vitamin D*: Insulin resistance and PCOS is said to be associated with low serum vitamin D levels. Further studies are required to evaluate the benefits of vitamin D supplementation in hirsutism.

11.9 Conclusion

The FDA, in 1998, defined permanent hair reduction as "the long-term, stable reduction in the number of hairs re-growing after a treatment regimen and does not imply the elimination of all hairs in the treatment area." For some patients, a successful outcome might be the conversion of dense, thick hair to fine, light hair, while for others, it might be a near-complete eradication of hair. The treatment of hirsutism must be tailored according to each patient. A combination therapy with anti-androgen and oral contraceptive pills, along with cosmetic treatment and lifestyle modifications, is the preferred line of management. The approach must be systematic and sometimes requires integrated management involving an endocrinologist and gynecologist.

References

1. Escobar-Morreale HF, Carmina E, Dewailly D, Gambineri A, Kelestimur F, Moghetti P, Pugeat M, Qiao J, Wijeyaratne CN, Witchel SF, Norman RJ. Epidemiology, diagnosis and management of hirsutism: A consensus statement by the Androgen Excess and Polycystic Ovary Syndrome Society. Hum Reprod Update. 2012 Mar–Apr;18(2):146–170

2. Archer JS, Chang RJ. Hirsutism and acne in polycystic ovary syndrome. Best Pract Res Clin Obstet Gynaecol. 2004 Oct;18(5):737–754

3. Azziz R, Carmina E, Sawaya ME. Idiopathic hirsutism. Endocr Rev. 2000;21:347–362

4. Tekin O, Avci Z, Isik B, et al. Hirsutism: Common clinical problem or index of serious disease? MedGenMed. 2004;6(4):56

5. Talaei A, Adgi Z, Mohamadi Kelishadi M. Idiopathic hirsutism and insulin resistance. Int J Endocrinol. 2013;2013:593197

6. Wankhade HV, Shah VH, Tomar SS, Singh PR. Clinical and investigative study of hirsutism. J Clin Diag Res. 2019 Jun;13(6)

7. Hafsi W, Badri TH.[Aug 26] In: StatPerals [Internet]. Treasure Island (FL): StatPearls Publishing, 2022.

8. Matheson E, Bain J. Hirsutism in women. Am Fam Physician. 2019 Aug 1;100(3):168–175

9. Agarwal NK. Management of hirsutism. Indian J Endocr Metab. 2013;17(Suppl S1):77–82

10. Rotterdam EA-SPCWG. Revised 2003 consensus on diagnostic criteria and long-term health risks related to polycystic ovary syndrome (PCOS). Hum. Reprod. 2004;19:41–47

11. Dewailly D, Gronier H, Poncelet E, Robin G, Leroy M, Pigny P, Duhamel A, Catteau-Jonard S. Diagnosis of polycystic ovary syndrome (PCOS): Revisiting the threshold values of follicle count on ultrasound and of the serum AMH level for the 250 definition of polycystic ovaries. Hum Reprod. 2011;26:3123–3129

12. Aswini R, Jayapalan S. Modified Ferriman-Gallwey score in hirsutism and its association with metabolic syndrome. Int J Trichology. 2017;9(1):7–13

13. Ferriman D, Gallwey JD. Clinical assessment of body hair growth in women. J Clin Endocrinol Metab. 1961;21:1440–1447

14. Hatch R, Rosenfield RL, Kin MH, Tredway D. Hirsutism: Implications, etiology, and management. Am J Obstet Gynecol. 1981;140:815–830

15. DeUgarte CM, Woods KS, Bartolucci AA, Azziz R. Degree of facial and body terminal hair growth in unselected black and white women: Toward a populational definition of hirsutism. J Clin Endocrinol Metab. 2006;91:1345–1350

16. Sachdeva S. Hirsutism: Evaluation and treatment. Indian J Dermatol. 2010;55(1):3–7

17. Mihailidis J, Dermesropian R, Taxel P, Luthra P, Grant-Kels JM. Endocrine evaluation of hirsutism. Int J Womens Dermatol. 2017 Feb 16;3(1 Suppl):S6–S10

18. Martin KA, Chang RJ, Ehrmann DA, Ibanez L, Lobo RA, Rosenfield RL, et al. Evaluation and treatment of hirsutism in premenopausal women: An endocrine society clinical practice guideline. J Clin Endocrinol Metab. 2008;93:1105–1120

19. Pasquali R, Gambineri A. Therapy in endocrine disease: Treatment of hirsutism in the polycystic ovary syndrome. Eur J Endocrinol. 2013 Dec 21;170(2):R75–90.

20. Wanitphakdeedecha R, Alster TS. Physical means of treating unwanted hair. Dermatol Ther. 2008 Sep–Oct;21(5):392–401

21. Jobanputra KS, Rajpal AV, Nagpur N G. Eflornithine. Indian J Dermatol Venereol Leprol. 2007;73:365–366

22. Ekback MP. Etiology and treatment of hirsutism. J Endocrinol Diabetes Obes. 2017;5(3):1110

23. Cosma M, Swiglo BA, Flynn DN, Kurtz DM, Labella ML, Mullan RJ. Clinical review: Insulin sensitizers for the treatment of hirsutism: A systematic review and metaanalyses of randomized controlled trials. J Clin Endocrinol Metab. 2008;93:1135–1142

24. Pazos F, Escobar-Morreale HF, Balsa J, Sancho JM, Varela C. Prospective randomized study comparing the long-acting gonadotropin-releasing hormone agonist triptorelin, flutamide, and cyproterone acetate, used in combination with an oral contraceptive in the treatment of hirsutism. Fertil Steril. 1999;71:122–128

25. Barrionuevo P, Nabhan M, Altayar O, Wang Z, Erwin PJ, Asi N, Martin KA, Murad MH. Treatment options for hirsutism: A systematic review and network meta-analysis. J Clin Endocrinol Metab. 2018 Apr 1;103(4):1258–1264

26. Lee CM. Laser-assisted hair removal for facial hirsutism in women: A review of evidence. J Cosmet Laser Ther. 2018 Jun;20(3):140–144.

27. Bhat YJ, Bashir S, Nabi N, Hassan I. Laser treatment in hirsutism: An update. Dermatol Pract Concept. 2020 Apr 20;10(2):e2020048

28. Sanchez LA, Perez M, Azziz R. Laser hair reduction in the hirsute patient: A critical assessment. Hum Reprod Update. 2002 Mar–Apr;8(2): 169–181

29. Arsiwala SZ, Majid IM. Methods to overcome poor responses and challenges of laser hair removal in dark skin. Indian J Dermatol Venereol Leprol. 2019;85:3–9

30. Somani N, Turvy D. Hirsutism: An evidence-based treatment update. Am J Clin Dermatol. 2014 Jul;15(3):247–266

CHAPTER 12: HAIR LOSS AND HAIR DISORDERS

Rachita Dhurat and Sandip Agrawal

12.1 Introduction

Hair loss, or alopecia, is the loss of hair from the head or body. Apart from a cosmetic concern, it is associated with psychological distress as patients usually complain of increased shedding of hair. Hair can be divided into three main groups according to their racial origin: Caucasian, Oriental, and African. These differ mainly in their appearance, geometry, mechanical properties, and water content. These differences in African hair explain why some types of cicatricial alopecia and hair diseases are more prevalent in or are almost exclusive to this ethnic group (1).

Granular pigments (eumelanin), which vary in color from black to dark red, give darker colors to the hair, while diffuse pigments (pheomelanin), which vary in color from bright red to pale yellow, give lighter colors to the hair. Afro-ethnic hair characteristically contains more eumelanin than pheomelanin and is, therefore, darker.

The hair follicles are asymmetrical, with an elliptical or oval cross-section and a curved hair follicle bulb. This elliptical shape with flattened and irregular hair shafts is responsible for lower resistance and a higher susceptibility to breakage when compared with Caucasian hair and Asian hair, which have straight hair follicles and round-shaped hair shafts with homogeneous diameters throughout the fiber. Black women have shorter hair when compared with other types of hair. Afro-ethnic hair grows more slowly than Caucasian hair (0.9 cm/month and 1.3 cm/month, respectively). Although African hair is drier, more brittle, and more susceptible to chemical and physical damage due to its spiral structure, it also has some advantages, especially in hot climates where it forms a natural barrier against the sun. Its spiral-curved form causes the air to cool up and easily circulate through the scalp, being part of the body's thermoregulatory mechanism (1).

Classification Alopecias are mainly classified as disorders involving the hair follicle and those involving the hair shaft (Table 12.1). Among disorders involving hair follicles, alopecias are subclassified as non-cicatricial (non-scarring) alopecia and cicatricial (scarring) alopecia. Hair follicles are lost permanently in cicatricial alopecia, while the damage is potentially reversible in non-cicatricial alopecias. According to the extent of involvement, alopecia can be **diffuse or localized** (2–4).

12.2 Diffuse Non-Scarring Hair Loss

Diffuse hair loss is a common complaint encountered by dermatologists in their daily clinical practice. Women present more frequently with this complaint. However, it can affect both sexes at any age. The common causes for diffuse hair loss include **androgenetic hair loss and telogen effluvium (TE)**.

12.2a Androgenetic Alopecia

Synonyms: male pattern alopecia, female pattern hair loss, patterned baldness. Androgenetic alopecia (AGA) is characterized by hair loss in a distinctive pattern that differs between men (Hamilton pattern) and women. In the early stages of androgenetic alopecia, the pattern may not be evident, and patients may present with diffuse hair loss. This presentation is far more common in women and can lead to diagnostic difficulty, with the main differential diagnosis being chronic telogen effluvium (5).

The Incidence of Baldness Men of Asian, Native American, and African backgrounds have a decreased frequency of frontal hair loss and less extensive alopecia as compared to Caucasians (6). Hamilton estimated that 30% of men developed androgenetic alopecia by the age of 30 and 50% by the age of 50 (7).

AGA in women has been termed female pattern hair loss (FPHL) because the androgen dependence of hair loss in all women with patterned alopecia has not been sufficiently demonstrated (8).

In women, there are two main peaks of onset of female pattern hair loss: the third decade and the second peak is from the age of about 40 through menopause (8). However, androgenetic alopecia in children and adolescents has been reported (9).

Etiology

As its name implies, AGA involves both genetic and hormonal factors. Genetics determine the density and the location of androgen-sensitive hair follicles on the scalp. After puberty, androgens transform these genetically programmed terminal hair follicles, predominantly of the frontoparietal scalp, into miniaturized follicles (10).

Clinical Features In men, there is a frontal hairline recession associated with thinning or balding on the crown or vertex (Figure 12.1). It has been well documented by Hamilton and Norwood (11, 12).

The various patterns of presentation that have been observed in women with FPHL are listed here:

- Diffuse central thinning with preservation of frontal margin (commonest) (13) (Figures 12.2 and 12.3)
- Frontal accentuation (Chrismas tree)—that is, a breach in frontal line (8)
- Diffuse thinning of hair over the entire scalp, often more noticeable thinning toward the back of the scalp (14)
- Diffuse thinning of hair over the parietal region (15)
- Male pattern (frontoparietal) (16)
- Bitemporal thinning is commonly associated with but not necessarily indicative of female pattern hair loss (17)
- There is no recession of the frontal hairline, although the hair on the frontal margin is miniaturized (i.e., finer and shorter)

Diagnosis The patterns of hair loss in male baldness are easily identifiable and are rarely confused with alternative causes of alopecia. A common clinical conundrum is that of an adult woman presenting with diffuse, non-scarring hair loss of the scalp. Evaluation of such cases is rather arduous, considering the various causes of hair loss in women. Women with mid-scalp widening are a straightforward case of FPHL. When women present with increased hair shedding but little or no

DOI: 10.1201/9780429243769-12

TABLE 12.1: Classification of Alopecia

	Hair Follicle Disorders				Hair Shaft Disorders
	Non-Cicatricial (Non-Scarring) *Reversible Damage*			Cicatricial (Scarring) *Permanent Loss of Hair Follicles*	
Diffuse		**Localized**			
Patterned	**Unpatterned**	**Patterned**	**Unpatterned**		
Androgenetic alopecia	Acute telogen effluvium	Pressure alopecia	Alopecia areata	LPP	Monolethrix
	Chronic telogen effluvium		Trichotillomania	DLE	Woolly hair
	Anagen effluvium		Tinea capitis	FFA	Trichothiodystrophy
	Diffuse alopecia areata		Traction alopecia	Folliculitis decalvans	Trichorrhexis nodosa
	Chemotherapy-induced alopecia		Syphilis	Morphea	Pili Torti
	Poisoning alopecia		Triangular alopecia	Pseudopelade of Brocq	
	Loose anagen syndrome			Congenital alopecia (e.g., aplasia cutis)	
	Congenital alopecia				

LPP: lichen planopilaris; DLE: discoid lupus erythematosus; FFA: frontal fibrosing alopecia.

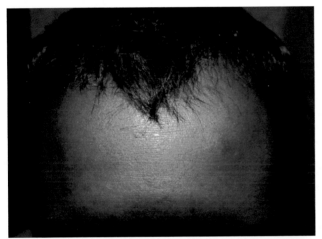

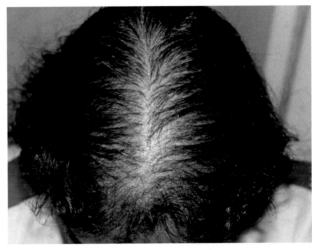

FIGURE 12.2 Female pattern hair loss: a 42-year-old female presented with loss of hair from vertex and midscalp, suggestive of FPHL Grade IV on Sinclair's five-point scale.

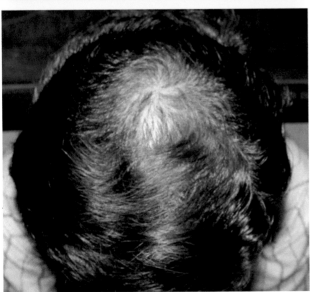

FIGURE 12.1 Male AGA: A 28-year-male presenting with M-shaped frontal recession with vertex thinning. The hairline has receded deeper into the frontal area and the temporal area. Diagnosis is AGA grade III vertex on the Norwood-Hamilton scale.

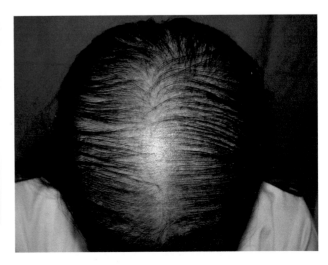

FIGURE 12.3 Female pattern hair loss: a 50-year-old woman presented with diffuse hair loss without obvious thinning on midscalp, FPHL grade 5 on Sinclair's five-point scale.

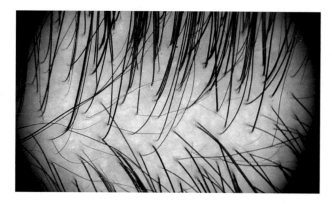

FIGURE 12.4 Trichoscopy shows hair diameter diversity of more than 20%.

reduction in hair volume over the mid-frontal scalp, various differential diagnoses should be considered, in particular acute and chronic telogen effluvium and diffuse alopecia areata. Hair diameter diversity of more than 10% on trichoscopy confirms the diagnosis of FPHL (18) (Figure 12.4). An endocrinal evaluation and evaluation of iron deficiency is required to rule out other comorbid conditions in females. In difficult cases, a biopsy is required (19, 20).

Management Minoxidil and finasteride/dutasteride are often prescribed for men with AGA (20). Minoxidil and finasteride/dutasteride both retard or stop hair loss and stimulate some hair regrowth; neither medication restores all lost hair or reverses complete baldness. Other non-minoxidil-based topical therapies used are latanoprost, bimatoprost, ketoconazole, and melatonin (20). Superiority of dutasteride over finasteride has been documented (21). The FDA has approved 5% minoxidil foam for women with FPHL (22). Hormonal treatment, such as oral medications that block the effects of androgens (e.g., spironolactone, cyproterone, finasteride, bicalutamide and flutamide), is also often tried in women (20).

A combination of low-dose oral minoxidil (0.25–2.5mg daily) and spironolactone (25 mg daily) has been shown to significantly improve hair growth, reduce shedding and improve hair density (23).

Procedural therapy includes platelet-rich plasma therapy (PRP), microneedling, hair transplantation, and scalp micropigmentation. Camouflage and low-level LASER therapy (LLLT) are also useful (20).

Cosmetic camouflages include colored hair sprays to cover thinning areas on the scalp, hair-bulking fiber powder, and hair wigs (24).

12.2b Telogen Effluvium

Telogen effluvium (TE), first described by Kligman in 1961 (25), refers to the loss of club hairs (telogen hair) (26). TE can be acute and chronic. Chronic diffuse telogen hair loss refers to telogen hair shedding persisting longer than six months (27). This is further subcategorized into a primary chronic TE (idiopathic) or be secondary to a variety of causes, including FPHL (28).

Acute TE is characterized by persistent excessive hair shedding, yet the loss of hair is replaced as rapidly as it sheds, so patients never become bald unless hair loss is more than 50%. It is a self-limiting, diffuse hair loss from the scalp that occurs around three months after a triggering event. Severe febrile

illness, pregnancy (telogen gravidarum), chronic systemic illness, a change in medication, a large hemorrhage, a crash diet or sudden starvation, accidental trauma, surgical operations, and severe emotional stress are the most common. In approximately one-third of cases, it is not possible to identify the precipitating event. Patients often do not relate these events to their recent illness (26, 29).

Chronic Diffuse Telogen Hair Loss Diffuse shedding of telogen hairs that persists beyond six months may be due to primary chronic telogen effluvium or may be secondary to the causes, such as iron deficiency, hypo- and hyperthyroidism, secondary syphilis, nutritional deficiencies, and systemic lupus (26).

Diagnosis On scalp examination, the pull test is diffusely positive both from occiputs and midscalp.

Although no specific trichoscopic criteria of telogen effluvium have been recognized, empty follicles, short regrowing upright and coiled hair, predominance of follicular units with single hair, and perifollicular discoloration (peripilar sign) are trichoscopic findings. A full blood count, iron studies, and thyroid function tests should be performed to exclude other causes of diffuse telogen hair loss (26, 29–31).

12.2c Loose Anagen Hair Syndrome

Loose anagen hair syndrome (32) is an uncommon cause of anagen hair loss. In this condition, anagen hair is sparse and easily pluckable and does not grow. It is a familial condition usually seen in young children. The main complaints are hairs are sparse, and they "do not grow." Hair can be pulled out easily without pain or breakage. Light microscopy shows anagen hair without an inner or an outer root sheath. The cuticle has a rippled or "floppy sock" appearance on scanning electron microscopy, and shafts may be triangular or grooved or have ridges. A biopsy demonstrates a lack of attachment of the hair cuticle with the IRS. The condition improves spontaneously over the years, particularly during adolescence, and at times even redevelops.

12.3 Patchy Non-Scarring Alopecia

12.3a Alopecia Areata

Alopecia areata (AA) is a common, non-scarring form of hair loss, which affects any hairy area of the body. The estimated incidence in the United States was found to be 20.9 per 100,000 person-years with a cumulative lifetime incidence of 2.1% (33). Hospital-based studies conducted from across the world estimated the incidence of AA to be between 0.57% and 3.8% (34–37). Patients with AA having a family history of the disease have been found to be between 0% and 8.6% (34, 37, 38). No significant difference in the incidence of AA was found between males and females in two population studies (33, 39). In children, the mean age of onset has been reported to be between ages five and ten years (40).

AA occurs as a result of a breach in the immune privilege of anagen hair follicles. It is mediated by the suppression of major histocompatibility complex (MHC) class I and the shutdown of pro-inflammatory mechanisms, including the action of antigen-presenting cells (APCs), mast cells, and natural killer cells. Disruption in these mechanisms leads to the collapse of immune privilege leading to the onset and progression of AA. The immune mechanism is mediated by CD8+ NKG2D+ T-cells through interleukin-15-positive feedback loop within

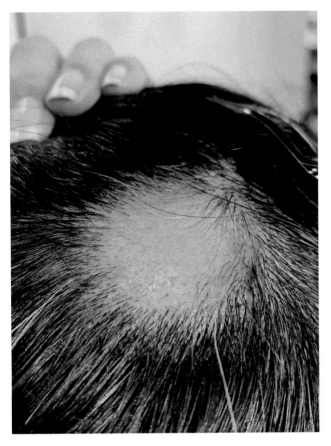

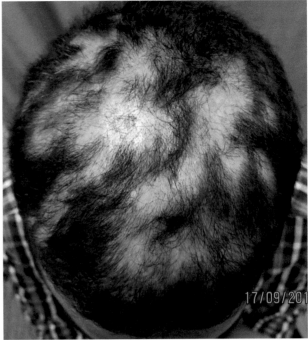

FIGURE 12.6 Reticular alopecia areata: A 28-year-old male presenting with multiple small patches of sudden hair loss and hair pull test positive.

FIGURE 12.5 A case of single patch alopecia areata.

follicular epithelial cells, mediated through the Janus kinase (JAK) signaling pathway. There is an accumulation of CD8+/CD4+ lymphocytes and APC around hair follicles, and an increase in the substance *P* mediates the transition from the anagen phase to the catagen phase resulting in characteristic nonscarring hair loss (41).

Clinical features: The scalp is the most commonly involved site, with or without the involvement of other body sites (34, 42). The most common site is the occipital region (43). Alopecia areata can be classified based on the extent or pattern of hair loss (44). The most common form is patchy (Figure 12.5) alopecia areata, which is seen in 75% of patients.

Alopecia areata can be classified according to its pattern, as follows:

*   *Reticular*—Hair loss is more extensive, and the patches coalesce (Figure 12.6).
*   *Ophiasis*—Hair loss is localized to the sides and lower back of the scalp.
*   *Sisaipho (ophiasis spelled backward)*—Hair loss spares the sides and back of the head. It may mimic androgenetic alopecia.
*   *Alopecia totalis*—100% Hair loss on the scalp.
*   *Alopecia universalis*—Complete loss of hair in all hair-bearing areas

Nail involvement, predominantly of the fingernails, is found in 6.8–49.4% of patients, most commonly in severe cases, with pitting being the most common finding.

Diagnosis Diagnosis is usually clinical, and a scalp biopsy is seldom needed, but it can be helpful when the clinical diagnosis is less certain.

Treatment The treatment of AA is challenging, and there is no FDA-approved therapy.

The various treatment options are tailored according to the pattern and extend of AA. None of them are reliably effective, especially for the treatment of severe AA, AT, and AU (45, 46).

1. *Topical or intralesional corticosteroids*
    For limited involvement, topical or intralesional corticosteroids are used. For adult patients having less than 50% scalp involvement, ILCSs, preferably triamcinolone acetinoide, are considered first-line therapy. Concentrations of 2.5 to 10 mg/mL are preferred. Transient atrophy, post-inflammatory hypopigmentation, and telengeictasias are the side effects.
2. *Contact sensitizers*
    Contact immunotherapy is one of the most effective treatments for extensive AA. Diphencyprone (DPCP) is most commonly used due to its stability in acetone. This acts by antigenic competition, nonspecific suppression of delayed hypersensitivity, and regularization of HLA expression in the lower portion of hair follicle epithelium.[125]
3. *Minoxidil* (Level of evidence 2)
    Minoxidil 2%–5% is mainly used as an adjuvant treatment with other forms of therapy.
4. *Anthralin*
    Short-duration contact therapy with anthralin 0.5%–1% is used as an alternative treatment. Seventy-five

percent of patients of patch AA and 25% of patients of AT showed a response with anthralin short-time contact therapy.[134]

5. *Systemic corticosteroids*
Systemic corticosteroids are the preferred option for rapid progressive and extensive AA.[139]
However, the relapse rate is high after stopping steroids.

Other treatment options include turban photochemotherapy (PUVA), cyclosporine, methotrexate, sulfasalazine, and camouflage. There is promising evidence regarding the effectiveness of JAK inhibitors tofacitinib, ruxolitinib, and baricitinib in AA (41).

12.3b Traction Alopecia (47)

Traction alopecia (TA) is caused primarily by pulling force being applied to the hair. It is commonly seen with certain hairstyles or braiding patterns that pull the hairline forcefully toward the vertex of the scalp.

It is an extremely common condition in black women, resulting from years of use of hairpieces and hairstyles. Sikh men are also susceptible to traction alopecia if the hair under the turban is tied too tightly for many years.

Usually, the areas of alopecia are symmetrical along the frontotemporal line. The involvement of the occipital region is unusual. The earliest sign of TA is the perifollicular erythema, which may progress to folliculitis if the trauma is continuous.

The presence of short hairs scattered along the frontotemporal line is a characteristic finding of TA and is called a fringe sign.

Less often, TA may affect the occipital region. In this case, the differential diagnosis with ophiasis alopecia areata is imperative. Ophiasis AA may be underdiagnosed in black women since there is a tendency to diagnose the condition in this population as TA.

Trichoscopy shows miniaturized hair and pinpoint white dots (visible acrosyringium). The hair may also show signs of breakage of the follicular shaft and sometimes display cylinders of the follicular sheath—which was freshly detached due to trauma (hair casts)

Patients and their parents should be instructed to avoid using tight hairstyles that exert too much traction upon the hair and scalp. The application of intralesional corticosteroids may be useful for reducing perifollicular inflammation in adults with early-stage TA. Topical and oral antibiotics are also reported as therapeutic options in cases of folliculitis. Minoxidil 2% and 5% are used in some studies to stimulate hair regrowth. In the advanced stages of TA, surgical treatment should be considered.

12.3c Pressure Alopecia (48)

Postoperative alopecia, or pressure alopecia, usually presents as non-scarring alopecia but can progress to scarring alopecia also. It is considered analogous to a healed pressure ulcer after prolonged immobilization of the head during surgery or while in intensive unit care. Pressure alopecia may be a presenting feature after three to four weeks of immobilization, or it may follow clinical features like swelling, tenderness, or ulceration. Regular head mobilization can prevent it.

12.3d Trichotillomania (49)

Trichotillomania (TTM) is an impulse control disorder characterized by unintentional but conscious pulling out of one's own hair on any part of the body. Trichotillomania is characterized by an overwhelming urge to repeatedly pull out one's own hair, resulting in repetitive hair pulling and subsequent hair loss.

Although common in children, it can be seen in any age group. Females are affected more in the adult age group, but in children, the male-to-female ratio is equal. The scalp is the most common site, although the eyebrows, beard, pubic, and hair at other body sites may be involved. Some affected individuals chew and/or swallow (ingest) the hair they have pulled out (trichophagy), which can result in gastrointestinal problems. Trichotillomania causes significant emotional distress and often impairs social and occupational functioning. Hair loss is usually asymmetrical and more toward the contralateral side of the dominant hand. Areas of alopecia in an artifactual pattern are seen on the scalp, either ill-defined or sharply demarcated. Broken-off hair and a black dot appearance may be seen within the patch. The margins of the scalp are spared when the condition is extensive so as to involve the entire scalp, and this is known as the tonsure pattern. The habit of pulling out hair is usually denied by patients. Hair can be pulled out unintentionally while watching television or reading or can be done consciously in a focused way. The disorder is labeled as an obsessive-compulsive disorder; however, less than 5% of patients may have severe psychiatric disorders (50, 51).

Diagnosis of trichotillomania is mainly based on history and clinical features; however, trichoscopy and rarely biopsy aid in diagnosis.

A wide variety of treatments are attempted clinically to alleviate TTM symptoms in adults, adolescents, and children, including cognitive and behavioral therapies, supportive counseling, support groups, hypnosis, medications such as selective serotonin reuptake inhibitors (fluoxetine), neuroleptics (haloperidol), tricyclic antidepressants (amitriptyline), monoamine oxidase inhibitors (isocarboxazid), mood stabilizers (lithium), and anxiolytics (clonazepam), as well as combined approaches (52).

12.3e Tinea Capitis

Tinea capitis, a fungal infection of the scalp hair, is seen most commonly in hot and humid areas, such as Africa, Southeast Asia, and Central America. *Microsporum* and *Trichophyton* are the main causative dermatophyte species. Clinically, two types of tinea capitis are seen: inflammatory and non-inflammatory. The inflammatory type (e.g., kerion) can result in scarring alopecia. Children between 3 and 14 years of age are the most affected age group; however, any age group may be affected. Diagnosis is clinical. Potassium hydroxide (KOH) examination of scales can be done. Trichoscopy also aids in diagnosis as it may show corkscrew hair, comma hair, zigzag hair, and broken hair. Treatment involves topical and systemic antifungals (Figure 12.7) (53, 54).

12.4 Cicatricial Alopecia

This type of alopecia may occur as a primary event when the follicle is the main target of the pathological process (primary scarring alopecia) or as a secondary event when the follicle acts as an "innocent bystander" in the course of a disease, which occurs outside the follicular unit (secondary scarring alopecia) (55).

The following is a brief review of the major primary scarring alopecias.

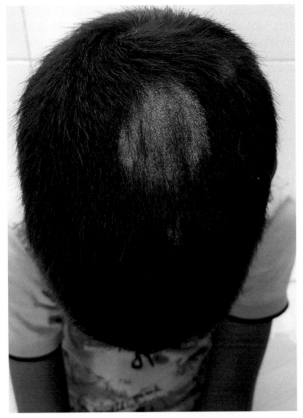

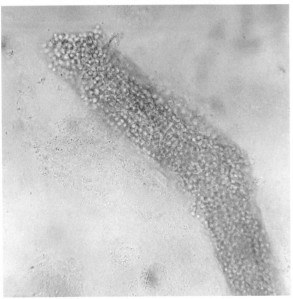

FIGURE 12.7 Tinea capitis: A six-year-old boy presented with three to four patches of localized hair loss, similar to that of alopecia areata, showing mild scaling, and Potassium hydroxide examination of scales was suggestive of endothrix.

12.4a Central Centrifugal Cicatricial Alopecia (1)

Central centrifugal cicatricial alopecia (CCCA) is defined as hair loss that starts at the vertex and middle region of the scalp and progresses centrifugally. It is most commonly seen in people of African descent, affecting more women than men. The prevalence increases with age, and the disease is more common at the end of the second and third decades of life (56, 57).

In 1968, LoPresti and colleagues first used the term "hot comb alopecia" to describe a variant of scarring alopecia that was associated with the use of hot metal combs by African American women. It was believed that the hot Vaseline used in some hair treatments caused chronic inflammation of the hair follicle, with its subsequent destruction and replacement with fibrous tissue. To date, the etiology of CCCA is controversial. The most likely theory is that it has a multifactorial origin, with possible predisposing factors being genetics, hair straightening chemicals, trauma caused by traction, and the spiral configuration of the hairs

CCCA may be classified as "early stage" (inflammatory) or "late stage" (cicatricial) (57). The hair loss starts at the crown or vertex of the scalp and gradually progresses centrifugally. As the disease progresses, it leaves an area of alopecia with irreversible loss of follicular ostia.

Biopsy is important to confirm the diagnosis. The absence of follicular ostia distinguishes CCCA from other non-cicatricial alopecia with similar morphology

To date, treatment recommendations are based on anecdotes or case reports. The main goal is to stop disease progression, especially in peripheral areas, and relieve symptoms by administering anti-inflammatory agents. Medium- or high-potency intralesional and topical corticosteroids are the first-line treatments (57, 58).

The combination of oral tetracycline (e.g., doxycycline or minocycline) with topical corticosteroids generally shows satisfactory results in cases with inflammation. Other second-line drugs include antimalarials, such as hydroxychloroquine (400 mg daily), cyclosporine, and mycophenolate mofetil, mainly used in patients with active, recalcitrant disease.

Topical minoxidil may be useful for stimulating viable hair follicles once the inflammation process is controlled. Hair transplantation is an option for the inactive stage for at least one year (1).

12.4b Lichen Planopilaris (59, 60)

Lichen planopilaris (LPP) occurs more frequently in Caucasians. It is usually seen in the third to seventh decade and is more common in females. The disease may present alone or in combination with other forms of lichen planus, such as cutaneous, nail, or mucosal lichen planus.

Although the pathogenesis of LPP remains unclear, the most accepted theory is that it is an autoimmune disorder in which activated T-lymphocytes attack the follicle.

In a few patients, areas other than the scalp may be involved. Violaceous erythematous follicular papules with slight scaling are seen in early lesions. Patches of smooth, skin-colored, scarring alopecia are seen in well-developed lesions (Figure 12.8). In active lesions, trichoscopy shows perifollicular scaling and perifollicular inflammation. In the later phase, pigment incontinence is visible as violaceous-blue interfollicular areas in trichoscopy. Large irregular white dots are seen in the fibrotic stage. Diagnosis is mainly clinical. In the early stages, biopsy may help diagnose to differentiate other causes of cicatricial alopecia. However, in advanced stages, it is difficult to differentiate different causes of cicatricial alopecia as only skin atrophy is present with loss of hair follicles.

Topical or intralesional corticosteroids and systemic immunosuppressants can be given in the active disease phase. Hair

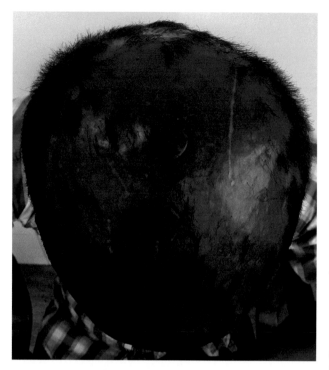

FIGURE 12.8 Lichen planopilaris: A 25-year-old male presented with multiple patches of hair loss showing smooth, shiny scalp skin with loss of follicular openings.

transplantation and camouflage treatment are other options for the inactive disease. Third-line drugs for the treatment of difficult-to-control LPP with aggressive evolution include retinoids, tetracyclines, griseofulvin, thalidomide, dapsone, topical tacrolimus, and minoxidil, although the effectiveness of the latter is still controversial.

12.4c Frontal Fibrosing Alopecia (61, 62)

This is a patterned cicatricial alopecia, considered to be a variant of lichen planopilaris, which superficially resembles AGA due to frontal recession. However, on close inspection, there is a loss of follicular orifices, perifollicular erythema, and hyperkeratosis at the marginal hairline. In contrast with AGA, the frontal hairline recedes in a straight line rather than bitemporally. It mostly affects postmenopausal women. The margin toward the hairy scalp is serrated and has numerous erythematous, follicular papules which involve the eyebrows as well. It can be rapidly progressive or self-limiting, so the course may be variable. Corticosteroids and minoxidil are used as topical treatments. Systemically, corticosteroids, retinoids, hydroxychloroquine, finasteride, and griseofulvin have been tried with variable responses.

12.4d Chronic Cutaneous Lupus Erythematosus (59)

Chronic cutaneous lupus erythematosus, or discoid (DLE) lupus, is commonly seen in adults. The lesions start with erythematous scaly patches that later are covered with adherent scales. These scales show "carpet tacks" on the undersurface after removal. In later stages, there is atrophic, depigmented scarring with telangiectases in the center and hyperpigmentation at the periphery of affected areas. Spontaneous remission may be seen in 30–40% of patients. Topical potent steroids

or intralesional steroids are the drugs of choice. Other topical agents used are tacrolimus (0.1%), tazarotene (0.05%), imiquimod (5%), and intralesional IFN-2α. Systemic agents, preferred in cases with rapid progression, are antimalarials, oral prednisolone, and isotretinoin.

12.4e Folliculitis Decalvans (63, 64)

Folliculitis decalvans is an inflammation of the hair follicle that leads to bogginess or induration of involved parts of the scalp along with pustules, erosions, crusts, ulcers, and scaling. Tufted hair follicles, in which hair emerges from a single follicular opening, are seen in advanced disease. African Americans are more frequently affected than white Americans.

Management involves a repeated culture of pustules to establish the identity and antibiotic sensitivity of the bacteria involved. No permanent cure has been found for this condition, but there are promising results in a regimen of dual therapy with rifampin 300 mg twice daily and clindamycin 300 mg twice daily.

12.5 Hair Shaft Disorder (65)

Hair shaft disorders are a diverse group of congenital and acquired abnormalities of the hair shaft. Some hair shaft disorders cause fragility of the hair shaft leading to increased hair breakage; others lack fragility but alter the appearance or texture of the hair. Hair shaft disorders can occur independently or in association with genetic or acquired diseases.

12.5a Chemotherapy-Induced Hair Loss (66)

Chemotherapy-induced hair loss, a side effect of anticancer treatment, has no definitive treatment, but topical minoxidil has been tried. Scalp cooling can minimize hair loss. As the condition is usually reversible, temporarily wearing a wig should be considered

Poisoning with heavy metals can also lead to diffuse alopecia. There are many case reports of alopecia with thallium poisoning.

12.6 Conclusion

Correct diagnosis of the type of alopecia and the severity of involvement are important for proper treatment. Clinical and trichoscopic features help us to reach a correct diagnosis.

Frequently Asked Questions

1. *Q: How is the type of hair loss identified?*
   A: Hair loss disorders can involve the hair follicle or the hair shaft. Among disorders involving hair follicles, alopecias are subclassified as non-cicatricial or non-scarring alopecia and cicatricial or scarring alopecia. Hair follicles are lost permanently in cicatricial alopecia, while the damage is potentially reversible in non-cicatricial alopecias. According to the extent of involvement, alopecia can be diffuse or localized. Clinical examination and trichoscopy are required to differentiate the type of hair loss.

2. *Q: What are the common disorders in the clinic?*
   A: The common disorders presenting in a clinic are telogen effluvium (TE) and androgenetic hair loss.

3. *Q: What is the most diagnostic feature of female pattern hair loss?*

   A: Hair diameter diversity of more than 10% on trichoscopy confirms the diagnosis of FPHL.

4. *Q: What other medication can we use for FPHL apart from minoxidil?*

   A: Among oral formulations, we can use low-dose oral minoxidil (0.25 mg–2.5 mg daily) and spironolactone (50 mg–100 mg daily), bicalutamide, dutasteride and finasteride. Procedural therapy includes platelet-rich plasma therapy (PRP), microneedling, hair transplantation, and scalp micropigmentation.

5. *Q: How does one diagnose acute telogen effluvium?*

   A: Acute TE is characterized by persistent excessive hair shedding. It is a self-limiting, diffuse hair loss from the scalp that occurs around three months after a triggering event. Severe febrile illness, pregnancy (telogen gravidarum), chronic systemic illness, a change in medication, a large hemorrhage, a crash diet or sudden starvation, accidental trauma, surgical operations, and severe emotional stress are the most common. In approximately one-third of cases, it is not possible to identify the precipitating event. On trichoscopy, multiple short upright regrowing hairs can be visualized.

References

1. Tanus A, Oliveira CCC, Villarreal DJV, Sanchez FAV, Dias MFRG. Black women's hair: The main scalp dermatoses and aesthetic practices in women of African ethnicity. An Bras Dermatol [Internet]. 2015 [cited 2019 Jul 10];90(4):450–465. Available from: www.ncbi.nlm.nih.gov/pubmed/26375213

2. Qi J, Garza LA. An overview of alopecias. Cold Spring Harb Perspect Med [Internet]. 2014 Mar 1 [cited 2019 Jul 14];4(3). Available from: www.ncbi.nlm.nih.gov/pubmed/24591533

3. Gupta M, Mysore V. Classifications of patterned hair loss: A review. J Cutan Aesthet Surg [Internet]. 2016 [cited 2019 Jul 14];9(1):3–12. Available from: www.ncbi.nlm.nih.gov/pubmed/27081243

4. Phillips TG, Slomiany WP, Allison R. Hair loss: Common causes and treatment. Am Fam Physician [Internet]. 2017 Sep 15 [cited 2019 Jul 15];96(6):371–378. Available from: www.ncbi.nlm.nih.gov/pubmed/28925637

5. Sinclair R. Diffuse hair loss. Int J Dermatol [Internet]. 1999 May [cited 2019 Jul 14];38 Suppl 1:8–18. Available from: www.ncbi.nlm.nih.gov/pubmed/10369535

6. Olsen EA, Messenger AG, Shapiro J, Bergfeld WF, Hordinsky MK, Roberts JL, et al. Evaluation and treatment of male and female pattern hair loss. J Am Acad Dermatol [Internet]. 2005 Feb [cited 2019 Jul 14];52(2):301–311. Available from: www.ncbi.nlm.nih.gov/pubmed/15692478

7. Orfanos CE. Androgenetic alopecia: Clinical aspects and treatment. In: Hair and Hair Diseases [Internet]. Berlin, Heidelberg: Springer; 1990 [cited 2019 Jul 14]. p. 485–527. Available from: www.springerlink.com/index/10.1007/978-3-642-74612-3_19

8. Olsen EA. Female pattern hair loss. J Am Acad Dermatol [Internet]. 2001 Sep [cited 2019 Jul 14];45(3):S70–80. Available from: www.ncbi.nlm.nih.gov/pubmed/11511856

9. Tosti A, Iorizzo M, Piraccini BM. Androgenetic alopecia in children: Report of 20 cases. Br J Dermatol [Internet]. 2005 Mar [cited 2019 Jul 14];152(3):556–559. Available from: www.ncbi.nlm.nih.gov/pubmed/15787828

10. Sinclair R, Torkamani N, Jones L. Androgenetic alopecia: New insights into the pathogenesis and mechanism of hair loss. F1000Research [Internet]. 2015 [cited 2019 Jul 14];4(F1000 Faculty Rev):585. Available from: www.ncbi.nlm.nih.gov/pubmed/26339482

11. Norwood OT. Male pattern baldness: Classification and incidence. South Med J [Internet]. 1975 Nov [cited 2019 Jul 15];68(11):1359–1365. Available from: www.ncbi.nlm.nih.gov/pubmed/1188424

12. Hamilton JB. Male hormone stimulation is prerequisite and an incitant in common baldness. Am J Anat [Internet]. 1942 Nov 1 [cited 2019 Jul 15];71(3):451–480. Available from: http://doi.wiley.com/10.1002/aja.1000710306

13. Ludwig E. Classification of the types of androgenetic alopecia (common baldness) occurring in the female sex. Br J Dermatol [Internet]. 1977 Sep [cited 2019 Jul 15];97(3):247–254. Available from: www.ncbi.nlm.nih.gov/pubmed/921894

14. Ekmekci T, Sakiz D, Koslu A. Occipital involvement in female pattern hair loss: Histopathological evidences. J Eur Acad Dermatology Venereol [Internet]. 2010 Mar [cited 2019 Jul 15];24(3):299–301. Available from: www.ncbi.nlm.nih.gov/pubmed/19703099

15. Camacho-Martínez FM. Hair loss in women. Semin Cutan Med Surg [Internet]. 2009 Mar [cited 2019 Jul 15];28(1):19–32. Available from: www.ncbi.nlm.nih.gov/pubmed/19341939

16. Redler S, Brockschmidt FF, Tazi-Ahnini R, Drichel D, Birch MP, Dobson K, et al. Investigation of the male pattern baldness major genetic susceptibility loci AR/EDA2R and 20p11 in female pattern hair loss. Br J Dermatol [Internet]. 2012 Jun [cited 2019 Jul 15];166(6):1314–1318. Available from: www.ncbi.nlm.nih.gov/pubmed/22309448

17. Venning VA, Dawber RP. Patterned androgenic alopecia in women. J Am Acad Dermatol [Internet]. 1988 May [cited 2019 Jul 15];18(5 Pt 1):1073–1077. Available from: www.ncbi.nlm.nih.gov/pubmed/3385027

18. Harries M, Tosti A, Bergfeld W, Blume-Peytavi U, Shapiro J, Lutz G, et al. Towards a consensus on how to diagnose and quantify female pattern hair loss—The 'Female Pattern Hair Loss Severity Index (FPHL-SI)'. J Eur Acad Dermatology Venereol [Internet]. 2016 Apr [cited 2019 Jul 15];30(4):667–676. Available from: www.ncbi.nlm.nih.gov/pubmed/26676524

19. Zhang X, Caulloo S, Zhao Y, Zhang B, Cai Z, Yang J. Female pattern hair loss: Clinico-laboratory findings and trichoscopy depending on disease severity. Int J Trichology [Internet]. 2012 Jan [cited 2019 Jul 15];4(1):23. Available from: www.ncbi.nlm.nih.gov/pubmed/22628986

20. Fabbrocini G, Cantelli M, Masarà A, Annunziata MC, Marasca C, Cacciapuoti S. Female pattern hair loss: A clinical, pathophysiologic, and therapeutic review. Int J women's dermatology [Internet]. 2018 Dec [cited 2019 Jul 15];4(4):203–211. Available from: www.ncbi.nlm.nih.gov/pubmed/30627618

21. Shanshanwal S., Dhurat R. Superiority of dutasteride over finasteride in hair regrowth and reversal of miniaturization in men with androgenetic alopecia: A randomized controlled open-label, evaluator-blinded study. Indian J Dermatol Venereol Leprol [Internet]. 2017 [cited 2019 Jul 15];83(1):47. Available from: www.ncbi.nlm.nih.gov/pubmed/27549867

22. Gupta AK, Foley KA. 5% Minoxidil: Treatment for female pattern hair loss. Skin Therapy Lett [Internet]. [cited 2019 Jul 15];19(6):5–7. Available from: www.ncbi.nlm.nih.gov/pubmed/25807073

23. Sinclair RD. Female pattern hair loss: A pilot study investigating combination therapy with low-dose oral minoxidil and spironolactone. Int J Dermatol [Internet]. 2018 Jan [cited 2019 Jul 15];57(1):104–109. Available from: http://doi.wiley.com/10.1111/ijd.13838

24. Saed S, Ibrahim O, Bergfeld WF. Hair camouflage: A comprehensive review. Int J women's dermatology [Internet]. 2016 Dec [cited 2019 Jul 15];2(4):122–127. Available from: www.ncbi.nlm.nih.gov/pubmed/28492024

25. Kligman AM. Pathologic dynamics of human hair loss. Arch Dermatol [Internet]. 1961 Feb 1 [cited 2019 Jul 15];83(2):175. Available from: http://archderm.jamanetwork.com/article.aspx?doi=10.1001/archderm.1961.01580080005001

26. Malkud S. Telogen effluvium: A review. J Clin Diagn Res [Internet]. 2015 Sep [cited 2019 Jul 15];9(9):WE01–3. Available from: www.ncbi.nlm.nih.gov/pubmed/26500992

27. Shrivastava S. Diffuse hair loss in an adult female: Approach to diagnosis and management. Indian J Dermatol Venereol Leprol [Internet]. 2009 [cited 2019 Jul 15];75(1):20. Available from: www.ncbi.nlm.nih.gov/pubmed/19172026

28. Sinclair R. Chronic telogen effluvium: A study of 5 patients over 7 years. J Am Acad Dermatol [Internet]. 2005 Feb [cited 2019 Jul 15];52(2 Suppl 1):12–16. Available from: www.ncbi.nlm.nih.gov/pubmed/15692504

29. Hughes EC, Gossman WG. Telogen effluvium [Internet]. StatPearls. StatPearls Publishing; 2019 [cited 2019 Jul 15]. Available from: www.ncbi.nlm.nih.gov/pubmed/28613598

30. Torres F, Tosti A. Trichoscopy: An update. G Ital Dermatol Venereol [Internet]. 2014 Feb [cited 2019 Jul 15];149(1):83–91. Available from: www.ncbi.nlm.nih.gov/pubmed/24566568

31. Rudnicka L, Olszewska M, Rakowska A, Slowinska M. Trichoscopy update 2011. J Dermatol Case Rep [Internet]. 2011 Dec 12 [cited 2019 Jul 15];5(4):82–88. Available from: www.ncbi.nlm.nih.gov/pubmed/22408709

32. Dhurat RP, Deshpande DJ. Loose anagen hair syndrome. Int J Trichology [Internet]. 2010 Jul [cited 2019 Jul 15];2(2):96–100. Available from: www.ncbi.nlm.nih.gov/pubmed/21712911

33. Mirzoyev SA, Schrum AG, Davis MDP, Torgerson RR. Lifetime incidence risk of alopecia areata estimated at 2.1% by Rochester epidemiology project, 1990–2009. J Invest Dermatol [Internet]. 2014 Apr [cited 2019 Jul 15];134(4):1141–1142. Available from: www.ncbi.nlm.nih.gov/pubmed/24202232

34. Guzmán-Sánchez DA, Villanueva-Quintero GD, Alfaro N, McMichael A. A clinical study of alopecia areata in Mexico. Int J Dermatol [Internet]. 2007 Dec 18 [cited 2019 Jul 15];46(12):1308–1310. Available from: www.ncbi.nlm.nih.gov/pubmed/18173532

35. Price VH. Alopecia areata: Clinical aspects. J Invest Dermatol [Internet]. 1991 May [cited 2019 Jul 15];96(5):68S. Available from: www.ncbi.nlm. nih.gov/pubmed/2022874

36. Sharma VK, Dawn G, Kumar B. Profile of alopecia areata in northern India. Int J Dermatol [Internet]. 2007 May 31 [cited 2019 Jul 15];35(1):22–27. Available from: http://doi.wiley.com/10.1111/j.1365-4362.1996.tb01610.x

37. Tan E, Tay Y-K, Goh C-L, Chin Giam Y. The pattern and profile of alopecia areata in Singapore-a study of 219 Asians. Int J Dermatol [Internet]. 2002 Nov [cited 2019 Jul 15];41(11):748–753. Available from: www.ncbi.nlm.nih.gov/pubmed/12452996

38. Yang S, Yang J, Liu JB, Wang HY, Yang Q, Gao M, et al. The genetic epidemiology of alopecia areata in China. Br J Dermatol [Internet]. 2004 Jul 1 [cited 2019 Jul 15];151(1):16–23. Available from: http://doi.wiley.com/10.1111/j.1365-2133.2004.05915.x

39. Safavi KH, Muller SA, Suman VJ, Moshell AN, Melton LJ. Incidence of alopecia areata in Olmsted County, Minnesota, 1975 through 1989. Mayo Clin Proc [Internet]. 1995 Jul [cited 2019 Jul 15];70(7):628–633. Available from: www.ncbi.nlm.nih.gov/pubmed/7791384

40. Rocha J, Ventura F, Vieira AP, Pinheiro AR, Fernandes S, Brito C. [Alopecia areata: A retrospective study of the paediatric dermatology department (2000–2008)]. Acta Med Port [Internet]. [cited 2019 Jul 15];24(2):207–214. Available from: www.ncbi.nlm.nih.gov/pubmed/22011591

41. Phan K, Sebaratnam DF. JAK inhibitors for alopecia areata: A systematic review and meta-analysis. J Eur Acad Dermatology Venereol [Internet]. 2019 May 10 [cited 2019 Jul 15];33(5):850–856. Available from: www.ncbi.nlm.nih.gov/pubmed/30762909

42. Tan E, Tay Y-K, Giam Y-C. A clinical study of childhood alopecia areata in Singapore. Pediatr Dermatol [Internet]. [cited 2019 Jul 15];19(4):298–301. Available from: www.ncbi.nlm.nih.gov/pubmed/12220271

43. Miteva M, Villasante A. Epidemiology and burden of alopecia areata: A systematic review. Clin Cosmet Investig Dermatol [Internet]. 2015 Jul [cited 2019 Jul 15];8:397. Available from: www.ncbi.nlm.nih.gov/pubmed/26244028

44. Madani S, Shapiro J. Alopecia areata update. J Am Acad Dermatol [Internet]. 2000 Apr [cited 2019 Jul 15];42(4):549–566; quiz 567–570. Available from: www.ncbi.nlm.nih.gov/pubmed/10727299

45. Darwin E, Hirt PA, Fertig R, Doliner B, Delcanto G, Jimenez JJ. Alopecia Areata: Review of epidemiology, clinical features, pathogenesis, and new treatment options. Int J Trichology [Internet]. 2018 [cited 2019 Jul 15];10(2):51–60. Available from: www.ncbi.nlm.nih.gov/pubmed/29769777

46. Hordinsky MK. Current treatments for alopecia areata. J Investig Dermatology Symp Proc [Internet]. 2015 Nov 1 [cited 2019 Jul 15];17(2):44–46. Available from: https://linkinghub.elsevier.com/retrieve/pii/S1087002416300417

47. Tanus A, Oliveira CCC, Villarreal DJV, Sanchez FAV, Dias MFRG. Black women's hair: The main scalp dermatoses and aesthetic practices in women of African ethnicity. An Bras Dermatol [Internet]. 2015 [cited 2019 Jul 15];90(4):450. Available from: www.ncbi.nlm.nih.gov/pubmed/26375213

48. Davies KE, Yesudian P. Pressure alopecia. Int J Trichology [Internet]. 2012 Apr [cited 2019 Jul 15];4(2):64–68. Available from: www.ncbi.nlm.nih.gov/pubmed/23180911

49. Papadopoulos AJ, Janniger CK, Chodynicki MP, Schwartz RA. Trichotillomania. Int J Dermatol [Internet]. 2003 May [cited 2019 Jul 15];42(5):330–334. Available from: www.ncbi.nlm.nih.gov/pubmed/12755966

50. Christenson GA, Mackenzie TB, Reeve EA. Familial trichotillomania. Am J Psychiatry [Internet]. 1992 Feb [cited 2019 Jul 15];149(2):283. Available from: www.ncbi.nlm.nih.gov/pubmed/1580914

51. Christenson GA, Mackenzie TB, Mitchell JE. Characteristics of 60 adult chronic hair pullers. Am J Psychiatry [Internet]. 1991 Mar [cited 2019 Jul 15];148(3):365–370. Available from: www.ncbi.nlm.nih.gov/pubmed/1992841

52. Franklin ME, Zagrabbe K, Benavides KL. Trichotillomania and its treatment: A review and recommendations. Expert Rev Neurother [Internet]. 2011 Aug 9 [cited 2019 Jul 15];11(8):1165–1174. Available from: www.ncbi.nlm.nih.gov/pubmed/21797657

53. Elghblawi E. Tinea capitis in children and trichoscopic criteria. Int J Trichology [Internet]. 2017 [cited 2019 Jul 15];9(2):47–49. Available from: www.ncbi.nlm.nih.gov/pubmed/28839385

54. Hay RJ. Tinea capitis: Current status. Mycopathologia [Internet]. 2017 Feb [cited 2019 Jul 15];182(1):87. Available from: www.ncbi.nlm.nih.gov/pubmed/27599708

55. Rongioletti F, Christana K. Cicatricial (scarring) alopecias. Am J Clin Dermatol [Internet]. 2012 Aug 1 [cited 2019 Jul 15];13(4):247–260. Available from: www.ncbi.nlm.nih.gov/pubmed/22494477

56. Callender VD, Onwudiwe O. Prevalence and etiology of central centrifugal cicatricial alopecia. Arch Dermatol [Internet]. 2011 Aug 1 [cited 2019 Jul 15];147(8):972. Available from: www.ncbi.nlm.nih.gov/pubmed/21844458

57. Whiting DA, Olsen EA. Central centrifugal cicatricial alopecia. Dermatol Ther [Internet]. 2008 Jul [cited 2019 Jul 15];21(4):268–278. Available from: www.ncbi.nlm.nih.gov/pubmed/18715297

58. Summers P, Kyei A, Bergfeld W. Central centrifugal cicatricial alopecia—an approach to diagnosis and management. Int J Dermatol [Internet]. 2011 Dec [cited 2019 Jul 15];50(12):1457–1464. Available from: www.ncbi.nlm.nih.gov/pubmed/22097988

59. Ross EK, Tan E, Shapiro J. Update on primary cicatricial alopecias. J Am Acad Dermatol [Internet]. 2005 Jul [cited 2019 Jul 15];53(1):1–37. Available from: www.ncbi.nlm.nih.gov/pubmed/15965418

60. Kang H, Alzolibani AA, Otberg N, Shapiro J. Lichen planopilaris. Dermatol Ther [Internet]. 2008 Jul [cited 2019 Jul 15];21(4):249–256. Available from: www.ncbi.nlm.nih.gov/pubmed/18715294

61. Tosti A, Piraccini BM, Iorizzo M, Misciali C. Frontal fibrosing alopecia in postmenopausal women. J Am Acad Dermatol [Internet]. 2005 Jan [cited 2019 Jul 15];52(1):55–60. Available from: www.ncbi.nlm.nih.gov/pubmed/15627081

62. Dhurat R, Shukla D, Dandale A, Ghate S, Agrawal S, Shanshanwal S. Early diagnosis and prompt treatment improves quality of life in patients with frontal fibrosing alopecia. Ski Appendage Disord [Internet]. 2019 Apr [cited 2019 Jul 15];5(3):172–176. Available from: www.ncbi.nlm.nih.gov/pubmed/31049342

63. Otberg N, Kang H, Alzolibani AA, Shapiro J. Folliculitis decalvans. Dermatol Ther [Internet]. 2008 Jul [cited 2019 Jul 15];21(4):238–244. Available from: www.ncbi.nlm.nih.gov/pubmed/18715292

64. Powell JJ, Dawber RP, Gatter K. Folliculitis decalvans including tufted folliculitis: clinical, histological and therapeutic findings. Br J Dermatol [Internet]. 1999 Feb [cited 2019 Jul 15];140(2):328–333. Available from: www.ncbi.nlm.nih.gov/pubmed/10233232

65. Mirmirani P, Huang KP, Price VH. A practical, algorithmic approach to diagnosing hair shaft disorders. Int J Dermatol [Internet]. 2011 Jan [cited 2019 Jul 15];50(1):1–12. Available from: www.ncbi.nlm.nih.gov/pubmed/21182495

66. Trüeb RM. Chemotherapy-induced hair loss. Skin Therapy Lett [Internet]. [cited 2019 Jul 15];15(7):5–7. Available from: www.ncbi.nlm.nih.gov/pubmed/20700552

CHAPTER 13: PERIORBITAL CONDITIONS IN ETHNIC SKIN

Milind Naik

13.1 Introduction

The face receives maximum attention when it comes to identity and as a sign of youth. Among the facial features, the periocular region is often a candid indicator of age. Periorbital aesthetic concerns, although global, often have certain specific ethnic considerations in a given continent or country.

Ophthalmologists are often consulted for periorbital concerns such as eyelid bags, dark circles under the eye, wrinkles around the eye, and under-eye hollows. The oculoplastic surgeon and the astute ophthalmologist are therefore integral parts of this service provider team. There is an increasing trend to seek non-surgical cosmetic corrections for aging changes as well as to enhance looks.[1] Moreover, many of the complications that arise out of these therapies lie in the purview of ophthalmology.

In this chapter, we describe the relevant periorbital anatomy and discuss the four commonest ethnic considerations in the periorbital region: wrinkles, hills and valleys, hyperpigmentation, and dermatochalasis.

13.2 Functional Periorbital Anatomy

To give aesthetically and functionally pleasing results, it is important to know the dynamic and functional anatomy of the periorbital region. The *eyebrow* is normally at the level of

the superior orbital rim in men and above it in women. The male eyebrow is rather flat, whereas the female eyebrow arches higher laterally (Figure 13.1). The *upper eyelid crease* is a critical surgical landmark and is formed by the cutaneous expansion of the levator aponeurosis. Table 13.1 summarizes the differences between upper eyelid anatomy in Asians (Oriental) and non-Asians (Caucasians) and is depicted in Figure 13.1. The eyelid crease is generally 7 to 8 mm above the lid margin in females and slightly lower in males.[2] The *eyelid fold* is formed by the preseptal skin and orbicularis muscle which is draped over the upper-lid crease. The *orbital septum* extends 360 degrees from the orbital rim, to fuse with the levator aponeurosis, outer tarsal borders, and canthal ligaments. In the Oriental eyelid, the septum is inserted low, and has implications in cosmetic lid surgery.[3] The *orbital fat* is contained within the orbit by the orbital septum.[4] The upper lid has two fat pads (medial and central), with the lacrimal gland occupying the lateral position (Figure 13.2). The lower eyelid has three fat pads (medial, central, and lateral). The inferior oblique muscle originates from the anterior medial orbital floor and separates the medial and central fat pad. A fascial lateral extension of the sheath of the inferior oblique inserts on the anterior lateral orbital rim and separates the central from the lateral fat pad.[5] The *lower-lid crease* is not as prominent as the upper and is formed by the cutaneous insertion of fibers from lower eyelid retractors. It is usually 2 to 3 mm below the medial eyelid margin and 5 to 6 mm below the lateral eyelid margin.[5]

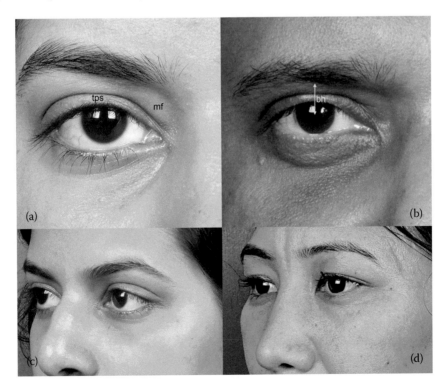

FIGURE 13.1 Differences between a female (a) and a male (b) periorbital region. The female eyebrow arches upward and outward, whereas the male eyebrow is flat, leading to a shorter brow height (bh). In a female, the eyelid crease is higher, leading to a broader tarsal plate show (tps). The medial fat pad (mf) in the upper eyelid is usually a cosmetic concern for the female. Note the differences between Caucasian (c) and Oriental (d) eyelid anatomy.

DOI: 10.1201/9780429243769-13

TABLE 13.1: Anatomic Differences between Caucasian and Asian Eyelids

Anatomic Feature	Caucasian Eyelid	Asian Eyelid
Preseptal fat pad location	Preseptal	Preseptal and pretarsal
Septum-levator fusion point	Above tarsus	As low as the pretarsal plane
Tarsal height	9–10.5 mm	6.5–8 mm
Medial lid crease origin	Medial eyelid	Medial canthus
Presence of crease	100%	50%

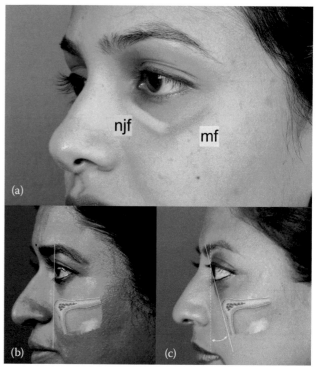

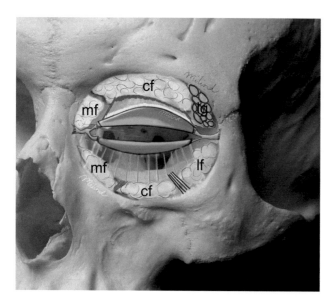

FIGURE 13.2 Periorbital fat pads, left orbit. The upper eyelid has two fat pads, central (cf) and medial (mf). The superior oblique tendon separates the two fat pads. Laterally, the upper lid has no fat pad since that space is occupied by the lacrimal gland (lg). The lower eyelid has three fat pads, medial (mf), central (cf), and lateral (lf). The central and medial fat pads are separated by the inferior oblique muscle. The central and lateral fat pad is separated by lateral raphe, a condensation within the capsulopalpebral fascia.

The junction of the lower eyelid and the cheek is defined by two skin folds.[5] The *nasojugal fold* runs from the medial canthus down toward the mid-cheek, and the *malar fold* runs from the lateral canthus toward the mid-cheek (Figure 13.3). The lower eyelid retractors fuse with the *orbital septum* approximately 5 mm inferior to their insertion on the tarsal plate.[6] The medial fat is paler and denser than the central fat pad. The lateral canthal angle is more acute than the medial canthal angle. It is normally 2 mm superior to the medial canthal position (Figure 13.3a).

The concept of negative vector plays an important role in lower-lid treatments. This assesses how far anteriorly the eyeball is placed in relation to the inferior orbital rim (Figure 13.3 b, c). In most patients, a line dropped vertically from the cornea touches the inferior orbital rim. In patients with a negative vector, the inferior orbital rim falls posterior to this line.[6] These patients may be at risk for lower-lid retraction or hollowed-out appearance post blepharoplasty. Patients of African ethnicity may have genetically prominent eyes and, therefore, a

FIGURE 13.3 The lower eyelid merges with the skin of the cheek, with no specific demarcation in youth. The nasojugal fold (njf) runs from the medial canthus along the orbital rim, and the malar fold (mf) runs from the lateral canthus along the orbital rim (a). These two folds deepen with age, giving a tired, hollowed-out look. In a normal person, the plane of the cornea lies behind or is in line with the plane of the inferior orbital rim (b). In patients with a prominent eye (c), the corneal plane is placed ahead of the orbital rim (negative vector). The negative vector provides less bony support to the lower eyelid soft tissues, thereby increasing the tendency to scar downward.

pre-existing negative vector. With this background, let us now discuss the four commonest ethnic considerations in the periorbital region: wrinkles, hills and valleys, hyperpigmentation, and dermatochalasis.

13.3 Periocular Wrinkles

Dynamic periorbital wrinkles are caused by contractions of the underlying muscles. The commonest muscles implicated in periocular wrinkles are shown in Figure 13.4. Botulinum toxin can relax the muscles underneath, thereby reducing the overlying wrinkles to provide a younger look.[7]

13.3.1 Crow's Feet

Crow's feet are fine or coarse rhytids (wrinkles) originating from the lateral canthus and project outward in a fan-like distribution (Figure 13.5). They are most prominent during the "dynamic" state of smiling or squinting. With age, they may turn into static lines. Several factors accelerate the development of crow's feet, including sun exposure, smoking, lack of subcutaneous fat, and redundant skin.

An assessment of crow's feet should be performed at rest and while the patient is smiling. Four types of crow's feet rhytids

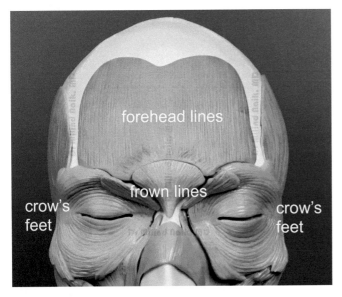

FIGURE 13.4 The muscles targeted for treatment of periocular wrinkles. Frontalis for horizontal forehead lines, procerus and corrugator supercilia for glabellar frown lines, and lateral raphe of orbicularis oculi for crow's feet. The corrugator lies deep below the orbicularis oculi.

were identified by Kane et al.[8] A dose of 5–15 units of botulinum toxin type A can be injected per side, subcutaneously, about 1 cm lateral to the lateral canthus (Figure 13.6). The dose can be altered based on gender, muscle function, and the extent of wrinkles. Injection given above the canthal line is close to the lacrimal gland and can induce dry eye in patients with reduced tear secretions.[9] Similarly, injection given too low to the lateral canthal line can weaken the zygomaticus major, thereby causing smile asymmetry.

13.3.2 Horizontal Forehead Lines

The frontalis muscle is responsible for raising the eyebrows and upper eyelids. This action, over time, results in the development of horizontal forehead lines. Initially dynamic in nature, these lines can become static with age. A dose of 10–20 units of botulinum toxin for women and 20–30 units for men is recommended for forehead wrinkles (Figure 13.7).[7] The injections are placed in two rows, starting at least 2 cm above the orbital rim, in order to avoid brow ptosis. Side effects include brow ptosis and blepharoptosis.

13.3.3 Glabellar Frown Lines

The glabellar frown lines are caused by the two corrugator supercilii muscles placed horizontally and the procerus muscle placed vertically. They collectively pull the brow medially and downward (Figure 13.8). The corrugator supercilii are horizontally oriented muscle that lie beneath the

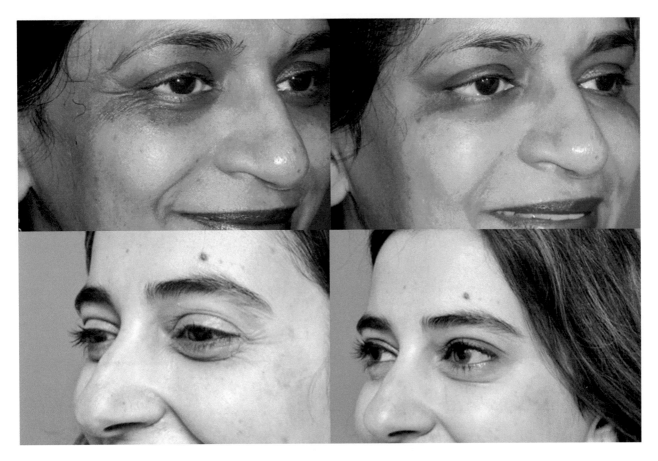

FIGURE 13.5 Crow's feet or lateral canthal rhytids can be treated with botulinum toxin injection. These dynamic lines become less prominent after the treatment, and the effect can last for three to four months.

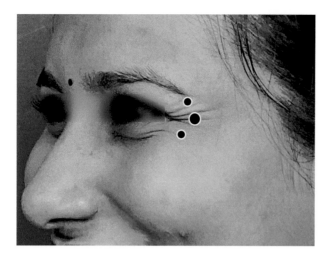

medial eyebrow, extending outward to about the mid-pupillary line. The procerus is a vertically oriented muscle that lies in between the eyebrows. The glabella is typically treated with five injection sites with a dose of 20–30 units for women and 30–40 units for men (Figure 13.9).[7] Personal anecdotal experience suggests that, unlike in the West, the Indian patient wants only a reduction in action rather than complete akinesia. Side effects include brow ptosis and blepharoptosis.

13.3.4 Brow Contouring

Apart from wrinkles, Botulinum toxin is also used for facial contouring by altering the balance between two facial muscles. For example, the brow can be reshaped by relaxing the frontalis muscle in the midline and relaxing the orbital part of orbicularis oculi superolaterally to achieve a laterally arching eyebrow (Figure 13.10).

13.4 Periocular Hills and Valleys

The soft tissue contour changes around the eye are best described as hollows and elevations. Hollows require fillers or fat, whereas elevations may require excision where there is an apparent

FIGURE 13.6 Sites for botulinum toxin injection to treat crow's feet. Usually, one injection 1 cm lateral to the lateral canthus in the subcutaneous plane is enough (5–10 units of botulinum toxin type A). Additional sites above or below this canthal line can be added based on the extent of the wrinkles.

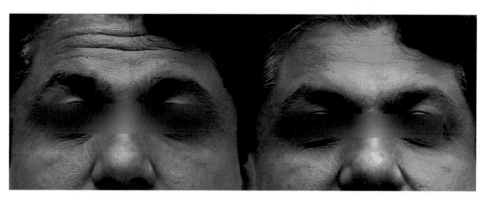

FIGURE 13.7   Pre- and post-botulinum toxin injection photographs showing the reduction in dynamic horizontal forehead lines.

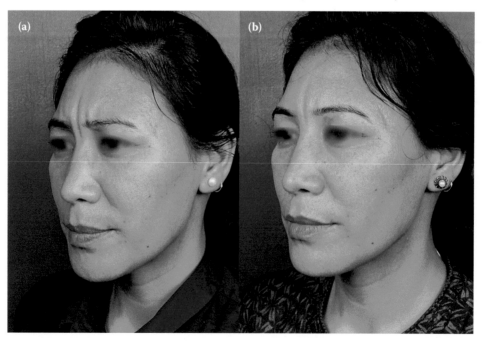

FIGURE 13.8   Vertical glabellar frown lines formed by the contraction of the corrugator supercilii muscle (a). Significant reduction in the lines following botulinum toxin injection (b). Often, patients are keen to treat the "frown expression" rather than the lines for a more pleasing appearance.

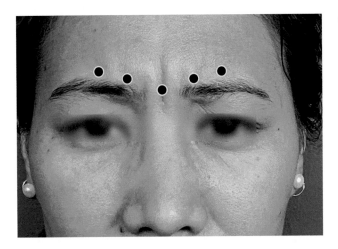

FIGURE 13.9 Botulinum toxin type A, 25 units, injected at five sites for the treatment of glabellar frown lines. The central point between the two eyebrows is for the procerus muscle, injected superficially. Two more points on either side, for the corrugator. The lateral most point reaches the mid-pupillary plane to target the tail of the corrugator. Corrugator injections are placed deep, staying above and beyond the orbital rim.

TABLE 13.2: A Simplified Classification of the Hills and Valleys of the Lower Eyelid

Valleys	Hills
Tear trough (orbital rim hollow)	Orbicularis roll
Eyelid crease hollow	Orbital fat prolapsed (fat bag)
Zygomatic hollow	Fluid bag
	Triangular malar mound

excess. These can be best understood as valleys (hollows) or hills (bags) and are more applicable to the lower-lid aging changes.[10]

13.4.1 The Valleys

Starting from the eyelid margin downward, the valleys include the eyelid crease hollow, tear trough, and zygomatic hollow (Table 13.2).

13.4.1.1 Eyelid Crease Hollow

The eyelid crease hollow is formed by the cutaneous attachment of the lower eyelid retractors and represents the surface marking of the lower border of the tarsus (Figures 13.11 and 13.12). It is less prominent than the upper eyelid crease and is bound superiorly by the pretarsal orbicularis roll and inferiorly by the orbital fat prolapse.

13.4.1.2 Tear Trough, or Orbital Rim Hollow

The tear trough hollow is an important feature of eyelid and midface aging. It is a depression along the medial lower eyelid, just lateral to the anterior lacrimal crest and limited inferiorly by the orbital rim.[10] This region corresponds anatomically with the location of the lacrimal sac, hence the term "tear trough" (Figure 13.11).

Tear trough hollow can result from several factors, including loss of subcutaneous fat, thinning of the skin over the orbital rim ligaments, and descent of the cheek. Partial bony resorption of the underlying orbital rim also contributes. While the term "tear trough" would be more appropriate for the younger age group (where it is not an aging change), in the older age group it is aptly termed the orbital rim hollow.

The *orbital rim hollow* corresponds with the location of the orbital rim or orbitomalar ligament. Medially, it is synonymous with the tear trough. Laterally, it follows the circular contour of the inferior orbital rim. In the mid-pupillary line, overlying the infraorbital foramen, the orbital rim hollow widens into a triangular pit (Figure 13.12).

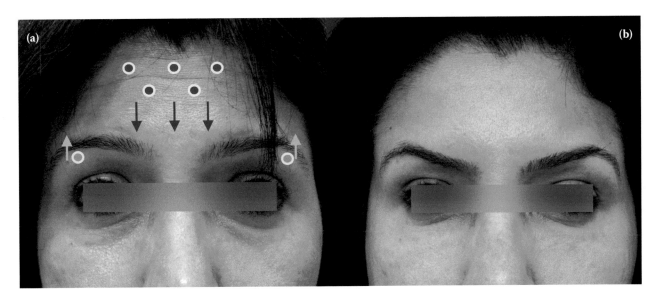

FIGURE 13.10 Brow contouring with botulinum toxin. The frontalis is relaxed in the center with 20–30 units of botulinum toxin type A (central red points), thereby moving the head of the brow downwards (a). The orbital orbicularis is relaxed supero-temporally along the eyebrow with 5–10 units of botulinum toxin type A to raise the tail of the brow (green points). This gives an arched, feminine eyebrow without surgery (b).

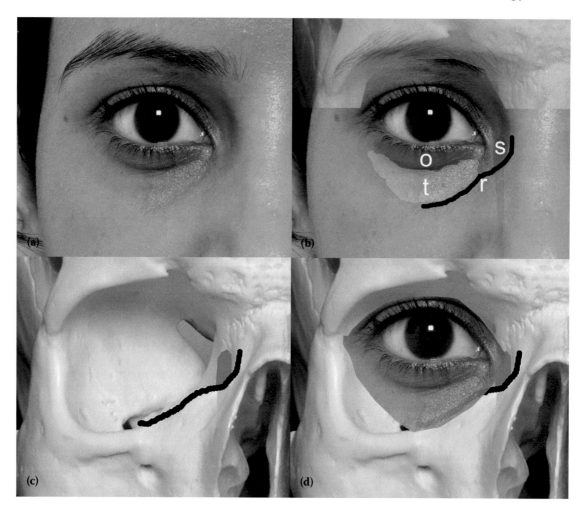

FIGURE 13.11 The right eye demonstrating the hills and valleys around the eye (a). Note the orbicularis roll (o) and the tear trough (t) in relation to the inferomedial orbital rim (r). The lacrimal sac (s) lies medially (bottom left and right), continuing below the orbital rim as the nasolacrimal duct. The tear trough, therefore, does not lie over the orbital rim but often lateral or superior to it.

13.4.1.3 Zygomatic Hollow

It corresponds to the location of the orbitozygomatic ligament (Figure 13.12). It lies along the origin of the levator labii superioris and zygomatic major and minor muscles. The zygomatic hollow is bound by the triangular malar fullness above and by the lateral cheek fat below.[10]

13.4.1.4 Significance of the Valleys

The *eyelid crease hollow* is an important landmark of diagnostic significance. It helps differentiate the two hills that are later described in this chapter: orbicularis roll (which lies above it) and fat bag (which lies below it). It does not require treatment.

Among all the valleys, the tear trough (orbital rim hollow) receives the maximum attention with respect to treatment modalities. Hyaluronic acid fillers and autologous fat transfer are the two commonly employed techniques to fill this valley (Figure 13.13). Several commercial preparations of hyaluronic acid fillers are available, along with recommendations for use.[11] For fillers as well as botulinum toxin, we now have consensus recommendations that are specific to Indian patients.[12] In the majority of cases, fillers are required in the medial half (medial to the mid-pupillary line). One of the widely discussed and

grave complications of filler injection is blindness caused by retrograde migration of the filler particles, thereby causing central retinal artery occlusion.[13] It is important for ophthalmologists and aestheticians to be aware of this complication.

The *zygomatic hollow* receives attention with respect to the filling of the malar volume loss. Filling the zygomatic hollow along with the tear trough restores the malar volume and thereby the malar prominence.

13.4.1.5 Brow Deflation

An important area of volume loss (which can be considered as a valley) in the upper eyelid is the loss of brow fat pad. This is most apparent in the central and lateral regions and often leads to an appearance of pseudo-dermatochalasis (Figure 13.14).

13.4.2 The Hills

Starting from the eyelid margin downward, the lower eyelid hills include the prominent orbicularis roll, orbital fat/fluid bag, and triangular malar mound (Table 13.3).[10]

13.4.2.1 Prominent Orbicularis Roll

The pretarsal lower eyelid orbicularis roll can be excessively prominent in few, causing a cosmetic concern. It becomes more prominent when the orbicularis contracts during facial

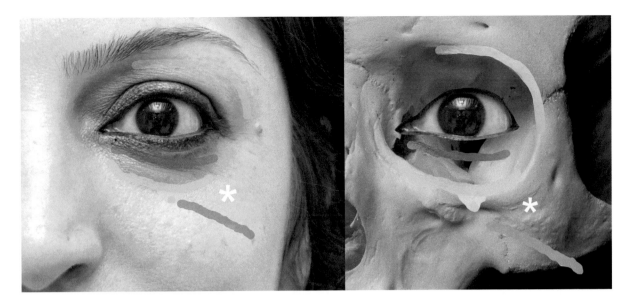

FIGURE 13.12 The left eye demonstrating the three periorbital hollows. The red line marks the eyelid crease hollow that divides the orbicularis roll (above) and fat bag (below). The green line marks the orbital rim hollow. Medially it represents the tear trough. Note the widened triangular pit along the mid-pupillary line. The orbital rim hollow marks the lower limit of the fat bag. The orbital rim hollow can sometimes be visible along the superior orbital rim (light green). The violet line represents the zygomatic hollow, which extends inferolaterally from the midpoint of the orbital rim hollow. The triangular area between the lateral half of the orbital rim hollow and the zygomatic hollow is termed as the triangular malar mound (asterisk).

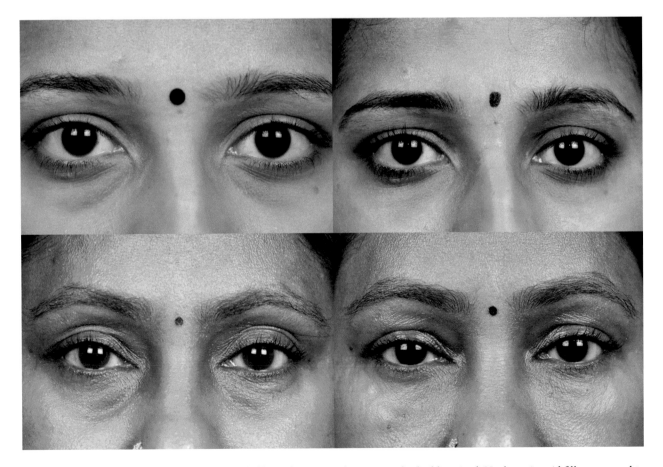

FIGURE 13.13 Tear troughs are under-eye hollows that can make a person look old or tired. Hyaluronic acid filler was used to fill the hollow. Note the improvement in the apparent pigmentation caused by the shadowing effect.

TABLE 13.3: Differentiating Features between the Lower Eyelid Fat Bag and Fluid Bag

Features	Fat Bag	Fluid Bag
Variability	Constant (increases slowly over the years)	Variable from day to day
Upper limit	Septal confluence hollow	Septal confluence hollow
Lower limit	Orbital rim hollow	May extend beyond the orbital rim hollow
Contour	Compartmentalized into central, medial, and lateral fat pads	Single, smooth contour
Changes with gaze	Increases in upgaze; decreases in downgaze	Similar in all gazes
Anatomic location	Orbital (behind orbital septum)	Subcutaneous (anterior to the septum)
Treatment	Fat excision or repositioning	No effective treatment available

expressions such as smiling, leading to near-complete closure of the palpebral aperture of the eye.

13.4.2.2 Orbital Fat Prolapse

This could be considered as the commonest lower-lid hill that presents to the ophthalmologist. Orbital fat prolapse is bound superiorly by the eyelid crease hollow and inferiorly by the orbital rim hollow.[10] The fat actually lies in a deeper plane, behind the orbital septum. The orbital fat seems more prominent with advancing age and also with upgaze (Figure 13.15). It appears to reduce the downgaze.

13.4.2.3 Fluid Bag, or Festoon

The fluid bag in the lower eyelid can mimic fat prolapse, and it requires experience to differentiate the two (Table 13.2). The fluid bag is in the subcutaneous plane, is bound superiorly by the eyelid crease hollow, but need not be bound inferiorly by the orbital rim and may extend beyond it.[10] It also does not show the typical compartmentalization like fat bags and appears

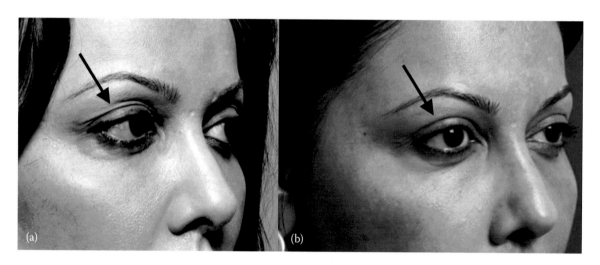

FIGURE 13.14 Pseudo-dermatochalasis caused by mild loss of brow fat pad (a). The apparent skin fold disappears (b) after filler injection into the brow fat pad, thereby avoiding a blepharoplasty.

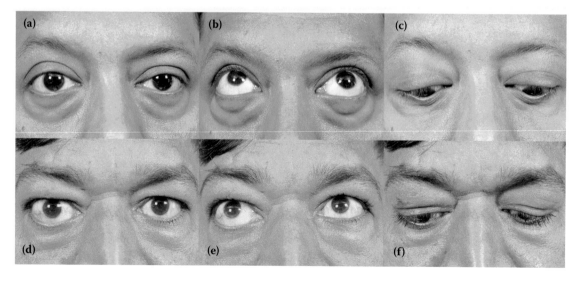

FIGURE 13.15 Differentiating lower eyelid fat bags (a–c) from fluid bags (d–f). Note the compartmentalization of the fat bags (a), increase in upgaze (b), and decrease in downgaze (c). Fat bags are bound inferiorly by orbital rim hollow. In comparison, a fluid bag is not compartmentalized, has indistinct borders, does not change much with gaze, and may not always be restricted by orbital rim hollow (d–f).

more or less the same in upgaze and downgaze (Figure 13.15). Fluid bags can have a bluish hue and may be worse in the morning hours, during the menstrual period, or even after a salty meal. Rarely, orbital fat and fluid may coexist.

13.4.2.4 *Triangular Malar Mound*

The triangular malar mound or malar festoon is a fluid bag located inferolateral to the orbital rim.[10] It is bound above, by the orbital rim hollow, and below, by the zygomatic hollow (Figure 13.16). Prominent triangular malar mounds often run in families and can be variable. It is often more prominent in patients with thyroid disorders due to the increased fluid retention in this region.[14] It may also have an allergic component. With the loss of skin elasticity, the malar mound can become an actual festoon.

13.4.2.5 *The Significance of the Hills*

For the prominent orbicularis roll, an injection of 1–2 units of botulinum toxin type A into the pretarsal orbicularis in the mid-pupillary plane is the best option. *Orbital fat prolapse* requires conservative fat removal or repositioning and is the surgically most amenable "hill" in the lower eyelid.[15] Fluid bags and triangular malar mounds are primarily areas of fluid retention and are difficult to treat. Several non-invasive, injectable, and surgical options are available for the treatment of malar fluid bags.[16, 17] When using hyaluronic acid fillers for the orbital rim hollow, patients with triangular malar mounds should

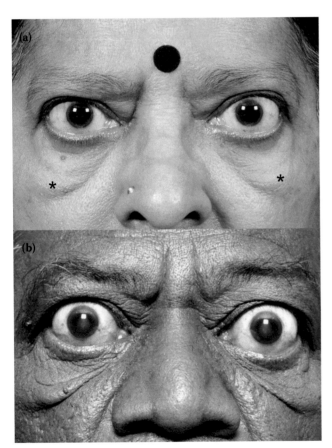

FIGURE 13.16 Pre-malar edema (asterisk) with active fluid festoon (a). Chronic partially collapsed fluid festoon in a patient with thyroid eye disease (b). Note the classic eye signs of thyroid eye disease.

preferably be avoided or the fillers should be injected deep since the gel can imbibe more fluid and give an unnatural look.

13.4.2.6 *Customized Approach*

The volumetric changes in the lower eyelid commonly present as a hill, a valley, or a combination of the two (Figure 13.17). It is useful to first establish an anatomic definition for the patient's symptom of "tired look." Is it the fat bag? Or is it the orbital rim hollow? Evaluating old photographs of the patient often helps understand chronological changes in the anatomy. It is always helpful to "rewind" the years by addressing the recent findings (fat or hollow) rather than give a new look to your patient.

13.5 The Dark Circles (Periocular Hyperpigmentation)

Periorbital hyperpigmentation, or dark circles, is another common cause of an aged or tired appearance. Under-eye hyperpigmentation has anatomical, internal, and environmental causes.[18] Often, the cause is multi-factorial.[19, 20]

Eyelid skin is the thinnest in the body and does not have fat under it. This allows fine blood vessels (capillaries) and eyelid muscle fibers to be almost "seen through," thereby giving a reddish-blue color to the skin. Compare it to the lighter color of the cheek skin, which is thicker, and has fat underneath it. Reduced sleep can lead to dilatation of these vessels, thereby increasing the "shade" of under-eye darkening.

The pigment in the skin around the eyes (melanin) may increase due to eye allergy, a hormonal influence on pigment cells, or a reaction to a topical cream or medication. Moreover, Indian skin is overall more pigmented, making these contrasts even more striking. Lifestyle-related causes include sun exposure, inadequate sleep, overuse of alcohol, and smoking.

Sometimes, the lower-eyelid contour can make it appear darker. For example, the dark shadows will be more obvious in the presence of lower-eyelid fat bags or a hollow.

Fluid accumulation within the thin lower eyelid skin is another cause of under-eye hyperpigmentation. Systemic causes include heart, kidney, or liver disease, Addison's disease, and circulatory disturbances that lead to fluid retention in the body. Post-inflammatory hyperpigmentation may also occur in patients with eczema or atopy.

The natural reasons why eyelid skin looks darker cannot be eliminated, but some remedies can be suggested. Sun protection with the use of physical and chemical sunscreens is important in the prevention of dark circles. Good hydration thickens the eyelid skin, thereby making it less transparent, and cold compresses help reduce the caliber of the blood vessels that are seen through the thin skin. Adequate sleep (minimum of eight hours) would ensure that the under-eye skin looks healthy.

Next, we need to target excessive pigment in the skin. The first step is to address any obvious precipitating cause if it can be identified, such as eye allergy, or an uncorrected/changed spectacle correction. Certain under-eye creams can reduce pigment production within the skin cells and can effectively reduce these dark areas. Hydroquinone is the best when it comes to skin-lightening creams. It is recommended to use them only under the direct supervision of a dermatologist. Non-invasive methods such as the use of intense pulsed light (IPL) and Q-switched lasers work by targeting excess pigment and vascularity, reducing hyperpigmentation. However, in

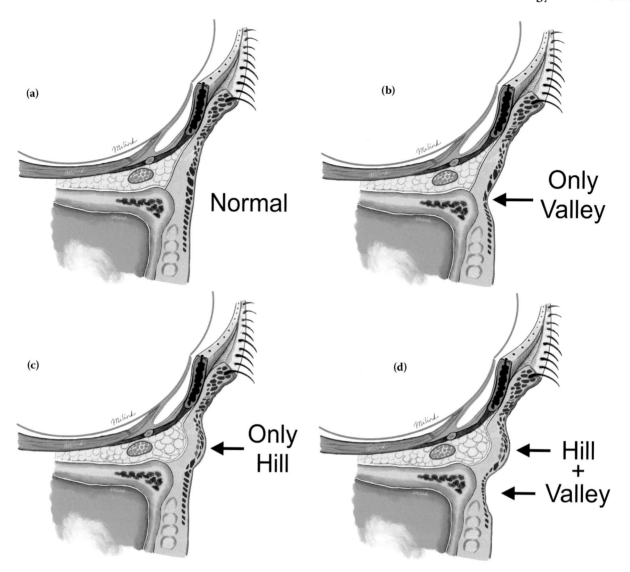

FIGURE 13.17 Common clinical scenarios with respect to lower eyelid hills and valleys. Normal anatomy in a youth is a smooth continuum from lids to cheek (a). "Only valley" is a scenario with a tear-trough deformity along the orbital rim (b) that requires fillers or fat. "Only hill" is a scenario with fat bag (c) that requires fat removal via a blepharoplasty. "Hill-valley-hill" is a scenario (d) that requires fat from the hill to be removed or transposed into the valley (fat reposition) or blepharoplasty with autologous fat transfer.

Indian skin, they are of limited value, considering the risks of post-inflammatory hyperpigmentation.

Lastly, the dark circles are caused by the hollows and fat bags under your eyes. These contour changes increase the dark circles by creating a shadowing effect. It requires the removal of the eyelid bags or filling of the hollow with fillers (Figure 13.13a,b).

In summary, good hydration, treatment of any eye allergy, skin-lightening creams, and effective treatment of under-eye contour changes (bags and hollows) can reduce dark circles significantly.

13.6 Dermatochalasis and Blepharochalasis

Excess eyelid skin is a slow aging change. In the upper lid, it overhangs the eyelid margin. In the lower eyelid, it may appear as excessive static wrinkles. Treatment may be required both for functional as well as aesthetic reasons. Upper eyelid blepharoplasty is most commonly performed for dermatochalasis, which represents excessive, overhanging inelastic upper eyelid skin due to aging (Figure 13.18). Blepharochalasis, on the other hand, represents excessive papery thin skin in the upper eyelid in young patients due to repeated episodes of edema and can also benefit from blepharoplasty (Figure 13.18). Less frequently, extensive upper eyelid xanthelasma may require a blepharoplasty-like excision.

13.6.1 Preoperative Evaluation

Preoperative patient evaluation for blepharoplasty should document medical and ocular evaluation. In addition to a complete eye examination, the evaluation of the periorbital area should take into account skin quality and quantity, underlying three-dimensional soft tissue contours, and the bony skeletal support. Ophthalmologic history should be obtained,

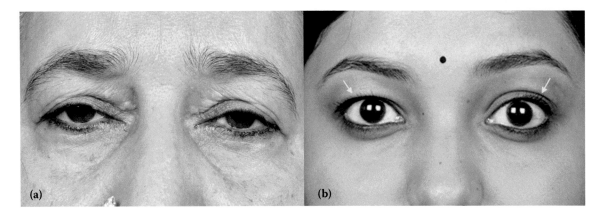

FIGURE 13.18 Common indications for upper blepharoplasty: Dermatochalasis is an aging change where the upper eyelid skin is in excess and overhangs the eyelid margin (a). Also note the xanthelasma medially. Blepharochalasis is a recurrent inflammatory eyelid edema occurring in young individuals that leads to stretching of the skin (b). Ptosis and lacrimal gland prolapse are other findings seen in blepharochalasis patients.

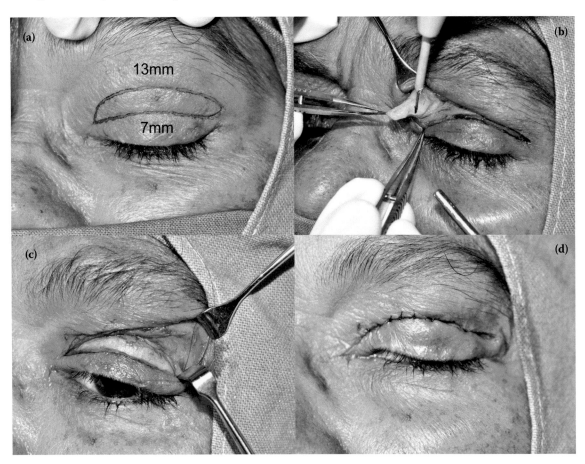

FIGURE 13.19 Upper eyelid blepharoplasty. The eyelid crease is marked 7–8 mm from the lashline and 13 mm from the brow (a). The incision is made with radiofrequency monopolar cautery (a). Medially, it converges towards the medial canthus, whereas laterally it stays parallel to the eyelid margin. Medial fat can be excised if excess (b). A minimally invasive lateral canthal resuspension can be done to raise the lateral canthus by fixing it to the periosteum of the lateral orbital rim (c). The wound is closed with interrupted 6-0 Vicryl sutures (d).

including vision, corrective lenses, allergic reactions, excess tearing, and dry eyes.

13.6.2 Blepharoplasty Surgery

Blepharoplasty may be performed under local or general anesthesia depending upon the surgical plan, patient preference, and need for concomitant operations. A simple upper or lower eyelid blepharoplasty can be performed under local anesthesia.

Upper eyelid blepharoplasty universally involves the removal of excess skin (Figure 13.19). A minimum of 20 mm of vertical lid height should be preserved for normal eye closure. Other

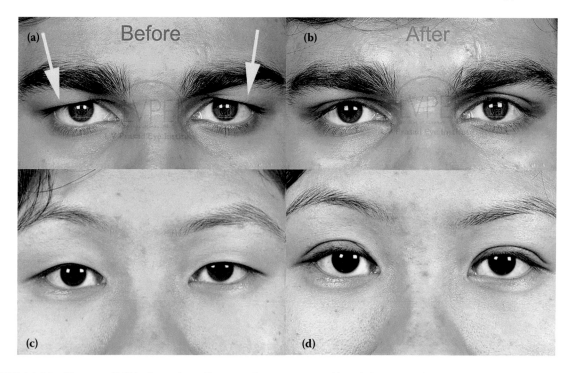

FIGURE 13.20 Upper eyelid blepharoplasty. Preoperative appearance (a) and three months post-operative appearance showing a well-defined lid fold (b). Upper eyelid anchor blepharoplasty in an Oriental eyelid. Preoperative appearance (c) and final post-operative appearance after three months showing a well-defined eyelid fold (d).

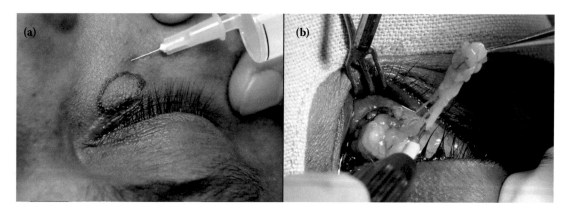

FIGURE 13.21 Transconjunctival blepharoplasty (surgeon's view). Injection of local anesthetic into the inferior conjunctival fornix (a). Stab incisions are placed over the palpebral conjunctiva to expose orbital fat, which is excised piecemeal while constantly checking the contour changes (b).

modifications during an upper blepharoplasty include conservative fat sculpting, reattachment of levator muscle if disinserted, lateral canthoplasty, and fixation of the prolapsed lacrimal gland (Figure 13.19).

A standard upper blepharoplasty involves only skin removal, with preservation of underlying orbicularis muscle and orbital soft tissue. Skin is excised above the supratarsal fold. This retains most of the definition of the existing lid fold and gives an aesthetically enhancing result (Figure 13.20 a,b) without "post-surgery appearance" or a hollowed-out orbit.

Anchor (invagination) blepharoplasty involves the creation of the upper eyelid crease by attaching the eyelid crease skin to the underlying levator aponeurosis. An anchor blepharoplasty includes minimal excision of the skin (2–3 mm), a strip of orbicularis (1–2 mm), and pretarsal fatty tissue. Anchor sutures are placed connecting the pretarsal skin to the aponeurosis. This technique is also used with some modification in the creation of eyelid fold in Oriental eyelids, also popularly called double eyelid surgery (Figure 13.20 c,d).

Any excess orbital fat may be safely excised through an upper eyelid blepharoplasty incision, most commonly required medially (Figure 13.19b). Overall, under-correction is preferred to prevent hollowing.

Lower eyelid blepharoplasty can be performed in two ways: transcutaneous and transconjunctival. The transconjunctival approach leaves no external scar and reduces the chances of eyelid retraction, scleral show, and postoperative ectropion than the transcutaneous method.[21, 22] The transcutaneous

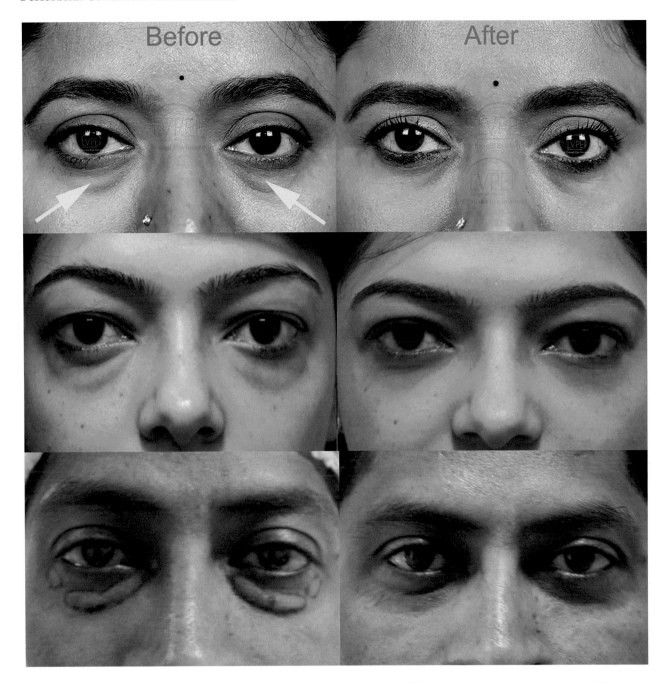

FIGURE 13.22 Preoperative (left) and postoperative (right) photographs following transconjunctival lower eyelid blepharoplasty with conservative fat excision. No external scar, no conjunctival sutures, and no scarring of the orbital septum are the advantages of the transconjunctival approach.

approach is preferred if there is excess skin that requires excision.[23] With the newer skin-tightening modalities available for the eyelid skin, the transconjunctival approach is the most popular.[21] Transconjunctival lower-lid blepharoplasty is often performed under local anesthesia (Figure 13.21). An incision is placed through the conjunctiva with a radiofrequency monopolar cautery or CO_2 laser. Gentle pressure on the eyeball prolapses the fat compartments, and the medial, central, and lateral fat pads are removed. The transoconjunctival incision heals by epithelization without any sutures. An excellent aesthetic outcome is achieved in most cases (Figure 13.22).

Lateral canthopexy can be combined with lower eyelid blepharoplasty.

13.7 Transcutaneous Lower-Lid Blepharoplasty

Transcutaneous lower-lid blepharoplasty is chosen when excess skin or orbicularis needs to be excised along with the prolapsed fat (Figure 13.23). In Caucasian patients, excess vertical skin in the lower lid can be dealt with skin-resurfacing techniques such as fractional laser resurfacing. In Indian skin,

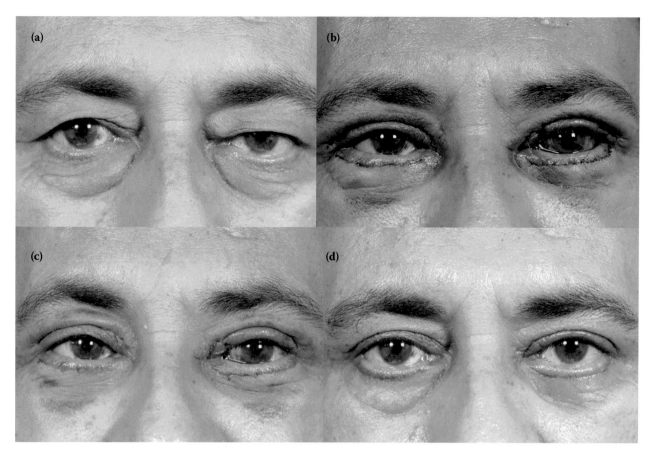

FIGURE 13.23 A middle-aged patient with upper eyelid dermatochalasis, left upper eyelid ptosis, excess lower eyelid skin, and lower-lid fat bags (a). The excess skin in the lower eyelid warrants an anterior approach to lower eyelid fat. He underwent a transcutaneous quad-blepharoplasty with conservative fat excision and left Müller muscle conjunctival resection for ptosis (b). Appearance on day 7 postoperative (c) and month 3 postoperative (d).

however, laser resurfacing can lead to post-inflammatory hyperpigmentation, and hence, a "skin pinch" technique to remove the skin is ideal in such a case.

13.8 Conclusion

The periocular region is the first to reveal aging changes on the face. Optimal use of botulinum toxin and fillers to enhance the periorbital and facial aesthetics is an art and science. The treatment of periocular hyperpigmentation is predominantly in the dermatologist's purview, and ophthalmologists play an important in treating periocular hollows to reduce the shadowing effect. Upper eyelid blepharoplasty is performed for dermatochalasis or blepharochalasis and predominantly involves skin excision. Lower eyelid blepharoplasty is commonly performed transconjunctivally but can be done via the anterior approach in cases of skin excess.

Clinical Pearls in Treating Periorbital Ethnic Skin

Asian (Indian)

- For wrinkle treatment, Indian patients prefer a reduction in lines rather than complete akinesia.
- When treating horizontal forehead lines with Botulinum toxin, place the injections at least 1.5 cm above the brow to avoid brow droop.

- When treating crow's feet with botulinum toxin, placing it too high can cause dry eye, whereas placing it too low can cause smile asymmetry.
- Treatment of glabellar frown lines with botulinum toxin has the highest chance of inducing ptosis as a complication. Place the injections well above the orbital rim.
- Tear trough hollow is the most commonly treated periorbital hollow or valley. Hyaluronic acid fillers are the most popular choice.
- A deflated eyebrow can present with apparent excess skin (pseudo-dermatochalasis), which may be perceived as an indication for blepharoplasty. Volumizing the brow is the correct solution.
- A prominent orbicularis roll in the lower eyelid can be safely treated with botulinum toxin injection without causing eyelid abnormality.
- Lower eyelid fat bags need to be differentiated from fluid bags as the treatment approach is completely different.
- Lower eyelid fat bags can be treated transconjunctivally in most cases to avoid external skin scars.
- Fluid festoons can either be eyelid or malar in location and are the most difficult to treat. Rule out thyroid disorders.
- Periocular pigmentation has anatomic and etiologic causes. Treatable aggravating factors need to be

addressed first before medical therapy that targets melanin.

- Upper eyelid blepharoplasty can be performed for dermatochalasis or blepharochalasis.
- Lower eyelid blepharoplasty is most commonly performed transconjunctival. Skin approach is rarely preferred when excess lower-lid skin needs to be simultaneously addressed.

Southeast Asian (Oriental)

- Crow's feet are relatively limited due to the thick eyelid skin. Similarly, glabellar lines are more likely to be static, with a requirement of a filler.
- The upper eyelid crease is very low set in Oriental eyelids, and this needs to be remembered for blepharoplasty and double eyelid surgery.
- For eyelid crease formation, excess upper eyelid fat has to be removed.

African

- Patients with African ethnicity have slightly prominent eyes, thereby posing a negative vector. This may have implications for lower eyelid surgical planning.
- For lower-lid blepharoplasty, it is best to use transconjunctival route to avoid hypertrophic lower-lid skin scars.

Frequently Asked Questions

1. *Q: What are the commonest periocular side effects of botulinum toxin injections?*

   A: Although rare, the side effects in order of frequency are ptosis and dry eye. Ptosis is most commonly associated with the treatment of glabellar frown lines. Contrary to popular belief, there is no satisfactory treatment of post-injection ptosis with topical eye drops. It usually wears off in two to four weeks. Dry eye is most commonly associated with treatment for crow's feet and can be caused by injection above the lateral canthal line.

2. *Q: How to discuss the side effect of blindness to a patient prior to periocular fillers?*

   A: Although blindness is extremely rare, it is important to discuss it with your patients. More likely, they would have read about it and would wonder why you avoided the topic.

   You can explain it to be an extremely rare event, as rare as a flight crash. Also, you take all precautions to avoid that possibility. However, since it is a globally observed rare event, even in the best of hands, the patient would find it listed as a complication on the consent form. Additionally, if you have taken fillers yourself, mentioning that helps build confidence.

3. *Q: Which patients require blepharoplasty?*

   A: In the upper eyelid, if the excess skin is hanging up to the lashline, it is a clear indication for surgery. For mild cases of the upper-lid skin fold, look for brow deflation, and treat that first. In the lower eyelid, moderate to severe fat bags (after differentiating them from fluid bags) are amenable to blepharoplasty. Mild fat bags can be camouflaged by fillers underneath them into the tear trough.

4. *Q: How to treat hypertrophic orbicularis roll in the lower lid?*

   A: Firstly, the word hypertrophy is a misnomer in this context. It is simply a prominent orbicularis roll. It can be treated with 1–2 units of botulinum toxin type A injection into the orbicularis of the lower eyelid. The injection is given at a single point, into the pretarsal muscle, in the mid-pupillary plane. Contrary to popular belief, lower eyelid ectropion will not happen with 2 units of toxin.

5. *Q: How to treat malar fluid bags?*

   A: Malar fluid bags are the hardest to treat. Firstly, they need to be investigated for the cause, the commonest being thyroid disorders. Most surgical options directly into the festoon area are likely to worsen it. Recent reports of doxycycline injections need to be observed for long-term results before advocating them. Conservative treatment options include control of thyroid hormone levels, head-end elevation during sleep, and cold compresses.

References

1. www.prnewswire.com/news-releases/aafprs-2018-annual-survey-reveals-key-trends-in-facial-plastic-surgery-300782534.html
2. Bosniak SL, Zilkha MC. Cosmetic blepharoplasty and facial rejuvenation. Lippincott-Raven; 1999.
3. Castanares S. Blepharoplasty for herniated intraorbital fat; anatomical basis for a new approach. Plastic and reconstructive surgery (1946). 1951 Jul;8(1):46.
4. Codner MA, Kikkawa DO, Korn BS, Pacella SJ. Blepharoplasty and brow lift. Plastic and reconstructive surgery. 2010 Jul 1;126(1):1e–7e.
5. Jordan D, Mawn L, Anderson RL. Surgical anatomy of the ocular adnexa: A clinical approach. Oxford University Press; 2012 Feb 29.
6. Jacono AA, Moskowitz B. Transconjunctival versus transcutaneous approach in upper and lower blepharoplasty. Facial Plast Surg. 2001;17:21–28.
7. Carruthers J, Fagien S, Matarasso SL, Botox Consensus Group. Consensus recommendations on the use of botulinum toxin type a in facial aesthetics. Plast Reconstr Surg. 2004 Nov;114(6 Suppl):1S–22S.
8. Kane MA 2003 Classification of crow's feet patterns among Caucasian women: The key to individualizing treatment. Plast Reconstr Surg. 112:S33–S39
9. Arat YO, Yen MT. Effect of botulinum toxin type a on tear production after treatment of lateral canthal rhytids. Ophthalmic Plast Reconstr Surg. 2007 Jan–Feb;23(1):22–24.
10. Naik MN. Hills and valleys: Understanding the under-eye. J Cutan Aesthet Surg. 2016;9:61–64
11. Matarasso S, Carruthers J, Jewell ML, Restylane Consensus Group. Consensus recommendations for soft-tissue augmentation with non-animal stabilized hyaluronic acid (Restylane). Plast Reconstr Surg. 2006 Mar;117(3 Suppl):3S–34S; discussion 35S–43S
12. Kapoor KM, Chatrath V, Anand C, Shetty R, Chhabra C, Singh K, Vedamurthy M, Pai J, Sthalekar B, Sheth R. Consensus recommendations for treatment strategies in indians using botulinum toxin and hyaluronic acid fillers. Plast Reconstr Surg Glob Open. 2017 Dec 28;5(12):e1574.
13. Beleznay K, Carruthers JDA, Humphrey S, Carruthers A, Jones D. Update on avoiding and treating blindness from fillers: A recent review of the world literature. Aesthet Surg J. 2019 May 16;39(6):662–674.
14. Kim BJ, Kazim M. Prominent premalar and cheek swelling: A sign of thyroid-associated orbitopathy. Ophthalmic Plast Reconstr Surg. 2006 Nov–Dec;22(6):457–460.
15. Naik M. Blepharoplasty and periorbital surgical rejuvenation. Indian J Dermatol Venereol Leprol. 2013;79:41–51
16. Chon BH, Hwang CJ, Perry JD. Treatment options for lower eyelid festoons. Facial Plast Surg Clin North Am. 2021 May;29(2):301–309.
17. Godfrey KJ, Kally P, Dunbar KE, Campbell AA, Callahan AB, Lo C, Freund R, Lisman RD. Doxycycline injection for sclerotherapy of lower eyelid festoons and malar edema: Preliminary results. Ophthalmic Plast Reconstr Surg. 2019 Sep/Oct;35(5):474–477.
18. Freitag FM, Cestari TF. What causes dark circles under the eyes? J Cosmet Dermatol. 2007 Sep;6(3):211–215.

19. Sheth PB, Shah HA, Dave JN. Periorbital hyperpigmentation: A study of its prevalence, common causative factors and its association with personal habits and other disorders. Indian J Dermatol. 2014 Mar;59(2):151–157.

20. Nouveau S, Agrawal D, Kohli M, Bernerd F, Misra N, Nayak CS. Skin hyperpigmentation in indian population: Insights and best practice. Indian J Dermatol. 2016 Sep–Oct;61(5):487–495.

21. Rizk SS, Matarasso A. Lower eyelid blepharoplasty: Analysis of indications and the treatment of 100 patients. PlastReconstr Surg. 2003;111:1299–306; discussion 1307–1308.

22. Zarem HA, Resnick JI. Minimizing deformity in lower blepharoplasty. The transconjunctival approach. ClinPlast Surg. 1993;20:317–321.

23. Adamson PA, Strecker HD. Transcutaneous lower blepharoplasty. Facial Plast Surg. 1996;12:171–183.

CHAPTER 14: PSYCHOLOGICAL CONCERNS IN ETHNIC SKIN

C. R. Satish Kumar

The connection between mind and body has been debated for many years. In recent years, researchers have provided evidence that a person's emotional state can have a huge influence on physical health[1] and immune function.[2] Stress, depression, anxiety, and other psychological variables are found to be the major contributing factors to skin diseases.[3,4] There is an established association between the central nervous system and skin.[5]

Stress has a great role to play in our daily life, influencing our mood, thoughts, behavior, and health. Stress plays an integral role in skin disease and the exacerbation of the disease.[6] In the recent past, researchers have established the link between chronic stress and dermatological disease, especially in conditions like psoriasis, alopecia areata, and atopic dermatitis.[7,8,9] These findings suggest that the perception of stress plays an important role in the maintenance and exacerbation of skin disease. Support for this comes from an Indian study in which major stressors, which include unemployment, health issues, and loss of person or belongings, were found to be the contributing factors in skin diseases, like psoriasis.[10]

Hans Seyle[11] proposed the general adaptation syndrome, laying the foundation for the first physiological theory of stress. He theorized that difficulty in coping with persistent adverse changes in the environment leads to the exhaustion of the coping resources in an individual. Since the individual fails to restrict the distressing stressors after repeated attempts will make him/her vulnerable to physiological disturbances.

Another proposed mechanism is that during persistent stress, an acute stress response is evoked (flight or fight) as a defense mechanism to combat stress. This is mediated by neuroendocrine, cellular, and molecular infrastructure located in the central nervous system and the periphery.[12] During adverse situations, stress response (flight or fight reactions) is triggered by the CNS, which arouses the sympathetic nervous system sending signals to adrenal glands to release stress hormones. As a result of the stress hormones evoked by the stressors, the skin suffers damage, leading to various complications.[13]

Resilience is an important area of discussion for stress response. Resilience refers to sustained positive functioning in the face of significant physical or psychological challenges.[14] Researchers have also proposed three distinct components of individual resilience: sustained engagement in desirable and valued activities, recovery from stressful experiences by returning to equilibrium, and personal growth in response to a physical or psychological challenge.[15]

Psychodermatology describes an association between dermatology and psychology. The incidence of psychological issues in skin diseases is high, estimated at about 30–60%.[16] Psychodermatology is separated into three classifications based on the association between dermatological and psychiatric disorders: (1) psychophysiological disorders caused by skin diseases triggering different emotional states (stress) but not directly combined with mental disorders (psoriasis, eczema), (2) primary psychiatric disorders responsible for self-induced skin disorders (trichotillomania) and (3) secondary psychiatric disorders caused by disfiguring skin (of ichthyosis, acne conglobata, vitiligo), which can lead to states of fear, depression, or suicidal thoughts.[17]

Skin color is a biological trait. It has been of prime significance in understanding the social and cultural background of the human race in the color of skin diseases. In this chapter, we will discuss the psychological factors (vulnerability) and adaptive features (resilience) in ethnic skin.

14.1 Disorders of Pigmentation

Disorders of pigmentation are the third most common presenting complaint in darker-skinned individuals.[18]

14.1.1 Vitiligo

This autoimmune disorder leads to loss of pigmentation in skin and mucous membranes. In dark-skinned individuals, the contrast between the actual dark-pigmented skin and the hypopigmented skin makes it markedly visible, which can negatively affect the perception of general health, worth, and desirability of an individual.[19] In an Indian study, it was seen that vitiligo patients had issues concerning their physical appearance, progression of white patches on exposed skin, ostracism, dietary restrictions, and difficulty in getting jobs, which was considered by them to be a significant barrier to getting married. Stigma and suicidal ideation was also reported by the patients, and the condition was perceived to be a serious illness.[20] Association between depression, anxiety spectrum disorders (anxiety and social anxiety), and vitiligo has been established in many studies.[21]

Gender differences in quality of life (QOL) is found in women with vitiligo.[22] A study in China showed that vitiligo patients experienced an impaired health-related QOL and disrupted marital relationships.[23] Another study in the Netherlands, conducted with 245 patients using the Skindex 29 and SF-36, showed that vitiligo patients had a low mental HRQOL.[24] The same researchers in 2008 showed that scores on the functioning scale of the Skindex-29 were significantly higher in patients with universal vitiligo, indicating more functional impairment in these patients compared with patients with general vitiligo.[25] These studies show that vitiligo leads to quality-of-life and functional impairments in patients.

In the case of vitiligo, resilience refers to the ability to cope with cosmetic disfigurement. The more positive an individual's self-concept is, the greater will his/her coping abilities be in relation to the impact of this disease.[26] Enhancing resilience will help these patients in treatment adherence and better adjustment in dealing with adverse conditions.

14.1.2 Melasma

Melasma is hyperpigmentation characterized by symmetric, poorly demarcated brown macules and patches that occur primarily on sun-exposed areas on the face and neck that affects female preferentially. Melasma has been found in patients of Hispanic, African American, Arab, South Asian, Southeast Asian, and East Asian descent, most prevalent in Latinos and most prevalent in those with darker skin types.[27] Cosmetic concerns associated with melasma include hyperpigmentation and an overall uneven skin tone.[28]

A survey study of Mexican women showed that 66% of participants developed melasma during pregnancy, and one-third

DOI: 10.1201/9780429243769-14

of these women had persistent pigmentation.[29] These pigmentations in pregnancy might cause many psychological issues. Melasma can be very distressing to patients and has been shown to impact a patient's QOL and self-esteem. These patients refuse to leave their house, feel inferior to others, and constantly think about melasma.[30] The melasma QOL (MELASQOL) survey is an instrument that was developed to identify impairments to a patient's life caused by the disease with greater emphasis on the emotional and psychosocial aspects.[31] Balkrishnan et al.[32] reported that the most affected domains by melasma were social life, recreation, leisure, and emotional well-being. The Spanish version of MELASQOL was developed by Dominguez et al.[33] to specifically target Latina women. Results showed that physical health, emotional well-being, social life, and money matters were most affected by melasma. These findings show that across different cultures, findings were similar in the QOL impairment in melasma patients.

14.1.3 Acne and Post-Inflammatory Hyperpigmentation

Acne is the most common skin disease in the general population, as well as in African Americans, Asians and Hispanics.[34,35] Acne is most frequently found in adolescents and young adults. Pomade acne, which is characterized by multiple comedones on the forehead and temples and along the hairline, is seen primarily in African American patients.[36]

Depression and anxiety have been found commonly among patients with acne.[37,38,39] A study showed emotional difficulties and social impairment, such as feelings of physical discomfort and anger.[40] The results of an Indian study showed a negative influence of acne vulgaris on patients' emotional states and that all psychiatric symptoms, such as somatization, obsession, sensitivity, depression, anxiety, hostility, phobia, paranoid ideation, and psychoticism, were associated with this skin disorder.[41] Social and emotional disturbances in patients with acne were found to be similar to that of psoriasis patients.[42] Acne vulgaris has a significant effect on the QOL and negative self-perceptions along with depression/anxiety symptoms.[43]

On the other hand, evidence shows negative correlations between resilience, depression, and QOL. These findings indicate that resilience enhancement techniques could help these patients cope with negative cognition and affect.[44,45] On these lines, a comparative study was conducted in India to study the perceived stress, optimism, and social appearance anxiety in patients with skin diseases. The result showed that perceived stress and social appearance anxiety were found to be highest in AA patients, followed by acne patients, and found least in melanosis patients. No significant difference was found in patients with melanosis, acne, and AA in regard to optimism.[46]

14.2 Hair/Scalp

14.2.1 Alopecia

Alopecia is a chronic skin disease in which people lose some or all of the hair on their head and their body. Certain types of scarring hair loss, such as traction alopecia or central centrifugal scarring alopecia, occur with increased frequency in darker-skinned populations, particularly women. Alopecia totalis refers to the loss of all hair on the head, and alopecia universalis refers to the loss of all head and body hair.[47]

Alopecia is psychologically devastating, leading to extreme psychological suffering in domains like personal, social, and work-related problems.[48] People with severe hair loss are more likely to experience psychological distress (Figures 14.1 and 14.2). It has been found that 40% of women with alopecia had marital problems due to hair loss, and about 63% had career-related problems. They have lower self-esteem, poor QOL, and poor body image.[49] Psychiatric disorders are more commonly found in alopecia patients; they are at higher risk for developing a serious depressive episode, anxiety disorder, social phobia, or paranoid disorder if treatment is not aimed in the early stages.[50] Additionally, these patients develop physical problems like loss of eyelashes and eyebrows, which lead to problems with identity and identity changes as these features help in defining an individual's facial identity.[51]

A study conducted on South African women with alopecia found a notable disease burden. Results showed psychological disturbances in self-image and interpersonal relationships.[52] Patients reported worries about the possibility of their children developing alopecia, their own condition worsening, and the cost burden. Another study conducted on Chinese patients showed that alopecia areata and androgenetic alopecia moderately affected QOL, including feelings of loss of self-confidence and low self-esteem. Additionally, it was seen that the Dermatology Life Quality Index (DLQI) score of alopecia areata patients was significantly higher than that of the androgenetic alopecia patients.[53]

A case study of a child with universal alopecia areata disease, vitiligo, and generalized anxiety disorder was conducted in which the psychological interventions focused on psychotherapy of infantile psychoanalytical orientation and the systematic parent orientation to reach the reduction of the symptoms and development of abilities for the confrontation of the chronic illness. Results showed the child presented positive adaptation to the illness, remission of the anxiety symptoms, and the development of resilient behaviors as a result of psychological interventions.[54]

14.2.2 Pseudofolliculitis Barbae (Razorbump)

Pseudofolliculitis barbae predominantly affects black men resulting in curved follicles. It is characterized by the development of itchy papules, pustules, and post-inflammatory hyperpigmentation. It typically results from shaving, most noticeable around the beard and neck. Not much data is available on the psychological issues in pseudofolliculitis barbae. Limited data suggest that due to the burden of the disease, the self-esteem and QOL of these patients are significantly affected.[55]

14.2.3 Perifolliculitis Capitis Abscedens et Suffodiens (Dissecting Cellulitis)

This condition occurs most frequently in adult African American men between the ages of 18 and 40.[56] This condition can lead to marked disfigurement, poor cosmetic appearance, and bad odor.[57] It has been observed that patients experience significantly improved QOL following surgical procedures.[58]

14.3 Others

14.3.1 Keloids

Keloids represent an exaggerated healing response to trauma, resulting in irregular deposition of collagen beyond the boundaries of the original injury. Keloid scars are mostly seen in Africans, Asians, and Hispanics.[59]

Keloids have a significant effect on the QOL since it has a major impact on the emotional well-being of patients. The

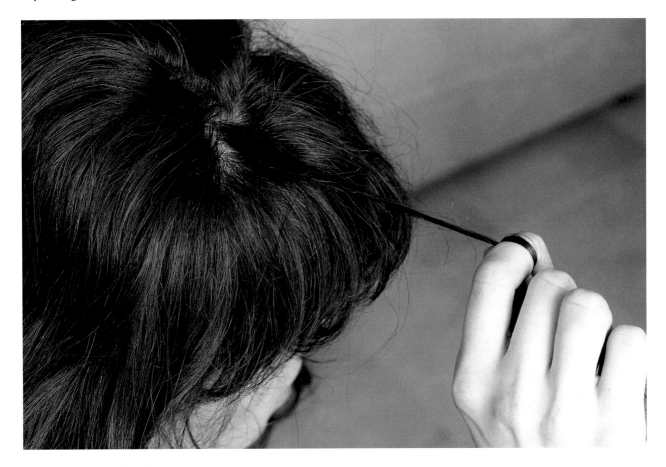

FIGURE 14.1 Trichotillomania.

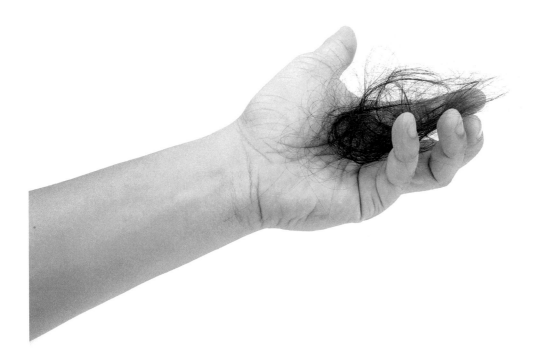

FIGURE 14.2 Alopecia.

HRQL reduction is comparable with the burden of major diseases like psoriasis, dermatitis, arthritis, and cancer.[60] In a study, almost half of them (48%) showed severe emotional symptoms, and about a quarter showed severe issues on the symptomatic and functional scale of the Skindex-29 questionnaire. They scored significantly lower on the SF-36 (generic instrument) dimensions, such as bodily pain, vitality, and social functioning, as well as on the mental component. It has been seen that itching and painful keloids were associated with the largest HRQL impairment, while cosmetic factors, such as color, thickness, pliability, and irregularity of the scar, were less related.[61]

Results from another study showed that the psychological scale was associated with pain and functional restrictions, although the correlations were lower. This study demonstrated for the first time an impairment of QOL in a large group of patients with keloid and hypertrophic scarring.[62] These results show that keloids cause disfiguration, discomfort (pain, itch), QOL impairment, and functional disability.

14.3.2 Sarcoidosis

Sarcoidosis is an idiopathic inflammatory disease that affects multiple organs and is associated with a variety of general and specific symptoms depending on the organs involved.[63] Evidence shows that fatigue is the most common complaint, and it is negatively related to the patient's QOL.[64–66] These patients go through severe stress, which is associated with the symptoms of the disease. Additionally, the depressive symptoms in these patients are associated with perceived stress, according to a Dutch study.[67] QOL impairment in sarcoidosis is generally manifested in domains such as physical, psychological, and social functioning.[68] A study showed that in sarcoidosis, the relationship between increased life stress and impairment in lung function throughout the study period. In addition, no consistent set of psychiatric symptoms was associated with the disease. These patients did, however, report many symptoms similar to patients with agoraphobia.[69]

14.3.3 Eczema

Eczema refers to a group of conditions characterized by red, itchy, and inflamed skin. Scratching is often associated with psychological factors, such as anger, irritation, impatience, relief, and anxiety. Scratching behavior becomes habituated, which means that the patients might develop scratching behavior in the absence of itching. In a study by Kamide,[70] it was seen that psychosocial factors were responsible for the exacerbation of atopic dermatitis in 29 (93.5%) of the 31 adult patients who required hospitalization. The most common psychosocial factors were excessive demands on the patient's time at work, school, home, and so on, taking examinations and mother-child relations, while few patients had mental disorders, such as panic disorder or depression.

QOL impairments correlate with disease severity, aberrant skin biophysiology, depression, anxiety, and stress symptoms in adolescents with AE.[71] Along these lines, results of a study showed that the rate of psychological disturbance in children with eczema was double in comparison with the control group. This difference was found significant for children with moderately severe and severe eczema but not for mild eczema. These findings suggest that school-going children with moderate and severe atopic eczema are at high risk of developing psychological disturbances, which may affect their academic and social development.[72]

14.3.4 Psoriasis

Psoriasis is one of the most common chronic inflammatory skin diseases affecting worldwide. The most common type of psoriasis is psoriasis vulgaris, also called plaque psoriasis. Evidence shows about 25% of patients have moderate to severe disease, and most of them require lifelong treatment.[73] Psoriasis often is associated with other medical conditions, especially in severe cases with a long history of the disease, making the burden of the disease even worse.[74]

In addition to somatic comorbidity, psoriasis can be associated with psychological disturbances. Patients with psoriasis show an increased risk of comorbid psychiatric disorders, such as depression, anxiety, and suicidal ideation.[75,76] Most patients depend on substances as a negative means of coping with the disease, which only worsens the condition even more. Evidence shows that substance dependence like alcohol consumption and nicotine abuse seems to be greater in psoriasis patients.[77] Psychosocial burden in psoriasis patients includes stigmatization in social situations and also the workplace, distortion of body image, and decreased self-esteem and self-concept.[78,79] These psychological factors definitely play a great role in health-related quality-of-life impairment (HrQoL).[80]

On the other hand, a very interesting study was conducted to study the association between childhood trauma and resilience in psoriasis patients by Crosta and colleagues.[81] They found that psoriatic patients had a significant prevalence of childhood trauma and a lower resilience level compared to healthy controls. Associations between traumatic experiences, low resilience, and reduced QOL in psoriatic subjects were found in their study.

14.3.4.1 Asian Obsession on Fairness and Fairness Products

In South Asia, dark skin is associated with labor and fieldwork in the sun, and it is associated with adverse moral and behavioral qualities, while white skin has a colonial notion of power and superiority.[82] The stereotype of white skin is also reflected in the South Asian film industry. Matrimonial columns and websites highlight the role of skin color in marriage preference by the partners.

The preference for fair skin in Asians has been targeted by fairness cream manufacturers. In Asian countries like India, Japan, Korea, China, and Thailand, skin fairness has been considered a cultural marker of class, wealth, and social status.[83] It is not just women, but lately, fairness creams have been launched exclusively for men. Survey shows that a large number of Indian men are already using them or interested in using them.[84] Advertisements project in society that fair skin is a necessary requisition for success in both the professional and the personal domain. They portray fair skin as a source of attractiveness toward the opposite sex and enhanced confidence in job interviews and job performance as well.

The increasing use of skin fairness products is considered a public health, environmental justice, and social justice issue due to the harmful health side effects and the potential reinforcement of racial and social inequalities.[85,86] An Indian study analyzed skin fairness product use among 1,992 women and men. They showed that 37.6% of the sample currently use skin fairness products, with women being twice more likely to use them. Additionally, 17% sample reported past experiences of adverse side effects, and adverts were the most common prompts for using fairness products.[87]

14.3.4.2 Body Dysmorphic Disorder

Body dysmorphic disorder is characterized by a distorted perception of one's body image.[88] Gender-specific body image perceptions exist. Women have preoccupation with body image distortion, especially with the breasts, hips, legs, and body weight, with particular emphasis on skin, hair, or nose,[89,90] while men have body image distortion, especially with the genitals, height, excess body hair, thinning hair, body build, and muscle size.[91]

In BDD, patients possess unrealistic expectations about the outcomes of cosmetic surgeries, and they frequently experience dissatisfaction after the surgery. (See footnote 91). Hence, BDD can be considered a contraindication to cosmetic surgeries and procedures.[92]

BDD patients manifest global functioning impairment, and due to their preoccupation with their body image defect, they exhibit compulsive behaviors such as mirror checking or self-mutilating surgery.[93]

Some studies have provided evidence that mild- to moderate-level BDD patients (who have no impairment in global functioning and have realistic psychosocial expectations) can benefit from cosmetic procedures. Thus, identifying the level of BDD based on emotional distress, avoidance behavior, and global functioning impairment may help in decision-making during cosmetic procedures.[94,95]

Sociocultural influences of idealistic images and the availability of quick-fix procedures are increasing mentalhealth issues. People with BDD most likely seek quick-fix procedures such as botox and dermal fillers. These people seek quick-fix procedures that ultimately do not solve the underlying psychological condition.[96] De Aquino, Haddad, and Ferreira[97] showed that the patient's experienced self-esteem sustainably improved after a BoNT-A and dermal filler treatment. Another study by Dayan, Arkins, Patel, and Gal[98] showed significant improvement in QOL and an increase in the overall experienced self-esteem, as well as self-worth based on looks, with the treatment of BoNT-A.

It is considered that patient satisfaction after BoNT-A treatment is not only due to improved aesthetic results but also due to the increased positive effect due to the treatment.[99] On these lines, Lewis and Bowler (See footnote 99) showed a positive influence on the patient's mood regardless of the patient's satisfaction with the aesthetic results after the treatment of BoNT-A for glabella frown lines.

14.4 Conclusion

Inflammatory, granulomatous, scarring, and pigmentary skin and hair diseases that are specific to skin-of-color patients have been found to have significant psychological disturbances in a majority of them and mental disorders in a few patients, which have shown to negatively impact the QOL of these patients. Since these conditions are considered cosmetic in nature, the burden of disease on QOL is generally not given importance in treating these patients. We understand from this chapter that the psychosocial effects of the disease at times may even be greater than the physical impact of the disorder, making it difficult for these patients to adapt to these changes in life.

Resilience is a developing area in the field of psychodermatology. In skin diseases, resilience is characterized by positive adaptation and recovery from the trauma. It is understood from this chapter that body image, self-esteem, and negative cognitions have been the major psychological aspects affecting the QOL of these patients. Resilient enhancement techniques bolster their adaptive coping styles to deal with their adversity, making them more accepting of their condition, improving their positive effect, and making them more optimistic about their health and future.

These diseases are not just cosmetic disfigurement, but they come along with severe psychological complications and QOL impairment. Hence, along with medical treatment, psychological intervention helps these patients cope with their condition. Such psychological interventions help the patient recover soon, adhere to medications, and help in adjusting to the adversities.

Frequently Asked Questions

1. *Q: How does my skin/health get affected by my emotions?*
   A: Researchers have provided evidence that a person's emotional state can have a huge influence on immune function. Stress, depression, anxiety, and other psychological variables are found to be the major contributing factors to skin diseases.

2. *Q: How do I understand what stressors affect my skin diseases?*
   A: There are two types of stress: eustress and distress. Distress is unpleasant, and it can evoke stress hormones such as cortisol resulting in many physical issues, including skin diseases.

3. *Q: What are the ways to manage/handle/cope with my stress?*
   A: Managing worries, negative moods, and any other unpleasant emotions like anger by practicing relaxation techniques or any psychotherapy is very important. Being ignorant and repressing unpleasant emotions can cause many psychological issues and health hazards.

4. *Q: How can I improve my self-care?*
   A: Being mindful of our thoughts, emotions, and behaviors is the first step in self-care. Practicing positive self-talks and meaningful and happiness activities are as important as goal-directed activities. Self-compassion and self-acceptance are important aspects of developing a strong core self-concept. A happy mind is required for a healthy body.

5. *Q: I had difficulty dealing with my emotions in the past, but currently, I am fine. Can my past difficulties still trouble me in the present?*
   A: Past emotional disturbances, when left unresolved, can still trouble the present emotional well-being. An individual can develop self-critical thoughts and self-defeating behaviors, which could lead to various psychiatric disorders and also somatic complaints in many people.

Notes

1 Peter Salovey et al.,"Emotional states and physical health," *American Psychologist* 55, no. 1 (March 2000): 110–121, https://doi.org/10A037// 0003-O66X.55.1.110.

2 John B. Jemmott III and Steven E. Locke, "Psychosocial factors, immunologic mediation, and human susceptibility to infectious diseases: How much do we know?" *Psychological Bulletin* 95, no. 1 (1984): 78–108, https://doi.org/10.1037/0033-2909.95.1.78.

3 Parker Magin, David Sibbritt and Kylie Bailey, "The relationship between psychiatric illnesses and skin disease: A longitudinal analysis of young Australian women," *Archives of Dermatology* 145, no. 8 (2009 Aug): 896–902, https://doi.org/10.1001/archdermatol.2009.155.

4 Shanu Kohli Kurd et al., "The risk of depression, anxiety, and suicidality in patients with psoriasis: A population-based cohort study," *Archives of Dermatology* 146, no. 8(2010): 891–895, https://doi.org/10.1001/archdermatol.2010.186.

5 Orest Hurko and Thomas T Provost, "Neurology and the skin. Neurology and medicine," *Journal of Neurology, Neurosurgery, and Psychiatry* 66, no. 4 (April 1999): 417–430.

6 Jack Green and Rodney D. Sinclair, "Perceptions of acne vulgaris in final year medical student written examination answers," *Australian Journal of Dermatology* 42, no. 2 (May 2001): 98–101.

7 Angelo Picari and Damiano Abeni, "Stressful life events and skin diseases: Disentangling evidence from myth," *Psychotherapy and Psychosomatics* 70, no. 3 (May 2001): 118–136, http://doi.org/10.1159/000056237.

8 Chris E. Griffiths and Helen L. Richards, "Psychological influences in psoriasis," *Clinical and Experimental Dermatology* 26, no. 4 (July 2001): 338–342, http://doi.org/10.1046/j.1365-2230.2001.00834.x.

9 Amit Garg et al.,"Psychological stress perturbs epidermal permeability barrier homeostasis: Implications for the pathogenesis of stress-associated skin disorders," *Archives of Dermatology* 137, no. 1 (February 2001): 53–59.

10 Sunil Dogra and Savita Yadav, "Psoriasis in India: Prevalence and pattern," *Indian Journal of Dermatology Venereology and Leprology* 76, no. 6 (2010): 595–601, https://doi.org/10.4103/0378-6323.72443.

11 Selye Hans, "Stress and the general adaptation syndrome," *British Medical Journal* 4667 (July 1950): 1384–1392.

12 George Chrousos, "Stress and disorders of the stress system," *Nature Reviews Endocrinology* 5, no. 7 (August 2009): 374–381, http://doi.org/10.1038/nrendo.2009.106.

13 Kenneth M. Hargreaves, "Neuroendocrine markers of stress," *Anesthesia Progress* 37, no. 2–3 (June 1990): 99–105.

14 Suniya S. Luthar, Dante Cicchetti and Bronwyn Becker, "The construct of resilience: A critical evaluation and guidelines for future work," *Child Development* 71, no. 3 (May 2000): 543–562, https://doi.org/10.1111/1467-8624.00164.

15 Alex Zautra, Anne Arewasikporn and Mary C. Davis, "Resilience: Promoting well-being through recovery, sustainability, and growth," *Research in Human Development* 7, no. 3 (July 2010): 221–238, https://doi.org/10.1080/15427609.2010.50443.

16 Caroline S. Koblenzer, "Psychosomatic concepts in dermatology. A dermatologist-psychoanalyst's viewpoint," *Archives of Dermatology* 119, no. 6 (June 1983): 501–512, https://doi.org/10.1001/archderm.1983.01650300055017.

17 Marta Kieć-Swierczyńska, et al., "The role of psychological factors and psychiatric disorders in skin diseases," *Medycyna Pracy* 57, no. 6 (February 2006): 551–555.

18 Ramendranath Halder et al., "Incidence of common dermatoses in a predominantly black dermatologic practice," *Cutis* 32, no. 4 (October 1983): 388–390.

19 Pearl Grimes, "White patches and bruised souls: Advances in the pathogenesis and treatment of vitiligo," *Journal of the American Academy of Dermatology* 51, no. 1 (August 2004): 5–7, https://doi.org/10.1016/j.jaad.2004.01.007.

20 Pooja Pahwa et al.,"The psychosocial impact of vitiligo in Indian patients," *Indian Journal of Dermatology, Venereology and Leprology* 79, no. 5 (September 2013): 679–685, https://doi.org/10.4103/0378-6323.116737.

21 Mahsa Saleki and Ameneh Yazdanfar, "Prevalence and frequency of depression in patients with vitiligo," *International Journal of Current Microbiology and Applied Sciences* 4, no. 3 (2015): 437–445.

22 Abdulrahman A.A. Amer and Xing-Hua Gao, "Quality of life in patients with vitiligo: An analysis of the dermatology life quality index outcome over the past two decades," *International Journal of Dermatology* 55, no. 6 (January 2016): 608–614, https://doi.org/10.1111/ijd.13198.

23 K-Y. Wang, K-H. Wang and Z-P. Zhang, "Health-related quality of life and marital quality of vitiligo patients in China," *Journal of the European Academy of Dermatology and Venereology* 25, no. 4 (April 2011): 429–435, https://doi.org/10.1111/j.1468-3083.2010.03808.x.

24 May W. Linthorst Homan et al., "The burden of vitiligo: Patient characteristics associated with quality of life," *Journal of the American Academy of Dermatology* 61, no. 3 (August 2009): 411–420, https://doi.org/10.1016/j.jaad.2009.03.022.

25 May W. Linthorst Homan et al., "Characteristics of patients with universal vitiligo and health-related quality of life," *Archives of Dermatology* 144, no. 8 (August 2008): 1062–1064.

26 Christian Kruger and Karin U. Schallreuter, "Cumulative life course impairment in vitiligo," *Current Problems in Dermatology* 44 (2013): 102–117, https://doi.org/10.1159/000350010.

27 Pearl Grimes, "Melasma. Etiologic and therapeutic considerations," *Archives of Dermatology* 131, no. 12 (December 1995): 1453–1457, https://doi.org/10.1001/archderm.131.12.1453.

28 Anthony Rossi and Maritza I. Perez, "Cosmetic concerns in melasma. Part 1: Pathogenesis and clinical considerations," *Cosmetic Dermatology* 24, no. 11 (November 2011): 511–513.

29 Roberto Arenas, "Melasma," in *Arenas R. Dermatología: Atlas, Diagnóstico y Tratamiento* (Mexico City, Mexico: Interamericana McGraw-Hill, 1996), 96.

30 J. Jiang et al., "The effect of melasma on self-esteem: A pilot study," *International Journal of Women's Dermatology* 4, no. 1 (March 2018): 38–42.

31 Rajesh Balkrishnan et al., "Development and validation of a health-related quality of life instrument for women with melasma," *British Journal of Dermatology* 149, no. 2 (September 2003): 572–577, https://doi.org/10.1016/S1098-3015(10)63963-0.

32 Balkrishnan et al., "Development and validation," 572–577.

33 Arturo R. Dominguez et al., "Melasma in Latina patients: Cross-cultural adaptation and validation of a quality-of-life questionnaire in Spanish language," *Journal of the American Academy of Dermatology* 55, no. 1 (August 2006): 59–66.

34 Halder et al., "Incidence of common dermatoses," 388–390.

35 Susan C. Taylor et al., "Acne vulgaris in skin of color," *Journal of the American Academy of Dermatology* 46, no. 2 (February 2002): 98–106, https://doi.org/10.1067/mjd.2002.120791.

36 Rebat Halder, Howard L. Brooks and Valerie D. Callender, "Acne in ethnic skin," *Dermatologic Clinics* 21, no. 4 (November 2003): 609–615.

37 M.M. Polenghi, S. Zizak and Enrico Molinari, "Emotions and acne," *Dermatology and Psychosomatics* 3, no. 1 (January 2002): 20–25, https://doi.org/10.1159/000051359.

38 Şebnem Aktan, Erol Özmen and B. Sanli, "Anxiety, depression, and nature of acne vulgaris in adolescents," *International Journal of Dermatology* 39, no. 5 (May 2000): 354–357.

39 Victoria Grahame et al., "The psychological correlates of treatment efficacy in acne," *Dermatology and Psychosomatics* 3, no. 3 (October 2002): 119–125, https://doi.org/10.1159/000066582.

40 Gavneet K. Pruthi and Nandita Babu, "Physical and psychosocial impact of acne in adult females," *Indian Journal of Dermathology* 57, no. 1 (March 2012): 26–29, https://doi.org/10.4103/0019-5154.92672.

41 Behnaz Behnam et al., "Psychological impairments in the patients with acne," *Indian Journal of Dermatology* 58, no. 1 (February 2013): 26–29, https://doi.org/10.4103/0019-5154.105281.

42 Rebecca Jane Lasek and M.M. Chren, "Acne vulgaris and the quality of life of adult dermatology patients," *Archives of Dermatology* 134, no. 4 (April 1998): 454–458.

43 Valerie D. Callender et al., "Racial differences in clinical characteristics, perceptions and behaviors, and psychosocial impact of adult female acne," *Journal of Clinical and Aesthetic Dermatology* 7, no. 7 (July 2014): 19–31.

44 Joslyn S. Kirby et al., "Association of resilience with depression and health-related quality of life for patients with hidradenitis suppurativa," *JAMA Dermatology* 153, no. 12 (November 2017), https://doi.org/10.1001/jamadermatol.2017.3596.

45 Leman Inanc, Sema Inanir and Ece Yazla, "Psychological resilience in patients with acne vulgaris," *Klinik Psikofarmakoloji Bulteni* 25, no. 1 (2015): 169–S170.

46 Priyanka Jain, "Perceived stress, Optimism and social appearance anxiety in patients with skin diseases: A comparative study," *IRA–International Journal of Management & Social Sciences* 3, no. 1 (April 2016), ISSN 2455-2267.

47 Nigel Hunt and Sue McHale, "The psychological impact of alopecia," *British Medical Journal* 331 (7522) (November 2005): 951–953, https://doi.org/10.1136/bmj.331.7522.951.

48 Nigel Hunt and Sue McHale, "Reported experiences of persons with alopecia areata," *Journal of Loss and Trauma* 10, no. 1 (January 2005): 33–50, https://doi.org/10.1080/15325020490890633.

49 Ina M. Hadshiew et al., "Burden of hair loss: Stress and the underestimated psychological impact of telogen effluvius and androgenetic alopecia," *Journal of Investigative Dermatology* 123, no. 3 (September 2004): 455–457, https://doi.org/10.1111/j.0022-202X.2004.23237.x.

50 John Y.M. Koo et al., "Alopecia areata and increased prevalence of psychiatric disorders," *International Journal of Dermatology* 33, no. 12 (January 1994): 849–850.

51 Hunt and McHale, "The psychological impact," 951–953.

52 Ncoza C. Dlova et al., "Quality of life in South African Black women with alopecia: A pilot study," *International Journal of Dermatology* 55, no. 8 (November 2015): 875–881, https://doi.org/10.1111/ijd.13042.

53 Min Zhang and Nan Zhang, "Quality of life assessment in patients with alopecia areata and androgenetic alopecia in the People's Republic of China," *Patient Preference and Adherence* 11 (January 2017): 151–155, https://doi.org/10.2147/PPA.S121218.

54 Marina Menezes, Mariana López and Josiane da Silva Delvan, "Psychotherapy of child with universal alopecia areata: Developing resilience," *Paidéia* 20, no. 46 (August 2010): 261–267.

55 Adebola Ogunbiyi, "Pseudofolliculitis barbae; current treatment options," *Clinical, Cosmetic and Investigational Dermatology* 12 (April 2019): 241–247, https://doi.org/10.2147/CCID.S149250.

56 Chad D. Housewright et al., "Excisional surgery (scalpectomy) for dissecting cellulitis of the scalp," *Dermatologic Surgery* 37, no. 8 (June 2011): 1189–1191.

57 Mairin A. Jerome and Donald Laub, "Dissecting cellulitis of the scalp: Case discussion, unique considerations, and treatment options," *Eplasty* 14 (June 2014): ic17.

58 Jugpal Arneja et al., "Management of fulminant dissecting cellulitis of the scalp in the pediatric population: Case report and literature review," *Canadian Journal of Plastic Surgery* 15, no. 4 (December 2007): 211–214, https://doi.org/10.1177/229255030701500406.

59 Chuma J. Chike-Obi, Patrick D. Cole and Anthony E. Brissett, "Keloids: Pathogenesis, clinical features, and management," *Seminars in Plastic Surgery* 23, no. 3 (August 2009): 178–184, https://doi.org/10.1055/s-0029-1224797.

60 Neil Aaronson et al., "Translation, validation, and norming of the Dutch language version of the SF-36 Health Survey in community and chronic disease populations," *Journal of Clinical Epidemiology* 51, no. 11(December 1998): 1055–1068.

61 Casimir Kouwenberg et al., "Emotional quality of life is severely affected by keloid disease: Pain and itch are the main determinants of burden," *Plastic and Reconstructive Surgery* 136, no. 4 (September 2015): 150–151, https://doi.org/10.1097/01.prs.0000472474.17120.84.

62 Oliver Seifert et al., "Quality of life of patients with keloid and hypertrophic scarring," *Archives of Dermatological Research* 297, no. 10 (May 2006), https://doi.org/433-38, 10.1007/s00403-006-0651-7.

63 Takashi Koyama et al., "Radiologic manifestations of sarcoidosis in various organs," *Radiographics* 24, no. 1 (January 2004): 87–104.

64 Christopher E. Cox et al., "Health related quality of life of persons with sarcoidosis," *Chest* 125, no. 3 (April 2004): 997–1004, PMID: 15006960.6.

65 Helen J. Michielsen et al., "Fatigue is associated with quality of life in sarcoidosis patients," *Chest* 130, no. 4 (October 2006): 989–949. PMID: 17035429, https://doi.org/10.1378/chest.130.4.989.

66 R.M. Wirnsberger et al., "Evaluation of quality of life in sarcoidosis patients," *Respiratory Medicine* 92, no. 5 (June 1998): 750–756, https://doi.org/10.1016/S0954-6111(98)90007-5.

67 Jolanda de Vries and M. Drent, "Relationship between perceived stress and sarcoidosis in a Dutch patient population," *Sarcoidosis Vasculitis and Diffuse Lung Diseases* 21, no. 1 (April 2004): 57–63.

68 Jolanda de Vries, Elyse E. Lower and M. Drent, "Quality of life in sarcoidosis: Assessment and management," *Seminars in Respiratory and Critical Care Medicine* 31, no. 4 (August 2010): 485–493, https://doi.org/10.1055/s-0030-1262216.

69 Elizabeth A. Klonoff and Mary Ellen Kleinhenz, "Psychological factors in sarcoidosis: The relationship between life stress and pulmonary function," *Sarcoidosis* 10, no. 2 (October 1993): 118–124.

70 Ryoichi Kamide, "Atopic dermatitis: Psychological care," *Japan Medical Association Journal* 45, no. 11(November 2002): 490–495.

71 Ellis Kam Lun Hon et al., "Quality of life and psychosocial issues are important outcome measures in eczema treatment," *Journal of Dermatological Treatment* 26, no. 1 (February 2014): 83–89, https://doi.org/10.3109/09546634.2013.873762.

72 C.M. Absolon et al., "Psychological disturbance in atopic eczema: The extent of the problem in school-aged children," *British Journal of Dermatology* 137, no. 2 (September 1997): 241–245.

73 Kristian Reich and Mrowietz Ulrich, "Treatment goals in psoriasis," *Journal der Deutschen Dermatologischen Gesellschaft* 5, no. 7 (August): 566–574, https://doi.org/10.1111/j.1610-0387.2007.06343.x.

74 Johannes Wohlrab et al., "Recommendations for detection of individual risk for comorbidities in patients with psoriasis," *Archives of Dermatological Research* 305, no. 2 (February 2013): 91–98, https://doi.org/10.1007/s00403-013-1318-9.

75 Peter Jensen et al., "Psoriasis and new-onset depression: A Danish nationwide cohort study," *Acta Dermato-Venereologica* 96, no. 1 (June 2015): 39–42.

76 Patryk Łakuta and Hanna Przybyła-Basista, "Toward a better understanding of social anxiety and depression in psoriasis patients: The role of determinants, mediators, and moderators," *Journal of Psychosomatic Research* 94 (March 2017): 32–38, https://doi.org/10.1016/jjPsychores.2017.01.007.

77 Sascha Gerdes et al., "Smoking and alcohol intake in severely affected patients with psoriasis in Germany," *Dermatology* 220, no. 1 (December 2009): 38–43, https://doi.org/10.1159/000265557.

78 Łakuta and Przybyła-Basista, "Towards a better," 32–38.

79 Helen L. Richards et al., "The contribution of perceptions of stigmatisation to disability in patients with psoriasis," *Journal of Psychosomatic Research* 50, no. 1 (January 2001): 11–15, https://doi.org/10.1016/S0022-3999(00)00210-5.

80 L.H.F. de Arruda and A.P.F. de Moraes, "The impact of psoriasis on quality of life," *British Journal of Dermatology* 144, no. 58 (May 2001): 33–36, https://doi.org/10.1046/j.1365-2133.2001.00034.x.

81 Maria Luigia Crosta et al., "Childhood trauma and resilience in psoriatic patients: A preliminary report," *Journal of Psychosomatic Research* 106 (March 2018): 25–28, https://doi.org/10.1016/j.jpsychores.2018.01.002.

82 Patricia Goon and Alison Craven, "Whose debt? Globalisation and white facing in Asia?" *Intersections: Gender, History and Culture in the Asian Context* 9 (August 2003), htpp://www.sshe.murdoch.edu.au/intersections/issue9/gooncraven.html.

83 Ophelia Dadzie and Antoine Petit, "Skin bleaching: Highlighting the misuse of cutaneous depigmenting agents," *Journal of the European Academy of Dermatology and Venereology* 23, no. 7 (April 2009): 741–750, https://doi.org/10.1111/j.1468-3083.2009.03150.x

84 Monica Chadha, "Indian men go tall, fair and handsome," last modified November 2, 2015, http://news.bbc.co.uk/go/pr/fr/-/2/hi/south_asia/4396122.stm.

85 Nadia Craddock, "Colour me beautiful: Examining the shades related to global skin tone ideals," *Journal of Aesthetic Nursing* 5, no. 6 (July 2016): 287–289, https://doi.org/10.12968/joan.2016.5.6.287.

86 Ami. R Zota and Bhavna Shamasunder, "The environmental injustice of beauty: Framing chemical exposures from beauty products as a health disparities concern," *American Journal of Obstetrics and Gynecology* 217, no. 4 (October 2017): 418.e1–418.e6, https://doi.org/10.1016/j.ajog.2017.07.020.

87 Hemal Shroff, Phillippa C. Diedrichs and Nadia Craddock, "Skin color, cultural capital, and beauty products: An investigation of the use of skin fairness products in Mumbai, India," *Frontiers in Public Health* 23, no. 5 (January 2018): 365, https://doi.org/10.3389/fpubh.2017.00365

88 Mohammad Alavi, Younes Kalafi, Gholam Reza Dehbozorgi and Ali Javadpour, "Body dysmorphic disorder and other psychiatric morbidity in aesthetic rhinoplasty candidates," *Journal of Plastic Reconstruction and Aesthetic Surgery* 64, no. 6 (June 2011): 738–741.

89 Rebecca Cogwell Anderson, "Body dysmorphic disorder: Recognition and treatment," *Plastic Surgical Nursing* 23, no. 3 (February 2003): 125–128.

90 Jacob K. Dey, Masaru Ishii, Maria Phillis, Patrick J. Byrne, Kofi D. Boahene and Lisa E. Ishie, "Body dysmorphic disorder in a facial plastic and reconstructive surgery clinic: Measuring prevalence, assessing comorbidities, and validating a feasible screening instrument," *JAMA Facial Plastic Surgery* 17, no. 2 (April 2015): 137–143.

91 Iliana E. Sweis, Jamie Spitz, David R. Barry Jr and Mimis Cohen, "A review of body dysmorphic disorder in aesthetic surgery patients and the legal implications," *Aesthetic Plastic Surgery* 41, no. 4 (August 2017): 949–954.

92 Kirsty Samantha Lee, Alexa Guy, Jeremy Dale and Dieter Wolke, "Adolescent desire for cosmetic surgery: Associations with bullying and psychological functioning," *Plastic and Reconstructive Surgery* 139, no. 5 (May 2017): 1109–1118, https://doi.org/10.1097/PRS.0000000000003252.

93 Panagiotis Ziglinas, Dirk Jan Menger and Christos Georgalas, "The body dysmorphic disorder patient: To perform rhinoplasty or not?" *European Archives of Otorhinolaryngology* 271, no. 9 (November 2014): 2355–2358, https://doi.org/10.1007/s00405-013-2792-6.

94 Paolo Giovanni Morselli and Filippo Boriani, "Should plastic surgeons operate on patients diagnosed with body dysmorphic disorders?" *Plastic and Reconstructive Surgery* 130, no. 4 (October 2012): 620–622, https://doi.org/10.1097/PRS.0b013e318262f65b.

95 Laura Bowyer, Georgina Krebs, David Mataix-Cols, David Veale and Benedetta Monzani, "A critical review of cosmetic treatment outcomes in body dysmorphic disorder," *Body Image* 19 (December 2016): 1–8, https://doi.org/10.1016/j.bodyim.2016.07.001.

96 "Here's why cosmetic clinics will screen botox patients for mental health problems," *Tech Times*, last modified April 30, 2019, www.techtimes.com/articles/242579/20190430/heres-why-cosmetic-clinics-will-screen-botox-patients-for-mental-health-problems.htm.

97 Marcello Simão de Aquino, Alessandra Haddad and Lydia Masako Ferreira, "Assessment of quality of life in patients who underwent minimally invasive cosmetic procedures," *Aesthetic Plastic Surgery* 37 (March 2013): 497–503.

98 Steven Dayan, John P. Arkins, Amit B. Patel and Thomas J. Gal, "A double-blind, randomized, placebo-controlled health-outcomes survey of the effect of botulinum toxin type a injections on quality of life and self-esteem," *Dermatologic Surgery* 36, no. 4 (December 2010): 2088–2097.

99 Michael B. Lewis and Patrick J. Bowler, "Botulinum toxin cosmetic therapy correlates with a more positive mood," *Journal of Cosmetic Dermatology* 8, no. 1 (March 2009): 24–26.

Bibliography

Aaronson, Neil, Martin Muller, Peter D.A. Cohen, Marie-Louise Essink-Bot, Minne Fekkes, Robbert Sanderman, Mirjam A.G. Sprangers, Adrienne te Velde and Erik Verrips. "Translation, validation, and norming of the Dutch language version of the SF-36 Health Survey in community and chronic disease populations." *Journal of Clinical Epidemiology* 51, no. 11 (December 1998): 1055–1068.

Absolon, C.M., David Cottrell, S.M. Eldridge and M.T. Glover. "Psychological disturbance in atopic eczema: The extent of the problem in school-aged children." *British Journal of Dermatology* 137, no. 2 (September 1997): 241–245.

Aktan, Şebnem, Erol Özmen and B. Sanli. "Anxiety, depression, and nature of acne vulgaris in adolescents." *International Journal of Dermatology* 39, no. 5 (May 2000): 354–357.

Alavi, Mohammad, Younes Kalafi, Gholam Reza Dehbozorgi, and Ali Javadpour. "Bodydysmorphic disorder and other psychiatric morbidity in aesthetic rhinoplasty candidates." *Journal of Plastic Reconstruction and Aesthetic Surgery* 64, no. 6 (June 2011): 738–741.

Amer, Abdulrahman A.A. and Xing-Hua Gao. "Quality of life in patients with vitiligo: An analysis of the dermatology life quality index outcome over the past two decades." *International Journal of Dermatology* 55, no. 6 (January 2016): 608–614. https://doi.org/10.1111/ijd.13198.

Anderson, Rebecca Cogwell. "Body dysmorphic disorder: Recognition and treatment." *Plastic Surgical Nursing* 23, no. 3 (February 2003): 125–128.

Arenas, Roberto. "Melasma." In: *Arenas R. Dermatología: Atlas, Diagnóstico y Tratamiento*, 96. Mexico City, Mexico: Interamericana McGraw-Hill, 1996.

Arneja, Jugpal S., Christopher N. Vashi, Eti Gursel and Joseph L Lelli. "Management of fulminant dissecting cellulitis of the scalp in the pediatric population: Case report and literature review." *Canadian Journal of Plastic Surgery* 15, no. 4 (December 2007): 211–214. https://doi.org/10.1177/229255030701500406.

Balkrishnan, Rajesh, Amy McMichael, Fabian Camacho, F. Saltzberg, T.S. Housman, S. Grummer, S.R. Feldman and M.M. Chren. "Development and validation of a health-related quality of life instrument for women with hermop." *British Journal of Dermatology* 149, no. 2 (September 2003): 572–577. https://doi.org/10.1016/S1098-3015(10)63963-0.

Behnam, Behnaz, Ramin Taheri, Raheb Ghorbani and Peyvand Allameh. "Psychological impairments in the patients with acne." *Indian Journal of Dermatology* 58, no. 1 (February 2013): 26–29. https://doi.org/10.4103/0019-5154.105281.

Bowyer, Laura, Georgina Krebs, David Mataix-Cols, David Veale and Benedetta Monzani. "A critical review of cosmetic treatment outcomes in body dysmorphic disorder." *Body Image* 19 (December 2016): 1–8. https://doi.org/10.1016/j.bodyim.2016.07.001.

Callender, Valerie D., Andrew F. Alexis, Selena Daniels, Ariane K. Kawata, Caroline T. Burk, Teresa K. Wilcox and Susan C. Taylor. "Racial differences in clinical characteristics, perceptions and behaviors, and psychosocial impact of adult female acne." *Journal of Clinical and Aesthetic Dermatology* 7, no. 7 (July 2014): 19–31.

Chadha, Monica. "Indian men go tall, fair and handsome." Last modified November 2, 2015. http://news.bbc.co.uk/go/pr/fr/-/2/hi/south_asia/4396122.stm.

Chike-Obi, Chuma J., Patrick D. Cole and Anthony E. Brissett. "Keloids: Pathogenesis, clinical features, and management." *Seminars in Plastic Surgery* 23, no. 3 (August 2009): 178–184. https://doi.org/10.1055/s-0029-1224797.

Christian, Kruger and Karin U. Schallreuter. "Cumulative life course impairment in vitiligo." *Current Problems in Dermatology* 44 (2013): 102–117. https://doi.org/10.1159/000350010.

Chrousos, George. "Stress and disorders of the stress system." *Nature Reviews Endocrinology* 5, no. 7 (August 2009): 374–381. http://doi.org/10.1038/nrendo.2009.106

Cox, Christopher E., James F. Donohue, Cynthia D. Brown, Yash P. Kataria and Marc A. Judson. "Health related quality of life of persons with sarcoidosis." *Chest* 125, no. 3 (April 2004): 997–1004. PMID: 15006960.6.

Craddock, Nadia. "Colour me beautiful: Examining the shades related to global skin tone ideals." *Journal of Aesthetic Nursing* 5, no. 6 (July 2016): 287–289. https://doi.org/10.12968/joan.2016.5.6.287.

Crosta, Maria Luigia, Clara De Simone, Salvatore Di Pietro, Maria Teresa Acanfora, Giacomo Caldarola, Lorenzo Moccia and Antonino Callea. "Childhood trauma and resilience in psoriatic patients: A preliminary report." *Journal of Psychosomatic Research* 106 (March 2018): 25–28. https://doi.org/10.1016/j.jpsychores.2018.01.002.

Dadzie Ophelia and Antoine Petit. "Skin bleaching: Highlighting the misuse of cutaneous depigmenting agents." *Journal of the European Academy of Dermatology and Venereology* 23, no. 7 (April 2009): 741–750. https://doi.org/10.1111/j.1468-3083.2009.03150.

Dayan, Steven, John P. Arkins, Amit B. Patel and Thomas J Gal. "A double-blind, randomized, placebo-controlled health-outcomes survey of the effect of botulinum toxin type a injections on quality of life and self-esteem." *Dermatologic Surgery* 36, no. 4 (December 2010): 2088–2097.

De Aquino Simão, Marcello, Alessandra Haddad and Lydia Masako Ferreira. "Assessment of quality of life in patients who underwent minimally invasive cosmetic procedures." *Aesthetic Plastic Surgery* 37 (March 2013): 497–503.

De Arruda, L.H.F. and A.P.F De Moraes. "The impact of psoriasis on quality of life." *British Journal of Dermatology* 144, no. 58 (May 2001): 33–36. https://doi.org/10.1046/j.1365-2133.2001.00034.x.

De Vries, Jolanda and M. Drent. "Relationship between perceived stress and sarcoidosis in a Dutch patient population." *Sarcoidosis Vasculitis and Diffuse Lung Diseases* 21, no. 1 (April 2004): 57–63.

De Vries, Jolanda, Elyse E. Lower and M. Drent. "Quality of life in sarcoidosis: Assessment and management." *Seminars in Respiratory and Critical Care Medicine* 31, no. 4 (August 2010): 485–493. https://doi.org/10.1055/s-0030-1262216.

Dey, Jacob K, Masaru Ishii, Maria Phillis, Patrick J, Byrne, Kofi D. Boahene and Lisa E. Ishie. "Body dysmorphic disorder in a facial plastic and reconstructive surgery clinic: Measuring prevalence, assessing comorbidities, and validating a feasible screening instrument." *JAMA Facial Plastic Surgery* 17, no. 2 (April 2015): 137–143.

Dlova, Ncoza C., Gabriella Fabbrocini, Carlo Lauro, Maria Spano, Antonella Tosti and Richard J. Hift. "Quality of life in South African Black women with alopecia: A pilot study." *International Journal of Dermatology* 55, no. 8 (November 2015): 875–881. https://doi.org/10.1111/ijd.13042.

Dogra, Sunil and Savita Yadav. "Psoriasis in India: Prevalence and pattern." *Indian Journal of Dermatology Venereology and Leprology* 76, no. 6 (2010): 595–601. https://doi.org/10.4103/0378–6323.72443.

Dominguez, Arturo R., Rajesh Balkrishnan, Allison R. Ellzey and Amit G. Pandya. "Melasma in Latina patients: Cross-cultural adaptation and validation of a quality-of-life questionnaire in Spanish language." *Journal of the American Academy of Dermatology* 55, no. 1 (August 2006): 59–66.

Garg, Amit, M.M. Chren, Laura Sands, Mary S. Matsui, Kenneth D. Marenus, Kenneth R. Feingold and Peter M. Elias. "Psychological stress perturbs epidermal permeability barrier homeostasis: Implications for the pathogenesis of stress-associated skin disorders." *Archives of Dermatology* 137, no. 1 (February 2001): 53–59.

Gerdes, Sascha, V.A. Zahl, Michael Weichenthal and U. Mrowietz. "Smoking and alcohol intake in severely affected patients with psoriasis in Germany." *Dermatology* 220, no. 1 (December 2009): 38–43. https://doi.org/10.1159/000265557.

Goon, Patricia and Alison Craven. "Whose debt? Globalisation and white facing in Asia?" *Intersections: Gender, History and Culture in the Asian Context* 9 (August 2003). http://www.sshe.murdoch.edu.au/intersections/issue9/gooncraven.html.

Grahame, Victoria., D.C. Dick, C.M. Morton, O. Watkins and K.G Power. "The psychological correlates of treatment efficacy in acne." *Dermatology and Psychosomatics* 3, no. 3 (October 2002): 119–125. https://doi.org/10.1159/000066582.

Green, Jack and Rodney D Sinclair. "Perceptions of acne vulgaris in final year medical student written examination answers." *Australian Journal of Dermatology* 42, no. 2 (May 2001): 98–101.

Griffiths, Chris E. and Helen L. Richards. "Psychological influences in psoriasis." *Clinical and Experimental Dermatology* 26, no. 4 (July 2001): 338–342. http://doi.org/10.1046/j.1365-2230.2001.00834.x.

Grimes, Pearl. "Melasma. Etiologic and therapeutic considerations." *Archives of Dermatology* 131, no. 12 (December 1995): 1453–1457. https://doi.org/10.1001/archderm.131.12.1453.

Grimes, Pearl. "White patches and bruised souls: Advances in the pathogenesis and treatment of vitiligo." *Journal of the American Academy of Dermatology* 51, no. 1 (August 2004): 5–7. https://doi.org/10.1016/j.jaad.2004.01.007.

Hadshiew, Ina M., Kerstin Foitzik, Petra C. Arck and Ralf Paus. "Burden of hair loss: Stress and the underestimated psychological impact of telogen effluvius and androgenetic alopecia." *Journal of Investigative Dermatology* 123, no. 3 (September 2004): 455–457. https://doi.org/10.1111/j.0022-202X.2004.23237.x.

Halder, Ramendranath, Pearl Grimes, C.I. McLaurin, M.A. Kress and J.A. Kenney. "Incidence of common dermatoses in a predominantly black dermatologic practice." *Cutis* 32, no. 4 (October 1983): 388–390.

Halder, Rebat, Howard L. Brooks and Valerie D. Callender. "Acne in ethnic skin." *Dermatologic Clinics* 21, no. 4 (November 2003): 609–615.

Hargreaves. Kenneth M. "Neuroendocrine markers of stress." *Anesthesia Progress* 37, no. 2–3 (June 1990): 99–105.

"Here's why cosmetic clinics will screen Botox patients for mental health problems." *Tech Times*. Last modified April 30, 2019.www.techtimes.com/articles/242579/20190430/heres-why-cosmetic-clinics-will-screen-botox-patients-for-mental-health-problems.htm.

Hon, Ellis Kam Lun, N.H. Pong, Terence C.W. Poon, Dorothy F. Chan, Ting F. Leung, Kelly Y.C. Lai, Y.K. Wing and Nai Ming Luk. "Quality of life and psychosocial issues are important outcome measures in eczema treatment." *Journal of Dermatological Treatment* 26, no. 1 (February 2014): 83–89. https://doi.org/10.3109/09546634.2013.873762.

Housewright, Chad D., Erica Rensvold, James Tidwell, Dennis Lynch and David F. Butler. "Excisional surgery (scalpectomy) for dissecting cellulitis of the scalp." *Dermatologic Surgery* 37, no. 8 (June 2011): 1189–1191.

Hunt, Nigel and Sue McHale. "The psychological impact of alopecia." *British Medical Journal* 331 (7522) (November 2005): 951–953. https://doi.org/10.1136/bmj.331.7522.951.

Hunt, Nigel and Sue McHale. "Reported experiences of persons with alopecia areata." *Journal of Loss and Trauma* 10, no. 1 (January 2005): 33–50. https://doi.org/10.1080/15325020490890633.

Hurko, Orest and Thomas T Provost. "Neurology and the skin. Neurology and medicine." *Journal of Neurology, Neurosurgery, and Psychiatry* 66, no. 4 (April 1999): 417–430.

Inanc, Leman, Sema Inanir and Ece Yazla. "Psychological resilience in patients with acne vulgaris." *Klinik Psikofarmakoloji Bulteni* 25, no. 1 (2015): 169–170.

Jain, Priyanka. "Perceived stress, Optimism and social appearance anxiety in patients with skin diseases: A comparative study." *IRA–International Journal of Management & Social Sciences* 3, no. 1 (April 2016). ISSN 2455-2267.

Jemmott III, John B. and Steven E. Locke. "Psychosocial factors, immunologic mediation, and human susceptibility to infectious diseases: How much do we know?" *Psychological Bulletin* 95, no. 1 (1984): 78–108. https://doi.org/10.1037/0033-2909.95.1.78.

Jensen, Peter, Ole Ahlehoff, Alexander Egeberg, Gunnar Gislason, Peter Riis Hansen and Lone Skov. "Psoriasis and New-onset Depression: A Danish Nationwide Cohort Study." *Acta Dermato-Venereologica* 96, no. 1 (June 2015): 39–42.

Jerome, Mairin A. and Donald Laub, "Dissecting cellulitis of the scalp: Case discussion, unique considerations, and treatment options." *Eplasty* 14 (June 2014): ic17.

Jiang, J., O. Akinseye, A. Tovar-Garza and A.G. Pandya. "The effect of hermop on self-esteem: A pilot study." *International Journal of Women's Dermatology* 4, no. 1 (March 2018): 38–42.

Kieć-Swierczyńska, Marta, Bohdan Dudek, Beata Krecisz, Dominika Swierczyńska-Machura, Wojciech Dudek, Adrianna Garnczarek and Katarzyna Turczyn. "The role of psychological factors and psychiatric disorders in skin diseases." *Medycyna Pracy* 57, no. 6 (February 2006): 551–555.

Kirby, Joslyn S., Muqadam Butt, Solveig Esmann and Gregor B.E. Jemec. "Association of resilience with depression and health-related quality of life for patients with hidradenitis suppurativa." *JAMA Dermatology* 153, no. 12 (November 2017). https://doi.org/10.1001/jamadermatol.2017.3596.

Klonoff, Elizabeth A. and Mary Ellen Kleinhenz. "Psychological factors in sarcoidosis: The relationship between life stress and pulmonary function." *Sarcoidosis* 10, no. 2 (October 1993): 118–124.

Koblenzer, Caroline S. "Psychosomatic concepts in dermatology. A dermatologist-psychoanalyst's viewpoint." *Archives of Dermatology* 119, no. 6 (June 1983): 501–512. https://doi.org/10.1001/archderm.1983.01650300055017.

Koo, John Y.M., William V.R. Shellow, Chris P. Hallman and Joel E. Edwards. "Alopecia areata and increased prevalence of psychiatric disorders." *International Journal of Dermatology* 33, no. 12 (January 1994): 849–850.

Kouwenberg, Casimir, Eveline Bijlard, Reiner Timman, Steven E.R Hovius, J.J.V. Busschbach and Marc A.M. Mureau. "Emotional quality of life is severely affected by keloid disease: Pain and itch are the main determinants of burden." *Plastic and Reconstructive Surgery* 136, no. 4 (September 2015): 150–151. https://doi.org/10.1097/01.prs.0000472474.17120.84.

Koyama, Takashi, Hiroyuki Ueda, Kaori Togashi, Shigeaki Umeoka, Masako Kataoka and Sonoko Nagai. "Radiologic manifestations of sarcoidosis in various organs." *Radiographics* 24, no. 1 (January 2004): 87–104.

Kurd, Shanu Kohli., Andrea B. Troxel, Paul Crits-Christoph and Joel M. Gelfand. "The risk of depression, anxiety, and suicidality in patients with psoriasis: A population-based cohort study." *Archives of Dermatology* 146, no. 8 (2010): 891–895. https://doi.org/10.1001/archdermatol.2010.186.

Łakuta, Patryk and Hanna Przybyła-Basista. "Toward a better understanding of social anxiety and depression in psoriasis patients: The role of determinants, mediators, and moderators." *Journal of Psychosomatic Research* 94 (March 2017): 32–38. https://doi.org/10.1016/jjPsychores.2017.01.007.

Lasek, Rebecca Jane and M.M. Chren. "Acne vulgaris and the quality of life of adult dermatology patients." *Archives of Dermatology* 134, no. 4 (April 1998): 454–458.

Lee, Kirsty Samantha, Alexa Guy, Jeremy Dale and Dieter Wolke. "Adolescent desire for cosmetic surgery: Associations with bullying and psychological functioning." *Plastic and Reconstructive Surgery* 139, no. 5 (May 2017): 1109–1118. https://doi.org/10.1097/PRS.0000000000003252.

Lewis, Michael B. and Patrick J. Bowler. "Botulinum toxin cosmetic therapy correlates with a more positive mood." *Journal of Cosmetic Dermatology* 8, no. 1 (March 2009): 24–26.

Linthorst, Homan May W., Mirjam A.G. Sprangers, John de Korte, Jan D. Bos and J. (Wietze) P.W. van der Veen. "Characteristics of patients with universal vitiligo and health-related quality of life." *Archives of Dermatology* 144, no. 8 (August 2008): 1062–1064. https://doi.org/10.1001/archderm.144.8.1062.

Linthorst, Homan May W., Phyllis I. Spuls, John de Korte, Jan D. Bos, Mirjam A. Sprangers and J. (Wietze) P.W. van der Veen. "The burden of vitiligo: Patient characteristics associated with quality of life." *Journal of the American Academy of Dermatology* 61, no. 3 (August 2009): 411–420. https://doi.org/10.1016/j.jaad.2009.03.022.

Luthar, Suniya S., Dante Cicchetti and Bronwyn Becker. "The construct of resilience: A critical evaluation and guidelines for future work." *Child Development* 71, no. 3 (May 2000): 543–562. https://doi.org/10.1111/1467-8624.00164.

Magin, Parker, David Sibbritt and Kylie Bailey. "The relationship between psychiatric illnesses and skin disease: A longitudinal analysis of young Australian women." *Archives of Dermatology* 145, no. 8 (2009 Aug): 896–902. https://doi.org/10.1001/archdermatol.2009.155.

McGarvey, Elizabeth L., L.D. Baum, Relana Pinkerton and L.M. Rogers. "Psychological sequelae and health-related alopecia among women with cancer." *Cancer Practice* 9, no. 6 (November 2001): 283–288.

Menezes, Marina, Mariana López and Josiane da Silva Delvan, "Psychotherapy of child with universal alopecia areata: Developing resilience." *Paidéia* 20, no. 46 (August 2010): 261–267.

Michielsen, Helen J., M. Drent, Tatjana Peros-Golubicic and Jolanda De Vries. "Fatigue is associated with quality of life in sarcoidosis patients." *Chest* 130, no. 4 (October 2006): 989–994. PMID: 17035429, https://doi.org/10.1378/chest.130.4.989.

Morselli, Paolo Giovanni and Filippo Boriani. "Should plastic surgeons operate on patients diagnosed with body dysmorphic disorders?" *Plastic and Reconstructive Surgery* 130, no. 4 (October 2012): 620–622. https://doi.org/10.1097/PRS.0b013e318262f65b.

Ogunbiyi, Adebola. "Pseudofolliculitis barbae; current treatment options." *Clinical, Cosmetic and Investigational Dermatology* 12 (April 2019): 241–247. https://doi.org/10.2147/CCID.S149250.

Pahwa, Pooja, Manju Mehta, Binod K. Khaitan, Vinod Kumar Sharma and M. Ramam. "The psychosocial impact of vitiligo in Indian patients." *Indian Journal of Dermatology, Venereology and Leprology* 79, no. 5 (September 2013): 679–685. https://doi.org/10.4103/0378-6323.116737.

Phillips, Amali. "Gendering colour: Identity, femininity and marriage in Kerala." *Anthropologica* 46, no. 2 (2004): 253–272. https://doi.org/10.2307/25606198.

Picardi, Angelo and Damiano Abeni. "Stressful life events and skin diseases: Disentangling evidence from myth." *Psychotherapy and Psychosomatics* 70, no. 3 (May 2001): 118–136. http://doi.org/10.1159/000056237.

Polenghi, M.M., S. Zizak and Enrico Molinari. "Emotions and acne." *Dermatology and Psychosomatics* 3, no. 1 (January 2002): 20–25. https://doi.org/10.1159/000051359.

Pruthi, Gavneet K. and Nandita Babu. "Physical and psychosocial impact of acne in adult females." *Indian Journal of Dermatology* 57, no. 1 (March 2012): 26–29. https://doi.org/10.4103/0019-5154.92672.

Reich, Kristian and Mrowietz Ulrich. "Treatment goals in psoriasis." *Journal der Deutschen Dermatologischen Gesellschaft* 5, no. 7 (August): 566–574. https://doi.org/10.1111/j.1610-0387.2007.06343.x.

Richards, Helen, L., Donal G. Fortune, Chris E. Griffiths and Chris J. Main. "The contribution of perceptions of hermophilesn to disability in patients with psoriasis." *Journal of Psychosomatic Research* 50, no. 1 (January 2001): 11–15. https://doi.org/10.1016/S0022-3999(00)00210.

Rossi, Anthony and Maritza I. Perez. "Cosmetic concerns in hermop, part 1: Pathogenesis and clinical considerations." *Cosmetic Dermatology* 24, no. 11 (November 2011): 511–513.

Ryoichi, Kamide. "Atopic dermatitis: Psychological care." *Japan Medical Association Journal* 45, no. 11 (November 2002): 490–495.

Saleki, Mahsa and Ameneh Yazdanfar. "Prevalence and frequency of depression in patients with vitiligo." *International Journal of Current Microbiology and Applied Sciences* 4, no. 3 (2015): 437–445.

Salovey, Peter, Alexander J. Rothman, Jerusha B. Detweiler and Wayne T. Steward. "Emotional states and physical health." *American Psychologist* 55, no. 1 (March 2000): 110–121. https://doi.org/10A037//0003-O66X.55.1.110.

Schneiderman, Neil, Gail Ironson, and Scott D. Siegel. "Stress and health: Psychological, behavioral, and biological determinants." *Annual Review of Clinical Psychology* 1 (2005): 607–628.

Seifert, Oliver, Gerhard Schmid-Ott, Peter Malewski and Ulrich Mrowietz. "Quality of life of patients with keloid and hypertrophic scarring." *Archives of Dermatological Research* 297, no. 10 (May 2006): https://doi.org/433-38, 10.1007/s00403-006-0651-7.

Selye, Hans. "Stress and the general adaptation syndrome." *British Medical Journal* 4667 (July 1950): 1384–1392.

Shroff, Hemal, Phillippa C. Diedrichs and Nadia Craddock. "Skin color, cultural capital, and beauty products: An investigation of the use of skin fairness products in Mumbai, India." *Frontiers in Public Health* 23, no. 5 (January 2018): 365. https://doi.org/10.3389/fpubh.2017.00365

Sweis Iliana E., Jamie Spitz, David R. Barry Jr and Mimis Cohen. "A review of body dysmorphic disorder in aesthetic surgery patients and the legal implications." *Aesthetic Plastic Surgery* 41, no. 4 (August 2017): 949–954.

Taylor Susan, C., Fran Cook-Bolden, Zakia Rahman and Dina Strachan. "Acne vulgaris in skin of color." *Journal of the American Academy of Dermatology* 46, no. 2 (February 2002): 98–106. https://doi.org/10.1067/mjd.2002.120791.

Vashi, Neelam A. and Howard I. Maibach. "Dermatoanthropology of ethnic skin and hair." Boston, USA: Springer, 2017.

Wang, K-Y., K-H. Wang and Z-P. Zhang. "Health-related quality of life and marital quality of vitiligo patients in China." *Journal of the European Academy of Dermatology and Venereology* 25, no. 4 (April 2011): 429–435. https://doi.org/10.1111/j.1468-3083.2010.03808.x.

Wirnsberger, R.M., Jolanda de Vries, Marinus H.M. Breteler, G.L van Heck, E.F.M. Wouters and M. Drent. "Evaluation of quality of life in sarcoidosis patients." *Respiratory Medicine* 92, no. 5 (June 1998): 750–756. https://doi.org/10.1016/S0954-6111(98)90007-5.

Wohlrab, Johannes, Gabriele Fiedler, Sascha Gerdes, Alexander Nast, Sandra Philipp, Marc Alexander Radtke, Diamant Thaçi, Wolfgang Koenig, Andreas Pfeiffer and Martin Härter. "Recommendations for detection of individual risk for comorbidities in patients with psoriasis." *Archives of Dermatological Research* 305, no. 2 (February 2013): 91–98. https://doi.org/10.1007/s00403-013-1318-9.

Zautra, Alex, Anne Arewasikporn and Mary C. Davis. "Resilience: Promoting well-being through recovery, sustainability, and growth." *Research in Human Development* 7, no. 3 (July 2010): 221–238. https://doi.org/10.1080/15427609.2010.50443.

Zhang, Min and Nan Zhang. "Quality of life assessment in patients with alopecia areata and androgenetic alopecia in the People's Republic of China." *Patient Preference and Adherence* 11 (January 2017): 151–155. https://doi.org/10.2147/PPA.S121218.

Ziglinas, Panagiotis, Dirk Jan Menger and Christos Georgalas. "The body dysmorphic disorder patient: To perform rhinoplasty or not?" *European Archives of Otorhinolaryngology* 271, no. 9 (November 2014): 2355–2358. https://doi.org/10.1007/s00405-013-2792-6.

Zota, Ami. R and Bhavna Shamasunder. "The environmental injustice of beauty: Framing chemical exposures from beauty products as a health disparities concern." *American Journal of Obstetrics and Gynecology* 217, no. 4 (October 2017): 418.e1–418.e6. https://doi.org/10.1016/j.ajog.2017.07.020.

Part III
Cosmeceuticals

CHAPTER 15: PHYSICAL PHOTOPROTECTION, COSMETIC CAMOUFLAGE, AND SUNSCREENS

Bhavjit Kaur

15.1 Introduction

Skin is the largest organ of the body, and it ages due to the interactions between *extrinsic*, or preventable (e.g., chemical products, ultraviolet, infrared sources, pollution, stress, poor nutrition, mechanical damage) and *intrinsic* (heredity and biological chronology) factors (1). Long-standing and repetitive exposure to UV radiation (UVR) from the sun is the most important environmental factor contributing to extrinsic aging and is referred to as photoaging (1). Photoaging is clinically and histologically distinct from the natural aging (chronological) of the skin. Photoaging also depends on the skin pigment (1). The effects of sunlight on the skin are profound and are estimated to account for up 80% to 90% (2) of the visible skin aging.

15.2 Sunlight

Photoaging could be contributed to solar energy (290–4,000 nm) that reaches earth after crossing the stratospheric ozone layer (Table 15.1): Ultraviolet rays (UV), infrared rays (IR), high-energy visible light (HEVL) (3–7).

Exposure to UVR is a known modifiable risk factor for skin cancer. Photoprotection is the foundation for the prevention of sunburn, photoaging, and all cancerous and precancerous skin lesions (8). UVA and UVB both play a role in photoaging and development of skin cancer and sunscreens with only UVB protective agents are not effective in blocking this effect (9). UVA is linked mainly with aging and pigmentation. It penetrates deep into the skin and produces free radical oxygen species resulting in DNA damage. UVB causes sunburn and DNA strand breaks. It induces pyrimidine dimer mutations associated with nonmelanoma skin cancers (6). For photoprotection, it is best to limit sun exposure between 10:00 a.m. and 4:00 p.m., specifically in children (10). When outside, one should seek out shaded areas under awnings or trees (11) and under oversized umbrellas/cabanas when around pools or on beaches (12).

15.2.1 Physical Means of Photoprotection

Clothing cannot provide complete photoprotection as it does not cover everything, but it is the basic and sometimes the most suitable means of photoprotection. Full-sleeved clothes (13) are a minimum to protect the skin from the harmful effects of UVR.

TABLE 15.1: Sunlight

	Visible Light		UV Rays			Infrared Rays		
% Age of sunlight reaching earth	38.9%	6.8%				54.3%		
		UVA	UVB	UVC	IRA	IRB	IRC	
Wavelength (nm)	380–780	320–400	280–320	200–280	760–1,440	1440–3,000	3000–1 mm	
	HEVL 400 to 760 nm	• 95% of total UVR reaching earth • Penetrates deeper than UVB • Involved in sun tanning, Tends to suppress the immune function Implicated in premature aging of the skin	• About 1,000 times as effective at inducing erythema in human skin as UVA • Blocked by glass and clouds • Primary cause of sunburn • Intensification of photoaging • Photo-carcinogenesis • Implicated in cataract formation	• Shortest wavelength • Most damaging UVR • Does not reach earth's surface	33% of solar energy that touches human skin	Does not penetrate deeply into the skin	Does not penetrate deeply into the skin	

DOI: 10.1201/9780429243769-15

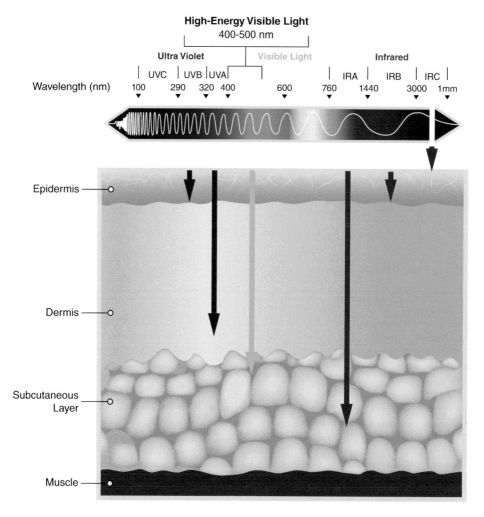

FIGURE 15.1 Photoprotection

The effectiveness of fabrics can be quantified as follows:

1. SPF (sun protection factor), the radiation dose needed to produce just noticeable erythema under fabric-covered skin; the radiation dose needed to produce just noticeable erythema of uncovered skin
2. UPF (ultraviolet protection factor), a concept originally standardized in Australia in 1996; the average effective UV irradiance transmitted without fabric, or the average effective UV irradiance transmitted through fabric

UPF quantifies how effectively a piece of clothing shields against the sun (11, 14). The higher the UPF rating, the more solar UVR gets blocked by the material and the less exposure to solar UVR you will receive.

15.2.2 The UPF of a Fabric Depends Upon
1. Fiber content, weave, and density: Tightly woven, denser, and thicker fabrics like denim and corduroy (11, 15) have higher UPF (4). Open-weave (11), thin, lightweight fabrics, including some silks and bleached cottons, provide lower protection (15)
2. Type of fiber: Synthetic and semi-synthetic fibers (such as polyester and rayon) offer the highest sun protection. Refined and bleached cotton or crepe offers minimum

protection (15, 16). Glossy fabrics (satin) reflect more UVR away from the skin than do matte fabrics, like linen, which tend to absorb UVR (11, 15)
3. Yarn and surface design (17)
4. Finishing processes (14, 17)
5. Fabric color: Colored fabric has greater UPF (4). Dark or bright colors (red or black) absorb more UVR than white or pastel shades. The more concentrated the hue, the better the UV defense (15). The presence of dyes increased protection considerably (16)
6. Presence of additives (14): UV absorbers and fluorescent whitening agents (4) and chemical treatment with bleaching agents result in increase in photoprotection (4)
7. The greater the distance of the fabric from the skin, the better the photoprotection (4). Stretching of the fabric lowers the UPF (11, 18)
8. Shrinkage of the fabric increases the UPF (4, 14)
9. Humidity lowers the UPF (18). Whether the fabric is wet or dry may increase or decrease UPF based on the type of fabric (6). For linen and viscose and polyester fabrics, UPF is significantly increased. For the cotton fabrics and the polyester + TiO_2 fabrics, UPF is significantly decreased (19)
10. Laundering and wear of the fabric over time lower the UPF (14, 17)

Fabrics are placed into classes from minimum to excellent based on the calculated label UPF value, which can range from 15 to 50+ (18). An average-weight cotton T-shirt gives only a sun protection factor (SPF) of 7 (14). Cover-up garments covering the arms, legs, and upper body; wide-brimmed hats (6 cm or greater, shading the face, neck, and ears); and sunglasses are also recommended for greater UV protection including in children (18, 20, 21). Hats do not provide protection against reflected or scattered UVR. Photoprotection by hats is also dependent on the material and weaving (6).

Sunglasses that block as close to 100% of both UVA and UVB (13) or at least 99% UV protection, also applicable to children (20), are recommended. Wraparound sunglasses block UVR from the side too (13).

15.3 Sunscreens

Sunscreens are pharmaceuticals (cosmetics in Europe) that provide photoprotection from the damage caused by UVA, UVB, IR (warmth), and HEVL (22).

15.3.1 Primary Photoprotection

1. Physical (inorganic) sunscreens are effective against UVA/UVB/HEVL radiation (9) and are mostly composed of zinc oxide and titanium dioxide. They can also comprise other ingredients—please see Table 15.2.

Features
- Thick and opaque in appearance
- Deflect or scatter UV light (13, 24)
- Absorb UV radiation (25, 26)

TABLE 15.2: Physical Sunscreen Ingredients

UVA		UVB	HEVL
340–400 nm	320–340 nm	Titanium dioxide	Iron oxide
UVA1	UVA2	Zinc oxide	Titanium dioxide
Zinc oxide	Titanium dioxide		Zinc oxide
	Zinc oxide		

Others:
Iron oxide, red veterinary petrolatum, kaolin
Calamine, ichthammol, talc, kaolin, talc, zinc oxide, calcium carbonate, and magnesium oxide

Newer forms of physical sunscreens have micronized particles and are easier to apply. Micronized zinc oxide and titanium dioxide can clump together over time, so they are often layered with dimethicone or silica to keep the sunscreen stable and smooth (6, 25, 27, 28).

2. Chemical (organic) sunscreens are effective against UVA or UVB or both and are mostly composed of one or more of many possible active ingredients (see Table 15.3).

Features
- Cosmetically acceptable
- Absorb UVA/UVB/both

The constituents of chemical sunscreens are unstable or photo-unstable. To overcome photo-instability, photo-stabilizers have been used as additives, including antioxidants, such as glutathione, vitamin C, vitamin E, and ubiquinone (29, 25, 30).

15.3.2 Secondary Photoprotection
15.3.2.1 IR Protection

Exposure to IR is felt as heat that could lead to the production of reactive oxygen species (ROS), which are responsible for IR-induced skin aging (31). IR targets the mitochondria and triggers a chain of reactions leading to overexpression of the matrix metalloproteinase (MMP) and depression of neocollagenesis. The antioxidant-rich ferment of *Thermus thermophilus* (microorganisms lodging around deep-sea hydrothermal vents) protects the skin against free radicals and provides photoprotection against UV and IR (32).

15.3.2.2 High-Energy Visible Light (HEVL) Protection

HEVL is high-energy, high-frequency light in the violet/blue band (400 to 500 nm) in the visible light spectrum. HEVL induces oxidative stress and activates MMPs and ROS in the skin. This effect is comparable to that produced by UVA and UVB combined (33). HEVL exposure could result in premature skin aging due DNA damage, skin pigmentation, wrinkles, reduced barrier function, and increased skin fragility (29). Results of a study showed that both UVA1 and visible-light-induced pigmentation in skin types IV–VI (34), but the pigmentation induced by visible light was darker and more sustained.

TABLE 15.3: Chemical and Other Sunscreen Ingredients

UVA		UVB (290–320)	UVA 2 and UVB
340–400 nm UVA1	320–340 nm UVA2	Para-aminobenzoic acid	Benzophenone
		Ensulizole	• Oxybenzone (benzophenone-3)
		Homosalate	• Sulisobenzone
Avobenzone	Ecamsule (Mexoryl SX)	Octyl salicylate	• Dioxybenzone
	Menthyl anthranilate	Trolamine salicylate	
		Padimate O	
		Octyl methoxycinnamate (octinoxate)	
		Cinoxate	
		Phenyl benzimidazole	
		4-Methylbenzylidene camphor	

Sources of HEVL include sunlight (major source), displays of flat digital screens televisions, smartphone screens, computers, tablets (35, 36), and residential and commercial lighting (37).

Liposhield HEV Melanin is fractionated melanin (Mel-HEV) (38). It is a bleached version of natural melanin, and it offers protection against HEV and ultraviolet (specifically UVA) (30) when applied topically. It absorbs harmful HEVL before it can penetrate the skin. Red visible light is deemed to have beneficial effects, and HEV Melanin is tailored so that red light can be transmitted to the skin (36). Physical sunscreen agents, such as iron oxide, titanium dioxide, and zinc oxide, can offer some visible light protection (28).

Pre-treatment with the antioxidants (39) or the addition of botanical antioxidants and DNA repair enzymes (40) can enhance photoprotection when compared with sunscreen alone. Antioxidants reduce the ROS produced from UVA radiation.(6) Genistein and N-acetyl, vitamins C and E, ferulic acid, coenzyme Q10, pycnogenol, silymarin, and idebenone are among the various antioxidants that can help in reducing photodamage (39, 40) and provide additional anticarcinogenic protection (41). They have been shown to augment protection against UV-induced epidermal thickening, overexpression of MMPs, and depletion of CD1a+ Langerhans cells (40). Topical antioxidants act from within the cell to decrease the scarcity of antioxidants (on sun exposure) and can remain active for several days after application (41).

Botanical substances like curcumin, resveratrol, green tea extract, carotenoids, and *Polypodium leucotomos* extract provide proven photoprotection (42). Polyphenols (flavonoids), lycopenes, fixed oils (almond, avocado, coconut, cottonseed, olive, peanut, sesame, and soybean) (43), volatile oils (oils from peppermint and tulsi, lavender, orange, eucalyptus, tea tree, and rose) (44), and silymarin, a flavinoid from milk thistle plants, shield skin by scavenging the from UV-induced ROS (6) and prevents lipid and lipoprotein oxidation. When topically applied, it decreases UVB-induced sunburn cells and promotes a reduction in the amount of UVB-induced pyrimidine dimers (6).

15.4 Characteristics of a Perfect Sunscreen

Model sunscreens must meet the following criteria: safe, cosmetically acceptable, and broad spectrum (effectively and efficiently blocking both UVB and UVA rays, which is possible with an agent that has an SPF of 30 or greater). A combination of physical and chemical agents—non-irritant, hypoallergenic, non-comedogenic (25), easily available in large quantities, affordable, non-toxic, with antioxidants and preferably natural (45), chemically inert, photostable ingredients—should remain on the superficial layers of the skin (46) even after swimming or sweating. Sunscreen should provide efficient protection against singlet oxygen and other ROS (27). A sunscreen should not only protect the skin from the sun but also minimize the cumulative health hazards from sun damage caused over time (9, 27, 46).

15.5 Sunscreen Labels

Sunscreen labels are often loaded with several claims of apparently high significance (47), and the information on the label is mostly not understood completely by the consumer (48).

SPF (sun protection factor, or sun*burn* protection factor) (49) quantifies the effectiveness of the sunscreen against UVB rays.

$$SPF = \frac{MED\ in\ sunscreen\ protected\ skin}{MED\ in\ sunscreen\ unprotected\ skin}.$$

MED (minimum erythematous dose) is the smallest amount of energy required for triggering the erythema.

For example, SPF 15 equals 150 minutes for erythema with a sunscreen or 10 minutes for erythema without a sunscreen (50).

SPF and percentage of sun's UVB rays curtained (50):

- SPF 15: 93%
- SPF 30: 97%
- SPF 50: 98%

No sunscreen can filter out 100% of the sun's UVB rays, so the term "sunblock" is misleading; it is important to wear protective clothing and seek shade (49).

Per EU recommendations, the manufacturers must display on their sunscreen label the following (24):

- Low protection—SPF 6 and 10
- Medium protection—SPF 15, 20, or 25
- High protection—SPF 30 or 50
- Very high protection—50+

Currently, there is no internationally agreed standard for testing and measuring UVA protection. The commonly used methods are persistent pigment darkening (PPD) and critical wavelength (22). Most countries have moved away from performing the in vivo PPD method and now use in vitro PPD methods to determine the UVA protection factor (50). The UVA protection of each sunscreen should be a third of the labeled SPF. The product that fulfills the EU requirements must have the UVA logo (uva) on the label (24, 50). The company "Boots" (51) was the first to develop the 0-to-5-star rating system in the European Union in 1992. This made it easy for consumers to understand the level of UVA protection when compared to UVB.

The star system was based on Diffey's UVA/UVB ratio (52) where 1 is the minimum sun protection and 5 is the ultra. Countries like the United States, Japan, Australia, and New Zealand have their own UV protection factor indices. In India, there are no guidelines currently for standardizing sunscreen agents (27).

A broad-spectrum sunscreen is one that can protect the skin from UVA (aging) rays and UVB (burning) rays (24). It should meet the standards for both UVB and UVA protection, with increasing SPF values indicating a proportional increase in UVA protection (50). The British Association of Dermatologists (24) recommends using an SPF 30 or higher with a UVA rating of 4 or 5 stars to provide a good standard of protection from the sun in addition to shade and clothing (50).

"Water resistant" and "very water resistant" indicate that sunscreen will remain effective for 40 mins and 80 mins, respectively. In Europe, in water-resistant and very-water-resistant sunscreen, the SPF protection must be 50% or more of its level on the label after two and four, respectively, 20-minute periods of submerging in water. The FDA, on the other hand, requires that the SPF should not be affected by immersion in water (53). Sunlight that enters the water may travel about 1,000 meters into the ocean under the right conditions, but there is rarely any significant light beyond 200 meters (54). These sunscreens have significantly better substantivity than sunscreens that make no claim of water resistance (24). Labeling the sunscreen as "sweatproof," "waterproof," (27, 50) or "all-day protection" (55) is misleading.

15.6 Application and Reapplication

Sunscreen should be applied generously to all bare skin to form a film. Arney (56). Cancer Research UK, advises that sunscreen should not be rubbed in. The correct way is to "pat it in" or "smooth it in" (56) (see Figure 15.2).

Sunscreen should be applied daily from 10:00 a.m. to 4:00 p.m. and at least 15–10 minutes before going out (24) or 30 minutes before going out and again just before going out (57). It should be reapplied to bare sites 15–30 minutes post-sun exposure to cover missed areas (52). All sunscreens, including "once a day" sunscreens, should be reapplied every two hours (24).

Photoprotection by sunscreen gets compromised (58), so sunscreens, including "once a day" sunscreens (24) should be reapplied every couple of hours, regardless of their SPF, because of the following reasons:

- Most people do not apply enough quantity of sunscreen.
- Eighty-five percent of the sunscreen can be removed from the skin by the following (52, 60):
  - Sweating
  - Any form of rubbing
  - Exposure to water
  - Towel-drying
- Sunrays can break down or clump up some sunscreen ingredients.
- Water-resistant sunscreens should be reapplied as follows (24):
  - Water resistant: Reapplied every 40 minutes if wet and every 2 hours if not wet

- Very water resistant: Reapplied every 80 minutes if wet and every 2 hours if not wet
- Immediately after towel-drying

Modern sunscreens may be more robust on the skin even after considerable exercise and water exposure for up to eight hours, so reapplication intervals may be longer than presently advocated, provided it is applied appropriately (61).

Aerosol spray sunscreen is easy to apply in a higher dosage, and consumers could be inclined to reapply more frequently. Sunscreen sprays need to be sprayed on the hand first and then rubbed into the face/neck area (61). Sprays are excellent for protecting the scalp from sun damage (55). Inhalation of spray sunscreens should be avoided (48, 49).

In a study in 2013 (62), skin aging was monitored from baseline to the end of the trial and was noticed to be 24% less in the daily sunscreen group than in the discretionary sunscreen group. It is advisable to apply sunscreen every day to obtain the maximal benefit of sunscreens (63). Sunscreen should be applied even when inside the house as UVA (UVA1) is transmitted through window glass (64). Window glass blocks virtually all UVB and at least half of all UVA (10). UVR gets through even on a cloudy, windy, and cool day. Clouds absorb UVB, but UVA can pass through (50, 64). According to the Cancer Council, Australia (65, 66), UVR may even be more intense due to reflection off the clouds. Cloudless skies allow practically 100% of UV to pass through, while overcast skies transmit 31% (57, 67). Wind can reduce the natural sun protection in the skin and may augment sunburn by allowing more of the sun's UVR to penetrate. Prolonged wind exposure will dry and slough-off the stratum corneum and the topical sunscreen protection, hence making the skin more vulnerable to photodamage (68).

15.7 Quantity

It is recommended that at least six to seven full teaspoons of sunscreen are needed to cover the body of an average adult (approximately 36 grams/two tablespoons/one shotglass/one ounce) (24, 65).

The recommended dose is 2 mg/cm^2 (24), or follow the "teaspoon rule" (25):

- More than half a teaspoon (3 mL)—each arm and face/neck (including ears)
- Little over one teaspoon (6 mL)—each leg, front of body, and back of body

One fingertip unit (1FTU) is a strip of product squeezed onto the index finger, from the distal crease to the fingertip. 3FTU is about 3 ml or more (author's experience) and is enough for the face (69).

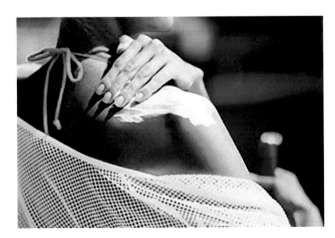

FIGURE 15.2 Reapplication of sunscreen within the first hour of exposure helps patients achieve even coverage with the necessary amount of product instead of every two hours (58). In reality, individuals do not apply the recommended dose (2 mg/cm^2) of sunscreen, and so the expected sun protection is rarely achieved (22). Some authors (59) recommend a double application of sunscreen prior to sun exposure optimizes sunscreen use compared to a single application. In one study (59), it was found that only 19% of the participants had applied 2 mg/cm^2 or more sunscreen after a double application; after a single application, none of them had done so.

- 3FTU for face
- 3FTU for ears and neck
- 3FTU for décolleté

Application of the above quantities of sunscreen is essential to reduce cutaneous photodamage (63). Lessening the amount applied greatly affects the SPF (70). Increased reapplication of sunscreen is noted among people who apply a UV detection sticker, but it does not change the sunburn rates (71).

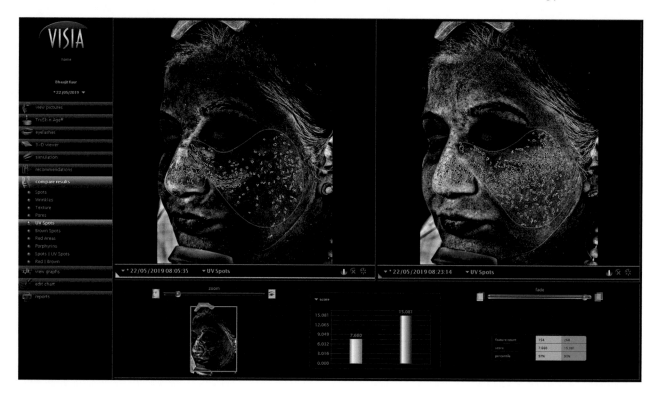

FIGURE 15.3 Forty-five minutes after sunscreen—also see even with the sunglasses removed the sunscreen versus no sunscreen.

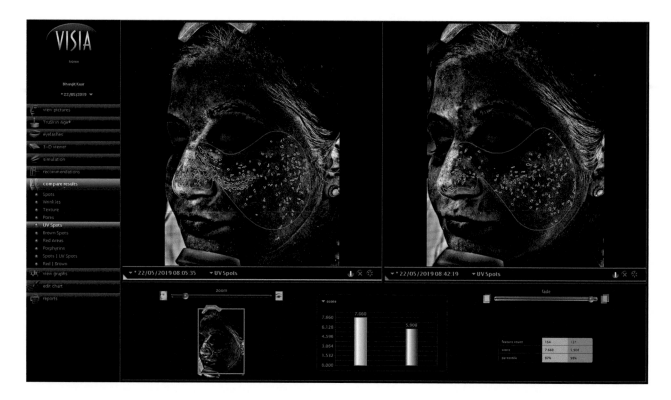

FIGURE 15.4 Forty-five minutes after sunscreen versus immediately after one layer of sunscreen, split face.

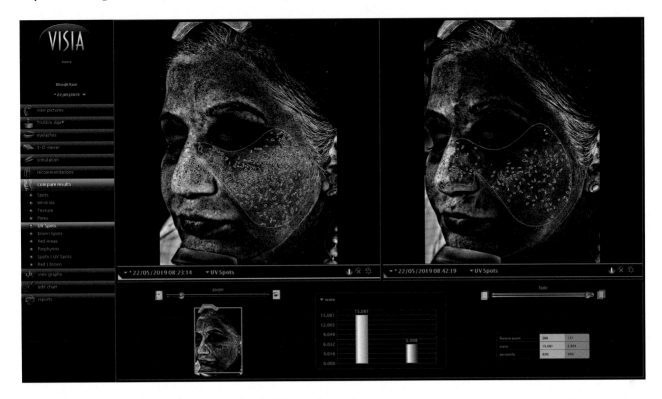

FIGURE 15.5 No sunscreen versus immediately after one layer of sunscreen.

The time interval between sunscreen application and dressing should be minimum of 8 minutes. When less sunscreen is used, the SPF is insensitive to the duration between application and dressing (72).

15.8 Shelf Life

Sunscreen could be used within three years after purchase (73) or before the expiration date on the container. Ingredients of the sunscreens are frequently photo-unstable, and they are able to react with the plastic package. This affects the efficiency of the sunscreens (74). Storing sunscreens in above 25°C in cars, in backpacks, or at the beach alters the composition faster than the normal expiration (75).

15.9 Advice for Children

Ideal parental sun protection efforts are overall low, predominantly in parents of darker-skinned children (76). It is estimated that 80% of sun damage occurs before the age of 18 years (77). Consistent use of a broad-spectrum sunscreen with an SPF of 15 or higher in the first 18 years of life has been expected to lower the risk of certain skin cancers by almost 80%, and pediatricians could play a major role in patient education regarding benefits of sunscreen application from an early age (78). Less than 25% to 50% of the lifetime UV dose was received before the age of 18–21, and the effect of UV damage is cumulative (79). There are many psychological, attitudinal, peer pressure, and social norms toward sun exposure and the use of photoprotection modalities (80), especially in adolescents.

In children younger than six months of age, sunscreen should be avoided (81). Sunscreen should only be applied if shade is not available and only to the small exposed parts of the body (10).

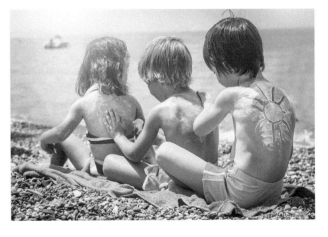

FIGURE 15.6 Photo 3/Istock/models/ArtMarie

Sources: Istock

In children six months of age and older, a physical sunscreen appropriate for sensitive skin should be used (9).

Sunscreen used for infants and children should be gentle, non-irritant, efficacious, hypoallergenic, and fragrance-free. Non-nanoparticle-sized mineral-based sunscreens (zinc oxide and titanium dioxide) may be a safer choice for children in addition to practicing sun avoidance or using protective clothing/hats (12, 68). In children, especially newborns, the skin is thin and immature. Newborns also lack a functioning acid mantle, so there is an increased risk of absorption and deeper penetration of chemicals in the sunscreen, making them more vulnerable to contact dermatitis (skin reactions, like rashes), allergies, or inflammation (82). Infants have an increased body-surface-area-to-body-weight ratio as compared to older children and adults, so they are at a greater risk of being affected by toxicity and side effects from the sunscreen (81). A patch test with the sunscreen should be done before complete application (82).

Sunscreen should be applied for children, just as it is recommended for adults. Sunscreen is not meant to allow your kids to spend more time in the sun (81).

15.10 Safety

There is limited information on the degree of absorption and systemic effect of most sunscreen ingredients. Therefore, further evaluation of the systemic exposure of sunscreen ingredients is warranted to better weigh any long-term risks of use (28). Since it is suggested that sunscreens are reapplied frequently throughout the day, it has been proposed that active sunscreen ingredients may be systemically absorbed and not remain on the stratum corneum (83). Further research is warranted to evaluate whether exposure to UV filters contributes to possible adverse effects on the developing organs of fetuses and children.

Titanium dioxide is solely deposited on the outermost surface of the stratum corneum and cannot be detected in the deeper stratum corneum layers, epidermis, or dermis (84). Zinc oxide is absorbed into the skin, although the extent of absorption is not known (83).

Benzophenone-3 has been found in 96% of urine samples, and several UV filters were present in 85% of Swiss breast milk samples (85). Octyl-methoxycinnamate and 3-(4-methylbenzylidene) camphor have been found in urine and plasma (86). To add to the controversy, a direct correlation was found between topically applied sunscreen's ingredients and endocrine disorders in children and young adults (12, 87), while some considered the alteration in thyroid and reproductive hormones were not related to sunscreen application (88). Plasma concentrations exceeding the threshold (0.5 ng/mL) recommended by the FDA was observed in studies (89, 90), with healthy volunteers applying sunscreens containing avobenzone, oxybenzone, octocrylene, and ecamsule under maximal-use conditions, but despite the findings, the authors did not recommend refraining from the use of sunscreens. Para-aminobenzoic acid (PABA) and trolamine salicylate are not considered safe anymore and are not currently used in sunscreens in the US market (91).

15.11 Adverse Reactions

Current research suggests that sunscreen ingredients are not hazardous to human health, but further studies assessing the risks of systemic absorption of various sunscreen agents in adults, children, and breastfeeding and pregnant women (28) are warranted. Physical sunscreens should be used where there are concerns about the use of chemical sunscreens.

In a study by Foley et al., 18.9% of volunteers in 1993 in Australia (92) developed an adverse reaction to sunscreen. Allergic inflammatory eruptions were noted, particularly in people with a history of atopy and contact urticarial (92). Anaphylaxis has been reported due to oxybenzone (93). Predisposing factors that can cause sunscreen allergy are unknown but are more likely to be sex, prior photodermatosis, use of sunscreen on damaged skin, working outdoors, and atopy (6). Para-aminobenzoic acid (including its esters), benzophenones, fragrances, and preservatives account for most of the reactions (55). Acneiform eruptions are also observed because of the vehicle rather than the ingredients within the

sunscreen; in such patients, gels or sprays should be recommended (94). Clinicians should consider contact and photocontact allergy, particularly in patients with photo-dermatoses and photo-aggravated dermatoses, and a patch test should be performed (95).

In addition to active compounds, sunscreens usually contain preservatives, emulsifiers, fragrances, and other additives. Allergic reactions were less common to the active sunscreen ingredients as compared to the other ingredients of the sunscreen. In the author's experience, the most common irritation complaint is stinging or burning of the eye area after sunscreen application. Irritant reactions (burning, pruritus, erythema, or stinging of skin) are more common than allergic contact dermatitis (96).

The likelihood of harm from the use of sunscreens containing nanoparticles (UV filters zinc oxide and titanium dioxide) is low (97) as nanoparticles do not penetrate beyond the stratum corneum (98). Review of literature by the Australian Therapeutic Goods Administration (99) determined that these nanoparticles nominally penetrate the stratum corneum and are unlikely to cause harm.

15.12 Contraindications

Most of the contraindications are due to PABA in some sunscreens, and PABA is not currently used in sunscreens in the US market (91).

Chemical sunscreen should not be used in patients who have the following:

- Ester local anesthetic hypersensitivity (e.g., benzocaine, procaine, tetracaine, PABA) (100)
- Skin disease, as the skin barrier may be compromised (e.g., severe eczema) (101)
- Hypersensitivity to aniline dyes, sulfonylurea, paraphenylenediamine, thiazide diuretic, and artificial sweeteners (e.g., saccharin and sodium cyclamate) (102)

15.13 Precautions

- Pregnant or breastfeeding (85)
- Children less than six months old, infants, and neonates (20, 21)
- Personal history of atopy (92)
- Atopic dermatitis (103)
- Patients with photosensitivity dermatitis, actinic reticuloid syndrome, and polymorphous light eruption (104)
- Avoid inhalation of spray sunscreens (48, 49). Inhalation might be specifically associated with increased brain exposure since the olfactory nerves can directly transport particles into the brain (105)
- Photo-dermatoses and photo-aggravated dermatoses (95)
- Seborrheic dermatitis may be aggravated by sunscreen agents (23)

15.14 Sunscreen for Lips and Eyes

Many individuals do not wear sunscreen on the eyelids and medial canthal areas due to the concern of stinging associated with sunscreen or fear of getting the sunscreen in the eyes. Once sunscreen is applied on the whole face (except the eyelids and area around eyes), individuals may feel safe to spend time in the sun; in such cases, unprotected areas are likely to receive enhanced cumulative UV doses. Most sunscreens are safe to be used on the eyelids and medial canthal areas. Mineral sunscreens made up of zinc or titanium dioxide are a favored choice as they do not sting.

Actinic cheilitis (AC) is a potentially malignant disorder of the lip, more prevalent in middle-aged individuals, probably caused by prolonged exposure to UVR (106). Protection from sun exposure should be encouraged to prevent the progression of AC. It is estimated that 95% of squamous cell carcinomas (SCC) of the lip originate from ACs. Low AC rates in women can be explained due to the use of more clothing or lipstick (105) that act as protective factors, while the predilection for men may reflect more prolonged occupational sun exposure and late retirement compared with women.

Stick sunscreens are lipid-soluble formula based and work best on eyes, nose, and lips as they are less messy and easy to apply (55). Tinted eye sunscreens are also available. Sunscreen should be reapplied following the same rule as for the rest of the face and body. It is not dangerous if sunscreen enters the eyes, but it should be flushed off the eyes as soon as possible (107, 108).

15.15 Sunscreen and Pollution

The literature review proposes that exposure to highly polluted environments, pollutants, and UVA has a deleterious synergy between them and could initiate skin aging and skin precancers and cancers (109). Pollutants are highly diverse chemical entities, including gases, such as ozone, nitrogen, and sulfur oxides, and particulate matter (PM) of different sizes and with different chemical constituents. PM is frequently combined with heavy metals or polycyclic aromatic hydrocarbons (PAHs). Numerous PAHs absorb photons in the UVA range and, at times, even in the visible range. On excitation by photons, PAHs can initiate a series of reactions resulting in the formation of ROS, which can damage cellular biomolecules (lipids, DNA, or proteins). By-products of UV-pollution reactions induce oxidative stress in the upper epidermis via the formation of lipid peroxidation products, with cascading consequences to deeper layers (109).

PM can penetrate the skin transepidermally and through hair follicles and induce skin aging by interacting with keratinocytes, melanocytes, and fibroblasts. Sunscreens and antioxidants can protect from potential damage from exposure to pollution, UVA, and HEVL (110). Newer sunscreens are available in combination with antioxidants like vitamin C. Antioxidants can also be used separately under sunscreen. The application of a cream reduces particle adhesion to the skin and thus protects the skin against pollution-induced oxidative and inflammatory pathways (111), which could in turn lead to skin aging and precancerous and cancerous lesions.

15.16 Controversies

Though sunscreens have an established role in preventing photoaging and many skin cancers caused by sun exposure (112), the long-term use of sunscreen is still controversial. According to Lindqvist (113), women who seek out the sun are at lower risk for cardiovascular disease (CVD) and noncancer/non-CVD diseases, such as diabetes, multiple sclerosis, and pulmonary diseases, than those who avoid sun exposure. Dr. Lindqvist (113) agreed that though there is an increased risk of skin cancers in the absence of sunscreen use, the skin cancers that occur in those exposing themselves to the sun have a better prognosis (114).

15.17 Sunscreen and Its Effect on Vitamin D ("Sunshine Vitamin")

Sunlight is the best source of vitamin D synthesis in the body. Sunlight availability is dependent on many factors, including but not limited to season, altitude, time of the day, and weather; these variables interfere with the amount of UVB reaching the skin and hence in vitamin D production (115). Vitamin D deficiency could cause rickets, osteomalacia, and osteoporosis and has been implicated in many chronic conditions, including lower immunity, infectious diseases, autoimmune diseases, cardiovascular diseases, diabetes, cancer (116), and dermatological and neurological diseases (115).

There are concerns that regular use of sunscreen may increase the risk of vitamin D deficiency. In a literature review, little evidence was found that sunscreen decreases 25(OH)D concentration when used in real-life settings (117), as covering the whole body with sunscreen is uncommon, and the majority do not apply the recommended (2 mg/cm^2) thickness of sunscreen and do not reapply.

When the sun is intense and the temperature is high enough to make the population use sunscreen, the vitamin D status is generally very satisfactory (115). In India, daily direct sun exposure of more than 45 minutes is required (116). Only short periods of sun exposure are needed to get the daily dose of vitamin D, which is 10 minutes for fair skin and 25 minutes for darker skin types (between 11:00 a.m. and 3:00 p.m., from March to September, in the UK) (118). This is if exposed body parts include forearms, lower legs, hands, and face (118).

Authors have used SPF<30 to SPF>50 to study the effect of sunscreen on vitamin D levels and have found no influence on serum 25-hydroxyvitamin D concentration (6, 119).

15.18 Effect on Ecosystems

UV filters in sunscreen or their by-products have been detected in freshwater, coastal, and marine ecosystems and in the Arctic. They have potential consequences on marine ecosystem (120). The substance 4-methylbenzylidene camphor poses a risk to algae, while benzophenone-3 and octyl methoxycinnamate are a risk to fishes and corals. This study is the first to report the occurrence of organic UV filters in the Arctic and provides a wider assessment of their potential negative impacts on the marine environment (120, 121).

An estimated 14,000 tons of sunscreen is thought to be deposited in oceans annually (122), probably damaging marine life. Hawaii and Palau have introduced bans on sunscreens that contain chemicals harmful (oxybenzone and octinoxate) to coral reefs and other marine life. The ban in Hawaii went into effect as a law on January 1, 2021 (122).

15.19 Oral Photoprotection

Apart from the value of SPF and UVA stars, the effectiveness of topical sunscreen depends on the amount applied, the frequency of application, the external conditions, exposure to water or sweat, the half-life of the constituents, and the degree of absorption through the skin, if any. Oral photoprotection, in contrast to topical sunscreen, is easy to use, has more uniform coverage, and is not affected by the various factors mentioned previously (123). Intake of oral agents like vitamins A, B3, C, D, and E; minerals like zinc and (123) selenium (27); polyphenols; *Polypodium leucotomos*; cocoa extract; green tea; and carotenoids, such as lutein, astaxanthin, and zeaxanthin, can increase systemic protection against the harmful effects of UV, visible, and infrared ranges. These agents are conferred with photoprotective and anti-photocarcinogenic properties. Protective mechanisms vary and include antioxidant, anti-inflammatory, and immunomodulatory effects (123). *Polypodium leucotomos* (PL) is rich in phenolic compounds. PL contains antioxidants like cinnamic, ferulic, and chlorogenic acids (124). PL extract (commercial name Fernblock, IFC Group, Spain) is a powerful antioxidant due to its high content of phenolic compounds. PL can be safely taken orally, or it can also be used topically. It inhibits the generation and release of ROS by UVR and there by influences the subsequent cascade of reactions at cellular and molecular levels; thus, the inhibition of carcinogenesis and photoaging is observed (124).

PL extract dispensed in a dose of 240 mg taken twice daily for 60 days was established as safe and effective for photoprotection. Additional studies using higher doses or longer duration may be warranted (125). Results of a double-blinded trial recommend the use of PL extract as an adjuvant treatment in photo-exacerbated conditions, such as melisma (126). It is essential to educate our patients that oral sunscreen could be taken but in addition to topical sunscreen and use of physical barriers, or else the risk of photo-cancers increases.

15.20 Sunscreen and Insect Repellents

In areas of endemic mosquito-borne disease, the use of mosquito repellents and physical barriers and changes in behavioral practices are essential components of personal protection approaches to reduce the risks of mosquito-borne diseases. The results of various studies on simultaneous or in combination use of sunscreen and insect repellent are controversial. This warrants more studies to increase effectiveness and decrease toxicity. Application of a combination product of sunscreen and insect repellent too often poses the risk of insect repellent toxicity, whereas application too intermittently could cause photodamage (127). When used as two separate products and sunscreen is applied and reapplied over insect repellent, then insect repellent protection times can be lowered substantially. The reapplication of a low-concentration repellent and sunscreen formulation may be a better option to provide the most effective protection from mosquitoes and UV rays while minimizing the risk of repellent toxicity (128). A study by Yiin et al. 2015 (129) suggested that applying sunscreen over insect repellent (insect repellents components such as *N*, *N*-diethyl-*m*-toulamide—DEET) on the skin leads to substantially higher absorption of DEET. It is recommended that should concurrent use of both be necessary, sunscreen should be applied first, followed by insect repellent after 15 minutes (129).

15.21 Camouflage and Cosmetics

The word "camouflage" is derived from the French word "camoufler," meaning "to blind." It is defined as a coverup by some means that alters or disguises the appearance (130). Common brands are Covermark, Dermablend, Dermacolor, Keromask, and Veil Cover. Camouflage creams are used to mask discoloration or scars on the skin. Most camouflage products contain ingredients providing sun protection to safeguard against photodamage; however, they should be used along with sunscreen for added sun protection (130). It is suggested that sunscreen should be applied before camouflage (130). Camouflage products are mostly waterproof and opaque and adhere to textured skin (131). Octyl methoxycinnamate, octocrylene, oxybenzone (132), avobenzone, titanium dioxide, and iron oxides are commonly found in some camouflage products (133). SPF protection may vary from less than 30 to 50 (134).

Cosmetics, especially foundation cream, also help to provide some degree of everyday sun protection. The SPF in cosmetics ranges from 4 to 30, and the opacity of the foundation makeup also provides UVA protection (54). Application of SPF moisturizers is inferior to sunscreens for sun protection (106).

15.22 Skin of Color and Use of Sunscreen

The largest part of the world's population is comprised of Asians. By 2050, nearly one-half of the U.S population will be non-white (135). Skin of color comprises Africans, African Americans, African Caribbeans, Asians (Chinese, Japanese, Indians, Pakistanis, Arabs, etc.), Native Americans (e.g., Navajo Indians), Hispanics, and mixed/multiple ethnic groups.

There is a misconception among many physicians and people that individuals with skin of color do not need to use sunscreen as dark skin is protected from photodamage and skin cancers (136, 137). Dark skin does offer some protection from UV rays, but people of color do experience tanning and sunburn, which shows UV-induced DNA damage has occurred. Though skin cancer comprises only 1% to 2% of all malignancies in people with darker skin, the mortality rates in this group are significantly higher when compared with their Caucasian counterparts (136). Exposure to the sun is also responsible for many skin conditions that present as hyperpigmentation or uneven skin tone. People with darker skin tones should use sunscreen like people with fairer skin (137).

15.23 Conclusion

Avoiding sun exposure and wearing sun-protective clothing are considered understandable essential approaches to prevent sun-related damage to the skin, but the application of sunscreen alone can show improvement in all photoaging parameters from baseline to as early as week 12, including improvement in skin clarity and texture in 100% of users (138).

Doctors should educate each patient about the hazardous effects of sun exposure. As professionals, we play a major role in educating our patients about the benefits and proper application technique of sunscreens and emphasizing reapplication every two hours. For job-holding women, reapplication seems unfeasible as they are wearing makeup, but some newer sunscreens can be applied over the makeup. Emphasis on reapplication, however, is very essential if the patient suffers from or is at risk of hyperpigmentation or having treatment for hyperpigmentation. Education should start from the preadolescent age groups to obtain maximal benefit.

More research is needed to study the harmful effects of systemically absorbed (89) sunscreen ingredients, sunscreen safety in pregnant and breastfeeding women, and the direct or indirect relationship to various skin cancers and certain other diseases.

Frequently Asked Questions

1. *Q: Should sunscreen be used every day?*
   A: Sunscreen should be applied daily, between 10:00 a.m. and 4:00 p.m., regardless of the weather and whether indoors or outdoors. Chemical sunscreen should not be used in pregnant or breastfeeding women.

2. *Q: How often should I use sunscreen?*
   A: It is recommended that sunscreen should be applied every two hours (if not wet), between 10:00 a.m. and 4:00 p.m. I tell my patients that they must apply sunscreen just before 10:00 a.m. and repeat this at 12:00 p.m. and 2:00 p.m. For working women, reapplication seems unfeasible as they are wearing makeup, but some newer sunscreens can be applied over the makeup. Emphasis on reapplication, however, is very essential in patients suffering from or at risk of hyperpigmentation.

3. *Q: What is the recommended dose of sunscreen?*
   A: It is easy to follow the "teaspoon rule" to calculate the amount of sunscreen for application:
   - More than half a teaspoon (3 mL)—each arm and face/neck (including ears)
   - Little over one teaspoon (6 mL)—each leg, front of body, and back of body

4. *Q: Which sunscreen is best for me?*
   A: The chosen sunscreen should provide protection of the skin from UVA and UVB, with a minimum SPF of 30 and in addition from infrared and HEVL radiation. If not available, then one should apply an antioxidant serum, such as vitamin C, at least five minutes before sunscreen application. A sunscreen that has both physical and chemical ingredients can also decrease the damage by HEVL.

5. *Q: What is the best way to apply sunscreen?*
   A: Sunscreen should be the last layer to be applied before makeup. Sunscreen should not be rubbed in. The correct way is to apply a film like a thin mask, wait 10–15 minutes and smooth it in, if needed. The application of a second layer to cover any missed areas of skin would be beneficial.

6. *Q: I have dark skin; Do I need to use sunscreen?*
   A: There is a false belief that dark skin provides complete protection from the harmful effect of sunlight. Dark skin does offer some protection from UVR, but people of color do experience mostly tanning and rarely sunburn, but it indicates that there is UV-induced DNA damage. The skin should be protected to decrease the risk of hyperpigmentation and skin cancer.

References

1. Fisher, G.J., Kang, S., Varani, J. "Mechanisms of photoaging and chronological skin aging," *Archives of Dermatological* 2002;138(11):1462–1470. Available from: https://jamanetwork.com/journals/jamadermatology/article-abstract/479061 [Accessed 2 December 2019]

2. Farage, M.A., Miller, K.W., Elsner, P., Maibach, H.I. "Intrinsic and extrinsic factors in skin ageing: A review," *International Journal of Cosmetic Science* 2008;30(2):87–95. Available from: https://onlinelibrary.wiley.com/doi/full/10.1111/j.1468-2494.2007.00415.x [Accessed 21 December 2019]

3. Barolet, D., Christiaens, F., Hamblin, M.R. "Infrared and skin: Friend or foe," *Journal of Photochemistry and Photobiology Biology* 2016;155:78–85. Available from: www.ncbi.nlm.nih.gov/pubmed/26745730 [Accessed 20 December 2019]

4. Rai, R., Srinivas, C.R. "Photoprotection," *Indian Journal of Dermatology, Venereology and Leprology* 2007;73(2):73–79. Available from: www.ijdvl.com/article.asp?2007/73/2/72/31889 [Accessed 2 December 2019]

5. Adithi, P., Khan, A.B., Roopesh, S.K. "Broad spectrum UVA & UVB photoprotectants: An overview," *Journal of Pharmaceutical Research* 2017;16(2):143. Available from: www.journalofpharmaceuticalresearch.org/index.php/kpc/article/view/116429/80895 [Accessed 11 December 2019]

6. Gabros, S., Zito, P.M. "Sunscreens and photoprotection," *Stat Pearls* 2019. Available from: www.ncbi.nlm.nih.gov/books/NBK537164/ [Accessed 22 January 2020]

7. Schroeder, P., Calles, C., Benesova, T., Macaluso, F., Krutmann, J. "Photoprotection beyond ultraviolet radiation-effective sun protection has to include protection against infrared A radiation-induced skin damage," *Skin Pharmacology and Physiology* 2010;23(1):15–17. Available from: www.ncbi.nlm.nih.gov/pubmed/20090404 [Accessed 13 January 2020]

8. Milch, J.M., Logemann, N.F. "Photoprotection prevents skin cancer: Let's make it fashionable to wear sun-protective clothing," *DO Cutis* 2017;99:89–92. Available from: https://pdfs.semanticscholar.org/0c99/a339202d78d713fb410a7341178b41d073a8.pdf [Accessed 21 December 2019]

9. Chien, A., Jacobe, H. "UV radiation and your skin," *Skin Cancer Foundation* 2019. Available from: www.skincancer.org/risk-factors/uv-radiation/ [Accessed 22 January 2020]

10. American Academy Of Pediatrics (AAP). "Ultraviolet light: A hazard to children. committee on environmental health," *Pediatrics* 1999;104(2). Available from: https://pediatrics.aappublications.org/content/104/2/328 [Accessed 3 January 2020]

11. Gies, P., McLennan, A. "What is sunsafe clothing?" *Skin Cancer.Org* 2015. Available from: www.skincancer.org/prevention/sun-protection/clothing/protection [Accessed 16 April 2019]

12. DiNardo, J.C., Downs, C.A. "Should we use products containing chemical UV absorbing sunscreen actives on children?" *Clinical Dermatology Research Journal* 2019;4:1. Available from: www.kitchenstewardship.com/wp-content/uploads/2019/03/Clinical-Research-Dermatology-Journal-Galley-Proof-March-13-2019.pdf [Accessed 3 January 2020]

13. USDOHHS US Department of Health and Human Services. The Surgeon General's Call to Action to Prevent Skin Cancer. "Reducing the risk of skin cancer." Office of the Surgeon General (US) Washington (DC) (2014). Available from: www.ncbi.nlm.nih.gov/books/NBK247163 [Accessed 19 January 2020]

14. Adam, J. "Sun-protective clothing," *Journal of Cutaneous Medicine and Surgery* 1998:3(1):50–53. Available from: www.ncbi.nlm.nih.gov/pubmed/9677262 [Accessed 13 December 2020]

15. Gohara, M., Morison, W., Sarnoff, D.S. "Clothing: Our first line defence," *Skin Cancer.Org* 2016. Available from: www.skincancer.org/prevention/sun-protection/clothing/clothing-our-first-line-of-defense [Accessed 6 January 2020]

16. Davis, S., Capjack, L., Kerr, N., Fedosejcvs, R. "Clothing as protection from ultraviolet radiation: Which fabric is most effective?" *International Journal of Dermatology* 1997;36(5):374–379. Available from: www.ncbi.nlm.nih.gov/pubmed/9199990. [Accessed 19 December 2019]

17. Hoffmann, K., Hoffmann, A., Hanke, D., Böhringer, B., Schindling, G., Schön, U., Klotz, M.L., Altmeyer, P. "Sun protection by optimally designed fabrics," *Hautarzt* 1998;49(1):10–16. Available from: www.ncbi.nlm.nih.gov/pubmed/9522187 [Accessed 21 January 2020]

18. ARPANSA. "The Australian and New Zealand standard for sun protective clothing," Australian Radiation Protection and Nuclear Safety Agency. 2019. Available from: www.arpansa.gov.au/our-services/testing-and-calibration/ultraviolet-services/labelling-sun-protective-clothing [Accessed 1 December 2019]

19. Gambichler, T., Hatch, KL., Avermaete, A., Altmeyer, P., Hoffmann, K. "Influence of wetness on the ultraviolet protection factor (UPF) of textiles: In vitro and in vivo measurements," *Photodermatology, Photoimmunology and Photomedicine* 2002;18(1):29–35. Available from: www.ncbi.nlm.nih.gov/pubmed/11982919 [Accessed 24 December 2019]

20. AAP Paediatricians. "Sun safety: Information for parents about sunburn & sunscreen," *American Academy of Paediatrics* 2019. Available from: www.healthychildren.org/English/safety-prevention/at-play/Pages/Sun-Safety.aspx [Accessed 13 January 2020]

21. USDOHHS, Appendix 5. US Department of Health and Human Services. The surgeon general's call to action to prevent skin cancer. Washington, DC: Office of the Surgeon General (US); 2014. Federal Departments, Agencies, and Policies. Available from: www.ncbi.nlm.nih.gov/books/NBK247166 [Accessed 19 January 2020]

22. Bens, G. "Sunscreen," *Advances in Experimental Medicine and Biology* 2014;810:429–463. Available from: www.ncbi.nlm.nih.gov/pubmed/25207381 [Accessed 25 January 2020]

23. InformedHealth.org [Internet]. "Non-melanoma skin cancer: How can you avoid too much sun?" Cologne, Germany: Institute for Quality and Efficiency in Health Care (IQWiG); Updated 2018 November 29. Available from: www.ncbi.nlm.nih.gov/books/NBK534634/[Accessed 26 January 2020]

24. BAD—British Association of Dermatologists. "Sunscreen fact sheet," 2013. Available from: www.bad.org.uk/for-the-public/skin-cancer/sunscreen-fact-sheet [Accessed 25 January 2020]

25. Kaimal, S., Abraham, A. "Sunscreens," *Indian Journal of Dermatology, Venereology and Leprology* 2011;22(77):238–243. Available from: www.ijdvl.com/text.asp?2011/77/2/238/77480 [Accessed 2 January 2020]

26. Cole, C., Shyr, T., Ou-Yang, H. "Metal oxide sunscreens protect skin by absorption, not by reflection or scattering," *Photodermatology, Photoimmunology and Photomedicine* January 2016;32(1):5–10. Available from: https://onlinelibrary.wiley.com/doi/full/10.1111/phpp.12214 [Accessed 2 January 2020]

27. Latha, M.S., Martis, J., Shobha, V., Sham Shinde, R., Bangera, S., Krishnankutty, B., Bellary, S., Varughese, S., Rao, P., Naveen Kumar, B.R. "Sunscreening agents: A review," *Journal of Clinical and Aesthetic Dermatology* 2013;6(1):16–26. Available from: www.ncbi.nlm.nih.gov/pmc/articles/PMC3543289/ [Accessed 2 January 2020]

28. Bissonnette, R. "Update on sunscreens," *Skin Therapy Letter* July–August 2008;13(6):5–7. Available from: www.ncbi.nlm.nih.gov/pubmed/18806906 [Accessed 24 January 2020]

29. Govindu, P.C.V., Hosamani, B., Moi, S., Venkatachalam, D., Asha, S., John, V.N., Sandeep, V., Gowd, K.H. "Glutathione as a photo-stabilizer of avobenzone: An evaluation under glass-filtered sunlight using UV-spectroscopy," *Photochemical & Photobiological Sciences* 2019 January 1;18(1):198–207. Available from: www.ncbi.nlm.nih.gov/pubmed/30421772/ [Accessed 6 January 2020]

30. Obagi, Z. Fractionated melanin—a major advance in sun protection. *Body Language* June 2015. Available from: www.bodylanguage.net/fractionated-melanin-a-major-advance-in-sun-protection/ [Accessed 10 January 2020]

31. Akhalaya, M.Y., Maksimov, G.V., Rubin, A.B., Lademann, J., Darvin, M.E. "Molecular action mechanisms of solar infrared radiation and heat on human skin," *Ageing Research Reviews* 2014;16:1–11. Available from: www.ncbi.nlm.nih.gov/pubmed/24742502. [Accessed 10 January 2020]

32. Eberlin, S., Costa, A., Pereira, A. Polettini A., Mendes, C., Weisz, L., Lage, R. "Effects of antioxidants in the protection of infrared radiation-induced matrix metalloproteinase-1 in human dermal fibroblast," *Journal of the American Academy of Dermatology* 2014;70(5) (Suppl 1):155. Available from: www.jaad.org/article/S0190-9622(14)00646-X/abstract [Accessed 26 December 2019]

33. Liebe, F., Kaur, S., Ruvolo, E., Kollias, N., Southall, M.D. "Irradiation of skin with visible light induces reactive oxygen species and matrix-degrading enzymes," *Journal of Investigative Dermatology* 2012;132(7):1901–1907. https://dx.doi.org/10.1038/jid.2011.476 [Accessed 24 December 2019]

34. Mahmoud, B.H., Ruvolo, E., Hexsel, C.L., Liu, Y., Owen, MR., Kollias, N., Lim, HW., Hamzavi, IH. "Impact of long-wavelength UVA and visible light on melanocompetent skin." *Journal of Investigative Dermatology* 2010 Aug;130(8):2092–2097. Available from: www.ncbi.nlm.nih.gov/pubmed/20410914 [Accessed 24 December 2019]

35. Taheri, M., Darabyan, M., Izadbakhsh, E., Nouri, F., Haghani, M., Mortazavi, S.A.R., Mortazavi, G., Mortazavi, S.M.J., Moradi, M. "Exposure to visible light emitted from smartphones and tablets increases the proliferation of Staphylococcus aureus: Can this be linked to acne?" *Journal of Biomedical Physics and Engineering* 2017;7(2):163–168. Available from: www.ncbi.nlm.nih.gov/pmc/articles/PMC5447253/ [Accessed 26 December 2019]

36. ZO Skin Health. "Is your smartphone damaging your skin?" *ZO-Lifestyle, Miscellaneous, Skin Conditions* 2017. Available from: https://zo-skinhealth.co.uk/zein-obagi-smartphone-hev-light-damage/ [Accessed 30 December 2019]

37. *HB Optical Laboratories.* "What is HEV (High Energy Visible) Light?" 2015. Available from: www.hboptical.com/blog/what-is-hev-high-energy-visible-light [Accessed 2 January 2020]

38. Liposhield® HEV Melanin. "Protectio.n from the adverse effects of High Energy Visible (HEV) Light," *Liposhield.com* Available from: www.liposhield.com/pdf/liposhield-study-overview.pdf [Accessed 2 January 2020]

39. Kang, S., Chung, J.H., Lee, J.H., Fisher, G.J., Wan, Y.S., Duell, E.A., Voorhees, J.J. "Topical N-acetyl cysteine and genistein prevent ultraviolet-light-induced signaling that leads to photoaging in human skin in vivo," *Journal of Investigative Dermatology* 2003:120(5):835–841. Available from: www.ncbi.nlm.nih.gov/pubmed/12713590 [Accessed 16 January 2020]

40. Matsui, M.S., Hsia, A., Miller, J.D., Hanneman, K., Scull, H., Cooper, K.D., Baron, E. "Non-sunscreen photoprotection: Antioxidants add value to a sunscreen," *Journal of Investigative Dermatology Symposium Proceedings* August 2009;14(1):56–59. Available from: https://doi.org/10.1038/jidsymp.2009.14 [Accessed 30 December 2019]

41. Pinnell, S.R., Yang, H., Omar, M., Monteiro-Riviere, N., DeBuys, H.V., Walker, L.C., Wang, Y., Levine, M. "Topical L-ascorbic acid: Percutaneous absorption studies," *Dermatologic Surgery* February 2001;27(2):137–142. Available from: www.ncbi.nlm.nih.gov/pubmed/11207686/ [Accessed 20 January 2020]

42. Rabinovich, L., Kazlouskaya, V. "Herbal sun protection agents: Human studies," *Clinics in Dermatology* 2018;36(3):369–375. Available from: https://doi.org/10.1016/j.clindermatol.2018.03.014 [Accessed 20 January 2020]

43. Kaur, C.D., Saraf, S. "In vitro sun protection factor determination of herbal oils used in cosmetics," *Pharmacognosy Research* 2010;2(1):22–25. Available from: https://pubmed.ncbi.nlm.nih.gov/21808534-in-vitro-sun-protection-factor-determination-of-herbal-oils-used-in-cosmetics/ [Accessed 20 January 2020]

44. Donglikar, M.M., Deore, S.L. "Sunscreens: A review," *Pharmacology Journals* 2016;8(3):171–179. Available from: www.phcogj.com/article/144 [Accessed 8 January 2020]

45. Pandika, M. "Looking to nature for new sunscreens," *ACS Central Science* 2018;4(7):788–790. Available from: https://pubs.acs.org/doi/10.1021/acscentsci.8b00433 [Accessed 8 January 2020]

46. Giacomoni, P.U., Teta, L., Najdek, L. "Sunscreens: The impervious path from theory to practice," *Photochemical and Photobiological Sciences* 2010;9(4):524–529. Available from: www.ncbi.nlm.nih.gov/pubmed/20354646/ [Accessed 14 December 2019]

47. Yang, E.J., Beck, K.M., Maarouf, M., Shi, V.Y. "Truths and myths in sunscreen labelling," *Journal of Cosmetic Dermatology* 2018;17(6):1288–1292. Available from: https://onlinelibrary.wiley.com/doi/abs/10.1111/jocd.12743 [Accessed 29 December 2019]

48. Kaur, B. "Sunscreens and their properties for skin protection from solar radiation," *Journal of Aesthetic Nursing* 2017;6(2). Available from: www.magonlinelibrary.com/doi/abs/10.12968/joan.2017.6.2.6 [Accessed 12 January 2020]

49. AAD. "How to use stick and spray sunscreens," *American Academy of Dermatologists* 2018. Available from: www.aad.org/public/skin-hair-nails/skin-care/sunscreen/how-to-use-stick-and-spray-sunscreens [Accessed 3 January 2020]

50. Ngan, V. "Sunscreen testing and classification," *DermanetNZ* 2012. Available from: www.dermnetnz.org/topics/sunscreen-testing-and-classification/ [Accessed 10 January 2020]

51. Boots. "UVA, UVB & SPF—What you need to know," *Boots Pharmacy.* Available from: www.boots.com/sun-and-holiday-inspiration/suncare-advice/spf-factors-uva-and-uvb#8Flw6oPSTLSX53g5.99 [Accessed 17 January 2020]

52. Diffey, B.L. "When should sunscreen be reapplied?" *Journal of the American Academy of Dermatology* 2001 Dec;45(6):882–885. Available from: www.ncbi.nlm.nih.gov/pubmed/11712033 [Accessed 26 January 2020]

53. Young, A.R., Claveau, J.A., Rossi, B. "Ultraviolet radiation and the skin: Photobiology and sunscreen photoprotection," *Journal of the American Academy of Dermatology* 2017;76(3;1):100–109. Available from: www.jaad.org/article/S0190-9622(16)30880-5/fulltext [Accessed 26 January 2020]

54. NOAA. "How far does light travel in the ocean?" *National Ocean Service.* Available from: https://oceanservice.noaa.gov/facts/light_travel.html [Accessed 4 January 2020]

55. Dale, W.B., Moon, S., Armstrong, F. "Comprehensive review of ultraviolet radiation and the current status on sunscreens," *Journal of Clinical and Aesthetic Dermatology* 2012;5(9):18–23. Available from: www.ncbi.nlm.nih.gov/pmc/articles/PMC3460660/#__sec5title [Accessed 11 January 2020]

56. Arney, K. "How to apply Sunscreen?" *NHS. UK. Video* 2018. Available from: www.nhs.uk/video/pages/how-to-apply-sunscreen.aspx [Accessed 26 January 2020]

57. NHS Choices. "Sunscreen and sun safety," *NHS choices* 2019. Available from: www.nhs.uk/live-well/healthy-body/sunscreen-and-sun-safety/#sunscreen [Accessed 26 January 2020]

58. Petersen, B., Wulf, H.C. "Application of sunscreen—theory and reality," *Photodermatology, Photoimmunology and Photomedicine* 2014;30:96–101. Available from: https://onlinelibrary.wiley.com/doi/full/10.1111/phpp.12099 [Accessed 26 January 2020]

59. Heerfordt, I.M., Torsnes, L.R., Philipsen, P.A., Wulf, H.C. "Sunscreen use optimized by two consecutive applications," *PLoS One* 2018;13(3):e0193916. Available from: www.ncbi.nlm.nih.gov/pmc/articles/PMC5874020/ [Accessed 26 January 2020]

60. Simon, S. "Choose the right sunscreen," *American Cancer Society* 2018. Available from: www.cancer.org/latest-news/choose-the-right-sunscreen.html [Accessed 26 January 2020]

61. Ou-Yang, H., Rzendzian, R.B. "Sunburn protection by sunscreen sprays at beach," *Cosmetics* 2017;4(1):10. Available from: www.mdpi.com/2079-9284/4/1/10/htm [Accessed 23 January 2020]

62. Hughes, M.C.B., Williams, G.M., Bake, P., Green, A.C. "Sunscreen and prevention of skin aging: A randomized trial," *Annals of Internal Medicine* 2013;158(11):781–790. Available from: www.ncbi.nlm.nih.gov/pubmed/23732711 [Accessed 23 January 2020]

63. Phillips, T.J., Bhawan, J., Yaar, M., Bello, Y., Lopiccolo, D., Nash, J.F. "Effect of daily versus intermittent sunscreen application on solar simulated UV radiation-induced skin response in humans," *Journal of the American Academy of Dermatology* 2000;43(4):610–618. Available from: https://dx.doi.org/10.1067/mjd.2000.107244 [Accessed 23 January 2020]

64. Marionnet, C., Pierrard, C., Golebiewski, C., Bernerd, F. "Diversity of biological effects induced by longwave UVA rays (UVA1) in reconstructed skin," *PLoS One* 2014;9(8). Available from: www.ncbi.nlm.nih.gov/pmc/articles/PMC4139344/ [Accessed 23 January 2020]

65. Cancer Council Australia. "Preventing skin cancer," *Cancer Council Australia*. Available from: www.cancer.org.au/preventing-cancer/sun-protection/preventing-skin-cancer/ [Accessed 22 January 2020]

66. Diffey, B.L. "Time and place as modifiers of personal UV exposure," *International Journal of Environmental Research and Public Health* 2018;15(6):1112. Available from: www.mdpi.com/1660-4601/15/6/1112 [Accessed 22 January 2020]

67. USEPA. "Sun safety. Calculating the UV index," *United States Environmental Protection Agency* 2017. Available from: www.epa.gov/sunsafety/calculating-uv-index-0 [Accessed 22 January 2020]

68. Tang, J.C., Hanke, C.W. "Against the wind," *Skin Cancer Foundation* 2017 May. Available from: www.skincancer.org/prevention/sun-protection/wind [Accessed 22 January 2020]

69. Taylor, S., Diffey, B. "Simple dosage guide for suncreens will help users," *British Medical Journal* 2002;324(7352):1526. Available from: www.ncbi.nlm.nih.gov/pmc/articles/PMC1123459/ [Accessed 22 January 2020]

70. Couteau, C., Diarra, H., Coiffard, L. "Effect of the product type, of the amount of applied sunscreen product and the level of protection in the UVB range on the level of protection achieved in the UVA range," *International Journal of Pharmaceutics* 2016;500(1–2):210–216. Available from: www.ncbi.nlm.nih.gov/pubmed/26806467 [Accessed 22 January 2020]

71. Hacker, E., Horsham, C., Ford, H., Hartel, G., Olsen, C.M., Pandeya, N., Janda, M. "UV detection stickers can assist people to reapply sunscreen," *Preventive Medicine* 2019;124:67–74. Available from: www.sciencedirect.com/science/article/pii/S0091743519301732 [Accessed 22 January 2020]

72. Beyer, D.M., Faurschou, A., Haedersdal, M., Wulf, H.C. "Clothing reduces the sun protection factor of sunscreens," *British Journal of Dermatology* 2010 February 1;162(2):415–419. Available from: www.ncbi.nlm.nih.gov/pubmed/19845666 [Accessed 27 January 2020]

73. Forney, R. "Does sunscreen become ineffective after its expiration date," *Skin Cancer.Org* 2019. Available from: https://blog.skincancer.org/2018/07/31/ask-the-expert-does-a-sunscreen-stay-effective-after-its-expiration-date/ [Accessed 27 January 2020]

74. Briasco, B., Capra, P., Mannucci, B., Perugini, P. "Stability study of sunscreens with free and encapsulated UV filters contained in plastic packaging," *Pharmaceutics* 2017;9:19. Available from: www.mdpi.com/1999-4923/9/2/19/pdf [Accessed 27 January 2020]

75. Singh, K.B.G., Dixit, S., Lee, A., Brown, P., Smith, S.D. "Assessment of attitudes towards sun-protective behaviour in Australians: A cross-sectional study," *Australasian Journal of Dermatology* 2016;57(2):102–107. Available from: https://onlinelibrary.wiley.com/doi/abs/10.1111/ajd.12334 [Accessed 27 January 2020]

76. Tan, M.G., Nag, S., Weinstein, M. "Parental use of sun protection for their children—does skin color matter?" *Paediatric Dermatology* 2018;35(2):220–224. Available from: https://onlinelibrary.wiley.com/doi/abs/10.1111/pde.13433 [Accessed 27 January 2020]

77. Wesson, K.M., Silverberg, N.B. "Sun protection education in the United States: What we know and what needs to be taught," *Cutis* 2003;71(1):71–74, 77. Available from: www.ncbi.nlm.nih.gov/pubmed/12553634?dopt=Abstract [Accessed 14 January 2020]

78. Truhan, A.P. "Sun protection in childhood," *Clinical Pediatrics (Phila)* 1991 December;30(12):676–681. Available from: www.ncbi.nlm.nih.gov/pubmed/?term=Truhan+AP.+Sun+protection+in+childhood.+Clin+Pediatr+(Phila)+1991%3B30(12)%3A676-81 [Accessed 23 January 2020]

79. Godar, D.E., Urbach, F., Gasparro, F.P., van der Leun, J.C. "UV doses of young adults," *Photochemistry and Photobiology* 2003 April;77(4):453–457. Available from: www.ncbi.nlm.nih.gov/pubmed/12733658?dopt=Abstract [Accessed 6 January 2020]

80. Dadlani, C., Orlow, S.J. "Planning for a brighter future: A review of sun protection and barriers to behavioral change in children and adolescents," *Dermatology Online Journal* 2008;14(9):1. Available from: https://escholarship.org/uc/item/6vs1r0r9 [Accessed 20 January 2020]

81. Sachs, H.C. "Should you put sunscreen on infants? Not usually," Consumer updates, *Food and Drug Administration* 2016. Available from: www.fda.gov/consumers/consumer-updates/should-you-put-sunscreen-infants-not-usually [Accessed 18 December 2019]

82. Linder, J. "Sun protection for infants," *Skin Cancer Foundation* 2013. Available from: www.skincancer.org/prevention/sun-protection/children/infants [Accessed 13 December 2019]

83. Gulson, B., McCall, M., Korsch, M., Gomez, L., Casey, P., Oytam, Y., Taylor, A., McCulloch, M., Trotter, J., Kinsley, L., Greenoak, G. "Small amounts of zinc from zinc oxide particles in sunscreens applied outdoors are absorbed through human skin," *Toxicological Sciences* 2010;118(1). Available from: www.ncbi.nlm.nih.gov/pubmed/20705894 [Accessed 4 January 2020]

84. Schulz, J., Hohenberg, H., Pflücker, F., Gärtner, E., Will, T., Pfeiffer, S., Wepf, R., Wendel, V., Gers-Barlag, H., Wittern, K.P. "Distribution of sunscreens on skin," *Adv Drug Deliv Rev* 2002 November;54(1):S157–163. Available from: www.ncbi.nlm.nih.gov/pubmed/12460721 [Accessed 9 December 2019]

85. Krause, M., Klit, A., Blomberg Jensen, M., Søeborg, T., Frederiksen, H., Schlumpf, M., Lichtensteiger, W., Skakkebaek, N.E., Drzewiecki, K.T. "Sunscreens: Are they beneficial for health? An overview of endocrine disrupting properties of UV-filters," *International Journal of Andrology* 2012 June;35(3):424–436. Available from: www.ncbi.nlm.nih.gov/pubmed/22612478 [Accessed 12 December 2019]

86. Janjua, N.R., Kongshoj, B., Andersson, A.M., Wulf, H.C. "Sunscreens in human plasma and urine after repeated whole-body topical application," *Journal of the European Academy of Dermatology and Venereology* 2008;22(4):456–461. Available from: www.ncbi.nlm.nih.gov/pubmed/18221342/ [Accessed 13 December 2019]

87. Wang, J., Ganley, C.J. "Safety threshold considerations for sunscreen systemic exposure: A simulation study," *Clinical Pharmacology and Therapeutics* 2019;105(1):161–167. Available from: www.ncbi.nlm.nih.gov/pmc/articles/PMC6312469/ [Accessed 2 January 2020]

88. Janjua, N.R., Kongshoj, B., Petersen, J.H., Wulf, H.C. "Sunscreens and thyroid function in humans after short-term whole-body topical application: A single-blinded study," *British Journal of Dermatology* 2007 May;156(5):1080–1082. Available from: https://onlinelibrary.wiley.com/doi/abs/10.1111/j.1365-2133.2007.07803.x [Accessed 13 December 2019]

89. Matta, M.K., Zusterzeel, R., Pilli, N.R., Patel, V., Volpe, D.A., Florian, J., Oh, L., Bashaw, E., Zineh, I., Sanabria, C., Kemp, S., Godfrey, A., Adah, S., Coelho, S., Wang, J., Furlong, L.A., Ganley, C., Michele, T., Strauss, D.G. "Effect of sunscreen application under maximal use conditions on plasma concentration of sunscreen active ingredients; a randomized clinical trial," *JAMA* 2019;321(21):2082–2091. Available from: https://jamanetwork.com/journals/jama/article-abstract/2733085 [Accessed 1 December 2019]

90. Benech-Kieffer, F., Meuling, W.J., Leclerc, C., Roza, L., Leclaire, J., Nohynek, G. "Percutaneous absorption of Mexoryl SX in human volunteers: Comparison with in vitro data," *Skin Pharmacol. Appl. Skin Physio* 2003;16(6):343–355. Available from: www.ncbi.nlm.nih.gov/pubmed/14528058 [Accessed 22 December 2019]

91. Doheny, K. "FDA proposes major changes to sunscreen rules," *Medscape* 2019. Available from: www.medscape.com/viewarticle/909428 [Accessed 19 December 2019]

92. Foley, P., Nixon, R., Marks, R., Frowen, K., Thompson, S. "The frequency of reactions to sunscreens: Results of a longitudinal population-based study on the regular use of sunscreens in Australia," *British Journal of Dermatology* 1993 May;128(5):512–518. Available from: www.ncbi.nlm.nih.gov/pubmed/8504041 [Accessed 16 December 2019]

93. Spijker, G.T., Schuttelaar, M.L., Barkema, L., Velders, A., Coenraads, P.J. "Anaphylaxis caused by topical application of a sunscreen containing benzophenone-3," *Contact Dermatitis* 2008;59:248–249. Available from: http://onlinelibrary.wiley.com/wol1/doi/10.1111/j.1600-0536.2008.01337.x/full [Accessed 13 January 2020]

94. Del Rosso, J.Q., Gold, M., Rueda, M.J., Brandt, S., Winkelman, W.J. "Efficacy, safety, and subject satisfaction of a specified skin care regimen to cleanse, medicate, moisturize, and protect the skin of patients under treatment for acne vulgaris," *Journal of Clinical and Aesthetic Dermatology* 2015;8(1):22–30. Available from: www.ncbi.nlm.nih.gov/pmc/articles/PMC3175800/ [Accessed 30 December 2019]

95. Schauder, S., Ippen, H. "Contact and photocontact sensitivity to sunscreens. Review of a 15-year experience and of the literature," *Contact Dermatitis* 1997;37(5):221–232. Available from: www.ncbi.nlm.nih.gov/pubmed/9412750 [Accessed 30 December 2019]

96. Nixon, R.L., Frowen, K.E., Lewis, A.E. "Skin reactions to sunscreens," *Australasian Journal of Dermatology* 1997 June;38(1):S83–85. Available from: www.ncbi.nlm.nih.gov/pubmed/10994480 [Accessed 13 December 2019]

97. Mohammed, Y.H., Holmes, A., Haridass, I.N., Sanchez, W.Y. Studier, H., Grice, J.E., Benson, H.A.E., Roberts, M.S. "Support for the safe use of zinc oxide nanoparticle sunscreens: Lack of skin penetration or cellular toxicity after repeated application in volunteers," *Journal of Investigative Dermatology* 2019 February;139(2):308–315. Available from: www.jidonline.org/article/S0022-202X(18)32655-1/fulltext [Accessed 4 January 2020]

98. Kimura, E., Kawano, Y., Todo, H., Ikarashi, Y., Sugibayashi, K. "Measurement of skin permeation/penetration of nanoparticles for their safety evaluation," *Biological and Pharmaceutical Bulletin* 2012;35: 1476–1486. Available from: www.ncbi.nlm.nih.gov/pubmed/22975498 [Accessed 4 January 2020]

99. "Therapeutic goods administration, literature review on the safety of titanium dioxide and zinc oxide nanoparticles in Sunscreens,"*Canberra (AUST): Australian Department of Health* 2017. Available from: www. tga.gov.au/literature-review-safety-titanium-dioxide-and-zinc-oxide-nanoparticles-sunscreens [Accessed 1 February 2020]

100. Ngan, V. "Allergy to PABA," *Dermanet NZ* 2002. Available from: https:// dermnetnz.org/topics/allergy-to-parabens/ [Accessed 27 January 2020]

101. Lim, H.W., Arellano-Mendoza, M., Stengel, F. "Current challenges in photoprotection," *Journal of the American Academy of Dermatology* 2017;76(3 Supp 1):S91–99

102. Mellowship, D. "Toxic beauty: The hidden chemicals in cosmetics and how they can harm us," *Octopus Publishing Group London e-book* 2009. Available from: https://books.google.co.uk/books?id=KYjXCIRNtjQC& pg=PT125&dq=sensitivity+to+artificial+sweeteners+and+sunscreen& hl=en&sa=X&ved=0ahUKEwjTnfmZnKLnAhUIbcAKHXkoCJIQ6AEI OzAC#v=onepage&q=sensitivity%20to%20artificial%20sweeteners%20 and%20sunscreen&f=false [Accessed 27 January 2020]

103. Simonsen, A.B., Koppelhus, U., Sommerlund, M., Deleuran, M. "Photosensitivity in atopic dermatitis complicated by contact allergy to common sunscreen ingredients," *Contact Dermatitis* 2016;74(1):56–58. Available from: www.ncbi.nlm.nih.gov/pubmed/26690280 [Accessed 27 January 2020]

104. Bilsland, D., Ferguson, J. "Contact allergy to sunscreen chemicals in photosensitivity dermatitis/actinic reticuloid syndrome (PD/AR) and polymorphic light eruption (PLE)," *Contact Dermatitis* 1993;29(2):70–73. Available from: www.ncbi.nlm.nih.gov/pubmed/8365179 [Accessed 25 January 2020]

105. Ruszkiewicz, JA., Pinkas, A., Ferrer, B., Peres, TV., Tsatsakis, A., Aschner, M. "Neurotoxic effect of active ingredients in sunscreen products, a contemporary review," *Toxicology Reports* 2017;4:245–259. Available from: www.ncbi.nlm.nih.gov/pmc/articles/PMC5615097/ [Accessed 25 January 2020]

106. Lopes, M.L., Silva, Júnior F.L., Lima, K.C., Oliveira, P.T., Silveira, É.J. "Clinicopathological profile and management of 161 cases of actinic cheilitis," *An Bras Dermatol* 2015;90(4):505–512. Available from: www.ncbi. nlm.nih.gov/pmc/articles/PMC4560539/ [Accessed 12 January 2020]

107. Lourenco, E.A.J., Shaw, L., Pratt, H., Duffy, G.L., Czanner G, Zheng, Y., Hamill, K.J., McCormick, A.G. "Application of SPF moisturisers is inferior to sunscreens in coverage of facial and eyelid regions," *Plos One* 2019;14(4). Available from: https://doi.org/10.1371/journal. pone.0212548 [Accessed 25 January 2020]

108. Boiko, S. "Ask the Expert: Can you safely use sunscreen around the eyes? If so then what kind is best?" *Skin Cancer.Org* 2018. Available from: www.skin-cancer.org/blog/sunscreen-around-your-eyes/ [Accessed 29 January 2020]

109. Marrot, L. "Pollution and sun exposure: A deleterious synergy mechanisms and opportunities for skin protection," *Current Medical Chemistry* 2017 September;25(40). Available online: www.researchgate.net/publication/319940336_Pollution_and_Sun_Exposure_A_Deleterious_ Synergy_Mechanisms_and_Opportunities_for_Skin_Protection [Accessed 4 January 2020]

110. Burke, K.E. "A new understanding of environmental damage to the skin and prevention with topical antioxidants," *Mechanisms of Ageing and Development* 2018 June;172:123–130. Available from: www.scien-cedirect.com/science/article/abs/pii/S0047637417302841?via%3Dihub [Accessed 25 January 2020]

111. Narda, M., Bauza, G., Valderas, P., Granger, C. "Protective effects of a novel facial cream against environmental pollution: In vivo and in vitro assessment," *Clinical, Cosmetic and Investigational Dermatology* 2018;11:571–578. Available from: www.ncbi.nlm.nih.gov/pmc/articles/ PMC6237134/ [Accessed 25 January 2020]

112. Mancebo, S.E., Hu, J.Y., Wang, S.Q. "Sunscreens," *Photodermatology, Dermatologic Clinics* 2014 July;32(3):427–438, Elsevier Inc. Available from: www.derm.theclinics.com/article/S0733-8635(14)00026-6/abstract [Accessed 11 January 2020]

113. Lindqvist, P.G., Epstein, E., Nielsen, K., Landin-Olsson, M., Ingvar, C., Olsson, H. "Avoidance of sun exposure as a risk factor for major causes of death: A competing risk analysis of the Melanoma in Southern Sweden cohort," *Journal of Internal Medicine* 2016;280(4):375–387. Available from: http://onlinelibrary.wiley.com/doi/10.1111/joim.12496/full [Accessed 25 January 2020]

114. Frellick, M. "Avoiding sun zas dangerous as smoking," *Medscape Medical News* 2016 March. Available from: www.medscape.com/viewarticle/860 805?pa=4SUlh%2F9D%2F6wmbVH%2B6z15J5PnaZqjVeAqRy79NwWb SIBYUH8uiwdOe9cXbzlZQBwccFrqow%2Bf2%2F37XuRaZT6JAA%3D %3D [Accessed 25 January 2020]

115. Mostafa, W.Z., Hegazy, R.A. "Vitamin D and the skin: Focus on a complex relationship: A review," *Journal of Advanced Research* 2015;6(6):793–804. Available from: www.ncbi.nlm.nih.gov/pmc/articles/PMC4642156/ [Accessed 13 December 2019]

116. Ritu G, Gupta, A. "Vitamin D deficiency in India: Prevalence, causalities and interventions," *Nutrients* 2014;6(2):729–775. Available from: www. ncbi.nlm.nih.gov/pmc/articles/PMC3942730/ [Accessed 12 December 2019]

117. Neale, R.E., Khan, S.R., Lucas, R.M., Waterhouse, M., Whiteman, D.C., Olsen, C.M. "The effect of sunscreen on vitamin D: A review," *British Journal of Dermatology* 2019 November;181(5):907–915. Available from: www.ncbi.nlm.nih.gov/pubmed/30945275 [Accessed 12 December 2019]

118. NHS UK. "How to get vitamin D from Sunlight,"*NHS UK* 2018 August. Available from: www.nhs.uk/live-well/healthy-body/how-to-get-vita-min-d-from-sunlight/ [Accessed 12 December 2019]

119. Singh, S., Jha, B., Tiwary, N.K., Agrawal, N.K. "Does using a high sun protection factor sunscreen on face, along with physical photoprotection advice, in patients with melasma, change serum vitamin D concentration in Indian conditions? A pragmatic pretest-posttest study," *Indian Journal of Dermatology, Venereology and Leprology* 2019;85(3):282–286. Available from: www.ijdvl.com/article.asp?issn=0378-6323;year=201 9;volume=85;issue=3;spage=282;epage=286;aulast=Singh [Accessed 7 December 2019]

120. Tsui, M.M., Leung, H.W., Wai, T.C., Yamashita, N., Taniyasu, S., Liu, W., Lam, P.K.S., Murphy, M.B. "Occurrence, distribution and ecological risk assessment of multiple classes of UV filters in surface waters from different countries," *Water Research* 2014 December 15;67:55–65. Available from: www.ncbi.nlm.nih.gov/pubmed/25261628?dopt=Abstract [Accessed 2 January 2020]

121. Tsui, M.M.P., Lam, J.C.W., Ng, T.Y., Ang, P.O., Murphy, M.B., Lam, P.K.S. "Occurrence, distribution, and fate of organic UV filters in coral communities," *Environmental Science and Technology* 2017 April 18;51(8):4182–4190. Available from: www.ncbi.nlm.nih.gov/ pubmed/28351139?dopt=Abstract [Accessed 2 January 2020]

122. Zachos, E., Rosen, E. "What sunscreens are best for you—and the planet? Harmful chemicals from sunscreen can damage coral. Here's how to protect both your skin and the reefs," *National Geographic* 2019 May. Available from: www.nationalgeographic.co.uk/environment/2019/05/ what-sunscreens-are-best-you-and-planet [Accessed 2 January 2020]

123. Parrado, C., Philips, N., Gilaberte, Y., Juarranz, A., González, S. "Oral photoprotection: Effective agents and potential candidates," *Frontiers of Medicine (Lausanne)* 2018;5:188. Available from: www.ncbi.nlm.nih. gov/pmc/articles/PMC6028556/ [Accessed 2 January 2020]

124. Parrado, C., Mascaraque, M., Gilaberte, Y., Juarranz, A., Gonzalez. S. "Fernblock (Polypodium leucotomos extract): Molecular mechanisms and pleiotropic effects in light-related skin conditions, photoaging and skin cancers, a review," *International Journal of Molecular Sciences* 2016 June 29;17(7). Available from: www.ncbi.nlm.nih.gov/pubmed/27367679 [Accessed 2 January 2020]

125. Nestor, M.S., Berman, B., Swenson, N. "Safety and efficacy of oral polypodium leucotomos extract in healthy adult subject," *Journal of Clinical and Aesthetic Dermatology* 2015;8(2):19–23. Available from: www.ncbi. nlm.nih.gov/pmc/articles/PMC4345929/ [Accessed 2 January 2020]

126. Goh, C.L., Chuah, S.Y., Tien, S., Thng, G., Vitale, M.A., Delgado-Rubin, A. "Double-blind, Placebo-controlled Trial to Evaluate the Effectiveness of *Polypodium Leucotomos* extract in the treatment of melasma in Asian skin: A pilot study," *Journal of Clinical and Aesthetic Dermatology* 2018;11(3):14–19. Available from: www.ncbi.nlm.nih.gov/pmc/articles/ PMC5868779/ [Accessed 2 January 2020]

127. Hexsel, C.L., Bangert, S.D., Hebert, A.A., Lim, H.W. "Current sunscreen issues: 2007 Food and Drug Administration sunscreen labelling recommendations and combination sunscreen/insect repellent products," *Journal of the American Academy of Dermatology* 2008 August;59(2):316–323. Available from: www.ncbi.nlm.nih.gov/pubmed/18485529 [Accessed 2 January 2020]

128. Webb, C.E., Russell, R.C. "Insect repellents and sunscreen: Implications for personal protection strategies against mosquito-borne disease," *Australian and New Zealand Journal of Public Health* 2009 October;33(5):485–490. Available from: https://onlinelibrary.wiley.com/ doi/full/10.1111/j.1753-6405.2009.00435.x [Accessed 22 January 2020]

129. Yiin, L.M., Tian, J.N., Hung, C.C. "Assessment of dermal absorption of DEET-containing insect repellent and oxybenzone-containing sunscreen using human urinary metabolites," *Environmental Science and Pollution Research International* 2015 May;22(9):7062–7070. Available from: www. ncbi.nlm.nih.gov/pubmed/25491253 [Accessed 12 January 2020]

130. Krishnaswamy, G., Kurian, S.S., Srinivas, C.R., Kumar, L.S. "Camouflage in xeroderma pigmentosum," *Indian Dermatol Online Journal* 2016;7(6):553–555. Available from: www.ncbi.nlm.nih.gov/pmc/articles/ PMC5134184/ [Accessed 5 January 2020]

131. Rayner, V.L. "Camouflage therapy," *Dermatologic Clinics* 1995;13(2):467–472. Available from: www.sciencedirect.com/science/article/abs/pii/S0733863518300937 [Accessed 5 January 2020]

132. Levy, L.L., Emer, J.J. "Emotional benefit of cosmetic camouflage in the treatment of facial skin conditions: Personal experience and review," *Clinical, Cosmetic and Investigational Dermatology* 2012;5:173–182. Available from: www.ncbi.nlm.nih.gov/pmc/articles/PMC3496327/#b33-ccid-5-173 [Accessed 5 January 2020]

133. Kryolan UK. "Dermacolor body camouflage," *Kryolan UK*. Available from: https://uk.kryolan.com/product/dermacolor-body-camouflage?ref=product-lines/dermacolor/foundation [Accessed 5 January 2020]

134. Colorescience UK. "Even up clinical pigment perfector SPF 50," *Colorescience UK* 2019. Available from: https://colorescienceuk.com/products/even-up-clinical-pigment-perfector-spf-50[Accessed 5 January 2020]

135. Vashi, N.A., Kundu, R.V. "Facial hyperpigmentation: Causes and treatment,"*British Journal of Dermatology*; Special Issue: *Ethnic Skin: A New Era for Studying Human Cutaneous Diversity* 2013 October;169(3):41–56. Available from: https://onlinelibrary.wiley.com/doi/full/10.1111/bjd.12536 [Accessed 5 January 2020]

136. Battie, C., Gohara, M., Verschoore, M., Roberts, W. "Skin cancer in skin of color: An update on current facts, trends, and misconceptions," *Journal of Drugs in Dermatology* 2013 February;12(2):194–198. Available from: www.ncbi.nlm.nih.gov/pubmed/23377393 [Accessed 5 January 2020]

137. Buchanan Lunsford, N., Berktold, J., Holman, D.M., Stein, K., Prempeh, A., Yerkes, A. "Skin cancer knowledge, awareness, beliefs and preventive behaviours among black and hispanic men and women," *Preventive Medicine Reports* 2018;12:203–209. Available from: www.ncbi.nlm.nih.gov/pmc/articles/PMC6199782/ [Accessed 5 January 2020]

138. Randhawa, M., Wang, S., Leyden, J.L., Cula, G.O., Pagnoni, A., Southall, M.D. "Daily use of a facial broad spectrum sunscreen over one-year significantly improves clinical evaluation of photoaging," *Dermatologic Surgery* 2016;0:1–8. Available from: www.dawsondermatology.com/docs/Daily%20Sunscreen%20Use%202016.pdf [Accessed 5 January 2020]

CHAPTER 16: CLEANSERS AND MOISTURIZERS

Jennifer David

16.1 Introduction

An intact epidermis is essential for maintaining homeostasis and providing an effective barrier to protect against irritants, environmental pollutants, and infectious organisms. The outermost layer of the epidermis, the stratum corneum, consists of flattened corneocyte cells (bricks) embedded in a lipid matrix (mortar) and forms the interface between the body and the external environment. The lipid matrix is composed of ceramides, cholesterol, and long-chain fatty acids maintained at an optimal ratio to mediate the permeability barrier against excessive water and electrolyte loss. The integrity of the skin's barrier function is objectively measured by the transepidermal water loss (TEWL), which is the evaluation of changes in the rate of passive evaporation (moisture loss) through the skin (1, 2).

Cleansing and moisturizing are the most basic steps in any skin care regimen. The role of a cleanser is to remove dirt, environmental pollution, excess sebum, and pathogens from the skin, whereas the function of a moisturizer is to minimize and repair any barrier damage induced by cleansing. The choice of one's cleansing and moisturizing agents can greatly affect the skin's barrier function and exacerbate or trigger underlying skin pathologies (atopic dermatitis, acne, post-inflammatory hyperpigmentation). Additionally, skin physiology varies between different ethnicities and can affect one's choice in selecting a cleaner and moisturizer.

16.2 Cleansers

Soaps as skin-cleansing agents were discovered thousands of years ago, and the widespread use of soap has been the single most important advancement in decreasing the spread of disease worldwide.(3) The advent of soap predates recorded history, going back thousands of years. Excavations of ancient Babylon uncovered cylinders from 2800 BCE with a soap-like substance inside, where the outside inscriptions detailed the process for making it. Additionally, ancient Egyptian texts dating back to c. 1500 BCE described similar recipes (3, 4).

The terms "soap" and "detergent" are commonly used interchangeably, but there are technical differences. Soap is a natural surfactant resulting from a reaction between a long-chain fatty acid and an alkali. Basic bar soap is formed by a process called saponification, where alkali salts (sodium hydroxide or potassium hydroxide) are made to react with fats (e.g., animal tallow or lard) or oils (e.g., coconut oil, olive oil, palm oil), resulting in sodium salts of fatty acids. The pH of basic soap is typically 9–10, which is far from the ideal skin pH of 5.4. Traditional soap's high pH, along with its inability to discern between lipids in the normal skin matrix and unwanted dirt/oil on the surface, leads to the disruption of the skin barrier. The dissolution of healthy lipids in the skin during cleansing accounts for the skin-tightening sensation that can sometimes be felt. Disrupting the skin barrier can cause or exacerbate skin conditions, such as atopic dermatitis, xerosis, acne, and psoriasis.

Attempts to diminish the irritancy of soaps led to the development of surfactants containing synthetic detergents in the 1940 and 1950s. A detergent is a cleansing or purifying surfactant that is often misconceived as being a more harsh skin-cleansing agent. Synthetic detergents (more commonly known as syndet bars) contain <10% of soap and have a pH ranging from 5.7 to 7.0, thus minimizing cutaneous alkalization. These properties make them less drying than traditional soap (4, 5).

Surfactants (shorthand for "surface acting agents") are chemical substances that trap dirt/oil and emulsify them upon exposure to water, allowing them to be washed away with very little mechanical force needed (Figure 16.1). There are various kinds of surfactants found in synthetic detergents, and because of their chemical makeup, they can be engineered to perform well under a variety of conditions. Surfactants are generally categorized into four major groups based on their net charge (Table 16.1 and Figure 16.2).

The head of the surfactant molecule is attracted to water (hydrophilic), and the tail is attracted to grease and dirt/oil (hydrophobic). When the detergent molecules meet dirt on the skin's surface, the tails are drawn into the dirt, but the heads still sit in the water. The attractive forces between the head groups and the water are so strong that the dirt is lifted away from the surface. The blob of dirt is now completely surrounded by detergent molecules and is broken into smaller pieces, which are washed away by the water.

- **Anionic Surfactants**
  - Anionic surfactants have a negative charge on their hydrophilic end and include natural soap surfactants (potassium cocoate). The negative charge helps the surfactant molecules lift and suspend soils in micelles. Because they are able to attack a broad range of soils, anionic surfactants are used frequently in soaps and detergents. Anionic surfactants create a lot of foam when mixed (6, 7).
  - Sulfates, sulfonates, and gluconates are examples of anionic surfactants.
- **Nonionic Surfactants**
  - Nonionic surfactants are neutral. They do not have any charge on their hydrophilic end. Nonionic surfactants are very good at emulsifying oils and are better than anionic surfactants at removing organic soils. Certain nonionic surfactants can be non-foaming or low-foaming. This makes them a good choice as an ingredient in low-foaming detergents (6, 7).
  - Examples of some common nonionic surfactants include ethoxylates, alkoxylates, and cocamides.
- **Cationic Surfactants**
  - Cationic surfactants have a positive charge on their hydrophilic end. They tend to be less irritating than anionic surfactants, and they have some disinfectant properties and thus are commonly used as preservatives. Cationic surfactants play a minor role in routine skin cleansers because they cannot be mixed with anionic surfactants. If positively charged cationic surfactants are mixed with negatively charged anionic surfactants, they will fall out of the solution and no longer be effective. Cationic and nonionic surfactants, however, are compatible (6, 7).

DOI: 10.1201/9780429243769-16

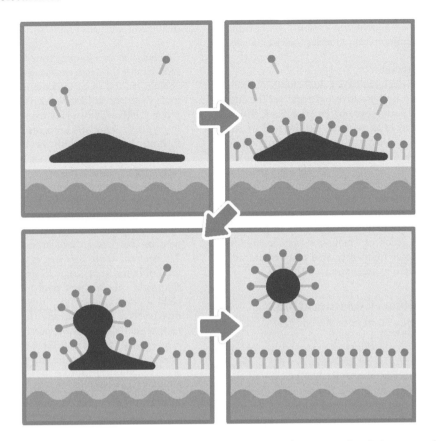

FIGURE 16.1 How surfactants work. The head of the surfactants molecule is attracted to water (hydrophilic) and the tail is attracted to grease and dirt/oil (hydrophobic). When the detergent molecules meet dirt on the skin surface, the tails are drawn into the dirt but the heads still sit in the water. The attractive forces between the head groups and the water are so strong that the dirt is lifted away from the surface. The blob of dirt is now completely surrounded by detergent molecules and is broken.

TABLE 16.1: Types of Surfactants and Their Properties

Surfactant Category	Types	Properties
Anionic (negative charge)	• Sodium lauryl sulfate (SLS)	• Good lathering
	• Sodium laureth sulfate (SLES)	• SLS can be a strong irritant where SLES has good cleansing power but less irritating
	• Cocoylisethionate	• Sodium cocylisethionate: very good skin tolerance
	• Sodium sterate	
	• Sodium tallowate	
Cationic (positive charge)	• Cetrimide	• Poorly tolerated alone
	• Sodium triethanolamine	• Strong antimicrobial properties
Nonionic (no charge)	• Cocoglucoside	• Poor lather
	• Lauryl glucoside	• Well tolerated
Amphoteric (positive and negative charge)	• Cocamidopropylbetaine	• Good lather
	• Cocoamphoacetate	• Well tolerated
	• Cocoamphodiacetate	

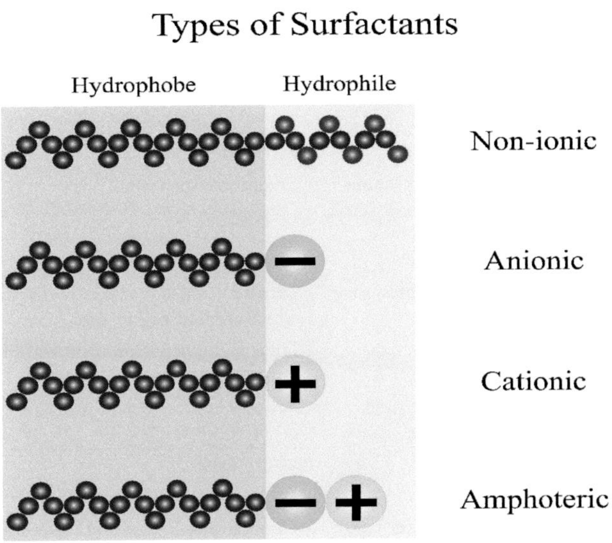

Types of Surfactants

Hydrophobe   Hydrophile

Non-ionic

Anionic

Cationic

Amphoteric

FIGURE 16.2 Types of surfactants.

- Examples of some common cationic surfactants include alkyl ammonium chlorides, cetrimide, and benzalkonium.
  - **Amphoteric Surfactants**
    - Amphoteric surfactants have a dual charge on their hydrophilic end, both positive and negative. The dual charges cancel each other out, creating a net charge of zero, referred to as zwitterionic. The pH of any given solution will determine how the amphoteric surfactants react. In acidic solutions, the amphoteric surfactants become positively charged and behave similarly to cationic surfactants. In alkaline solutions, they develop a negative charge, similar to anionic surfactants (6, 7).
    - Amphoteric surfactants are often used in personal care products, such as shampoos and cosmetics. Examples of some frequently used amphoteric surfactants are betaines and amino oxides.

16.3 Additional Considerations

16.3.1 Acid-Base Balance

Healthy skin leans more on the acidic side, with a pH of 5.5. This acid mantle discourages the colonization of bacteria/fungi and promotes the retention of moisture in the skin. When bathing occurs regularly, the pH of a cleanser has a significant impact on the skin's acid mantle. A cleansing product with a pH of 4 to 7 is recommended to avoid this disruption (8, 9).

16.3.2 Bar versus Liquid

There has been much debate regarding the use of bar versus liquid skin cleansers, especially in regard to infection control in communal spaces. Some infection control experts contend that when bar soaps are stored in contact with moisture, the resulting jelly mass at its base may harbor live pathogens. A study in the early 1990s by the Dial Corporation studied whether or not bacteria from a used bar of soap transferred to the skin. In short, it was determined that no, it does not. In this regard, both hand bar soaps and liquid hand soaps were determined equally safe when dealing with bacteria (10–12).

Cleansing Bar Subtypes (Table 16.2):

- *Combination bars (combars)* are milder than true soaps but induce more thorough cleansing than syndets. They usually contain natural soaps in combination with milder surfactants. Synthetic surfactants tend to blunt the irritancy of the product, although the pH remains high at 9–9.5 (5).
- *Superfatted soap bars* are a result of incomplete saponification (neutralization) by leaving unreacted fatty acids or oils in the product or by adding fatty alcohols, fatty acids, or esters during the manufacturing process. Common additives include lanolin, mineral oil, olive oil, cocoa butter, and other neutral fats. The amount of fat varies from 5% to 15% (most soaps ordinarily contain <2% fat); supperfatting typically enhances a soap's mildness, moisturization, and lather (5).
- *Transparent soap bars* are manufactured with a high level of humectants, such as glycerin (at least 10% more than other soaps), that tend to solubilize the soaps to yield a clear appearance. These products still contain high levels of active soap and an alkaline pH but are typically rendered mild by the presence of glycerin and a low level of total fatty matter (5).
- *Syndet bars* have skin-cleansing properties due to the presence of mild surfactants, and added moisturizers make them less irritating to the skin. The pH typically ranges from 5.7–7.0; thus, the disruption of the skin's acid mantle is minimal.

Liquid cleansers are complex formulations that contain a combination of surfactants and have a higher percentage of water, which offers the advantage of being able to incorporate a number of additives to help optimize skin health. However, they also carry the risk of contamination and thus need preservatives. This increases the risk of allergic reaction and can make chemical stability challenging (13).

16.3.3 Preservatives

Parabens and formaldehyde releasers (e.g., diazolidinyl urea, Quaternium-15, DMDM hydantoin) are the major classes of preservatives. Both classes have reported incidents of allergic and contact sensitivity and dermatitis. Some compounds are

TABLE 16.2: Categories of Bar Soaps

Soap	Superfatted Soap	Combar	Syndet Bar
• pH 9–10	• pH 9–10	• pH 7	• pH 5–7
• Saponification of fats (animal tallow or plant oils) and alkali salt (sodium hydroxide or potassium hydroxide)	• Traditional soap with	• Combine traditional soap + synthetic detergents	• Synthetic detergents in bar form mixed with moisturizers
• Not hard water soluble a soap scum	• Excess oil added (contain 5–15% fat where regular soap is <2%)	• Milder than true soaps	• Hard water soluble ◊ no soap scum
• Disrupts skin barrier tight feeling after washing	• Enhanced mildness, moisturization, and lather	• More thorough cleansing than syndets	• Mild and less irritation
• Disrupts skin barrier tight feeling after washing			
Product Type	***Product Type***	***Product Type***	***Product Type***
—Homemade soap	—Basics bar soap (Beiersdorf)	—Dial (Dial Corporation)	—Cetaphil bar (Galderma)
—Ivory bar soap (Procter & Gamble)	—Roge Cavaills Extra-Mild Superfatted Soap Milk (Pharmarcie LLC)	—Lever2000	—Dove bar (Unilever)
		—Irish Spring (Colgate Palmolive)	—Olay bar (Procter & Gamble)
			—CeraVe bar (L'Oreal)

more allergenic than others and cause greater numbers of reactions. One example is Quaternium-15, which is the sixth-most common allergen in cosmetic products (14–16).

16.3.4 Enhancers

Specialty additives help differentiate soaps and make them unique for marketing purposes. Cleansers in general should have a short contact time with the skin to minimize stratum corneum damage/irritation; thus, this does not allow enough time for added ingredients to remain on the skin and penetrate.

- *Perfumes*: Usually the most expensive ingredient; important factor for consumers; high incidence of allergic reactions
- *Sensory modifiers*: Beads or coarse grains for texture and mechanical exfoliation
- *Medications*: Active ingredients such as salicylic acid, sulfur, or benzoyl peroxide for the treatment of acne
- *Botanical ingredients* (aloe vera/lavender/chamomile): No special benefits in a rinse-off product
- *Vitamin E*: Moisturizing agent added for marketing purposes but no clinical benefit in a rinse-off product
- *Antibacterial ingredient*: Contains antimicrobial agents, such as triclosan, triclocarban, benzalkonium chloride, or carbanile, to inhibit the growth of bacteria and, thereby, odor.

16.3.5 Choosing a Product

Cleansing with water and a bar soap or liquid cleanser will affect the moisture skin barrier. Soap will bring about the greatest changes to the barrier and increase skin pH. Liquid cleansers are gentler, effecting less disruption of the barrier, with minimal change to skin pH, and can provide people with a cleanser that is a combination of surfactant classes, moisturizers, and acidic pH in order to minimize disruption to the skin barrier.

Choosing the correct cleanser for your skin type will depend on a few factors:

1. *What's your preferred vehicle—liquid soap, bar soap, or soap-free?*
   a. Bar formulations have fewer preservatives than liquid ones and thus are ideal for those sensitive to preservatives.
2. *Face wash versus body wash?*
   a. Face washes are typically gentler and are recommended for face and body use for those with sensitive skin.
3. *What's your predominant skin type (oily, dry, combination, sensitive)?*
   a. Gel or foam cleansers are better suited for removing excess oil and are ideal for hot, humid climates and oily and acne-prone skin.
   b. Creamy cleansers are more hydrating and ideal for dry skin and cooler climates.
4. *Are there associated skin problems/diseases?*
   a. Acne-prone skin can benefit from additives, such as salicylic acid or benzoyl peroxide.

The development of novel cleansers and additives for competitive marketing has created an overwhelming plethora of

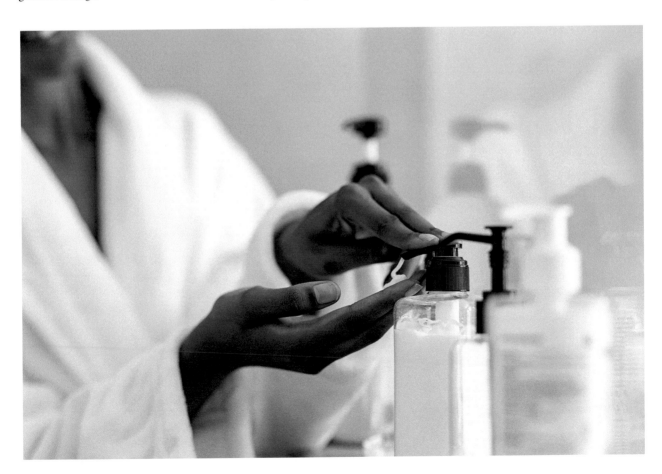

FIGURE 16.3

options for consumers, yet the final goal remains the same, provide an effective cleansing experience with minimal disruption to the skin barrier.

Tips for selecting a gentle, hydrating, and effective cleanser:

- Look for mild surfactants listed in the top half of the ingredient list. These include amphoteric compounds (chiefly, cocamidopropyl betaine, plus others in the betaine family and related compounds), nonionic compounds (such as cocamide diethanolamine, also called cocamide DEA), and hydrophobically modified (HM) polymers.
- Check for hydrating ingredients (e.g., glycerin, oils) that can help minimize irritation potential.

16.4 Moisturizers

Moisturizers are substances designed to improve and maintain the skin barrier and are designed to either impart or restore hydration to the stratum corneum. They function to raise the cutaneous water content through occlusion or humectancy, smooth the rough surface with an emollient, or increase the skin's own natural moisturizing factor (NMF). Moisturizers also serve as vehicles for the delivery of active ingredients that aid in skin rejuvenation, provide antioxidant properties, and deliver photoprotection. The water content of keratinocytes in the basal layer is about 70% and decreases to about 15–20% as mature keratinocytes reach the desquamating layers (9, 17, 18).

16.4.1 Occlusives

Occlusives increase the water content of the skin by slowing the evaporation of water from the surface of the skin. These ingredients are often greasy and are most effective when applied to damp skin. A well-structured occlusive must have molecules that can align and form a tight barrier. Short straight alkyl chains are the most efficient at aligning in the manner. The most effective occlusive moisturizers are petrolatum and mineral oil. Mineral oil is often used because of its favorable texture, but it is not as effective at preventing the evaporation of water as many other occlusives. Lanolin is expensive and potentially irritating. Silicone derivatives (dimethicone and cyclomethicone) are not greasy but have a limited moisturizing effect (17).

16.4.2 Humectants

Humectants are substances that attract moisture into the stratum corneum from the dermis or the environment. A humidity of 70% or higher is required for humectants to attract water from the atmosphere into the epidermis. Examples of humectants include glycerin, honey, sodium lactate, urea, propylene glycol, sorbitol, hyaluronic acid, pyrrolidone carboxylic acid, and gelatin (17).

16.4.3 Emollients

Emollients are ingredients that remain in the stratum corneum to act as lubricants. They help maintain the soft, smooth, and pliable appearance of the skin. Emollients are often thought of as "filling in the crevices" between corneocytes that are in the process of desquamation. By providing increased

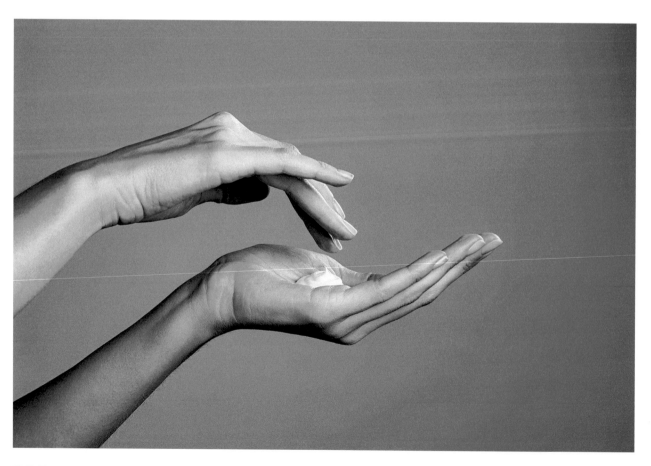

FIGURE 16.4

cohesion of cells, they flatten the curled edges of the individual corneocytes and create a smooth surface with less friction and greater light refractions. Long-chain saturated fatty acids and fatty alcohols are often used as emollients, such as stearic, linoleic, linolenic, oleic, and lauric acids (18).

The formulation of a moisturizer is important. Moisturizing lotions are water-in-oil combinations. Heavier creams are oil-in-water formulations. Oil-only preparations include petrolatum jelly, which, in its natural state, occludes the skin 99%.

16.4.4 Preservatives

Moisturizers utilize the same aforementioned preservatives used in cleansing agents to prevent the growth of harmful bacteria and fungi. The exception would be pure petroleum jelly, which, in its natural state, does not.

16.4.5 Enhancers

Specialty additives also help differentiate moisturizers and make them unique for marketing purposes.

- Ceramides enhance skin barrier and moisture retention
- Hydroxy acids (salicylic acid and glycolic acid) are exfoliants that facilitate the shedding of top-layer corneocytes
- Retinol has anti-aging effects by stimulating collagen synthesis
- Vitamin E (tocopherol) has antioxidant, moisturizing, and anti-aging effects
- Vitamin C (ascorbic acid) and ferulic acid have strong antioxidant, anti-aging (collagen synthesis), and skin-lightening effects (melanin inhibition)

16.4.6 Choosing a Product

As we mature, the skin's ability to retain moisture declines. These intrinsic changes, along with environmental factors, such as dry climate, cold temperatures, and frequent washing, lead to persistent dry, flaky skin. To be effective at replenishing moisture and maintaining a healthy skin barrier, an ideal moisturizer should be a combination of humectant, occlusive, and emollient agents.

Differentiating between moisturizers starts with understanding the key components, which can be found on the ingredient label in both lotions and creams. Water is often the first ingredient. Typically, a lotion contains more water-soluble

moisturizers, which are typically humectants. In a cream-based moisturizer, occlusives and emollients tend to be the primary moisturizers. Knowing which agents are in what category can be confusing; see Table 16.3 for a list of the most common humectants, occlusives, and emollients, according to their International Nomenclature Cosmetic Ingredients (INCI) name.

Choosing the correct moisturizer for your skin type will depend on a few factors:

1. *What's your preferred vehicle (lotion, cream, or petrolatum base)?*
   a. Petrolatum formulations have fewer preservatives than lotions and creams.
   b. Creams are heavier than lotions and are ideal for cold seasons.
   c. Lotions are lighter and ideal for warmer seasons.
2. *Face moisturizer versus body?*
   a. Make sure products for the face are non-comedogenic (i.e., they won't clog the pores and cause acne).
3. *What's your predominate skin type (oily, dry, combination, sensitive)?*
   a. Lotions are ideal for hot, humid climates or oily or acne-prone skin.
   b. Creams or petrolatum are ideal for dry skin and cooler climates.
4. *Associated skin problems/diseases?*
   a. Acne-prone skin can benefit from additives such as salicylic acid, retinol, or benzoyl peroxide.
   b. Disorders of hyperpigmentation benefit from having antioxidants, retinol, and hydroxy acids.

16.4.7 Clinical Pearls in Treating Skin of Color

The term "skin of color" identifies individuals of particular racial and ethnic groups (Asians, African Americans, Caribbean people, Latinos, Middle Eastern people, and Southeast Asians) who share similar cutaneous characteristics and disorders, as well as reaction patterns to those disorders. Understanding skin physiology and how that differs in ethnic skin types allows for recognizing the effects ingredients in cleansers and moisturizers may have on the skin. While we know there are differences in the architecture of the stratum corneum between different ages, body sites, and skin color, the data is often conflicting, limited by small sample sizes and difficulty in obtaining objective measurements. While there are flaws in some reports, studies have started to rely on objective measurements to accurately report racial differences in skin properties. These have included transepidermal water loss (TEWL), ceramide level, and stratum corneum thickness (Table 16.4).

16.4.7.1 Stratum Corneum Thickness

Investigators in the 1970s studied differences in the thickness, density, and compactness of the stratum corneum when comparing skin of color with white skin by counting the number of tape strips required to completely remove the

TABLE 16.3: Common Moisturizing Agents

Humectants	Moisturizers Emollients	Occlusives
• Acetamide MEA	• Acetylated lanolin	• Acetylated lanolin alcohol
• Ammonium lactate	• C15–15 alcohols	• Caprylic/capric triglyceride
• Copper PCA	• Dimethicone copolyol	• Cetyl ricinoleate
• Glucuronic acid	• Hexyl laurate	• Dimethicone
• Glycerin	• Isopropyl myristate	• Hydrogenated lanolin
• PCA	• Lanolin	• Mineral oil
• Propylne glycol	• PPG-20 cetyl ether	• Myristyl myristate
• Sodium PCA		• Petrolatum
• Sorbitol		• Soybean lipid
• Urea		• Squalane
• Xylose		• Vegetable oil

TABLE 16.4: Racial Differences in the Skin

	Transepidermal Water Loss	Ceramide Level	Stratum Corneum Cohesion
Black skin	++	+	+++
Caucasian skin	+	++	++
Asian skin	+++	+++	++

TABLE 16.5: Common Skin Conditions in Various Ethnic Groups in the United States

Blacks[25]		Hispanics[26]		Arabs[27]		South Asians[28]	
Acne	27.7%	Acne	20.0%	Acne	37.7%	Acne	37.0%
Eczematous dermatitis	23.4%	Eczematous dermatitis	19.3%	Eczematous dermatitis	25.5%	Eczematous dermatitis	22.0%
Pigmentary disorders	9.0%	Photoaging	16.8%	Fungal infection	20.0%	Fungal infection	20.0%
Seborrheic dermatitis	6.5%	Tinea/onychomycosis	9.9%	Condyloma/warts	20.0%	Condyloma/warts	8.0%
Alopecia	5.3%	Melasma	8.2%	Melasma	14.5%	Moles	8.0%
Fungal infections	4.3%	Condyloma/warts	7.1%	Keloid	10.7%		
Condyloma/warts	2.4%	Hyperpigmentation	6.0%	Psoriasis	4.7%		
Tinea versicolor	2.2%	Seborrheic keratosis	4.5%	Vitiligo	2.0%		
Keloids	2.1%	Acrochordon	4.2%				
Pityriasis rosea	2.0%	Seborrheic dermatitis	3.2%				
Urticaria	2.0%	Alopecia	2.3%				
		Psoriasis	0.8%				

stratum corneum. They found the black subjects required a greater number of tape stripings than white subjects despite histological evidence showing no significant difference in skin thickness between the groups, thus leading to the conclusion that the stratum corneum in black skin is more cohesive (19).

16.4.7.2 TEWL

Other studies reported that the composition of lipids varied between racial groups, with the lowest ceramide level found in African Americans, followed by Caucasians, Hispanics, and Asians (20, 21). Ceramide levels were inversely proportional to TEWL and directly proportional to water content, suggesting that darker skin has poor water retention capacity and the highest evaporative water loss (21).

When studying prevalence in skin disorders that affect the normal skin barrier, atopic dermatitis has been found to be more prevalent in African American and Asian/Pacific Islander individuals than Caucasians (22).

16.4.7.3 Ceramide Level

Early studies comparing living and cadaveric skin from the abdomen, back, and thigh found black skin to have slightly higher levels of epidermal lipid and sterol content relative to Caucasian skin. These data, however, were limited by a small sample size and the fact that measurements were made from both living and deceased subjects at different anatomical sites (23). More recently, Sugino et al. measured ceramide levels in the stratum corneum of four different races and found the highest levels to be in Asian skin. Significantly less ceramide was noted in Caucasian skin, and the lowest level was found in black skin (22). This was similarly observed by Hellemans et al., who quantified ceramide levels after hydrolysis and analysis of corresponding sphingolipid bases, showing the least amount of lipid in the stratum corneum of black skin (24).

While the data available get us closer to understanding the unique physiology of pigmented skin, the literature on the characteristics of the subjects with skin of color remains limited. Several groups over the past decades have attempted to pinpoint the underlying differences in skin structure and function in different ethnic skin types. However, most of these studies have been of small scale, and in some studies, interindividual differences in skin quality overwhelm any racial differences (25). Additional large-scale studies are still needed.

Researchers have also examined the rates of common skin disorders between different minority groups. Table 16.5 shows acne and eczema being the most common skin diagnoses seen in black, Latin American, Arab American, and South Asian American population in the United States (25–30). When choosing a skin care regimen these factors should be taken into consideration. Asking a patient if they have a history of acne-prone skin or eczema-prone skin will help you guide them to the cleansing and moisturizing agents that are best for their skin.

16.5 Conclusion

While additional studies are still needed to dig deeper into the racial variabilities of pigmented skin, current data established some quantifiable parameters showing the difference in TEWL, ceramide levels, and stratum corneum cohesion between black, Asian, and Caucasian skin. While the current industry is flooded with skin care products that are marketed toward specific ethnicities, head-to-head comparative studies are lacking. Future research looking at specific skin moisturizers and how they perform in ethnic skin will allow for the development of targeted therapies and individualized skin care regimens.

Frequently Asked Questions

1. *Q: How often should I wash my face?*
   A: Anyone over the age of 12 produces enough sebum to warrant washing their face at least twice a day, especially if they have acne-prone skin. Some people may opt to only splash their face with cool water in the morning, but one should not skip using a gentle cleanser with water every evening to wash away the dirt, pollution, and oils that build up during the day.
2. *Q: What are surfactants?*
   A: Surfactants are the primary component of cleaners. The word "surfactant" means "surface active agent." As the name implies, surfactants stir up activity on the surface you are cleaning to help trap dirt and remove it from the surface.
3. *Q: Should I rotate my cleansers and moisturizers?*
   A: Yes. You should rotate your skin care products with each season. During the cold winter months, creamy

hydrating cleansers and cream-based moisturizers are better for retaining skin moisture. During the hot summer months, foam/gel-based cleansers and lotion-based moisturizers are better for cleansing excess oil/sweat and light moisturizing.

4. *Q: If I have oily skin, do I still need to moisturize?*
   A: The short answer is yes. However, the type of moisturizer you use is important. You want to use lotion vehicles and look for the words "oil-free" and "non-comedogenic" on the label. You should avoid heavy ointments, balms, or cleansing oils.

5. *Q: Do I need different products for specific areas of the body?*
   A: Yes. Areas of the body such as the hands have a very thick stratum corneum, so occlusive balms are helpful for preventing dry, cracked skin. If you have acne-prone skin, you should avoid heavy creams and occlusive balms on the face, but they're okay for your hands. The eye area is more delicate and has a thinner stratum corneum than the skin on the rest of the face; thus, this area is more sensitive and will be the first area to break out into an itchy rash if you're sensitive/allergic to a product.

References

1. Harding, CR. "The stratum corneum: Structure and function in health and disease." *Dermatologic Therapy* vol. 17 Suppl 1 (2004): 6–15

2. Elias, PM. "Epidermal lipids, barrier function, and desquamation." *Journal of Investigative Dermatology* vol. 80 Suppl (1983): 44s–49s

3. Spitz, L. "Soap history, marketing and advertising." In: *Soap Technology from the 1900s American Oil Chemists' Society*, edited by Spitz, L, 1–47. Champaign, IL, 1990.

4. Stanislaus, IVS, Meerbott, PB. "Historical review." In: *American Soap Makers Guide*, edited by Baird, HC, 1–11. New York: Henry Carey Baird & Co., 1928.

5. Abbas, S et al. "Personal cleanser technology and clinical performance." *Dermatologic Therapy* vol. 17 Suppl 1 (2004): 35–42.

6. Baumann, L. "Cleansers." In: *Cosmeceuticals and Cosmetic Ingredients*, edited by Bauman, L, 19–21. New York: McGraw Hill, 2014.

7. Nix, DH. "Factors to consider when selecting skin cleansing products." *Journal of Wound, Ostomy, and Continence Nursing: Official Publication of the Wound, Ostomy and Continence Nurses Society* vol. 27,5 (2000): 260–268

8. Yosipovitch, G, Maibach, H. "Skin surface pH: A protective acid mantle." *Cosmetics Toiletries Magazine* vol. 111 (1996): 101–102

9. Harry, RG. "Moisturizers." In: *Harry's Cosmeticology*, eight edition, edited by Rieger, M. New York: Chemical Publishing Company, 2000

10. Larson, EL et al. "Quantity of soap as a variable in handwashing." *Infection Control: IC* vol. 8,9 (1987): 371–375

11. Heinze, JE. "Bar soap and liquid soap." *JAMA* vol. 251,24 (1984): 3222–3223

12. Heinze, JE, Yackovich F. "Washing with contaminated bar soap is unlikely to transfer bacteria." *Epidemiology and Infection* vol. 101,1 (1988): 135–142

13. Kirsner, RS, Froelich, CW. "Soaps and detergents: Understanding their composition and effect." *Ostomy/Wound Management* vol. 44,3A Suppl (1998): 62S–69S; discussion 70S

14. Soni, MG et al. "Safety assessment of propyl paraben: A review of the published literature." *Food and Chemical Toxicology: An International Journal Published for the British Industrial Biological Research Association* vol. 39,6 (2001): 513–532

15. Fransway, AF, Schmitz, NA. "A problem of preservation in the 1990s: (II). Formaldehyde and formaldehyde-releasing biocides: Incidences of crossreactivity and the significance of the positive response to formaldehyde." *American Journal of Contact Dermatitis* vol. 2 (1991):78–88

16. Marks, JG et al. "North American Contact Dermatitis Group patch test results for the detection of delayed-type hypersensitivity to topical allergens." *Journal of the American Academy of Dermatology* vol. 38,6 Pt 1 (1998): 911–918

17. Bolognia, J, Jorizzo, JL, Schaffer, JV. "Chapter 125. Skin barrier." In: *Dermatology*, third edition, edited by Bolognia, J, Jorizzo, J, Rapini, R, 1969–1975. Philadelphia: Elsevier Saunders, 2003 (2012).

18. Buamann, L. "Moisturizing agents." In: *Cosmeceuticals and Cosmetic Ingredients*, edited by Bauman, L, 21–23. New York: McGraw Hill, 2015.

19. Weigand, DA et al. "Cell layers and density of Negro and Caucasian stratum corneum." *Journal of Investigative Dermatology* vol. 62,6 (1974): 563–568

20. Muizzuddin, N et al. "Structural and functional differences in barrier properties of African American, Caucasian and East Asian skin." *Journal of Dermatological Science* vol. 59,2 (2010): 123–128

21. Kaufman, BP et al. "Atopic dermatitis in diverse racial and ethnic groups-Variations in epidemiology, genetics, clinical presentation and treatment." *Experimental Dermatology* vol. 27,4 (2018): 340–357

22. Sugino, K, Imokawa, G, Maibach, H. "Ethnic difference of stratum corneum lipid in relation to stratum corneum function." *Journal of Investigative Dermatology* vol. 100 (1993):597

23. Reinertson, RP, Wheatley, VR. "Studies on the chemical composition of human epidermal lipids." *Journal of Investigative Dermatology* vol. 32,1 (1959): 49–59

24. Hellemans, L et al. "Characterization of stratum corneum properties in human subjects from a different ethnic background." *Journal of Investigative Dermatology* vol. 124,4 (2005): A62

25. Halder, RM et al. "Cutaneous diseases in the black races." *Dermatologic Clinics* vol. 21,4 (2003): 679–687, ix

26. Sanchez, MR. "Cutaneous diseases in Latinos." *Dermatologic Clinics* vol. 21,4 (2003): 689–697

27. El-Essawi, D et al. "A survey of skin disease and skin-related issues in Arab Americans." *Journal of the American Academy of Dermatology* vol. 56,6 (2007): 933–938

28. Shah, SK et al. "A survey of skin conditions and concerns in South Asian Americans: A community-based study." *Journal of Drugs in Dermatology* vol. 10,5 (2011): 524–528

29. Graham-Brown, R. "Soaps and detergents in the elderly." *Clinics in Dermatology* vol. 14,1 (1996): 85–87

30. Rawlings, AV. "Ethnic skin types: Are there differences in skin structure and function?" *International Journal of Cosmetic Science* vol. 28,2 (2006): 79–93

CHAPTER 17: TOPICAL ANTI-ACNE AGENTS

Maya Vedamurthy

17.1 Introduction

Topical agents for treating acne are abundant and varied as the presentation of the acne itself, ranging from OTC products to prescription medication. However, the choice of the product depends on the physician's knowledge, the severity of acne, and skin type.

Acne is a common skin disorder that affects 79–95% of adolescents, especially in Western civilization.[1] Acne has a significant impact on a patient's quality of life, lowering self-esteem and affecting psychosocial development.[2]

17.2 Treatment of Acne (Table 17.1)

Effective treatment is chosen based on many variables, like the age of the patient, genetics, gender, severity of the lesion, and area involved, and usually, combination therapies give better results. However, topical treatments are preferred for mild to moderate acne, while systemic therapies are reserved for moderate to severe acne. Adjuvant or procedural therapies are add-ons to improve the outcome of treatment for acne at all stages.

17.2.1 Do Topicals Work in the Treatment of Acne?

Topical anti-acne agents are the agents of choice in mild to moderate acne. Retinoids and antimicrobials, such as benzoyl peroxide, are the mainstays of therapy in mild to moderate acne and the maintenance phase. Topical agents are available as gels, creams, lotion, pledgets, soap, and washes. Any topical agent requires six to eight weeks to show results but can be used for prolonged periods to prevent relapses.

17.3 Classification of Anti-Acne Agents

Topical anti-acne agents are classified based on their activity against acne (Table 17.2).

Active anti-acne ingredients have one or more of the following effects against acne.

17.3.1 Antimicrobial Agents

Propionibacterium acnes is the primary pathogen implicated in acne.[3] It is a gram-positive anaerobe that has a role in inciting inflammation in acne.[4] Antibacterial agents work potentially against *P. acnes* and possess surface-acting capability (Tables 17.3 and 17.4). They help prevent inflammatory lesions and hence are useful in the treatment of mild to moderate acne. However, antibacterials are not recommended as monotherapy and are best used in combination with benzoyl peroxide or

TABLE 17.2: Anti-Acne Agents

1. Antimicrobial—activity against *P. acnes*
2. Antioxidants—to decrease inflammation
3. Anti-inflammatory—to inhibit lipase production by *P. acnes*
4. Keratolytic/comedolytic—to exfoliate stratum corneum
5. Restoring normal keratinization and skin cell maturation
Miscellaneous
—Novel
—OTC products
—Mechanical

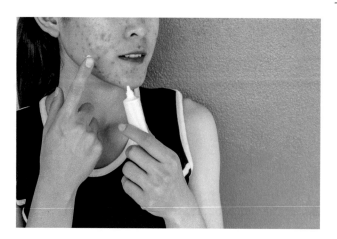

FIGURE 17.1   Acne.

TABLE 17.1: Aims of Treatment

1. Reduce ductal hypercornification
2. Decrease *P. acnes* population
3. Control sebum production
4. Anti-inflammatory effect
5. Reduce scar formation

TABLE 17.3: Topical Antibacterial Agents

1. Clindamycin
2. Nadifloxacin
3. Lincomycin
4. Triclosan
5. Benzoyl peroxide
6. Erythromycin
7. Clarithromycin
8. Azithromycin
9. Dapsone
10. Metronidazole
11. Minocycline

TABLE 17.4: Strength of Recommendation of Topical Antibacterial in Acne Management

	Strength of Recommendation	Level of Evidence
Benzoyl peroxide	A	I, II
Topical antibacterial (clindamycin, macrolides)	A	I, II
Dapsone	A	I, II
Azelaic acid	A	

DOI: 10.1201/9780429243769-17

retinoid to increase efficacy and decrease the development of resistant bacteria.

Antimicrobial agents are present in the form of cream, gel, lotion, washes, and soap.

17.3.2 How to Choose an Anti-Acne Agent

Clindamycin and nadifloxacin are the preferred topical antibacterial agents, which are thought to act against biofilms, are less resistant and have a protective effect against gram-negative folliculitis. The macrolide group, like clarithromycin, erythromycin, and azithromycin, is not preferred topically in the Indian market due to the risk of developing bacterial resistance. Lincomycin 2% has a role to play in certain circumstances. Triclosan is an antibacterial usually present in washes and soap but not recommended generally due to its carcinogenic potential.

17.3.2.1 Benzoyl Peroxide

Benzoyl peroxide is an antimicrobial agent effective against *P. acnes* through the release of free oxygen radicals.[5]

Benzoyl peroxide (BP) exhibits marked suppression of *P. acnes* and reduced proliferation and emergence of resistant strains. Hence, it can be considered a component of first-line therapy and long-term maintenance therapy. The microsphere formulation is known to reduce "facial shine" and skin oiliness in acne patients.

Benzoyl peroxide is available in two strengths, 2.5% and 5%. It is present in the form of gels, washes, and soaps. We have newer formulations in a concentration of 3.5% and 5% as creams and wash in the concentration of 7% incorporated into porous microspheres. The irritation potential of benzoyl peroxide is concentration-dependent. As benzoyl peroxide is converted to benzoic acid within hours of application, the microsponge technology allows slower and more progressive delivery of BP into the skin, which is responsible for its sustained therapeutic effects.

Topical dapsone is available as a 5% gel. It is a sulfone agent that works in inflammatory acne. The mechanism of action is not well understood, and its ability to kill *P. acnes* has not been well studied.

Azelaic acid is available as a 20% gel. It is used as an adjunctive therapy because of its mildly effective antibacterial, comedolytic, and anti-inflammatory agent. It is a valuable agent for treating post-inflammatory dyspigmentation. Topical metronidazole in gel formulation is found helpful in acne treated with steroids. It has antibacterial and anti-inflammatory effects.

17.3.3 Side Effects of Antibacterials and Their Management

All antibacterials have some side effects but with varying degrees.

Topical clindamycin is linked to pseudomembranous colitis, although the clinical relevance is low as systemic absorption of clindamycin after topical application is only 8% at its highest.[6] In order to reduce systemic exposure to clindamycin as much as possible, the topical application of clindamycin phosphate is to be preferred over clindamycin hydrochloride salt.[7]

Skin irritation is common with benzoyl peroxide and is known to occur with higher concentrations. Benzoyl peroxide can cause bleaching of clothing and bed linens.

About 5% of patients complain of burning and erythema with azelaic acid.

Dapsone is excreted in human milk and is considered pregnancy category C. Glucose-6-phosphate dehydrogenase testing is not required before starting topical dapsone.

Anti-inflammatory agents in topical acne therapy:

1. Tea tree oil
2. Nicotinamide
3. Zinc

17.3.3.1 Tea Tree Oil

Tea tree oil is considered to have antibacterial and antifungal properties. Terpene 4-ol, alpha terpineol, and alpha-pinene are said to have intrinsic antibacterial and anti-inflammatory effects. Tea tree oil is available in the form of gel, wash, and soap. Tea tree oil can produce allergic contact dermatitis.

17.3.3.2 Zinc

Zinc salt has been used as a topical anti-acne agent since 1970. Zinc salt is said to have anti-inflammatory and sebosuppressive effects.[8] Zinc is usually combined with antibacterial agents as it reduces bacterial resistance. Zinc is available as creams and washes for the treatment of acne.

17.3.3.3 Nicotinamide

Nicotinamide is a water-soluble agent used topically in acne and rosacea. Topical 4% nicotinamide gel is said to have anti-inflammatory properties, and its anti-acne effect is comparable to topical clindamycin.

17.4 Hydroxyl Acid

Hydroxyl acid is divided into alpha-hydroxy and beta-hydroxy acids. Both hydroxyl acids are available in the form of gels, washes, and chemical peels. Glycolic, lactic, and citric acids are a group of alpha-hydroxy acids effective in acne by thinning the stratum corneum and producing epidermolysis.

Salicylic acid is the only beta-hydroxy acid found helpful in acne. It is available as cleansers, astringents, lotions, and chemical peels. It has comedolytic, exfoliative, and anti-inflammatory properties, which are useful as an anti-acne agent.

Hydroxy acids tend to produce excessive dryness of the skin, which may be addressed by using suitable moisturizers.

17.5 Topical Retinoids

Topical retinoids play a significant role in the treatment of acne. They target the primary lesion, which is the microcomedo.[9] Therefore, they inhibit the formation of microcomedones and reduce the number of mature comedones. They promote normal desquamation of follicular epithelium, which prevents the development of a propitious microenvironment for *P. acnes*.

The available topical retinoids are tretinoin, adapalene, tazarotene, isotretinoin, motretinide, retinaldehyde, and retinoyl B-glucuronide.[10] Usually, the commercial preparations available are in the form of cream, gel, and lotions. The most commonly used topical retinoids are tretinoin, adapalene, and tazarotene. Topical retinoids can be used as monotherapy and in combination with antibiotics. They are used not only inactive phase of acne but also in the maintenance phase. Retinoids should be applied once daily and preferably in the evening or at night. The most common side effects are retinoid dermatitis, which can be avoided by using small amounts of less concentration or beginning treatment as short contact therapy. Tazarotene and tretinoin appear to have similar irritation potential, while adapalene and retinol have less irritation potential.

Tretinoin and adapalene are pregnancy category C, while tazarotene is category X, and women should be counseled regarding these risks before starting treatment with retinoids.

Retinol has better tolerability than tretinoin and is hence used in cosmeceuticals but lacks sufficient biological activity.

Tazarotene 0.1% is available in foam form to treat moderate to severe acne, mainly over the trunk. It is approved for patients over 12 years of age. It is the first retinoid in foam formulation. Tazarotene is also helpful in the prevention and management of post-inflammatory hyperpigmentation and scarring secondary to acne vulgaris. Tazarotene lotions 0.045% are also available for use over larger areas, such as the trunk in people nine years of age or older.

A fourth topical retinoid, trifarotene 0.005% cream, has been approved for the treatment of acne in patients over nine years old.

17.6 Combination Therapies

A combination helps to enhance compliance with the treatment regimen, as it decreases the risk of bacterial resistance and improves the tolerance of these agents.

Fixed combinations are available with antibiotics and retinoids or benzoyl peroxide. The antibiotics commonly used in combination are clindamycin, erythromycin, and dapsone with adapalene, tretinoin, or benzoyl peroxide

17.7 Anti-Acne Agents in Special Categories

17.7.1 Children

Three topical combination anti-acne agents with retinoids as one of them are recommended as follows in children.

- Adapalene 0.1%/BP 2.5% approved for use in patients ≥9 years of age.
- Clindamycin phosphate 1–2%/tretinoin 0.025% gel approved for use in children ≥12 years of age.
- Tretinoin 0.05% micronized tretinoin gel for children ≥10 years.
- All other retinoids are approved in patients ≥12 years of age.

17.7.2 Pregnancy

Acne in pregnant women is challenging as most effective anti-acne agents are contraindicated or not recommended. Based on the pregnancy risk categories, the following agents may be used effectively and safely (Table 17.5).

17.8 Novel Approaches in the Treatment of Acne

The conventional anti-acne agents cause discomfort in irritation, dryness, and itching, reducing patient compliance and, thereby, the effectiveness. A novel drug delivery system can overcome the disadvantages of conventional formulations while preserving the efficacy, so we have the following newer formulation to suit the need of acne patients.[12]

17.8.1 Liposomal Formulation of Retinoids

Tretinoin incorporated in liposomes shows comedolytic activity five to ten times higher than conventional formulations and has better local tolerability.

TABLE 17.5: Treatment Recommendatiosn in Pregnancy[11]

Types of Acne	Anti-Acne Agent	FDA Pregnancy Drug Class
Non-inflammatory comedonal	Azelaic acid	B
Inflammatory Mild to moderate	Benzoyl peroxide	C
	Azelaic acid	B
	Topical erythromycin	B
	Topical clindamycin or a combination of the above	B
	Glycolic acid	N (not rated)

17.8.1.1 Niosomes

Niosomes are the second-generation drug that has overcome the disadvantages of formulating conventional liposomes. Niosomes have the advantages of biodegrading non-toxicity and non-immunogenicity. Erythromycin has been successfully incorporated into a topical niosomal gel that has distinct advantages over the conventional formulation.

17.8.2 Microsponges

Microsponges are porous polymeric systems that carry active ingredients in the target area of the skin in a more predictable manner. They have good stability over a wide pH range and are compatible with a large number of active ingredients.

17.8.3 Microspheres

Microspheres are solid spherical particles manufactured by microencapsulation technique, with inert, natural, or synthetic polymers deposited around solid and liquid micronized particles, with the drug being homogenously distributed throughout the core. With this technique, the drug is deposited to act as a reservoir without the risk of degradation. They also have a lower potential for transdermal penetration and systemic exposure. Tretinoin and benzoyl peroxide microspheres have shown beneficial results.

17.8.4 Mechanical Treatments[13]

Multiple over-the-counter products are available for the treatment of acne. As they are non-prescription products, patients tend to start using them when acne is mild. Some of these products tend to worsen acne.

17.8.4.1 Scrubs

Scrubs are available as gels, lotion, or creams, which are used as face washes. They contain different types of abrasive material, such as polyethylene heads, aluminum oxide, or ground fruit pits, and are often in a colorful presentation. They are meant to remove comedones; on the contrary, they disrupt epidermal barrier function and cause irritant dermatitis.

17.8.4.2 Washcloth/Cleaning Cloth

These cloths are meant to exfoliate the skin. However, some have an active anti-acne agent like topical antibiotics or BP incorporated, which are deposited on the skin.

17.8.4.3 Cosmetic Adhesive Pads/Strip-Off Pads

Adhesive pads are gradually used to remove corneocytes, dirt, or loose open comedones. They are more popularly used for areas such as the nose.

17.8.4.4 Brushes

Circular rotating brushes are more popularly used for truncal acne to act as exfoliators. Small brushes with fine bristles are used on facial skin. However, they have the potential to cause skin irritation.

17.8.4.5 Heating Devices

The principle with these devices is that heat activates heat shock proteins of *P. acnes*, causing the destruction of bacteria. It is an electronic heating device to treat acne vulgaris.

17.9 Procedural Therapies in Acne

Many procedures are offered in a dermatologist's office to treat acne effectively. They are as follows:

1. Microdermabrasion
2. Cryotherapy
3. Blue light
4. Chemical peels
5. Lasers

All these procedures help in targeting the pathophysiology of acne at different levels. They are valuable adjuvants in the management of acne.

17.10 Newer/Emerging Topical Anti-Acne Agents

Research on new microbiological targets has explored the potential of newer therapeutic agents and alternative treatments for acne.[14]

Taurine bromamine has anti-inflammatory and antibactericidal activity against *P. acnes* that is comparable to clindamycin. Data have suggested it to be an agent of choice in antibiotic-resistant acne.

A Japanese experimental study has shown chlorhexidine gluconate ointment to be a useful anti-acne agent due to its antibacterial activity and dissolving action of its base on free fatty acids.

L-ascorbyl 2-phosphate (APS) 5% lotion, a stable form of vitamin C derivative, has shown to possess anti-inflammatory and antioxidant properties and appears to be safe and effective in the treatment of acne.

A lot of interest has been shown in complementary and alternative medications like rose extract, herbs containing icariin, and resveratrol, although significant human studies are lacking. Many newer molecules are on the horizon and may serve as useful adjuncts in the management of acne.

TABLE 17.6: Cutaneous Side Effects from Topical Anti-Acne Agents and Potential Drug Delivery

Common Topical Acne Treatments	Cutaneous Side Effects	Drug Delivery
Retinoids	Retinoid dermatitis	Microsponges, liposomes, nanoemulsions, aerosol foams
Benzoyl peroxide	Itching redness, hair and clothing discoloration	Polymers, fullerenes
Clindamycin phosphate	Irritation, allergic contact dermatitis	Aerosol sprays, polymers, nanoemulsions
Erythromycin	Burning, allergic contact dermatitis	Aerosol sprays, polymers, nanoemulsions
Salicylic acid	Dryness, redness, peeling	Polymers, microsponges

Topical minocycline foam 4% has been formulated to overcome the side effects of systemic administration of the drug. It improves inflammatory and non-inflammatory acne and is useful for truncal acne. It is used to treat moderate to severe acne in adults and children over nine years old.

A novel first-in-class topical anti-androgen in the form of an androgen receptor inhibitor is approved for acne therapy. The molecule clascoterone (cortexolone 17α-propionate) is approved for use in patients over 12 years of age.

17.11 Conclusion

New insights into the pathogenesis of acne coupled with the fear of systemic adverse events with effective anti-acne medications like antibiotics, isotretinoin, and hormonal agents have led to the discovery of newer topical agents and formulations to treat acne safely across all ages. The newer topical anti-acne agents are not only safe but are also effective, mainly when used early in the course of the disease. This also improves compliance and satisfaction of acne patients, making it a worthwhile treatment option in the management of this chronic disorder.

Frequently Asked Questions

1. *Q: How is acne caused?*
   A: Acne occurs when the oil glands (pores) in the skin get blocked. Hormones make the oil glands produce more oil and the dead skin cells and sebum that accumulate to form a plug. Bacteria multiply quickly in these clogged pores and cause inflammation that leads to redness and swelling, resulting in acne.
2. *Q: Does diet play a role?*
   A: Diet does play an important role in acne. Food with a high glycemic index, such as processed and refined foods, including white bread, sweetened baked goods, candies, instant oats, boxed cereals, and animal milk, as well as a high glycemic load, worsens acne. Low-fat milk and skim milk are said to aggravate acne more than whole milk. Skim milk shows higher spikes of Insulin than whole milk and also has higher levels of casein protein that contains a protease that prevents IGF-1 degradation, thereby increasing its absorption and triggering acne. Alcohol consumption can also lead to the worsening of acne. A paleolithic diet and food rich in fish, vegetables, fruits, zinc, vitamin D, and omega-3 fatty acids are encouraged.
3. *Q: What is bodybuilder acne?*
   A: Bodybuilders and young gym enthusiasts tend to take high-protein foods, protein supplements, growth hormones, and anabolic steroids to build up their muscles. Whey ("fast protein") is digested quickly in two hours. It increases the insulin surge, which causes stimulation of sebaceous glands leading to acne. Bodybuilder acne presents itself as a severe form of acne with large, deep, solid, painful lumps or cysts under the skin.
4. *Q: Does acne occur in all age groups?*
   A: Yes, acne is more common in teenagers, but it can also be seen in the first year of life, mid-childhood between one to seven years of age, adulthood, and late adulthood.
5. *Q: How to prevent acne scarring?*
   A: It is a common consequence of acne in the majority of patients with acne lesions. There is a genetic tendency

for scarring. Early diagnosis and appropriate treatment prevent acne scarring as the duration of inflammation relates to scar production; hence, a delay in treatment more likely results in scarring.

6. *Q: Why does acne fluctuate?*

   A: Although acne has a genetic tendency, other factors play a role, like hormones, diet, stress, sunlight, and other external causes, like sweating, cosmetics, and parlor activities, like facials, that can cause a flare-up of acne. Some over-the-counter products contain steroids, and this can cause or worsen acne.

7. *Q: Is washing with cold or hot water good for acne?*

   A: Cold water causes constriction of pores and makes the skin appear better, while hot water opens the pores and stimulates excess oil secretion. It is often the aggressive cleaning products that can aggravate acne or cause skin irritation.

8. *Q: Can acne appear on other sites of the body?*

   A: Yes, moderate or severe forms of acne can occur on the trunk other than the face and warrants early and aggressive treatment.

9. *Q: Should I avoid wearing cosmetics and sunscreens if I have acne?*

   A: No, one can wear cosmetics or sunscreens even if one has acne. Your dermatologist will help you choose suitable products. Generally, it is advisable to wear oil-free or non-comedogenic products, which are usually mentioned on the product label itself. It is advisable to choose a mild cleanser, an oil-free moisturizer, and non-comedogenic makeup.

References

1. Cordain L, Lindeberg S, Hurtado M, Hill K, Eaton SB, Brand-Miller J. Acne vulgaris: A disease of Western civilization. Archives of Dermatology. 2002 Dec 1;138(12):1584–1590.
2. Magin P, Adams J, Heading G, Pond D, Smith W. Psychological sequelae of acne vulgaris: Results of a qualitative study. Canadian Family Physician. 2006 Aug 1;52(8):978–979.
3. Cove JH, Cunliffe WJ, Holland KT. Acne vulgaris: Is the bacterial population size significant? British Journal of Dermatology. 1980 Mar;102(3):277–280.
4. Tochio T, Tanaka H, Nakata S, Ikeno H. Accumulation of lipid peroxide in the content of comedones may be involved in the progression of comedogenesis and inflammatory changes in comedones. Journal of Cosmetic Dermatology. 2009 Jun;8(2):152–158.
5. Cunliffe WJ, Dodman B, Ead R. Benzoyl peroxide in acne. Practitioner. 1978 Mar;220(1317):479.
6. Abdellatif AA, Tawfeek HM. Transfersomal nanoparticles for enhanced transdermal delivery of clindamycin. AAPS PharmSciTech. 2016 Oct 1;17(5):1067–1074.
7. Van Hoogdalem EJ. Transdermal absorption of topical anti-acne agents in man; review of clinical pharmacokinetic data. Journal of the European Academy of Dermatology and Venereology. 1998 Sep;11:S13–19.
8. Katsambas A, Dessinioti C. New and emerging treatments in dermatology: Acne. Dermatologic Therapy. 2008 Mar;21(2):86–95.
9. Chivot M. Retinoid therapy for acne. American Journal of Clinical Dermatology. 2005 Feb 1;6(1):13–19.
10. Gollnick H, Cunliffe W, Berson D, Dreno B, Finlay A, Leyden JJ, Shalita AR, Thiboutot D. Management of acne: A report from a Global Alliance to Improve Outcomes in Acne. Journal of the American Academy of Dermatology. 2003 Jul 1;49(1):S1–37.
11. Chien AL, Qi J, Rainer B, Sachs DL, Helfrich YR. Treatment of acne in pregnancy. Journal of the American Board of Family Medicine. 2016 Mar 1;29(2):254–262.
12. Sibinovska N, Komoni V, Netkovska AK, Vranic E, Crcarevska SM, et al. Novel approaches in treatment of acne vulgaris. Macedonian Pharmaceutical Bulletin. 2016;62(2):3–16.
13. Decker A, Graber EM. Over-the-counter acne treatments: A review. Journal of Clinical and Aesthetic Dermatology. 2012 May;5(5):32.
14. Arshdeep, De D. What's new in management of acne. IJDVL. 2013;79:279–287.

CHAPTER 18: LIGHTENING FORMULATIONS

Susan C. Taylor and Amanda A. Onalaja-Underwood

18.1 Introduction

Skin color is determined by several chromophores, including oxyhemoglobin, reduced hemoglobin, and carotenoids, with melanocytes and melanin being the most important in determining skin color. Hypermelanosis is skin color that is darker than normal as a result of increased melanin in the epidermis, dermis, or both. There are many disorders characterized by hypermelanosis (Table 18.1). Skin-lightening agents are frequently used to reduce or eliminate hypermelanosis.

Agents that lighten skin color modulate different signaling steps in the pigmentation pathway. The production of melanin pigment, brownish-black eumelanin, and reddish-yellow pheomelanin by melanocytes defines melanogenesis. The melanocyte is a dendritic cell that is embryonically derived from neuroectoderm that produces melanin in specialized organelles called melanosomes utilizing three synthetic enzymes (1). Tyrosinase catalyzes the rate-limiting step in melanogenesis. Differences in pigmentation among populations are not due to a difference in the number of melanocytes, as all people have similar numbers of melanocytes. Rather, there are differences in the size, shape, density, aggregation, and transfer of melanosomes, with individuals with darker skin having larger melanosomes containing larger quantities of eumelanin (2). The abnormal production of melanin by intrinsic or extrinsic factors is manifested as hypermelanosis or hyperpigmentation.

Lightening formulations act via a variety of mechanisms, including regulating melanocyte activation, inhibiting melanogenesis, inhibiting melanosome transfer to keratinocytes, and removing epidermal pigment (Table 18.2) (33). In this chapter, we review the most common lightening agents and their indications and mechanisms of action. Furthermore, we provide clinical pearls in treating and advising patients of color on the use of lightening formulations and review frequently encountered questions.

18.2 Indications

Patients of color requesting skin-lightening agents may have a variety of motivations, including achieving or maintaining an even skin tone, attaining an overall lighter skin color, or reducing or eliminating hypermelanosis. Hypermelanosis may negatively impact the quality of life (4). In some societies, lighter skin color is preferred, and a darker skin tone may be equated to a lower socioeconomic status. In this case, patients desire a lighter skin tone to appear beautiful and of a higher social status (5, 6).

When evaluating patients with hypermelanosis, evaluation to identify an underlying systemic cause is a critical initial step. For example, diffuse cutaneous pigmentation may suggest metabolic disease (e.g., Addison's disease, hemochromatosis, hyperthyroidism), drug-induced hypermelanosis (with or

TABLE 18.1: Disorders of Hypermelanosis

Hypermelanosis Disorders	Description
Acanthosis nigricans	Velvety plaques over the neck and flexures
Café-au-lait macules	1 to 20 cm tan to brown macules, epidermal, present at birth or early childhood
Ephelides	1 to 2 mm sharply defined macules, red or tan to light brown
Lichen planus pigmentosus	Symmetrically distributed brown to gray-brown macules on sun-exposed areas of the head and neck and flexural areas
Melasma	Symmetrically distributed light-brown, brown, or gray macules on the forehead and malar face
Nevus of Ota	Mottled blue-gray macules over the zygomatic and temporal areas; scleral pigmentation can also be seen
Pigmented contact dermatitis	Diffuse or patchy brown pigmentation on the forehead and cheeks
Post-inflammatory hyperpigmentation	Irregular, darkly pigmented macules and patches
Solar lentigines	Pigmented, well-defined macules; light brown, brown, or gray

TABLE 18.2: Agents Used in Skin-Lightening Formulations

Regulates melanocyte activation

Broad-spectrum sunscreen	Blocks with zinc oxide, titanium dioxide, and iron oxide and impedes melanocyte stimulation, blocking UVB, UVA, and visible light

Reduction in melanin synthesis

Hydroquinone	Inhibits tyrosinase and melanin synthesis
Arbutin	Derivative of hydroquinone found in cranberries, blueberries, wheat, and pears; competitively and reversely binds tyrosinase
Azelaic acid	Reversibly inhibits tyrosinase and melanin production
Cysteamine	Inhibits tyrosinase and peroxidase, which are integral to melanin biosynthesis
Kojic acid	Inactivates tyrosinase by chelating copper atoms
Vitamins C and E	Inhibits tyrosinase
Licorice extract	Has been shown to prevent UVB-induced pigmentation and to inhibit tyrosinase activity, superoxide anion production, and cyclo-oxygenase activity

Reduces melanin transfer

Niacinamide	Inhibits 35–68% of melanosome transfer in melanocyte culture
Soy extract	Inhibits the protease-activated receptor 2 pathway that is necessary to regulate keratinocyte phagocytosis of melanosomes and melanosome transfer

Removal of epidermal pigment

Retinol	Increases cell turnover and interferes with epidermal melanin dispersion

DOI: 10.1201/9780429243769-18

without photosensitivity), or a malignant process (e.g., diffuse melanosis cutis) (7–11). Treatment of an underlying metabolic disorder, malignancy, or discontinuation of an offending drug must occur for the resolution of the hypermelanosis.

Likewise, for localized hypermelanosis, as observed in PIH, identification and treatment of the underlying inflammation or minimizing cutaneous injury is key to the prevention of PIH or ameliorating the worsening of hypermelanosis. Melasma induced by oral contraceptive pills or estrogen replacement therapy may partially respond to the discontinuation of these hormones. Once an underlying disorder is treated or ruled out, then therapy with a lightening formulation can be initiated. There are a wide array of skin-lightening formulations that offer varying degrees of efficacy. Overall, these formulations function best in treating epidermal-melanin-induced hypermelanosis and are not efficient in removing pigmentation in the dermal layer of the skin as this is usually the result of melanin-laden macrophages with minimal tyrosinase activity (12).

18.3 Classification

18.3.1 Lightening Formulations That Regulate Melanocyte Activation

18.3.1.1 Broad-Spectrum Sunscreen

The foundation for the treatment of hypermelanosis consists of photoprotection with sunscreen agents. Furthermore, it will assist in maintaining the positive effect of any lightening formulation. Success in lightening hyperpigmentation depends on meticulous avoidance of sun exposure and the application of sunscreen every two hours. Sunscreens containing zinc oxide, titanium dioxide, and iron oxide have been determined to regulate melanocyte activation by impeding melanocyte stimulation by scattering UVB, UVA, and visible light (13). Studies have demonstrated improvement in hypermelanosis with the use of sunscreen alone (14). A broad-spectrum sunscreen with an SPF of 30 or more should be judiciously applied after the lightening formulation. Tinted sunscreens that contain visible light-blocking iron oxide are preferable and offer the widest spectrum of wavelength protection; however, their opaque color gives them the disadvantage of being less cosmetically appealing. In addition to sunscreen, patients should be advised of other methods of photoprotection, including using a hat or other clothing to protect their skin. Oral agents, such as *Polypodium leucotomos*, has been demonstrated to exhibit a variety of antioxidant and photoprotective properties (15, 16). Patients should be cautioned that sun exposure can reverse any benefit obtained from a lightening formulation.

18.3.2 Lightening Formulations That Reduce Melanogenesis

18.3.2.1 Hydroquinone (HQ)

Hydroquinone (HQ) formulations remain the gold standard of hypermelanosis treatment in the United States (17). The efficacy of HQ is due to its inhibition of mushroom tyrosinase, degradation of melanosomes, melanocyte destruction by the production of free radicals, and inhibition of DNA and RNA synthesis (12, 18). HQ is available at 2% concentration in over the counter cosmetic products in the United States and 4% concentration by prescription. Concentrations of 6–10% may be compounded in the US and have been used to treat refractory cases (19). Studies reveal that an improvement in hypermelanosis may require 4–12 weeks of twice-daily treatment, but treatment duration may extend to 12 months (20).

HQ, in synergy with other lightening agents, such as retinoids, has been used to treat pigmentary disorders such as melasma. Kligman and Willis proposed a compounded formulation of 0.1% tretinoin, 5% hydroquinone, and 0.1% dexamethasone for the treatment of melasma, ephelides, and post-inflammatory hyperpigmentation (21). Currently, a triple combination treatment for melasma containing 0.05% tretinoin, 0.01% fluocinolone acetonide, and 4% hydroquinone has been demonstrated to achieve favorable results (22). In general, combination formulations of HQ are used once nightly.

More immediate side effects of HQ include local irritation, contact dermatitis, a halo of hypopigmentation on normal skin around treated lesions (which resolves spontaneously with cessation of HQ), and brown nail discoloration (12). Exogenous ochronosis (EO) is a side effect of long-term hydroquinone use. It is commonly seen in patients from the African diaspora who utilize HQ-containing formulations for prolonged periods of time. EO is an accumulation of homogentisic acid in the dermis and can be observed with various concentrations of HQ, including 1–2% (23–25).

Additionally, nephropathy, renal tubular cell adenomas, hepatocellular adenomas, and mononuclear cell leukemia have been described in rodent models that have been given large doses of oral HQ (26). Although the human carcinogenicity potential of topical application has not been established, it may be cytotoxic to melanocytes. HQ is currently banned in Europe, Japan, and Australia, and a ban was once considered in the United States (27).

18.3.2.2 Arbutin

Arbutin is a competitive inhibitor of the tyrosinase enzyme rather than an inhibitor of tyrosinase synthesis as compared to HQ (28). Two derivatives of arbutin, a naturally occurring plant derivative of HQ, are available for the treatment of hypermelanosis, α-arbutin, and deoxyarbutin. Deoxyarbutin, a synthetic form of arbutin, inhibits mushroom tyrosinase in vitro and has demonstrated significant improvement in overall skin lightening. α-Arbutin is the synthetic isomer of arbutin and has been reported to be non-melanocytotoxic (29, 30).

Reflecting its modest efficacy in skin lightening, in the United States arbutin is frequently compounded with other topical skin-lightening agents, including kojic acid, vitamin C, and/or niacinamide. In Japan, α-arbutin in concentrations up to 3% are sold in skin-lightening products (27). As there is a paucity of controlled clinical trials on the safety and efficacy of α-arbutin and deoxyarbutin, there are no evidence-based recommendations for treatment or maintenance regimens (31).

Side effects of arbutin include contact dermatitis, as reported in Japan (32–34), and a paradoxical hyperpigmentation felt to be due to prolonged exposure to high doses of arbutin (28). The potential for deoxyarbutin agent to decay into HQ raises concerns with regard to the safety of the agent used in skin-lightening products (e.g., stability of the shelf life of the compound). Thus, the Scientific Committee on Consumer Safety, as managed by the European Commission, has concluded that the use of deoxyarbutin in facial cream products is not safe (35).

18.3.2.3 Azelaic Acid (AzA)

AzA is a dicarboxylic acid produced by the *Malassezia furfur* species of fungi that is available in the United States as a 20% cream, or as a 15% foam or gel. Its mechanisms of action include tyrosinase inhibition, inhibition of DNA synthesis in active melanocytes, and inhibition of melanocyte mitochondrial oxidoreductases of the respiratory chain (36–38). AzA may be melanocytotoxic and play a role in tinea versicolor induced hypopigmentation (39, 40). Studies have reported that 20% AzA cream applied twice daily is effective in the treatment of facial hyperpigmentation, epidermal melasma, PIH of Fitzpatrick skin phototype IV–VI (41, 42).

Side effects of AzA include burning, pruritus, erythema or tingling These side effects are deemed mild and self-limiting and does not necessitate cessation of the agent (43, 44).

18.3.2.4 Cysteamine

The thiol compound cysteamine inhibits both enzymes, tyrosinase, and peroxidase, which are integral to melanin biosynthesis (45, 46). A randomized, double-blind, vehicle-controlled trial of 5% cysteamine cream in 50 melasma patients demonstrated statistically significant improvement in the MASI score and melanin index at four months as compared to placebo (47). These results were replicated by Farshi and colleagues, who demonstrated statistically significant improvement in MASI scores using cysteamine cream in subjects with epidermal melisma (48). In both trials, cysteamine cream was applied once daily and removed three hours after application. The suggested maintenance therapy is twice weekly (47, 48).

Side effects of cysteamine cream may include irritation and erythema, although they have been deemed self-limiting, and the formulation is reportedly well tolerated (47, 49).

18.3.2.5 Kojic Acid

Kojic acid is a fungal metabolite of *Aspergillus*, which inhibits melanin production by chelating copper at the active site of tyrosinase (50). Kojic acid, in concentrations of 1–4%, is often combined with other ingredients, such as 2% HQ and 10% glycolic acid, and manufactured as soaps, creams, or gels. Kojic acid products are typically used twice daily for four to eight weeks or until the patient has achieved the desired results (51, 52).

The side effects of kojic acid in lightening formulations include erythema and contact dermatitis (53). This agent is considered to have significant sensitizing potential since a relatively high frequency of contact dermatitis has been observed in patients using kojic-acid-containing products, even at 1% concentration (50, 53, 54).

18.3.2.6 Vitamins C and E

The water-soluble vitamin ascorbic acid, commonly known as vitamin C, inhibits melanin synthesis by chelating copper at the active site of tyrosinase (3). Clinical studies have demonstrated the efficacy of topical 5% ascorbic acid in melisma (55, 56).

Tocopheryl acetate, known as vitamin E, is a fat-soluble vitamin that exerts its skin-lightening effects by inhibiting tyrosinase, increasing intracellular glutathione, and interfering with lipid peroxidation of melanocyte membranes (3, 57). Studies done with a facial lotion containing 0.5% tocopheryl acetate, 4% niacinamide (vitamin B3), 0.5% panthenol (vitamin B5) have shown to improve skin tone and texture (58).

The use of topical vitamin C is well tolerated and can be used daily for a long duration without many side effects. With regard to topical vitamin E, the most common adverse event is a transient, mild burning sensation; however, there are a few case reports of vitamin E causing contact dermatitis and erythema multiforme (59–62).

18.3.2.7 Licorice Extract

Licorice is obtained from the root of the *Glycyrrhiza glabra* plant (63). Licorice extract contains liquiritin and glabridin,

both of which have skin-lightening effects (64). Glabridin prevents UVB-induced pigmentation and inhibits tyrosinase activity, superoxide anion production, and cyclooxygenase activity (3, 65). This suggests that glabridin extract has an inhibitory influence on both melanogenesis and skin inflammation. However, there are no controlled clinical trials in humans on the efficacy of glabridin on skin lightening.

Liquiritin is a flavonoid that, when used twice daily as a liquiritin cream in a study evaluation with melasma, demonstrated that the pigmentation intensity was markedly reduced in 70% of subjects. The lightening effect of liquiritin is related to its ability to disperse melanin. Mild irritation is a side effect of licorice extract use but resolves with the continuation of treatment (66).

18.3.3 Lightening Formulations That Inhibit Melanosome Transfer to Keratinocytes

18.3.3.1 Niacinamide

Niacinamide (also called nicotinamide) is a biologically active form of niacin (vitamin B3) that is found in root vegetables and in yeast (67). It causes suppression of melanosome transfer from melanocytes into keratinocytes, which is the mechanism for the reduction in cutaneous pigmentation (68, 69).

Niacinamide can be used topically in concentrations up to 5% daily, and it is generally well tolerated; however, in some rare cases, mild skin irritation has been described (70, 71).

18.3.3.2 Soy

Soybeans are legumes that are rich in biologically active ingredients, such as serine protease inhibitors (64). Protease-activated receptor (PAR)-2, found only on keratinocytes, is a G-protein-coupled receptor that plays a role in melanosome transfer (64). The soy-derived serine protease inhibitors, soybean trypsin inhibitor and Bowman-Birk inhibitor, prevent PAR-2 cleavage, affect cytoskeletal and cell surface organization, and reduce keratinocyte phagocytosis (72). This suggests that modulation of PAR-2 activation by soy extracts results in changes in pigment production and deposition (73). Hence, soy is a commonly used skin-lightening ingredient in moisturizers and cosmeceuticals that is generally used twice daily and has demonstrated significant improvement in hyperpigmentation, skin tone, and appearance (74). Although the adverse effects and safety profile of soy-based lightening formulations are not well documented in the literature, it is seemingly well tolerated.

18.3.4 Lightening Formulations That Remove Epidermal Pigment

18.3.4.1 Retinoids

Retinoids (vitamin A derivatives) include natural compounds, such as retinal (vitamin A aldehyde) and retinol (vitamin A alcohol), and synthetic topical compounds, such as 0.01–0.1% tretinoin (retinoic acid), 0.1–0.3% adapalene, and 0.05–0.1% tazarotene. Topical isotretinoin is not available in the United States. The skin-lightening properties of retinoids include keratolytic activity and interference with epidermal melanin dispersion (75, 76). Both retinol and retinal are thought to be able to penetrate the skin and be converted into retinoic acid once intracellular, which forms the basis for their efficacy (77). Studies performed with a 0.1% retinol cream applied nightly have revealed significant improvements in overall mottled pigmentation and photodamage, as well as other signs of aging (e.g., crow's feet, wrinkles, and cheek wrinkles). Retinoids have also been shown to reduce epidermal pigmentation (78, 79).

Skin irritation (retinoid dermatitis) is an expected side effect of retinoid use and is characterized by erythema, scaling, peeling, dryness, burning, and stinging (76). Application of a pea-sized amount of product every other day for a month and then titrating up to once daily application over time will allow the patient to build a tolerance to the product and improve compliance.

18.4 Clinical Pearls in Treating Ethnic Skin/Skin of Color

Dyschromia is the fifth most common diagnosis in African Americans and the tenth in Hispanic patients seen by dermatologists (80). Treatment modalities are individualized to patients by skin type, location of the dyschromia, and by proxy, racial/ethnic group (81). Treating the skin of patients of color requires a delicate balance between clearing the condition, preserving natural pigmentation, and minimizing side effects. Thus, the proper diagnosis and treatment with a lightening formulation by a dermatologist knowledgeable in treating skin of color are important for a successful outcome.

Patients of Southeast and East Asian Descent

* Cupping, coin rubbing, and moxibustion are three ancient healing techniques that complement acupuncture therapy through the use of heat to stimulate circulation and promote healing. Patients that regularly practice these techniques may develop ecchymoses, hemosiderin deposition, or post-inflammatory hyperpigmentation. Parents may be accused of child abuse by healthcare professionals unaware of these practices.
* A common cultural practice among certain Southeast Asian cultures is the application of black henna tattoos, which may contain high concentrations of the allergen para-phenylenediamine (PPD). A brisk contact allergic dermatitis may result in long-lasting PIH.

Patients of African Descent

* PIH occurs from pathophysiological responses to inflammation, cutaneous irritation or injury, and subsequent melanocyte lability. The inflammatory skin disorder acne is the most common cause of PIH in this patient population. Additionally, dermatologic procedures (e.g., electrodesiccation, microdermabrasion, chemical peels, and laser hair removal treatments) commonly result in PIH when in the hands of those less experienced with darker skin types.

Patients of Hispanic Descent

* Melasma occurs more frequently in people of Latin descent when compared to the general population in the United States. In addition to sunscreen use, treatments for melasma include skin-lightening formulations such as hydroquinone, topical retinoids, and combination formulations of the two with a steroid. Additionally, certain laser and light therapies and oral medications have been demonstrated to be safe and effective with melasma as well.

Frequently Asked Questions

1. Q: *Should patients exfoliate their skin before using a lightening formulation?*
   A: Gentle chemical exfoliating of the skin may assist in the penetration of the lightening formulation. However, this should be done several days before the application of the lightening formula, and special care is needed to avoid traumatizing the skin.
2. Q: *Can you use skin-lightening products while you are pregnant?*
   A: It is not advisable to use prescription or OTC skin-lightening creams during conception or pregnancy. Additionally, hormonal changes in pregnancy can cause hypermelanosis. Thus, the use of sunscreen every two hours during sun exposure is advisable.
3. Q: *Is skin lightening permanent?*
   A: Using a topical lightening formulation will not remove melanin permanently. New melanin is continually being produced by melanocytes. However, to maintain the skin-lightening effects of hypermelanosis, sun protection should be practiced regularly.
4. Q: *Are systemic treatments available to lighten skin?*
   A: Tranexamic acid (TXA), a synthetic form of lysine, inhibits the plasminogen-plasmin pathway and melanin synthesis by decreasing arachidonic acid. Thus, TXA reduces MSH and pigment production. Oral TXA has not been approved by the US FDA for the treatment of hypermelanosis. However, available data in the literature indicates that oral TXA 250 mg twice daily can improve melasma after 8–12 weeks of treatment (82).

References

1. D'Mello SA, Finlay GJ, Baguley BC, Askarian-Amiri ME. Signaling pathways in melanogenesis. International Journal of Molecular Sciences. 2016;17(7).
2. Taylor SC. Skin of color: Biology, structure, function, and implications for dermatologic disease. Journal of the American Academy of Dermatology. 2002;46(2 Suppl Understanding):S41–62.
3. Ebanks JP, Wickett RR, Boissy RE. Mechanisms regulating skin pigmentation: The rise and fall of complexion coloration. International Journal of Molecular Sciences. 2009;10(9):4066–4087.
4. Maymone MBC, Neamah HH, Wirya SA, Patzelt NM, Secemsky EA, Zancanaro PQ, et al. The impact of skin hyperpigmentation and hyperchromia on quality of life: A cross-sectional study. Journal of the American Academy of Dermatology. 2017;77(4):775–778.
5. Alrayyes SF, Alrayyes SF, Farooq Dar U. Skin-lightening practices behind the veil: An epidemiological study among Saudi women. Journal of Cosmetic Dermatology. 2020 Jan;19(1):147–153.
6. Ladizinski B, Mistry N, Kundu RV. Widespread use of toxic skin lightening compounds: Medical and psychosocial aspects. Dermatologic Clinics. 2011;29(1):111–123.
7. Stulberg DL, Clark N, Tovey D. Common hyperpigmentation disorders in adults: Part I. Diagnostic approach, le au lait macules, diffuse hyperpigmentation, sun exposure, and phototoxic reactions. American Family Physician. 2003;68(10):1955–1960.
8. Stefanato CM, Bhawan J. Diffuse hyperpigmentation of the skin: A clinicopathologic approach to diagnosis. Seminars in Cutaneous Medicine and Surgery. 1997;16(1):61–71.
9. Pepine M, Flowers FP, Ramos-Caro FA. Extensive cutaneous hyperpigmentation caused by minocycline. Journal of the American Academy of Dermatology. 1993;28(2 Pt 2):292–295.
10. Sasidharanpillai S, Abdul Latheef EN, Kumar PJ, Sathi PP, Manakkad SP, Jishna P, et al. Anaplastic large cell non Hodgkin's lymphoma presenting as diffuse cutaneous hyperpigmentation. Indian Journal of Dermatology, Venereology and Leprology. 2018;84(3):316–320.
11. Di Tullio F, Mandel VD, Scotti R, Padalino C, Pellacani G. Imatinib-induced diffuse hyperpigmentation of the oral mucosa, the skin, and the nails in a patient affected by chronic myeloid leukemia: Report of a case and review of the literature. International Journal of Dermatology. 2018;57(7):784–790.

12. Katsambas AD, Stratigos AJ. Depigmenting and bleaching agents: Coping with hyperpigmentation. Clinics in Dermatology. 2001;19(4):483–488.

13. Kullavanijaya P, Lim HW. Photoprotection. Journal of the American Academy of Dermatology. 2005;52(6):937–958; quiz 59–62.

14. Sarkar R, Garg VK, Jain A, Agarwal D, Wagle A, Flament F, et al. A randomized study to evaluate the efficacy and effectiveness of two sunscreen formulations on Indian skin types IV and V with pigmentation irregularities. Indian Journal of Dermatology, Venereology and Leprology. 2019;85(2):160–168.

15. Nestor M, Bucay V, Callender V, Cohen JL, Sadick N, Waldorf H. Polypodium leucotomos as an adjunct treatment of pigmentary disorders. Journal of Clinical and Aesthetic Dermatology. 2014;7(3):13–17.

16. Nestor MS, Berman B, Swenson N. Safety and efficacy of oral Polypodium leucotomos extract in healthy adult subjects. Journal of Clinical and Aesthetic Dermatology. 2015;8(2):19–23.

17. Arndt KA, Fitzpatrick TB. Topical use of hydroquinone as a depigmenting agent. JAMA. 1965;194(9):965–967.

18. Parvez S, Kang M, Chung HS, Cho C, Hong MC, Shin MK, et al. Survey and mechanism of skin depigmenting and lightening agents. Phytotherapy Research: PTR. 2006;20(11):921–934.

19. Skin bleaching drug products for over-the-counter human use; Proposed rule. In: Administration USFaD, editor. Office of the Federal Register, National Archives and Records Administration; 2006. p. 51146–51155. https://www.federalregister.gov/d/E6-14263

20. Ennes SBP, Paschoalick RC, Alchorne MMDA. A double-blind, comparative, placebo-controlled study of the efficacy and tolerability of 4% hydroquinone as a depigmenting agent in melasma. Journal of Dermatological Treatment. 2000;11(3):173–179.

21. Kligman AM, Willis I. A new formula for depigmenting human skin. Archives of Dermatology. 1975;111(1):40–48.

22. Grimes PE, Bhawan J, Guevara IL, Colon LE, Johnson LA, Gottschalk RW, et al. Continuous therapy followed by a maintenance therapy regimen with a triple combination cream for melasma. Journal of the American Academy of Dermatology. 2010;62(6):962–967.

23. Bhattar PA, Zawar VP, Godse KV, Patil SP, Nadkarni NJ, Gautam MM. Exogenous Ochronosis. Indian Journal of Dermatology. 2015;60(6):537–543.

24. Findlay GH, Morrison JG, Simson IW. Exogenous ochronosis and pigmented colloid milium from hydroquinone bleaching creams. The British Journal of Dermatology. 1975;93(6):613–622.

25. Tan SK. Exogenous ochronosis—successful outcome after treatment with Q-switched Nd:YAG laser. Journal of Cosmetic and Laser Therapy: Official Publication of the European Society for Laser Dermatology. 2013;15(5):274–278.

26. Whysner J, Verna L, English JC, Williams GM. Analysis of studies related to tumorigenicity induced by hydroquinone. Regulatory Toxicology and Pharmacology: RTP. 1995;21(1):158–176.

27. Draelos ZD. Skin lightening preparations and the hydroquinone controversy. Dermatologic Therapy. 2007;20(5):308–313.

28. Maeda K, Fukuda M. Arbutin: Mechanism of its depigmenting action in human melanocyte culture. Journal of Pharmacology and Experimental Therapeutics. 1996;276(2):765–769.

29. Boissy RE, Visscher M, DeLong MA. DeoxyArbutin: A novel reversible tyrosinase inhibitor with effective in vivo skin lightening potency. Experimental Dermatology. 2005;14(8):601–608.

30. Zhu W, Gao J. The use of botanical extracts as topical skin-lightening agents for the improvement of skin pigmentation disorders. Journal of Investigative Dermatology Symposium Proceedings. 2008;13(1):20–24.

31. Woolery-Lloyd H, Kammer JN. Overview of cosmetic concerns in skin of color. In: Alexis AF, Barbosa VH, editors. Skin of Color: A Practical Guide to Dermatologic Diagnosis and Treatment. New York, NY: Springer; 2013. p. 221–236.

32. Oiso N, Tatebayashi M, Hoshiyama Y, Kawada A. Allergic contact dermatitis caused by arbutin and dipotassium glycyrrhizate in skin-lightening products. Contact Dermatitis. 2017;77(1):51–53.

33. Numata T, Tobita R, Tsuboi R, Okubo Y. Contact dermatitis caused by arbutin contained in skin-whitening cosmetics. Contact Dermatitis. 2016;75(3):187–188.

34. Matsuo Y, Ito A, Masui Y, Ito M. A case of allergic contact dermatitis caused by arbutin. Contact Dermatitis. 2015;72(6):404–405.

35. Sccs, Degen GH. Opinion of the Scientific Committee on Consumer safety (SCCS)—Opinion on the safety of the use of deoxyarbutin in cosmetic products. Regulatory Toxicology and Pharmacology: RTP. 2016;74:77–78.

36. Mazurek K, Pierzchala E. Comparison of efficacy of products containing azelaic acid in melasma treatment. Journal of Cosmetic Dermatology. 2016;15(3):269–282.

37. Leibl H, Stingl G, Pehamberger H, Korschan H, Konrad K, Wolff K. Inhibition of DNA synthesis of melanoma cells by azelaic acid. Journal of Investigative Dermatology. 1985;85(5):417–422.

38. Lemic-Stojcevic L, Nias AH, Breathnach AS. Effect of azelaic acid on melanoma cells in culture. Experimental Dermatology. 1995;4(2):79–81.

39. Nazzaro-Porro M, Passi S. Identification of tyrosinase inhibitors in cultures of Pityrosporum. Journal of Investigative Dermatology. 1978;71(3):205–208.

40. Galadari I, el Komy M, Mousa A, Hashimoto K, Mehregan AH. Tinea versicolor: Histologic and ultrastructural investigation of pigmentary changes. International Journal of Dermatology. 1992;31(4): 253–256.

41. Farshi S. Comparative study of therapeutic effects of 20% azelaic acid and hydroquinone 4% cream in the treatment of melasma. Journal of Cosmetic Dermatology. 2011;10(4):282–287.

42. Lowe NJ, Rizk D, Grimes P, Billips M, Pincus S. Azelaic acid 20% cream in the treatment of facial hyperpigmentation in darker-skinned patients. Clinical Therapeutics. 1998;20(5):945–959.

43. Thiboutot D, Thieroff-Ekerdt R, Graupe K. Efficacy and safety of azelaic acid (15%) gel as a new treatment for papulopustular rosacea: Results from two vehicle-controlled, randomized phase III studies. Journal of the American Academy of Dermatology. 2003;48(6):836–845.

44. Ziel K, Yelverton CB, Balkrishnan R, Feldman SR. Cumulative irritation potential of azelaic acid gel compared to metronidazole gel after repeated applications to healthy skin. Journal of Drugs in Dermatology: JDD. 2005;4(6):727–731.

45. Qiu L, Zhang M, Sturm RA, Gardiner B, Tonks I, Kay G, et al. Inhibition of melanin synthesis by cystamine in human melanoma cells. Journal of Investigative Dermatology. 2000;114(1):21–27.

46. Kasraee B. Peroxidase-mediated mechanisms are involved in the melanocytotoxic and melanogenesis-inhibiting effects of chemical agents. Dermatology (Basel, Switzerland). 2002;205(4):329–339.

47. Mansouri P, Farshi S, Hashemi Z, Kasraee B. Evaluation of the efficacy of cysteamine 5% cream in the treatment of epidermal melasma: A randomized double-blind placebo-controlled trial. British Journal of Dermatology. 2015;173(1):209–217.

48. Farshi S, Mansouri P, Kasraee B. Efficacy of cysteamine cream in the treatment of epidermal melasma, evaluating by Dermacatch as a new measurement method: A randomized double blind placebo controlled study. Journal of Dermatological Treatment. 2018;29(2):182–189.

49. Kasraee B, Mansouri P, Farshi S. Significant therapeutic response to cysteamine cream in a melasma patient resistant to Kligman's formula. Journal of Cosmetic Dermatology. 2019;18(1):293–295.

50. Serra-Baldrich E, Tribo MJ, Camarasa JG. Allergic contact dermatitis from kojic acid. Contact Dermatitis. 1998;39(2):86–87.

51. Lim JT. Treatment of melasma using kojic acid in a gel containing hydroquinone and glycolic acid. Dermatologic. 1999;25(4):282–284.

52. Garcia A, Fulton JE, Jr. The combination of glycolic acid and hydroquinone or kojic acid for the treatment of melasma and related conditions. Dermatologic Surgery. 1996;22(5):443–447.

53. Garcia-Gavin J, Gonzalez-Vilas D, Fernandez-Redondo V, Toribio J. Pigmented contact dermatitis due to kojic acid. A paradoxical side effect of a skin lightener. Contact Dermatitis. 2010;62(1):63–64.

54. Nakagawa M, Kawai K, Kawai K. Contact allergy to kojic acid in skin care products. Contact Dermatitis. 1995;32(1):9–13.

55. Espinal-Perez LE, Moncada B, Castanedo-Cazares JP. A double-blind randomized trial of 5% ascorbic acid vs. 4% hydroquinone in melasma. International Journal of Dermatology. 2004;43(8):604–607.

56. Dayal S, Sahu P, Yadav M, Jain VK. Clinical efficacy and safety on combining 20% trichloroacetic acid peel with topical 5% ascorbic acid for melasma. Journal of Clinical and Diagnostic Research: JCDR. 2017;11(9):Wc08–Wc11.

57. Shimizu K, Kondo R, Sakai K, Takeda N, Nagahata T, Oniki T. Novel vitamin E derivative with 4-substituted resorcinol moiety has both antioxidant and tyrosinase inhibitory properties. Lipids. 2001;36(12): 1321–1326.

58. Jerajani HR, Mizoguchi H, Li J, Whittenbarger DJ, Marmor MJ. The effects of a daily facial lotion containing vitamins B3 and E and provitamin B5 on the facial skin of Indian women: A randomized, double-blind trial. Indian Journal of Dermatology, Venereology and Leprology. 2010;76(1):20–26.

59. Goldman MP, Rapaport M. Contact dermatitis to vitamin E oil. Journal of the American Academy of Dermatology. 1986;14(1):133–134.

60. Parsad D, Saini R, Verma N. Xanthomatous reaction following contact dermatitis from vitamin E. Contact Dermatitis. 1997;37(6):294.

61. Thiele JJ, Ekanayake-Mudiyanselage S. Vitamin E in human skin: Organ-specific physiology and considerations for its use in dermatology. Molecular Aspects of Medicine. 2007;28(5–6):646–667.

62. Saperstein H, Rapaport M, Rietschel RL. Topical vitamin E as a cause of erythema multiforme-like eruption. Archives of Dermatology. 1984;120(7):906–908.

63. Nazari S, Rameshrad M, Hosseinzadeh H. Toxicological effects of Glycyrrhiza glabra (Licorice): A review. Phytotherapy Research: PTR. 2017;31(11):1635–1650.

64. Taylor S, Woolery-Lloyd H. Pigmentation disorders in skin of color: The role of natural substances. Seminars in Cutaneous Medicine and Surgery. 2008;27(3 Suppl):14–15.

65. Yokota T, Nishio H, Kubota Y, Mizoguchi M. The inhibitory effect of glabridin from licorice extracts on melanogenesis and inflammation. Pigment Cell Research. 1998;11(6):355–361.

66. Amer M, Metwalli M. Topical liquiritin improves melasma. International Journal of Dermatology. 2000;39(4):299–301.

67. Wohlrab J, Kreft D. Niacinamide—mechanisms of action and its topical use in dermatology. Skin Pharmacology and Physiology. 2014;27(6):311–315.

68. Hakozaki T, Minwalla L, Zhuang J, Chhoa M, Matsubara A, Miyamoto K, et al. The effect of niacinamide on reducing cutaneous pigmentation and suppression of melanosome transfer. British Journal of Dermatology. 2002;147(1):20–31.

69. Navarrete-Solís J, Castanedo-Cázares JP, Torres-Álvarez B, Oros-Ovalle C, Fuentes-Ahumada C, González FJ, et al. A double-blind, randomized clinical trial of niacinamide 4% versus hydroquinone 4% in the treatment of melasma. Dermatology Research and Practice. 2011;2011:379173.

70. Kimball AB, Kaczvinsky JR, Li J, Robinson LR, Matts PJ, Berge CA, et al. Reduction in the appearance of facial hyperpigmentation after use of moisturizers with a combination of topical niacinamide and N-acetyl glucosamine: Results of a randomized, double-blind, vehicle-controlled trial. British Journal of Dermatology. 2010;162(2):435–441.

71. Berson DS, Osborne R, Oblong JE, Hakozaki T, Johnson MB, Bissett DL. Niacinamide. In: Farris PK, editor. Cosmeceuticals and Cosmetic Practice. John Wiley & Sons, Ltd.; 2013. p. 103–112.

72. Paine C, Sharlow E, Liebel F, Eisinger M, Shapiro S, Seiberg M. An alternative approach to depigmentation by soybean extracts via inhibition of the PAR-2 pathway. Journal of Investigative Dermatology. 2001;116(4):587–595.

73. Seiberg M, Paine C, Sharlow E, Andrade-Gordon P, Costanzo M, Eisinger M, et al. Inhibition of melanosome transfer results in skin lightening. Journal of Investigative Dermatology. 2000;115(2):162–167.

74. Wallo W, Nebus J, Leyden JJ. Efficacy of a soy moisturizer in photoaging: A double-blind, vehicle-controlled, 12-week study. Journal of Drugs in Dermatology: JDD. 2007;6(9):917–922.

75. Ortonne JP. Retinoid therapy of pigmentary disorders. Dermatologic Therapy. 2006;19(5):280–288.

76. Kang HY, Valerio L, Bahadoran P, Ortonne JP. The role of topical retinoids in the treatment of pigmentary disorders: An evidence-based review. American Journal of Clinical Dermatology. 2009;10(4):251–260.

77. Bailly J, Crettaz M, Schifflers MH, Marty JP. In vitro metabolism by human skin and fibroblasts of retinol, retinal and retinoic acid. Experimental Dermatology. 1998;7(1):27–34.

78. Tucker-Samaras S, Zedayko T, Cole C, Miller D, Wallo W, Leyden JJ. A stabilized 0.1% retinol facial moisturizer improves the appearance of photodamaged skin in an eight-week, double-blind, vehicle-controlled study. Journal of Drugs in Dermatology: JDD. 2009;8(10):932–936.

79. Grimes P, Callender V. Tazarotene cream for postinflammatory hyperpigmentation and acne vulgaris in darker skin: A double-blind, randomized, vehicle-controlled study. Cutis. 2006;77(1):45–50.

80. Davis SA, Narahari S, Feldman SR, Huang W, Pichardo-Geisinger RO, McMichael AJ. Top dermatologic conditions in patients of color: An analysis of nationally representative data. Journal of Drugs in Dermatology: JDD. 2012;11(4):466–473.

81. Kang SJ, Davis SA, Feldman SR, McMichael AJ. Dyschromia in skin of color. Journal of Drugs in Dermatology: JDD. 2014;13(4):401–406.

82. Del Rosario E, Florez-Pollack S, Zapata L, Jr., Hernandez K, Tovar-Garza A, Rodrigues M, et al. Randomized, placebo-controlled, double-blind study of oral tranexamic acid in the treatment of moderate-to-severe melasma. Journal of the American Academy of Dermatology. 2018;78(2):363–369.

CHAPTER 19: ANTI-AGING AGENTS FOR ETHNIC SKIN

Sumayah Taliaferro, Awa Bakayoko, and Valerie D. Callender

19.1 Introduction

The desire to preserve youthfulness exists across the globe. Central to the universal desire to maintain healthy, beautiful skin is the goal of delaying visible signs of aging. Differences in facial aging can be observed in different ethnic groups. It is well established that there are two pathways through which facial aging occurs: intrinsic and extrinsic. Intrinsic aging of the skin occurs due to soft tissue volume loss, fat atrophy, and loss of skeletal support that occurs naturally with age. Extrinsic changes occur due to chronic sun exposure, manifesting as wrinkles, mottled pigmentation, and decreased elasticity.[1] Those with fair complexions tend to experience extrinsic signs of skin aging, while darker-skinned individuals tend to observe intrinsic signs of skin aging. Darker-skinned individuals also tend to experience more pigmentary changes. Several natural ingredients and manufactured products have been identified to tackle signs of both intrinsic and extrinsic aging. This chapter reviews many of these agents, including sunscreens, antioxidants, botanicals, skin-lightening agents, and manufactured products, to address their anti-aging properties and hyperpigmentation with a specific focus on agents commonly used for ethnic skin.

19.2 Classification

19.2.1 Sunscreens

UV exposure to the skin ignites a host of biological effects that lead to key features of aging skin, which include wrinkling, skin laxity, loss of moisture, dyschromia, and skin cancer. Photoaging of the skin, the most common type of extrinsic aging, occurs due to cellular DNA damage from UV light. UV radiation also increases proinflammatory cytokines. Sunscreens remain the main essential agents to prevent photoaging of the skin. Skin of color, which has naturally inherent sun protection from melanin, also exhibits notable effects of photodamage with aging when sun protection is not routine. Recommended sunscreens should offer protection against UVA and UVB (broad coverage), and data now suggests that protection against visible and infrared light may offer anti-aging benefits as well. UVB (290–320 nm wavelength) affects the DNA of cells, most notably forming cyclobutane pyrimidine dimers, sometimes referred to as the "signature mutations" of UV damage and UVB "fingerprint mutations." UVB also indirectly causes oxidative damage to skin cells through the formation of reactive oxygen species (ROS). UVA (320–400 nm) contributes greatly to photoaging. On a cellular level, UVA penetrates deeper than UVB, passing through the dermal-epidermal junction and into the dermis, where it upregulates the expression of matrix metalloproteinases (MMPs). The resulting accelerated breakdown of collagen yields early wrinkling and sagging skin. UVA also generates ROS that damage cells, specifically through what are now known as the "UVA fingerprint mutations."[2, 3] Furthermore, UV light exerts an immunosuppressive effect on skin, which decreases the routine protective mechanisms of inhibiting cellular death of abnormal cells. As a result, the proliferation of dysplastic cells may go unchecked and increase the formation of malignant neoplasms. Visible light (400–700 nm) may also contribute to hyperpigmentation and to certain other extrinsic factors of aging.[4] Table 19.1 consists of a list of active sunscreen ingredients approved by the FDA.

19.2.2 Retinoids

Retinoids have substantial data to support their role in anti-aging of the skin. Retinoids have been shown to histologically and clinically reverse and halt skin aging. Data show that retinoids decrease collagen breakdown and increase new collagen production. Derived from all-trans-retinol, vitamin A has several forms. Keratinocytes in human skin convert retinyl palmitate to retinol. Retinol is converted into retinaldehyde, which in turn transforms to retinoic acid (tretinoin), the active ingredient. On a cellular level, tretinoin has been shown to stimulate collagen synthesis. It increases TGF-beta and procollagen and inhibits MMPs. Reported changes in the histology of skin treated with retinoic acid include epidermal thickening, an increase in the granular layer of the epidermis, decreased melanin content, compaction of the stratum corneum, and increased collagen deposition in the papillary dermis.

Clinically, tretinoin has proven efficacy in the improvement of fine lines, coarse wrinkling, skin roughness, skin laxity, and hyperpigmentation. Tretinoin decreases skin atrophy, a hallmark feature of aging skin, and has been shown to improve dyschromia associated with photoaging of the skin due to its ability to increase epidermal cell turnover.

Tretinoin may also enhance skin hydration by increasing glycosaminoglycan synthesis and thereby improving the water-binding capacity of the skin. Both tretinoin and tazarotene, synthetic retinoids, are the gold standard topical retinoids for the treatment of aging skin. Research on adapalene for anti-aging

TABLE 19.1: Active Sunscreen Ingredients Approved by the FDA

Chemical Sunscreen	Protection Level
Avobenzone	Mostly UVA
Cinoxate	Mostly UVB
Dioxybenzone	UVB, substantial UVA
Ecamsule (Mexoryl)	UVA, partial UVB
Homosalate	UVB
Menthyl anthranilate	UVB, substantial UVA
Octocrylene	UVB, partial UVA
Octyl methoxycinnamate (octinoxate)	UVB, partial UVA
Octyl salicylate	UVB
Oxybenzone	UVB, substantial UVA
(PABA) aminobenzoic acid	UVB
Padimate O	UVB
Phenylbenzimidazole	UVB
Sulisobenzone	UVB, substantial UVA
Trolamine salicylate	UVB
Physical Sunscreen/Sunblock	**Protection Level**
Titanium dioxide	UVB, substantial UVA
Zinc oxide	UVA and UVB

DOI: 10.1201/9780429243769-19

purposes is not as extensive, but significant data exists showing that it also reduces the signs of photoaging of the skin.[5–9]

19.2.3 Alpha- and Beta-Hydroxy Acids

Among the alpha-hydroxy acids are glycolic, lactic, malic, and citric acids. Alpha-hydroxy acids have been shown to increase collagen synthesis, improve skin cell turnover, and even improve hydration. Specifically, alpha-hydroxy acid increases type 1 collagen mRNA. It has been found to increase hyaluronic acid in the dermis and epidermis and may yield a humectant effect to improve the barrier function of the skin. Alpha-hydroxy acids may contribute greatly to anti-aging, particularly when combined with other agents. For example, it enhances the beneficial effect of tretinoin.[10, 11] Alpha-hydroxy acids may also enhance the effect of hydroquinone and improve hyperpigmentation associated with aging.

19.2.4 Antioxidants

Antioxidants are scavengers of free radicals that prevent oxidation and cellular damage. There is a growing abundance of data *in vivo* and *in vitro* and clinical data supporting the use of antioxidants to protect against UV-induced skin damage.

19.2.4.1 Vitamin C

Vitamin C (ascorbic acid) is the most popular antioxidant for the skin. Best known for its treatment of hyperpigmentation and its cytoprotective effects, vitamin C is considered a crown jewel agent of anti-aging. L-ascorbic acid, the biologically active form of vitamin C, decreases with age. Systemically, humans must acquire ascorbic acid. Thus, it is a required nutrient in the diet. The effects of topically applied vitamin C are much greater on skin aging than ingestion of vitamin C. However, the challenges of topical vitamin C include its difficulty in penetrating the skin and stabilizing it in solution because it is water soluble and photosensitive. While L-ascorbic acid is the biologically active form, ascorbyl palmitate is a fat-soluble form of ascorbic acid found in cosmeceuticals.

Ascorbic acid is a cofactor for collagen synthesis and upregulates collagen formation.[12, 13] Vitamin C also decreases the production of matrix metalloproteinases.[14] It has also been found to yield anti-inflammatory effects. A study by Alster and West[15] demonstrated that ascorbic acid reduced erythema in patients post-CO_2 laser treatments. Furthermore, cytoprotective data indicate inhibition of activator protein-1, a gene transcription factor that induces UV-related keratinocyte death. Vitamin C decreases hyperpigmentation of the skin by inhibiting tyrosinase and decreasing melanogenesis. Its benefits of improving and preventing dyschromia of aging skin are well-supported. Discoloration with aging is a deep concern for people of all ethnicities, but particularly those with darker skin types who may have delayed wrinkling of the skin and more often insidious or rapid hyperpigmentation and other dyschromias with time. L-ascorbic acid is often found with vitamin E (α-tocopherol), as it may help to regenerate the oxidized forms of α-tocopherol.

19.2.4.2 Vitamin E

Vitamin E is a lipid-soluble antioxidant that is naturally located in the stratum corneum of healthy skin. Produced by sebaceous glands, it is the main antioxidant found in the human epidermis. Environmental damage depletes vitamin E in the epidermis. Vitamin E is photoprotective from UV and infrared light, displays anti-inflammatory and excellent moisturizing properties, and may function as a preservative in skin products. There are various forms of vitamin E, including tocopherols and tocotrienols. A-tocopherol is the most abundant vitamin E in humans. Conversion capability is an important factor for effective topical agents. For example, in one report, the acetate form of vitamin E, even when well absorbed into the skin, did not convert to the biologically active α-tocopherol. A-tocopherol has been shown to improve rhytids, skin roughness, facial lines, and wrinkle depth.[16]

19.2.4.3 Ubiquinone (Co-enzyme Q10)

Ubiquinone is a potent endogenous antioxidant found in the cells of the body, including the skin. Tissue levels of ubiquinone decrease with age. It is lipophilic and decreases skin roughness, improves facial lines, and increases hydration.[17] Idebenone is a more soluble synthetic product derived from ubiquinone.

19.2.4.4 Niacinamide (Nicotinamide)

Niacin (vitamin B3) has two forms—niacinamide (nicotinamide) and nicotinic acid. It is thought that the two forms readily convert from one form to the other, and both exert biological actions, although nicotinic acid may be more active than niacinamide. Niacinamide increases NADP and NADPH, which have significant antioxidant effects. Niacinamide has been shown to improve the barrier function of the skin by thickening the stratum corneum, stimulating the differentiation of keratinocytes, and increasing the synthesis of ceramides.[18] Nicotinamide has also been reported to stimulate collagen synthesis and increase filaggrin and involucrin. It decreases excessive dermal glycosaminoglycans. Niacinamide also improves dyschromia associated with photoaging of the skin. One mechanism it reduces hyperpigmentation is by decreasing the transfer of melanosomes from melanocytes to keratinocytes.[19]

19.2.4.5 Alpha-Lipoic Acid (ALA)

Alpha-lipoic acid is an antioxidant that restores glutathione levels, which naturally decline with age. This agent has also been found to improve glucose metabolism. Thus, it is a helpful supplement for diabetes, as it may decrease or help prevent diabetic complications. When applied topically, it may improve the aging of the skin by increasing epidermal thickness.[20]

19.2.5 Polyphenol/Flavonoid Antioxidants
19.2.5.1 Tea

The active ingredients in tea (*Camellia sinensis*) are green tea polyphenols (GTP), epigallacatechin, and epicatechin-3-gallate. Green tea exhibits antioxidant and anti-inflammatory activity. Tea polyphenols and tea polysaccharides are key bioactive components of green tea. Data indicate that it inhibits metalloproteinases, which are activated by UV radiation. UV exposure may lead to an overexpression of cyclooxygenase (COX-2), which results in an increase in proinflammatory prostaglandin products. GTPs inhibit UV-induced COX-2 and prostaglandins. Green tea has been shown to specifically decrease cyclobutane pyrimidine dimers. It may also improve skin elasticity.[21] Topically applied tea polyphenols exert anti-aging effects by enhancing moisture retention, stimulating fibroblast proliferation, absorbing UVA and UVB, and inhibiting tyrosinase. The inhibition of tyrosinase regulates melanogenesis and aids in the correction of hyperpigmentation and dyschromias common in aging skin.[22] Research further shows green tea to be among several polyphenols that deliver significant anticarcinogenic and chemopreventive effects. Variations exist in the bioavailability of polyphenols, which impacts efficacy. Penetration into the skin may be limited unless enhanced by vehicles that increase delivery through the skin, such as cream-based and lipid-soluble topical products.

19.2.5.2 Resveratrol

Resveratrol is a polyphenolic compound found in the skin and seeds of grapes. While its richest sources are black grapes and red wine, it is also found in cocoa, mulberry fruit, tomatoes, and peanuts. It displays anti-inflammatory effects and notable antiproliferative activity, which makes it protective against some cancers. Cellular studies show that it is preventative and reduces all stages of carcinogenesis in the skin (initiation, promotion, and progression of tumor formation).[23, 24]

19.2.5.3 Pomegranate

Pomegranate is known for its antioxidant and healing properties. An animal study demonstrated protection against photoaging with pomegranate juice concentrated powder, illustrating its cytoprotective, moisturizing, anti-inflammatory, and antioxidant properties. Future studies may further show its positive effects on skin aging.[25]

19.2.5.4 Curcumin

Curcumin, a component of turmeric and a bioactive polyphenol, possesses several beneficial effects on aging. It is increasingly recognized for its anti-aging action, which includes anticancer, anti-inflammatory, antimicrobial, and antioxidant actions. The effects of curcumin, specifically on skin aging, include its direct antioxidant photoprotective effects.[26]

19.2.5.5 Ginkgo Biloba

Ginkgo biloba contains flavonoids (e.g. ginkgetin) and polyphenols. Studies indicate that it may increase the growth of procollagen and fibroblasts in the skin. It has been shown to have photoprotective and anti-inflammatory effects as well. One mechanism of action may be the downregulation of COX-2.[27]

19.2.5.6 Ginseng

Ginseng may yield antioxidant and anti-inflammatory effects through its active ingredient, ginsenoside. A study indicated red ginseng improved wrinkles and increased collagen synthesis.[28]

19.2.5.7 Soy

Topical soy has anti-aging benefits related to its ability to improve thinning skin through collagen production and its antioxidant properties. In vitro studies show that soy stimulates collagen production. Specific studies indicate that soy also increases elastin synthesis. Soy may deliver antioxidant effects due to its isoflavone ingredients, genistein and daidzein.[29]

The hypopigmenting effects of soy result from a decreased phagocytosis of melanosomes and slowed melanosome transfer, which yields a reduction in pigment production. Soy proteins, such as soybean trypsin inhibitor, inhibit the protein-activated receptor 2 (PAR-2) pathway involved in melanin transfer to keratinocytes.[30]

19.2.5.8 Silymarin

Silymarin is a flavonoid derived from milk thistle. Silymarin has shown anti-turmeric activity in laboratory animals. In a murine study, silibinin, a main component of silymarin, inhibits UV cellular damage when used topically or ingested.[31] It displays antiglycation activity as well.

19.2.5.9 Polypodium Leucotomos

Polypodium leucotomos is a natural extract from a tropical fern plant that originated in Central and South America and has photoprotective effects. Animal and human studies confirm its photoprotective and anti-aging benefits orally and topically. Specifically, *P. leucotomos* has demonstrated reduced dermal elastosis. It downregulates COX-2 (elevations in COX-2 have been associated with skin cancers due to UV exposure). It reduces UVB immunosuppression and oxidative DNA damage. A study showed that *P. leucotomos* protects against morphological changes seen in fibroblasts after UV exposure. Overall, it exerts cytoprotective effects on UV-exposed skin and minimizes photoaging, including hyperpigmentation.[32] Statistically significant improvements were noted in patients in a small study who were treated with *P. leucotomos* orally for melasma,[33] a helpful finding particularly relevant in skin of color for whom melasma and post-inflammatory hyperpigmentation occur with greater frequency in aging skin.

19.2.5.10 Bakuchiol

Bakuchiol is a botanical plant derived from seeds of the *Psoralea corylifolia* plant, indigenous to Asia and India. It is often touted as a more natural alternative to retinol because it has similar anti-aging properties and a gentler effect on the skin. It has shown efficacy in treating fine lines and also enhances the radiance of the skin. Used for years in Ayurvedic medicine, this ingredient is earning an important place in dermatology and anti-aging medicine.[34]

19.2.6 Hormonal Agents
19.2.6.1 Topical Estrogen

Estriol and estradiol have been shown to increase collagen fibers, especially collagen III. Topically applied estrogen may yield improvements in wrinkling and firmness of the skin. Studies also show that estrogen may increase skin hydration. Specifically, an increase in mucopolysaccharides, hyaluronic acid, and overall water content in the skin has been demonstrated as a result of topical applications of estrogen.[35] Initially received with enthusiasm, topical estrogen treatment is now viewed with caution regarding the potential increased risk for breast cancer.

19.2.6.2 Topical Melatonin

Melatonin is a neuroendocrine hormone of the pineal gland known for its function in regulating the sleep cycle. Skin and hair follicles are involved in melatonin synthesis, and melatonin receptors are found on the skin and hair follicles. Recent research indicates new roles for melatonin in anti-aging. Melatonin has demonstrated anti-inflammatory effects and antioxidant benefits. It may stimulate tissue regeneration. Another valued effect is its role in the preservation of mitochondrial function and cardiolipin. Overall, melatonin provides anti-aging benefits through direct and indirect antioxidant activity.[36]

19.2.7 Growth Factors

Growth factors are made up of biological compounds, such as cytokines and regulatory proteins, which are necessary for wound healing. Growth factors influence signaling pathways that control cellular functions, such as cell differentiation and maturation. Thus, growth factors are integral for tissue repair, remodeling, and regeneration.[37]

Endogenous growth factors decrease with age. Intrinsic and extrinsic aging is characterized by a thinning of the dermis and epidermis, diminished cell turnover, and reduced cell hydration, all effects associated with reduced fibroblast activity and slowed collagen synthesis. As the skin ages, there is also a decline in enzymes that upregulate collagen production and an increase in enzymes that inhibit collagen biosynthesis. Fibroblast growth factors in topical formulations have demonstrated anti-aging activity. The cellular effects include the regeneration of collagen, thickening of the epidermis, stimulation of fibroblast growth, and increased angiogenesis.[38]

TGF-β, derived from cultured fibroblasts, is found in topical cosmeceuticals. In tissue, the transforming growth factor (TGF-β) is active in promoting collagen synthesis, stimulating the formation of granulation tissue, improving wound strength, and stabilizing the dermal-epidermal junction. Other growth factors include vascular endothelial growth factor (VEGF), hepatocyte growth factor, IL-6, IL-8, platelet-derived growth factor, and granulocyte colony-stimulating factor. There are a growing number of cosmeceuticals containing growth factors. Products may contain a single growth factor or several. They may be synthetic or cultured from fibroblasts. One brand suggests that growth factors are most effective in producing favorable anti-aging biological effects when there is a physiologically diverse and balanced mixture of growth factors, such as those derived from cultured fibroblasts.[39] It is challenging to quantify growth factor content and to compare efficacy among products. Kinetin is a plant growth factor. Kinetin has been shown to decrease aging of fibroblasts and may have antioxidant properties. When introduced, it gained recognition for being gentle on the skin, displaying minimal irritation compared to retinoids.

19.2.8 Peptides

Peptides are chains of amino acid sequences that induce cellular activity which leads to increased collagen production.

19.2.8.1 Argireline

Argireline, a synthetic hexapeptide (made of a fragment of SNAP-25), has been identified as an anti-aging agent with demonstrable anti-wrinkle effects. It inhibits the release of neurotransmitters at the neuromuscular junction and has been touted as a topical alternative to cosmetic injectable neurotoxin. It has also been shown to increase type I collagen fibers.[40, 41]

19.2.9 Anti-Aging Minerals
19.2.9.1 Copper

Copper, a trace element required for wound healing, is a cofactor of superoxide dismutase. Copper is also a cofactor for another enzyme, lysyl oxidase, which is involved in collagen and elastin production. Copper also aids in collagen synthesis by downregulating MMPs and decreasing collagenase activity. Peptides complexed with copper may help with skin firmness and decrease fine lines and hyperpigmentation.[42]

19.2.9.2 Selenium

Selenium, an essential trace element with antioxidant properties, may specifically exert photoprotective activity and provide a protective role in certain skin diseases, such as psoriasis and eczema. However, some data is inconsistent, and there are concerns about toxicity.[43]

19.2.10 Nutraceuticals Targeting Advanced Glycation End Products
19.2.10.1 Carnosine

Carnosine, a dipeptide anti-senescence agent, inhibits the glycosylation of proteins and DNA. Carnosine exhibits antioxidant, cell-rejuvenating, and metal-chelating effects. Its anti-aging effects have been demonstrated in oral form, and a few studies show its efficacy on skin cells. Topical carnosine in a combination mixture with peptides showed cytoprotective effects on human skin fibroblasts.[44, 45]

19.3 Clinical Pearls in Treating Ethnic Skin

One of the most common signs of photoaging in ethnic skin is hyperpigmentation. Thus, addressing hyperpigmentation

TABLE 19.2: Agents Targeting Hyperpigmentation in Aging Skin

Agent	Source	Mechanism of Action	Indication	Use/Dosage
Aloesin	Aloe vera plant	Competitively inhibits tyrosinase and modulates melanogenesis	Hyperpigmentation	Often in topical form, in combination with other skin-lightening ingredients
Arbutin	β-D-glucopyranoside derivative of hydroquinone; derived from plant leaves (bearberry, blueberry, cranberry, pear trees) and wheat	Competitively inhibits tyrosinase in a dose-dependent manner in cultured melanocytes; inhibits melanosome maturation[46]	Hyperpigmentation	Often in topical form, in combination with other skin-lightening ingredients
Azelaic acid	Organic, naturally occurring compound—a dicarboxylic acid, which inhibits tyrosinase, derived from *Malassezia furfur* (*P. ovale*)	The *Pityrosporum* species oxidizes unsaturated fatty acids to dicarboxylic acids. Dicarboxylic acids competitively inhibit tyrosinase. Azelaic acid has antibacterial and anti-inflammatory effects. Also, it has antiproliferative and cytotoxic effects on melanocytes. It may selectively inhibit hyperactive melanocytes and has been utilized in the treatment of lentigo maligna[47–49]	Acne, rosacea, hyperpigmentation	Available in topical formulations in concentrations of 10–20%; applied sparingly to affected areas of skin once or twice daily

Anti-Aging Agents for Ethnic Skin

Agent	Source	Mechanism of Action	Indication	Use/Dosage
Cysteamine	A biological chemical compound	Inhibits tyrosinase and peroxidase	Used in a topical formulation to treat hyperpigmentation, melasma, and lentigines; used systemically in the treatment of nephropathic cystinosis[50]	Applied to hyperpigmented areas for 15–30 minutes, then washed off; used daily as tolerated
Hydroquinone	Chemical aromatic organic compound; a natural source includes the bombardier beetle	Inhibits tyrosinase	Hyperpigmentation, melasma *Hydroquinone, the most efficacious and commonly used tyrosinase inhibitor, is considered the gold standard for the treatment of hyperpigmentation Despite concerns about its potential carcinogenic effects, many experts regard it as important in the armamentarium of treatment of hyperpigmentation. With appropriate use, it appears that its benefits outweigh potential risks[51–53]	Available in topical OTC products 1–2%; prescription cream 4%; may be compounded in higher percentages (6–12%) Available in combination cream with tretinoin and fluocinolone; typically applied sparingly to hyperpigmented areas of skin nightly for 1–3 months
Kojic acid	A fungal metabolite agent derived from species of *Aspergillus*, *Penicillum*, and *Acetobacter*	Inhibits the production of free tyrosinase; also acts as an antioxidant	Hyperpigmentation	Clinically, used in topical concentrations ranging from 1–4%; provides enhanced skin hypopigmenting effects in combination with other skin-lightening ingredients[54]
Licorice	Licorice compounds include glabridin, lichochalcone A, and liquirtin, derived from the root of *Glycyrrhiza glabra*[55]	Inhibits tyrosinase	Hyperpigmentation	Liquirtin is available as a topical applied in a dose of 1 g per day for one month for efficacy
Lignin peroxidase	An enzyme derived from fungi (e.g., *Phanerochaete chrysosporium*) that degrade lignin[56]	Melasma, hyperpigmentation	Decreases eumelanin; breaks down melanin	Lignin peroxidase was available as a specifically branded product with a two-part dispenser. The melanozyme is not active until it is oxidized. One side of the dispenser contains hydrogen peroxide (0.012%), termed the activator
Mequinol	A derivative of HQ; mequinol (4-hydroxyanisole) is a hydroquinone monomethyl ether	Acts as a substrate for tyrosinase and is thought not to be as toxic to the melanocyte as HQ[57]	Hyperpigmentation associated with photoaging, solar lentigo	2% topical (often combined with tretinoin)
N-acetylglucosamine (NAG)	A monosaccharide derivative of glucose and chitin; a component of bacterial and fungal cell walls and outer shells of insects and crustaceans	Inhibits conversion of pro-tyrosinase to tyrosinase. In vitro findings suggest that NAG affects the expression of genes involved in pigmentation	Hyperpigmentation, anti-aging, skin dryness[58, 59]	Available in topical cosmetic skin care products
Tranexamic acid	A synthetic amino acid of lysine	An antifibrinolytic that binds to receptor sites on plasminogen, decreasing the conversion of plasminogen to plasmin, which helps prevent the breakdown of fibrin	In systemic form, it is used to prevent excessive bleeding and blood loss. In gynecology, it is used to treat heavy bleeding, and in hematology, it is used to treat blood disorders. Recently, in dermatology, it has been shown to significantly improve resistant melasma[60]	250 mg twice daily for three months. While efficacy is notable, potential side effects have led to cautious oral use. Increased risk of thromboembolism, allergic reactions, and changes in vision. Tranexamic acid is also available in topical form for the treatment of melasma and hyperpigmentation
Vitamin C	Food-derived (mainly citrus) or synthetic (chemically identical)	Acts as a co-factor for collagen synthesis to upregulate collagen formation; inhibits tyrosinase	Hyperpigmentation, antioxidant effects, photoprotection, wound healing, immune support	A range of concentrations (5–30%); applied topically daily

is important in the overall anti-aging strategy for people of color. Table 19.2 includes a list of agents that specifically target hyperpigmentation in aging skin. Incorporating topical vitamin C and tretinoin (or other retinol products) early in skin care regimens aid in correcting and preventing excessive melanogenesis. Appropriate use of hydroquinone and other pigment correctors (e.g., kojic acid, arbutin, azelaic acid) is essential in the armamentarium of treatment of melasma and other forms of hyperpigmentation. Greater efficacy is often achieved with the combined use of products. For example, a regimen including an exfoliating cleanser, vitamin C, and sunscreen in the morning and tretinoin and niacinamide at night may improve hyperpigmentation more significantly than either product used alone.

19.4 Indications for Agents

TABLE 19.3: Indications for Agents

Agent	Indications
Sunscreen	• Photoaging • Prevention of skin cancer • Hyperpigmentation
Retinoids	• Aging skin • Acne • Hyperpigmentation
Alpha- and beta-hydroxy acids	• Aging skin • Hyperpigmentation • Acne
Vitamin C	• Antioxidant effect (skin repair) • Hyperpigmentation • Aging skin (collagen promoting)
Vitamin E	• Antioxidant effect (skin repair) • Dry skin
Ubiquinone	• Antioxidant effect (skin repair) • Dry skin
Niacinamide	• Antioxidant effect (skin repair) • Hyperpigmentation • Skin hydration • Collagen synthesis
Alpha-lipoic acid	• Antioxidant effect (skin repair)
Camellia sinensis (tea)	• Antioxidant effect (skin repair) • Hyperpigmentation
Resveratrol	• Antioxidant effect (skin repair) • Anticancer (cytoprotection)
Pomegranate	• Antioxidant effect (skin repair) • Skin hydration • Anticancer (cytoprotection)
Curcumin	• Antioxidant effect (skin repair) • Antimicrobial effects • Anticancer (cytoprotective)
Ginkgo biloba	• Enhanced cognitive performance (oral form) • Aging skin (may boost collagen)
Ginseng	• Antioxidant effect (skin repair) • Anti-inflammatory effects • Aging skin (may boost collagen)
Soy (in topical form)	• Photoaging • Hyperpigmentation • Reduction of unwanted hair
Silymarin	• Antioxidant effect (skin repair) • Radiodermatitis • Anticancer *Indications for oral use include liver protection.*
Polypodium leucotomos	• Prevention of sunburn • Antioxidant effect • Anticancer • Hyperpigmentation • Vitiligo • Improvement of inflammatory skin disease, such as eczema and psoriasis
Bakuchiol	• Prevention of wrinkles (collagen-stimulating effects)
Topical estrogen	• Menopause symptoms • Aging skin • Wound healing

Agent	Indications
Topical melatonin	• Aging skin • May aid in the treatment of alopecia and restoring pigment to gray hair
Growth factors	• Promotion of collagen formation
Peptides	• Promotion of collagen formation
Argireline	• Promotion of collagen formation • Treatment of wrinkles (rhytids)—botulinum-toxin-like effect
Copper	• Promotion of collagen formation • Wound healing • Photoprotection • Antioxidant effect[61]
Selenium	• Antioxidant effect • Photoprotection[43] • Anti-inflammatory • Anticancer[62]
Carnosine	• Antioxidant effect • Cytoprotective effects[44, 63]

19.5 How to Use and Dosage

TABLE 19.4: Use and Dosages of Agents

Agent	Use/Dosage
Sunscreen	The American Academy of Dermatology recommends 2 mg of sunscreen per square centimeter, which corresponds to approximately one ounce for the full body. Sunscreens should be applied 15 to 30 minutes prior to sun exposure and reapplied every two hours.
Retinoids	Recommended use of tretinoin, the prototypic retinoid is a pea size to the affected area applied nightly, as tolerated, 20 to 30 minutes after cleansing the skin. Retinoid use should begin with lower concentrations and be followed by a gradual increase in concentration based on tolerability.
Alpha- and beta-hydroxy acids	Various concentrations exist in over-the-counter products.
Vitamin C	Concentrations of 5–30% are used in topical form.
Vitamin E	The recommended daily requirement of vitamin E orally is 30 IU or 15 mg a day. A dose of 100 IU is often the starting dose for antioxidant benefits. Topical vitamin E is available in various concentrations, such as cream or ointment (e.g., 30 units/g or 100 units/g) or oil (e.g., 70,000 IU/2.5 fl. oz.).
Ubiquinone	Oral doses range from 20 to 200 mg/day. Currently, no specific guidelines indicate optimal concentrations for topical ubiquinone. However, higher levels of quinone in the skin have been demonstrated after the application of Q10-containing cream.
Niacinamide	The recommended concentration of topical niacinamide is 5% or less.
Alpha-lipoic acid	There is no established oral or topical dose. Oral doses range from 50 to 600 mg daily or as high as 1,800 mg daily.
Camellia sinensis (tea)	Optimal topical concentrations have not been established. However, studies show improvement of photoaging with 6–10% topical formulations.[21, 64] Oral doses range from 300 to 1,000 mg once to twice daily.
Resveratrol	Optimal topical concentrations have not been established. Oral doses of resveratrol range from 100 mg to 3,000 mg daily.
Pomegranate	The recommended oral dose is 700 mg daily. Optimal concentrations of topical preparations are unclear at this time and may range from 10% to 40%.
Curcumin	Optimal concentrations in topical form have not been established. However, in oral and topical form, its effects appear to be dose-dependent. Orally, 500–1500 mg per day of curcuminoids is recommended for their antioxidant and anti-inflammatory effects.
Ginseng	Average recommended doses range from 40 to 240 mg for oral supplementation but up to 600 mg/day, depending on the desired effect.
Soy (in topical form)	Concentrations of 1–5% are often used in topical form.[29]
Silymarin	Optimal topical doses have not been established. Oral doses may range from 200 to 800 mg daily.
Polypodium leucotomos	Typical doses range from 360 to 480 mg daily. Higher doses of 960 to 1,200 mg are also used.
Bakuchiol	Concentrations of 0.5–2% are typically used topically.
Topical estrogen	Various concentrations and formulations exist, varying in the vehicle and configuration of estradiol.[65]
Topical melatonin	The recommended dosage of 3% topical melatonin is 15 mg applied once daily.
Growth factors	Optimal topical doses have not been established.
Peptides	Optimal topical doses have not been established; However, results have been observed with 0.1% (w/w) concentrations.[66, 67]
Argireline	Currently available in a 10% preparation.
Copper	Optimal topical doses have not been established. Oral supplementation ranges from 2 to 3 mg daily.
Selenium	Optimal topical concentrations of 0.02–0.05%.[62]
Carnosine	Optimal topical doses have not been established.

19.6 Side Effects

TABLE 19.5: Side Effects of Agents

Agent	Side Effects
Sunscreen	Contact dermatitis to chemical sunscreens, such as oxybenzone, are well recognized. Fragrance, lanolin, formaldehyde releasers, preservatives, and other ingredients in sunscreens may also cause allergic reactions.
Retinoids	Dryness, irritation, peeling of the skin, and photosensitivity.
Alpha- and beta-hydroxy acids	Photosensitivity, peeling and irritation of skin. May be formulated with parabens, which can cause contact dermatitis.
Vitamin C	Application of vitamin C for long durations is generally regarded as safe. Minor irritations (stinging, burning, redness) may occur but are uncommon. While topical vitamin C is indicated for all skin types, it should be used cautiously in acne-prone skin. Vehicles of topical vitamin C are aimed at stabilizing the active ingredient and for optimal absorption into the skin. Many hydrophilic bases are oily or acnegenic.
Vitamin E	Rare possible side effects include local skin irritation, such as redness, burning, or stinging.
Ubiquinone	Local skin irritation, while rare, is possible with topical coQ10.
Niacinamide	Skin irritation, such as redness, may occur, but skin issues are infrequent.
Alpha-lipoic acid	Possible local skin irritation, though uncommon.
Camellia sinensis (tea)	Possible local skin irritation.
Resveratrol	Very few topical side effects are noted except for redness or skin irritation from possible hypersensitivity. High oral doses may cause gastrointestinal upset.
Pomegranate	Pomegranate sensitivities are well recognized.
Curcumin	Yellowing of the skin and skin irritation are reported in topical form. The most noted oral side effects are gastrointestinal.
Ginkgo biloba	When taken orally, side effects include GI upset and increased risk of bruising.
Ginseng	When taken orally, side effects include increased bleeding risk, especially when combined with other blood thinners. It may affect insulin levels and lower the seizure threshold.
Soy (in topical form)	Rashes may occur in those with sensitivities to soy. It does not appear to induce hormonal side effects in topical form.
Silymarin	Oral gastrointestinal side effects (nausea, diarrhea, etc.) are reported.
Polypodium leucotomos	Considered very safe. Reports of any adverse effects are very limited.
Bakuchiol	Skin irritation may occur with concentrations above 1%.
Topical estrogen	Possible side effects include local irritation and hyperpigmentation.
Topical melatonin	Considered very safe. Reports of any adverse effects are very limited.
Growth factors	Possible local skin irritation.
Peptides	Possible local skin irritation.
Argireline	Some minimal concerns for cytotoxicity exist.
Copper	When taken orally, side effects include GI upset. Very high oral doses can cause hepatic and renal damage.
Selenium	Possible skin irritation and dry skin. High oral doses are associated with cardiac and renal toxicity.
Carnosine	Possible local skin irritation.

19.7 Choosing a Product

As discussed ealier, there are a plethora of products that can be used to tackle visible signs of aging. When choosing the correct product, it is important to have a systematic approach to specific skin concerns to target. Table 19.3 summarizes the indications for the use of these anti-aging agents. Information on dosages and how to use these ingredients are listed in Table 19.4. Side effects have been reported with the use of several of these ingredients, ranging from local irritation to contact dermatitis. These side effects are discussed further in Table 19.5.

A robust skin care regimen includes sunscreen, a collagen stimulator, and antioxidants. Choosing the best sunscreen includes numerous variables, but current guidelines recommend a sun protection factor of 30 or above. Mineral sunscreens are best for sensitive skin. However, mineral-based sunscreens are often not cosmetically elegant for darker skin tones. These factors must be considered, as ultimately, the best sunscreen will be the one that individuals actually use.

Ingredients with collagen-stimulating effects are considered essential in the arsenal of anti-aging skin care. Retinol has the strongest scientific data and is thus recommended the most, but it has high reports of irritation. Fortunately, when retinol is not tolerated, other products may provide boosts in collagen. These include growth factors, peptides, alpha-hydroxy acids, vitamin C, and bakuchiol.

Vitamin C (L-ascorbic acid) is perhaps the most widely studied antioxidant for topical use. A growing body of evidence exists for many other antioxidants discussed in this chapter. Each may offer unique benefits.

Frequently Asked Questions

1. *Q: What type of vitamin C should one use?*
   A: Pure ascorbic acid is most preferred but is fragile and easily breaks down with exposure to light and air. Thus, stabilized forms, such as sodium ascorbyl phosphate and magnesium ascorbate, are often used in topical products. Serums are best absorbed through the skin compared to

creams and lotions. Recommended concentrations of vitamin C are between 8% and 20%. Some experts recommend 30% if tolerated. Higher concentrations have a greater propensity for irritation, possibly without added efficacy.

2. Q: *What are the concerns with topical hydroquinone?*

A: For years, hydroquinone has been considered the gold standard for the treatment of hyperpigmentation and is the most commonly used tyrosinase inhibitor. Hydroquinone is a metabolite of benzene. Thus, concerns about its safety may have originally emerged from the recognized carcinogenicity of benzene. Animal studies have indicated a potential carcinogenic risk, but human data is limited to a few case reports suggesting possible risk. Exogenous ochronosis is a rare but notable adverse effect of the long-term use of topical hydroquinone.

3. Q: *I am allergic to sunscreens; which sunscreen is best to use?*

A: Topical sunscreens come in the form of chemical ingredients or physical barrier protectors. It is best to use a physical barrier sunscreen containing zinc oxide or titanium dioxide if you are sensitive to certain sunscreens. Currently, there are novel formulations of physical barrier sunscreens that include the use of nanoparticles of titanium dioxide and/or zinc oxide that do not leave a white/gray hue in darker-skinned individuals.

4. Q: *Can cosmetic procedures be combined with cosmeceuticals?*

A: Yes. The best outcomes typically occur in patients who use professional-grade skin care products to help to maintain facial rejuvenation achieved by chemical peels and lasers. Sun protection, skin-lightening agents, vitamin C, and other antioxidants are often essential aftercare ingredients used after aesthetic treatments. The effects of retinoids, growth factors, and anti-aging peptides provide a synergistic effect to enhance the outcomes of dermal fillers and botulinum toxin treatments. Body products containing retinol and collagen-building ingredients are often recommended after body contouring laser procedures.

5. Q: *Can these products also be used on the body for anti-aging?*

A: Yes, anti-aging ingredients are beneficial for skin all over the body. Several beauty brands have recognized the restorative effects of antioxidants, retinoids, alpha- and beta-hydroxy acids, and anti-aging peptides for body use. Exfoliants are now popular for the scalp, body, and feet. Skin-lightening agents are also used for underarms, inner thighs, elbows, and knees in darker skin types. Retinol is showing up in body washes and body lotions to offer more youthful, even-toned skin.

19.8 Conclusion

There are multiple anti-aging agents that can be used to address the visible signs of aging in ethnic skin. The type of agents used largely depends on the individual goals of the patient. The most common visible anti-aging goal in people of color includes the treatment of hyperpigmentation, which must include the use of photoprotection to prevent further pigmentary changes and skin-lightening agents. These agents can be used synergistically for optimal results and can be combined with aesthetic procedures such as chemical peels and

select lasers. In addition, these anti-aging agents are generally safe to use and are effective in addressing the special needs of skin-of-color patients.

References

1. Davis EC, Callender VD. Aesthetic dermatology for aging ethnic skin. Dermatol Surg. 2011 Jul;37(7):901–917.
2. Agar NS, Halliday GM, Barnetson RS, Ananthaswamy HN, Wheeler M, Jones AM. The basal layer in human squamous tumors harbors more UVA than UVB fingerprint mutations: A role for UVA in human skin carcinogenesis. Proc Natl Acad Sci U S A. 2004 Apr 6;101(14):4954–4959.
3. Halliday GM, Agar NS, Barnetson RS, Ananthaswamy HN, Jones AM. UV-A fingerprint mutations in human skin cancer. Photochem Photobiol. 2005 Jan–Feb;81(1):3–8.
4. Porges SB, Kaidbey KH, Grove GL. Quantification of visible light-induced melanogenesis in human skin. Photodermatol. 1988 Oct;5(5):197–200.
5. Griffiths CE, Russman AN, Majmudar G, Singer RS, Hamilton TA, Voorhees JJ. Restoration of collagen formation in photodamaged human skin by tretinoin (retinoic acid). N Engl J Med. 1993 Aug 19;329(8):530–535.
6. Kligman LH, Duo CH, Kligman AM. Topical retinoic acid enhances the repair of ultraviolet damaged dermal connective tissue. Connect Tissue Res. 1984;12(2):139–150.
7. Weiss JS, Ellis CN, Headington JT, Voorhees JJ. Topical tretinoin in the treatment of aging skin. J Am Acad Dermatol. 1988 Jul;19(1 Pt 2):169–175.
8. Bagatin E, Gonçalves HS, Sato M, Almeida LMC, Miot HA. Comparable efficacy of adapalene 0.3% gel and tretinoin 0.05% cream as treatment for cutaneous photoaging. Eur J Dermatol. 2018 Jun 1;28(3):343–350.
9. Phillips TJ, Gottlieb AB, Leyden JJ, Lowe NJ, Lew-Kaya DA, Sefton J, Walker PS, Gibson JR; Tazarotene Cream Photodamage Clinical Study Group. Efficacy of 0.1% tazarotene cream for the treatment of photodamage: A 12-month multicenter, randomized trial. Arch Dermatol. 2002 Nov;138(11):1486–1493.
10. Kligman AM. The computability of combinations of glycolic acid and tretinoin in acne and photodamaged facial skin. J Geriatr Dermatol. 1995;3 (Suppl A):25A–28A
11. Kim SJ, Won YH. The effect of glycolic acid in cultured human skin fibroblasts: Cell proliferative effect and increased collagen synthesis. J Dermatology. 1998 Feb;25(2):85–89.
12. Antoniou C, Kosmadaki MG, Stratigos AJ, Katsambas AD. Photoaging: Prevention and topical treatments. Am J Clin Dermatol. 2010;11(2):95–102.
13. Fitzpatrick RE, Rostan EF. Double-blind, half-face study comparing topical vitamin C and vehicle for rejuvenation of photodamage. Dermatol Surg. 2002 Mar;28(3):231–234.
14. Humbert PG, Haftek M, Creidi P, Lapière C, Nusgens B, Richard A, Schmitt D, Rougier A, Zahouani H. Topical ascorbic acid on photoaged skin. Clinical, topographical and ultrastructural evaluation: Double-blind study vs. placebo. Exp Dermatol. 2003 Jun;12(3):237–244.
15. Alster TS, West TB. Effect of topical vitamin C on postoperative carbon dioxide laser resurfacing erythema. Dermatol Surg. 1998 Mar;24(3):331–334.
16. Gallardo V, Muñoz M, Ruíz MA. Formulations of hydrogels and lipogels with vitamin E. J Cosmet Dermatol. 2005 Sep;4(3):187–192.
17. Knott A, Achterberg V, Smuda C, Mielke H, Sperling G, Dunckelmann K, Vogelsang A, Krüger A, Schwengler H, Behtash M, Kristof S, Diekmann H, Eisenberg T, Berroth A, Hildebrand J, Siegner R, Winnefeld M, Teuber F, Fey S, Möbius J, Retzer D, Burkhardt T, Lüttke J, Blatt T. Topical treatment with coenzyme Q10-containing formulas improves skin's Q10 level and provides antioxidative effects. Biofactors. 2015 Nov–Dec;41(6):383–390.
18. Tanno O, Ota Y, Kitamura N, Katsube T, Inoue S. Nicotinamide increases biosynthesis of ceramides as well as other stratum corneum lipids to improve the epidermal permeability barrier. Br J Dermatol. 2000 Sep;143(3):524–531.
19. Bissett DL, Miyamoto K, Sun P, Li J, Berge CA. Topical niacinamide reduces yellowing, wrinkling, red blotchiness, and hyperpigmented spots in aging facial skin. Int J Cosmet Sci. 2004 Oct;26(5):231–238.
20. Matsugo S, Bito T, Konishi T. Photochemical stability of lipoic acid and its impact on skin ageing. Free Radic Res. 2011 Aug;45(8):918–924
21. Chiu AE, Chan JL, Kern DG, Kohler S, Rehmus WE, Kimball AB. Double-blinded, placebo-controlled trial of green tea extracts in the clinical and histologic appearance of photoaging skin. Dermatol Surg. 2005 Jul;31(7 Pt 2):855–860; discussion 860.
22. Wei X, Liu Y, Xiao J, Wang Y. Protective effects of tea polysaccharides and polyphenols on skin. J Agric Food Chem. 2009 Sep 9;57(17):7757–7762.
23. Aggarwal BB, Bhardwaj A, Aggarwal RS, Seeram NP, Shishodia S, Takada Y. Role of resveratrol in prevention and therapy of cancer: Preclinical and clinical studies. Anticancer Res. 2004 Sep–Oct;24(5A):2783–2840.

24. Chedea VS, Vicaş SI, Sticozzi C, Pessina F, Frosini M, Maioli E, Valacchi G. Resveratrol: From diet to topical usage. Food Funct. 2017 Nov 15;8(11):3879–3892.

25. Abdellatif AAH, Alawadh SH, Bouazzaoui A, Alhowail AH, Mohammed HA. Anthocyanins rich pomegranate cream as a topical formulation with anti-aging activity. J Dermatolog Treat. 2020 Feb 5:1–8.

26. Agrawal R, Kaur IP. Inhibitory effect of encapsulated curcumin on ultraviolet-induced photoaging in mice. Rejuvenation Res. 2010 Aug;13(4):397–410.

27. Kim SJ, Lim MH, Chun IK, Won YH. Effects of flavonoids of Ginkgo biloba on proliferation of human skin fibroblast. Skin Pharmacol. 1997;10(4):200–205.

28. Cho S, Won CH, Lee DH, Lee MJ, Lee S, So SH, Lee SK, Koo BS, Kim NM, Chung JH. Red ginseng root extract mixed with Torilus fructus and Corni fructus improves facial wrinkles and increases type I procollagen synthesis in human skin: A randomized, double-blind, placebo-controlled study. J Med Food. 2009 Dec;12(6):1252–1259.

29. Kang S, Chung JH, Lee JH, Fisher GJ, Wan YS, Duell EA, Voorhees JJ. Topical N-acetyl cysteine and genistein prevent ultraviolet-light-induced signaling that leads to photoaging in human skin in vivo. J Invest Dermatol. 2003 May;120(5):835–841.

30. Hermanns JF, Petit L, Piérard-Franchimont C, Paquet P, Piérard GE. Assessment of topical hypopigmenting agents on solar lentigines of Asian women. Dermatology. 2002;204(4):281–286.

31. Mallikarjuna G, Dhanalakshmi S, Singh RP, Agarwal C, Agarwal R. Silibinin protects against photocarcinogenesis via modulation of cell cycle regulators, mitogen-activated protein kinases, and Akt signaling. Cancer Res. 2004 Sep 1;64(17):6349–6356.

32. Nestor MS, Berman B, Swenson N. Safety and efficacy of oral Polypodium leucotomos extract in healthy adult subjects. J Clin Aesthet Dermatol. 2015 Feb;8(2):19–23.

33. Goh CL, Chuah SY, Tien S, Thng G, Vitale MA, Delgado-Rubin A. Double-blind, placebo-controlled trial to evaluate the effectiveness of *Polypodium Leucotomos* extract in the treatment of melasma in Asian skin: A pilot study. J Clin Aesthet Dermatol. 2018 Mar;11(3):14–19.

34. Dhaliwal S, Rybak I, Ellis SR, et al. Prospective, randomized, double-blind assessment of topical bakuchiol and retinol for facial photoageing. Br J Dermatol. 2019;180(2):289–296.

35. Thornton MJ. Estrogens and aging skin. Dermatoendocrinol. 2013 Apr 1;5(2):264–270.

36. Day D, Burgess CM, Kircik LH. Assessing the potential role for topical melatonin in an antiaging skin regimen. J Drugs Dermatol. 2018;17(9):966–969.

37. de Araújo R, Lôbo M, Trindade K, Silva DF, Pereira N. Fibroblast growth factors: A controlling mechanism of skin aging. Skin Pharmacol Physiol. 2019;32(5):275–282.

38. Fitzpatrick RE, Rostan EF. Reversal of photodamage with topical growth factors: A pilot study. J Cosmet Laser Ther. 2003 Apr;5(1):25–34.

39. Sundaram H, Mehta RC, Norine JA, Kircik L, Cook-Bolden FE, Atkin DH, Werschler PW, Fitzpatrick RE. Topically applied physiologically balanced growth factors: A new paradigm of skin rejuvenation. J Drugs Dermatol. 2009 May;8(5 Suppl Skin Rejuenation):4–13.

40. Wang Y, Wang M, Xiao XS, Pan P, Li P, Huo J. The anti wrinkle efficacy of synthetic hexapeptide (Argireline) in Chinese Subjects. J Cosmet Laser Ther. 2013 Apr 22.

41. Wang Y, Wang M, Xiao XS, Huo J, Zhang WD. The anti-wrinkle efficacy of Argireline. J Cosmet Laser Ther. 2013 Aug;15(4):237–241.

42. Ogen-Shtern N, Chumin K, Cohen G, Borkow G. Increased pro-collagen 1, elastin, and TGF-β1 expression by copper ions in an ex-vivo human skin model. J Cosmet Dermatol. 2020 Jun;19(6):1522–1527.

43. McKenzie RC. Selenium, ultraviolet radiation and the skin. Clin Exp Dermatol. 2000 Nov;25(8):631–636.

44. Hipkiss AR, Brownson C. Carnosine reacts with protein carbonyl groups: Another possible role for the anti-ageing peptide? Biogerontology. 2000;1(3):217–223.

45. Garre A, Martinez-Masana G, Piquero-Casals J, Granger C. Redefining face contour with a novel anti-aging cosmetic product: An open-label, prospective clinical study. Clin Cosmet Investig Dermatol. 2017 Nov 13;10:473–482.

46. Maeda K, Fukuda M. Arbutin: Mechanism of its depigmenting action in human melanocyte culture. J Pharmacol Exp Th. 1996 Feb;276(2):765–769

47. Kircik LH. Efficacy and safety of azelaic acid (AzA) gel 15% in the treatment of post-inflammatory hyperpigmentation and acne: A 16-week, baseline-controlled study. J Drugs Dermatol. 2011;10(6):586–590.

48. Lowe NJ, Rizk D, Grimes P, Billips M, Pincus S. Azelaic acid 20% cream in the treatment of facial hyperpigmentation in darker-skinned patients. Clin Ther. 1998;20(5):945–959.

49. Vereecken P, Heenen M. Recurrent lentigo maligna melanoma: Regression associated with local azelaic acid 20%. Int J Clin Pract. 2002 Jan–Feb;56(1):68–69.

50. Farshi S, Mansouri P, Kasraee B. Efficacy of cysteamine cream in the treatment of epidermal melasma, evaluating by Dermacatch as a new measurement method: A randomized double blind placebo controlled study [published correction appears in J Dermatolog Treat. 2020 Feb;31(1):104]. J Dermatolog Treat. 2018;29(2):182–189.

51. Davis EC, Callender VD. Postinflammatory hyperpigmentation: A review of the epidemiology, clinical features, and treatment options in skin of color. J Clin Aesthet Dermatol. 2010 Jul;3(7):20–31.

52. Taylor SC, Burgess CM, Callender VD, Fu J, Rendon MI, Roberts WE, Shalita AR. Postinflammatory hyperpigmentation: Evolving combination treatment strategies. Cutis. 2006 Aug;78(2 Suppl 2):6–19.

53. Puizina-Ivić N, Mirić L, Carija A, Karlica D, Marasović D. Modern approach to topical treatment of aging skin. Coll Antropol. 2010 Sep;34(3):1145–1153.

54. Draelos ZD, Yatskayer M, Bhushan P, et al. Evaluation of a kojic acid, emblica extract, and glycolic acid formulation compared with hydroquinone 4% for skin lightening. Cutis 2010;86:153–158.

55. Draelos ZD. A split-face evaluation of a novel pigment-lightening agent compared with no treatment and hydroquinone. J Am Acad Dermatol. 2015 Jan;72(1):105–107. Epub 2014 Oct 16. Erratum in: J Am Acad Dermatol. 2015 Jun;72(6):1096.

56. Quay ER, Chang YC, Graber E. Evidence for anti-aging South Korean cosmeceuticals. J Drugs Dermatol. 2017 Apr 1;16(4):358–363.

57. Fleischer AB Jr, Schwartzel EH, Colby SI, Altman DJ. The combination of 2% 4-hydroxyanisole (Mequinol) and 0.01% tretinoin is effective in improving the appearance of solar lentigines and related hyperpigmented lesions in two double-blind multicenter clinical studies. J Am Acad Dermatol. 2000 Mar;42(3):459–467.

58. Bissett DL, Robinson LR, Raleigh PS, Miyamoto K, Hakozaki T, Li J, Kelm GR. Reduction in the appearance of facial hyperpigmentation by topical N-acetyl glucosamine. J Cosmet Dermatol. 2007 Mar;6(1):20–26.

59. Bissett DL, Farmer T, McPhail S, Reichling T, Tiesman JP, Juhlin KD, Hurley GJ, Robinson MK. Genomic expression changes induced by topical N-acetyl glucosamine in skin equivalent cultures in vitro. J Cosmet Dermatol. 2007 Dec;6(4):232–238.

60. Bala HR, Lee S, Wong C, Pandya AG, Rodrigues M. Oral tranexamic acid for the treatment of melasma: A review. Dermatol Surg. 2018;44(6):814–825.

61. Duncan C, White AR. Copper complexes as therapeutic agents. Metallomics. 2012;4(2):127–138.

62. Burke KE. Photodamage of the skin: Protection and reversal with topical antioxidants. J Cosmet Dermatol. 2004;3(3):149–155.

63. Boldyrev AA, Gallant SC, Sukhich GT. Carnosine, the protective, anti-aging peptide. Biosci Rep. 1999;19(6):581–587.

64. Gianeti MD, Mercurio DG, Campos PM. The use of green tea extract in cosmetic formulations: Not only an antioxidant active ingredient. Dermatol Ther. 2013;26(3):267–271.

65. Rzepecki AK, Murase JE, Juran R, Fabi SG, McLellan BN. Estrogen-deficient skin: The role of topical therapy. Int J Womens Dermatol. 2019;5(2):85–90. Published 2019 Mar 15.

66. Gorouhi F, Maibach HI. Role of topical peptides in preventing or treating aged skin. Int J Cosmet Sci. 2009;31:327–345.

67. Hantash BM, Jimenez F. A split-face, double-blind, randomized and placebo-controlled pilot evaluation of a novel oligopeptide for the treatment of recalcitrant melasma. J Drugs Dermatol. 2009 Aug;8(8):732–735.

CHAPTER 20: COSMECEUTICALS IN HAIR CARE

Malavika Kohli and Banani Choudhury

20.1 Background

Definition

Albert Klingman defined a cosmeceutical as follows (1):

- It is a scientifically designed product intended for external application to the human body.
- It produces a useful, desired result.
- It has desirable aesthetic properties.
- It meets rigid chemical, physical, and medical standards.

A major breakthrough came in the field of peptides through the invention of a yeast peptide in wound healing, back in 1930. Subsequently, through the enzymatic hydrolysis of the yeast *Saccharmyces cerevesiae*, a low-molecular-weight protein fraction could be extracted, which was shown to stimulate collagen synthesis, angiogenesis, and granulation in the wound. To date, 500 peptide extracts have been identified from this particular yeast for skin and hair care.

20.2 How Do They Differ from Cosmetics and Drugs?

Broadly, cosmeceuticals are functional cosmetics (2).

For example, a product that eliminates wrinkles is a drug, whereas a product that minimizes the appearance of wrinkles is a cosmetic, even though both of them have the same products. "Cosmeceutical" is a term coined approximately two decades ago by Albert Kligman to refer to topically applied products that are not merely cosmetics that adorn or camouflage yet are not true drugs that have undergone rigorous placebo-controlled studies for safety and efficacy.

Classification (3)

- Peptides form a large group of hair cosmeceuticals.
- The most commonly available molecule is acetyl tetrapeptides (available in most Indian brands), but the most commonly researched molecule is GHK-Cu.

Peptide classification: Broadly peptides can be classified as per their molecular structure:

1. Biomimetic peptides
   - CG-Wnt
   - CG-Nokkin (oligopeptide-54)
   - CG-Keramin2 (decapeptide-10)
2. GHK-Cu peptides
3. Acetyl tetrapeptide

20.3 Other Cosmeceuticals Available for Hair Care

20.3.1 Decoding the Cosmeceuticals Available in the Market

Capixyl is the combination of biomimetic peptides (acetyl tetrapetides3) combined with red clover extract rich in biochanin A.

This combination has a synergistic effect. Biochanin A (an isoflavone derived from red clover) has a direct action on 5-alpha-reductase, which modulates DHT (dihydrotestosterone), reduces inflammation (reduction of IL1 alpha and IL8) at the follicle bed, and stimulates the ECM (extracellular matrix) protein synthesis in the vicinity of the hair follicle (4–6).

Acetyl-tetrapepdtide-3 is a pure peptide obtained by solid phase peptide synthesis (signal peptide found in matrix portion of collagen and fibrin, also in growth fraction isolated from human plasma). It has a role in ECM component stimulation, like collagen III and VII and laminin (4, 7).

Procapil is the trademark name for the patented compound biotinoyl tripeptide 1 (Glycyl-Hystidyl-Lysine: GHK)

It is a combination of a vitaminized matrikine with apigenin and oleanolic acid. Matrikines refer to peptides originating from the fragmentation of matrix proteins and presenting biological activities, especially tissue repair process. It acts by improving scalp microcirculation and counter follicular aging and atrophy (8–13).

Most hair lotions have the following few ingredients, which have a synergistic effect with peptides on hair growth and cycle (14). They are listed in the following paragraphs.

Oleanolic acid is extracted from olive tree leaves and inhibits 5-alpha-reductase (14)

Apigenin is a flavonoid extracted from citrus fruits that causes vasodilatation and increases scalp microcirculation (14)

Ginkgo biloba has antioxidant and anti-inflammatory properties.

Saw palmetto extract is an extract made from berries of an American dwarf tree. It is rich in fatty acids and phytosterols (beta sitosterols), beta carotene, and polysaccharides and is believed to block DHT.

Aminexil (pyrrolidino diaminopyrimidine oxide 1.5%) is a molecule that helps perifollicular inflammation and prevents and improves fibrosis.

Melatonin acts as a direct radical scavenger against environmental stress factors like UV rays.

Caffeine possess two activities, indirect via 5-alpha-reductase activity and direct by stimulating hair growth parameters.

Other substances include amino acids/proteins, creatine, adenosine, cococin, glycine, taurine, cysteine, dextran, hydrolyzed vegetable protein and collagen, niacinamide, pyridoxine, tocopherol, biotin, ascorbic acid, calcium pantothenate, and folate. They are believed to strengthen hair and repair damaged hair. They are specifically formulated (low molecular weight and liposomal formulation) to penetrate the hair cortex, and higher-molecular-weight components coat the hair shaft to lubricate the hair follicle.

Some of the hair lotions are labeled *stem cell lotions* (15). They have the molecules like redensyl, unitrienol T 27 (biomolecule complex for sebum regulation), dexpanthenol, coQ 10, and AnaGain.

They work on hair bulge stem cells by stimulating the germinative cells in outer root sheath cells (ORSc), thereby triggering a new hair cycle. They also increase dermal papilla fibroblast metabolism, thereby increasing anagen hair growth.

AnaGain is a patented molecule introduced by Mibelle Biochemistry. It is an organic pea sprout extract and helps to

DOI: 10.1201/9780429243769-20

stimulate the hair life cycle (according to DNA microarray analysis of plucked hair).

PhytoCellTec Malus Domestica is a patented liposomal preparation of apple stem cell cells that are claimed to increase the longevity of skin and hair cells and delay the senescence of hair follicles.

Auxina Tricogena (patented botanical product) increases scalp circulation and increases metabolism in hair follicles, thereby activating stem cells.

Officinalis plant extract enhances vascular supply to dermal papillae cells.

Redensyl (DHQG, EGCG2) targets ORCs hair follicle stem cells to protect from apoptosis and activate the metabolism of dermal papillary fibroblast.

Crescina HFSC is a combination of Swiss-patented compounds that work by activating hair follicle stem cells. The study of HF stem cells started with the identification of epidermal stem cells in the hair follicle bulge region as quiescent "label-retaining cells." Bulge cell molecular markers like keratin 15, CD 34 (mice), and CD 200 (human) allowed isolation of bulge cells from follicles (16–20).

Stemoxydine is one of the other molecules that work on tissue hypoxia theory. It is a potent P4H inhibitor (prolys 4 hydroxylase) and has the ability to induce hypoxia-like signaling. Based on in vitro studies, it is hypothesized that induction of hypoxia signaling is important to maintain hair follicle stem cell functionality.

Stemoxydine is one of the other molecules that work on tissue hypoxia theory. It is a potent P4H inhibitor (prolys 4 hydroxylase) and has the ability to induce hypoxia-like signaling. Based on in vitro studies, it is hypothesized that induction of hypoxia signaling is important to maintain hair follicle stem cell functionality.

Most hair lotions have the combination of Procapil and AnaGain or AnaGain and Capixyl or Capixyl and Procapil alone. Acetyl tetrapeptide and biochanin alone or in combination with Capixyl/Procapil are available.

These cosmeceuticals are also available in combination with topical finasteride and minoxidil.

Understanding the mechanism of action of peptides in hair loss and thinning has gained momentum after understanding new horizons in the pathogenesis of androgenetic alopecia, which has been discussed by Antonella Tosti et al. (21) recently.

1. Wnt/b-catenin pathway: Hair follicle regeneration begins when signals from mesenchymal-derived dermal papillae cells (DPC) reach epidermal stem cells in the bulge region. Activation of Wnt signalling, particularly Wnt 10b, is essential for hair follicle development and hair cycling and growth.
2. Micro-inflammation
3. Prostagandin imbalance
4. Oxidative stress
5. Loss of extracellular matrix

Hair peptides act on dermal papilla mesenchymal cells (modified fibroblasts), thereby strengthening the anchorage of the hair follicle, as shown in Figure 20.1. In addition, by stimulating the hair stem cells in the bulge region when the chemical signal comes in the anagen phase, they help in the transition of the telogen phase to the anagen phase. Androgen receptors are also located at the dermal papillae, making the peptides useful in androgenetic alopecia (21).

Biomimetic peptides are a combination of short-chain peptides derived from the extracellular matrix. They act on hair follicle morphogenesis through different signaling pathways.

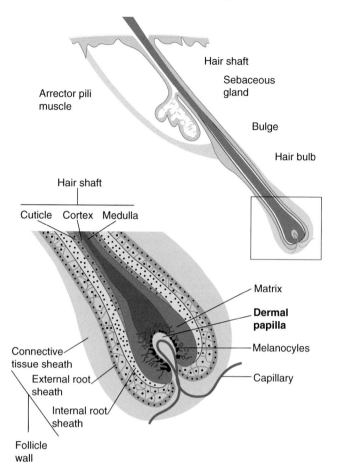

FIGURE 20.1 Hair morphology.

Hair follicle morphogenesis depends on Wnt, Shh, Notch, BMP, and other signaling pathways as they interplay between epithelial and mesenchymal cells, as mentioned in Figures 20.2 and 20.3 (22–28).

The Wnt pathway plays an essential role during hair follicle induction, Shh is involved in morphogenesis and late-stage differentiation, Notch signaling determines stem cell fate, and BMP is involved in cellular differentiation. *The Wnt pathway is considered to be the master regulator during hair follicle morphogenesis.* Signal crosstalk between epithelial and mesenchymal cells takes place mainly through primary cilia. Primary cilia formation is initiated with epithelial laminin-511 interaction with dermal β-1 integrin, which also upregulates the expression of downstream effectors of the Shh pathway in dermal lineage. These peptides have an individual mode of action, as enumerated in Figures 20.4 and 20.5.

- **CG-Wnt**
  - Stimulates hair placode formation
  - Generates *de novo* hair through activated catenin signal
- **CG-Nokkin (oligopeptide-54)**
  - Strong BMP blocker—promotes hair growth and inhibits depigmentation
  - Stimulates the formation of healthier hair
  - Helps blood circulation in the scalp and revitalizes hair follicles
- **CG-Keramin2 (decapeptide-10)**
  - Downregulates DKK-1

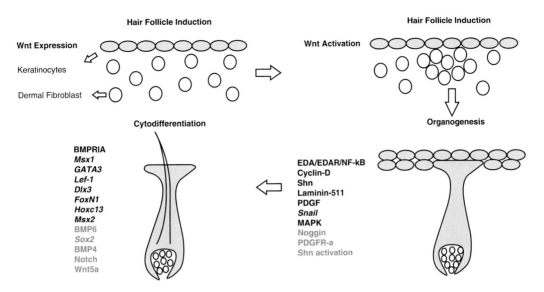

FIGURE 20.2 Hair morphogenesis: Stages of hair follicle morphogenesis. HFs (hair follicles) are formed by the interaction between epithelium (keratinocytes) and underlying dermal fibroblasts. Comprehensive lists of signaling molecules (capitals) and transcription factors (italics) are provided for each stage.

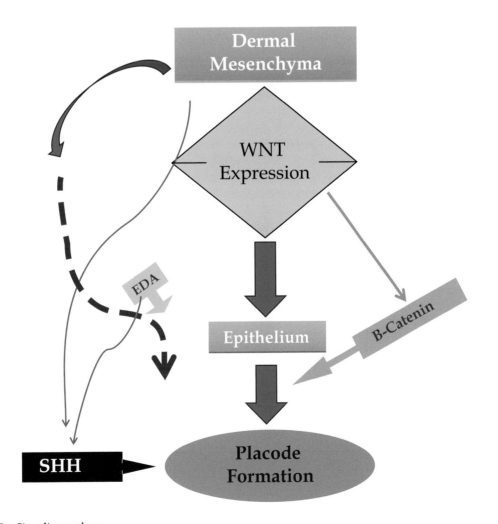

FIGURE 20.3 Signaling pathway.

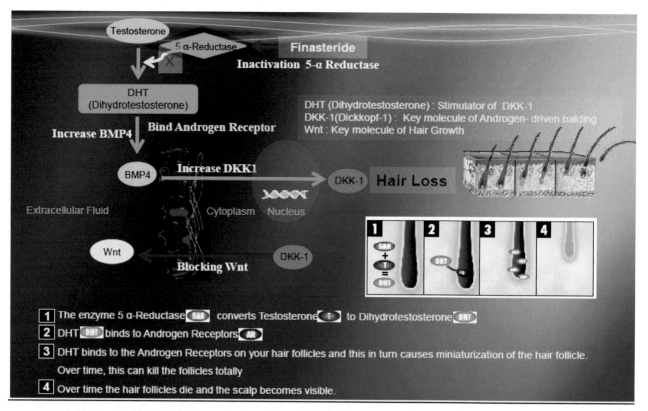

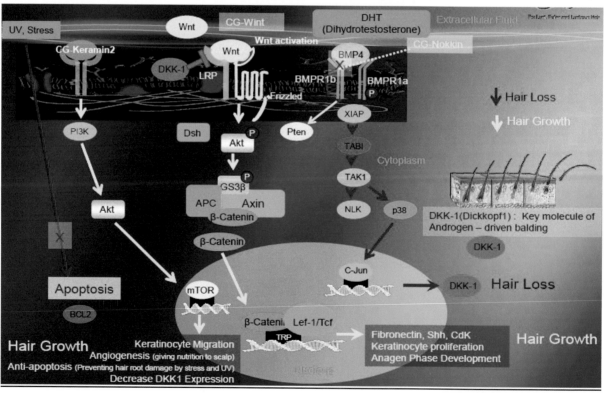

FIGURES 20.4 and 20.5   Effects of biomimetic peptides in androgenetic alopecia.

- Promotes new hair cell proliferation and migration—induces strong hair follicles and hair shafts

Signaling molecules and pathways indicated in black are either expressed or activated in keratinocytes, while gray ones are associated with dermal fibroblast.

20.4 Where Do Cosmeceuticals Score in Hair Care (29–31, 21)

Hair cosmeceuticals can be used for all the indications of hair loss and thinning.

1. Androgenetic alopecia
   - Patients with hypersensitivity or contraindication to minoxidil
   - Young reproductive age group with a risk of taking finasteride
   - Cyclical and supportive role with minoxidil
   - Co-prescription with nutraceuticals
2. Telogen effluvium: Acute and chronic of different etiologies
3. Alopecia areata

20.4.1 Clinical Situations Frequently Encountered in Day-to-Day Practice

1. *Dry frizzy hair*: Lots of young girls use different shampoos available over the counter/salon and keep experimenting with shampoos and hair care products. Some of these products, over long-term usage, can give rise to dry hair, and patients then complain about frizzy and unmanageable hair. Hair cosmeceuticals, along with active ingredients, have dexpanthenol, CoQ, amino acids, and proteins; topical biotin helps in coating the outer hair cortex and helps in hair nourishing.
2. *Hair textural change*: Dietary deficiency and drastic dietary change, PCOS-related hair textural change, and post-menopausal hormonal change can cause hair textural deterioration. Hair cosmeceutical lotions can improve hair texture by acting on hair root stem cells and increasing microcirculation to the hair, thereby nourishing hair quality.
3. *Chemically treated hair*: These patients form a large group in practice. Most of the patients do hair-smoothening treatments that contain formaldehyde or no formaldehyde, depending on the type of smoothening treatment. To keep the longevity of hair treatments, they are advised to use sulfate-free shampoos, which may not be able to clean the scalp, thus causing dry, flaky scalp. Dry, flaky scalp is a major cause of acute hair fall. In this group of patients, hair cosmeceuticals are ideal to use. If issues of hair fall or textural change happen due to chemical treatments, there is a new generation of hair lotions that are alcohol-free and water-based, which makes them ideal for chemically treated hair. Some of the hair peptides have additional sebum-regulating ingredients that, when applied on the scalp, help in sebum control and inflammation.
4. *Volume and density*: Hair cosmeceuticals have the benefit of stimulating new hair growth (by acting on germinative hair cells in the bulge area), along with making existing hair roots stronger by virtue of increased extracellular matrix formation around the hair roots, thereby increasing hair anchorage strength. So over a period of time, patients start noticing increased density and volume of hair.
5. *Inability to grow long hair*: There are patients encountered who complain about this, which happens due to a short anagen cycle or hair breakage (dry, frizzy hair or chemically treated hair). Hair cosmeceutical lotions (peptides) can increase the duration of the anagen phase by stimulating the fibroblast cells in dermal papillae, thereby increasing the anagen hair growth. Also, ingredients like apigenin, caffeine, and adenosine increase scalp microcirculation, which works synergistically with hair peptides to strengthen anagen hair. Compared to minoxidil, which needs supervision, monitoring, and follow-up, hair cosmeceuticals chosen by a dermatologist for a particular patient can be used at home for a long term without any irritation/allergy/hypersensitivity, which allows better compliance and helps patients stick to their routine of daily usage.

ADJUNCTIVE TREATMENT OF COSMECEUTICALS WITH OTHER TOPICALS AND NUTRACEUTICALS

We often use hair cosmeceuticals with topical minoxidil and topical finasteride in combination, particularly in androgenetic alopecia.

After obtaining trichoscopy images, we grade the hair thinning severity and prescribe hair peptides (Capixyl/Procapil) with additional anti-DHT effect (biochanin A) in rotation with minoxidil 2% or 5% (with or without finasteride).

Oral finasteride/dutasteride and natural botanical flavonoids (saw palmetto/sitosterols) can be added depending on the severity and after counseling patients.

In telogen effluvium cases, the authors prefer oral nutraceuticals in rotational format along with topical cosmeceutical lotions.

20.5 How to Increase the Efficiency of Peptide Penetration

Most peptide sequences have been incorporated with palmitic acid, trifluoroacetic acid, and elaidic acid to enhance penetration to the scalp.

Also, liposomal formulations help in easy and deeper penetration to the target tissue.

20.6 Tests for Efficacy

20.6.1 Physical Examination of the Scalp

Physical examination of the scalp covers the following: assessment of ponytail volume, visible hair thinning, thinning of a hair shaft, intensity of sebaceous secretions, and scalp rash (if any).

There are many tools to measure the tests of the efficacy of cosmeceutical peptides in the functioning of hair.

- Hair pull test
- Hair pluck test
- Trichoscopy: Assessment of hair density, diameter, proportion of vellus and terminal hairs, ratio and

distribution of hairs in follicular units, proportion of anagen and telogen hairs in the androgen-dependent and androgen-independent scalp regions, ratio of the terminal and vellus hairs in the parietal and occipital scalp surface (any inflammation)

- Photo trichogram: Anagen/telogen ratio
- Morphological changes in the hair (sampled by pulling out or biopsy): immunofluorescence finding of markers collagen IV and laminin 5 in hair root sheath in the telogen hair bulb and keratinocyte multiplication and optimum dermo-epidermal adhesion on outer root sheath in anagen hair
- DNA assay

20.6.1.1 Dosage

Most hair cosmeceuticals are prescribed by dermatologists per the etiology of hair fall and thinning.

Most lotions require a twice-a-day application and daily application for three to four months and maintenance application per requirement.

No hypersensitivity or side effects have been noticed by the authors so far, and patient acceptability is also high due to the non-sticky base of the solutions.

20.7 Conclusion

Natural processes within the body are modulated almost exclusively by the interaction of specific amino acid sequences, either as peptides or as subsections of proteins. With respect to skin and hair, proteins and peptides are involved in the modulation of cell proliferation, cell migration, inflammation, angiogenesis, melanogenesis, and protein synthesis and regulation. The creation of therapeutic or bioactive peptide analogs of specific interactive sequences has opened the door to a diverse new field of pharmaceutical and active cosmetic ingredients for the skin care and hair care industry.

Peptides in cosmeceuticals are one of the new, popular options to treat hair loss issues. Some of the cosmeceuticals work as supportive molecules to take care of damaged cuticles of treated/colored/salon-treated hair.

Most studies related to hair lotion ingredients into hair care products are in vitro. As we all know, these results do not always translate into in vivo actions. For any active ingredient to work, it must be absorbed in a stable form into the viable dermis. It is not an easy task to penetrate the barrier of the skin. Double-blinded, placebo-controlled drug study data is lacking, as it is with all cosmeceuticals, as a result of regulatory concerns by the industry.

It is imperative for us to stay abreast of the different ingredients and composition of hair lotions and their mechanism of action on hair follicles. The practical application of when, why, and on whom to use different products will enable dermatologists to improve the methodology of product selection and, ultimately, improve patients' clinical results. In choosing an effective cosmeceutical regimen, it is critical to match patients and their problems with the appropriate products. Most patients have multiple needs, and they should be matched with products that offer ingredients with multifactorial benefits.

This chapter attempts to understand the formulations and decodes the complex functioning of the hair cosmeceuticals available in the market.

Frequently Asked Questions

1. Q: *A young girl aged 25 years comes to the clinic and says, "I have had hair fall for the last three months. Please prescribe some medicines and lotions to stop hair fall."*
A: After taking a detailed history of the causes of acute hair loss, we will rule out ferritin, B12, and D3 deficiencies. We take a detailed dietary history regarding protein intake, dietary fads, period history (to rule out hormonal imbalance), any chemical treatments, and hair-styling/grooming techniques

    Next, we do trichoscopy to assess scalp condition and pattern of hair fall.

    We supplement with oral nutraceuticals if there is any deficiency and counsel the patient if it's a case of acute telogen effluvium.

    Among hair cosmeceuticals, we prefer using peptides with additional apigenin and caffeine to increase scalp health (increasing scalp microcirculation) for acute hair fall as they help in hair follicle anchorage by virtue of increased ECM production and stop shedding initially, followed by regrowth of hair.

2. Q: *When will I see results and, what is the maintenance strategy with hair cosmeceuticals?*
A: Hair cosmeceutical lotions take six weeks to show their effect, and maintenance is for three to four months in the case of acute telogen effluvium and nine to twelve months in chronic telogen effluvium and AGA with regular follow-ups.

    Counseling plays a huge role in hair concern consults. So proper counseling regarding the nature of the disease and the course of the disease process and the regular use of hair lotion are imperative for a good outcome.

3. Q: *A 55-year-old female patient presented with hair fall and patterned hair loss. How do we proceed with treating the case?*
A: After taking a detailed history and doing a trichoscopy, we follow the following treatment plan:
If the hair shedding is acute with patterned hair thinning, then we start with hair peptides with additional biochanin A (due to its property of 5-alpha-reductase inhibition).

    After four to six weeks, we start peptides with minoxidil combinations alternately with hair peptide lotions alone for another six to eight weeks, and then we review the patient with trichoscopy.

    Maintenance plan: continue with only minoxidil or a combination of minoxidil and peptides, depending on improvement.

    Rotational nutraceuticals and oral antiandrogens can be supplemented with hair cosmeceutical lotion to have synergistic benefits.

    If there is any contraindication to minoxidil or if there is a difficulty in follow-up, we prefer molecules like Stemoxydine, Redensyl, AnaGain, and hair stem follicle cell (HSFC) lotions in case of patterned hair loss.

4. Q: *How safe are hair cosmeceuticals lotions if they need to be used longer—for example, for one to two years or for a whole lifetime?*
A: Hair peptides and cosmeceuticals are safe to use long-term under a dermatologist's guidance and supervision.

    Hair peptides are excellent in maintenance in chronic telogen effluvium patients and in weaning off minoxidil intolerance or resistance. Oral minoxidil, along with hair cosmeceuticals, is the ideal solution for these patients

5. *Q: A 38-year-old female patient, a mother of two, comes with frontal thinning of hair along with loss of hair volume.*

A: Trichoscopy plays a huge role in this case to rule out chronic telogen effluvium (CTE) or CTE progressing to patterned hair loss (female pattern hair loss).

Depending on trichoscopy findings, hair cosmeceuticals (CTE) or minoxidil with hair cosmeceuticals (female pattern baldness) can be prescribed.

Trichoscopy has been an invaluable objective tool in understanding patterns of hair loss, grading the severity, allowing early diagnosis and prognosis of the disease process, monitoring treatment, and planning a maintenance course.

In day-to-day practice, trichoscopy helps physicians give an affirmative diagnosis and reassure patients to allay their fear of hair loss. In patients who are skeptical about their hair improvement status following treatments, trichoscopy is an objective tool to reassure them.

References

1. Klingman AM. Cosmetics a dermatologists look into future: Promises and problems. Dermatol Clin. 2000;18:699–709.
2. Verma A, Gautam S, Devi R, Singh N. Cosmeceuticals: Acclaiming its most fascinating position in personal care industry. Indian J. Pharm. Sci. 2016;8:506–518.
3. Dureja H. Cosmeceuticals: An emerging concept. Indian J Pharmacol. 205;37(3):155–159.
4. Uno H, Kurata S, Uno H, Kurata S. Chemical agents and peptides affect hair growth. J Invest Dermatol. 1993;101(1 Suppl):143S–147.
5. Medjakovic S, Jungbauer A. Red clover isoflavones biochanin A and formononetin are potent ligands of the human aryl hydrocarbon receptor. J Steroid Biochem Mol Biol. 2008;108(1–2):171–177.
6. Thors L, Burston JJ, Alter BJ, McKinney MK, Cravatt BF, Ross RA, et al. Biochanin A, a naturally occurring inhibitor of fatty acid amide hydrolase. Br JPharmacol. 2010;160(3):549–560.
7. Loing E, Lachance R, Ollier V, Hocquaux M. A new strategy to modulate alopecia using a combination of two specific and unique ingredients. J Cosmet Sci.2013;64:45–58.
8. Pickart L. The human tri-peptide GHK and tissue remodeling. J Biomater Sci Polymer Edn. 2008;19(8):969–988.
9. Pickart L, Freedman JH, Loker WJ, Peisach J, Perkins CM, Stenkamp RE, et al. Growth-modulating plasma tripeptide may function by facilitating copper uptake into cells. Nature. 1980;288(5792):715–717.
10. Maquart FX, Pickart L, Laurent M, Gillery P, Monboisse JC, Borel JP. Stimulation of collagen synthesis in fibroblast cultures by the tripeptide-copper complex glycyl-L-histidyl-L-lysine-Cu2+. FEBS Lett. 1988;238(2):343–346.
11. Wegrowski Y, Maquart FX, Borel JP. Stimulation of sulfated glycosaminoglycan synthesis by the tripeptide-copper complex glycyl-L-histidyl-L-lysine-Cu2+. Life Sci. 1992;51(13):1049–1056.
12. Maquart FX, Bellon G, Pasco S, Monboisse JC. Matrikines in the regulation of extracellular matrix degradation. Biochimie. 2005;87(3–4):353–360.
13. Siméon A, Emonard H, Hornebeck W, Maquart FX. The tripeptide-copper complex glycyl-L-histidyl-L-lysine-Cu2+ stimulates matrix metalloproteinase-2 expression by fibroblast cultures. Life Sci. 2000 Sep 22;67(18):2257–2265.
14. Garre A, Piquero J. Efficacy and safety of a new hair loss lotion containing Oleanolic acid, Apigenin, Botinyl Tripeptide 1, Diaminopyrimidine oxide, adenosine, biotin and Ginkgo Biloba in patients with Androgenetic alopecia and telogen effluvium in six months open label prospective clinical study. JCosmo Trichol. 2010;4(1):132.
15. Plikus MV, Baker RE, Chen CC, Fare C, de la Cruz D, Andl T, et al. Self-organizing and stochastic behaviors during the regeneration of hair stem cells. Science. 2011;332:586–589.
16. Tsai SY, Bouwman BA, Ang YS, Kim SJ, Lee DF, Lemischka IR, et al. Single transcription factor reprogramming of hair follicle dermal papilla cells to induced pluripotent stem cells. Stem Cells. 2011;29:964–971.
17. Tanimura S, Tadokoro Y, Inomata K, Binh NT, Nishie W, Yamazaki S, et al. Hair follicle stem cells provide a functional niche for melanocyte stem cells. Cell Stem Cell. 2011;8:177–187.
18. Ohyama M, Terunuma A, Tock CL, Radonovich MF, Pise-Masison CA, Hopping SB, et al. Characterization and isolation of stem cell-enriched human hair follicle bulge cells. J Clin Invest. 2006;116:249–260.
19. Gude D. Hair follicle stem cells: A new arena. J Cosmo Trichol. 2011; 2(1):125–126.
20. Sonthalia S, Daulatabad D, Tosti A. Hair restoration in androgenetic alopecia: Looking beyond minoxidil, finasteride and hair transplantation. J Cosmo Trichol. 2016;2:1000105.
21. Leirós GJ, Attorresi AI, Balañá ME. Hair follicle stem cell differentiation is inhibited through cross-talk between Wnt/ß-catenin and androgen signalling in dermal papilla cells from patients with androgenetic alopecia. Br J Dermatol. 2012;166:1035–1042.
22. Fu J, Hsu W. Epidermal Wnt controls hair follicle induction by orchestrating dynamic signaling crosstalk between the epidermis and dermis. J Invest Dermatol. 2013;133:890–898.
23. Kishimoto J, Burgeson RE, Morgan BA. Wnt signaling maintains the hair-inducing activity of the dermal papilla. Genes Dev. 2000;14:1181–1185.
24. Hajem N, Chapelle A, Bignon J, Pinault A, Liu JM, Salah-Mohellibi N, et al. The regulatory role of the tetrapeptide AcSDKP in skin and hair physiology and the prevention of ageing effects in these tissues-a potential cosmetic role. Int J Cosmet Sci. 2013;35:286–298.
25. Messenger AG, Elliott K, Temple A, Randall VA. Expression of basement membrane proteins and interstitial collagens in dermal papillae of human hair follicles. J Invest Dermatol. 1991;96:93–97.
26. Randall VA, Thornton MJ, Hamada K, Messenger AG. Androgen action in cultured dermal papilla cells from human hair follicles. Skin Pharmacol. 1994;7:20–26.
27. Mokos ZB, Mosler EL. Advances in a rapidly emerging field of hair follicle stem cell research. Coll Antropol. 2014;38:373–378.
28. Gnedeva K, Vorotelyak E, Cimadamore F, Cattarossi G, Giusto E, Terskikh VV, et al. Derivation of hair-inducing cell from human pluripotent stem cells. PLoS One. 2015;10:e0116892.
29. Kubanov AA, Gallyamova YA, Korableva OA. A randomized study of biomimetic peptides efficacy and impact on the growth factors expression in the hair follicles of patients with telogen effluvium. J App Pharm Sci. 2018;8(04):015–022.
30. Lu GQ, Wu ZB, Chu XY, Bi ZG, Fan WX. An investigation of crosstalk between Wnt/β-catenin and transforming growth factor-β signaling in androgenetic alopecia. Medicine (Baltimore). 2016 Jul;95(30):e4297. Lupo MP, Cole AL. Cosmeceutical peptides. Dermatol Ther. 2007 Sep–Oct;20(5):343–349.
31. Rinaldi F, Marzani B, Pinto D, Sorbellini E. Randomized controlled trial on a PRP-like cosmetic, biomimetic peptides based, for the treatment of alopecia areata. J Dermatolog Treat. 2019.

CHAPTER 21: LIP, NAIL, AND EYE CARE

Sahana P. Raju and Mukta Sachdev

21.1 Introduction

An aesthetically pleasing appearance forms one of the top priorities in today's world. Skin care tops the list, with maximum importance being given to healthy and glowing skin. Our lips, eyes, and nails require certain specific methods of care as well, which will be described in this chapter.

21.2 Lip Care

21.2.1 Specific Anatomical Considerations

Lips form the junction between the mucosa of the oral cavity and the stratum corneum of the outer skin. They are covered by a thin layer of stratum corneum, leading to poor barrier function and increased transepidermal water loss. They also have a rich capillary supply, leading to the characteristic pigmentation (1).

21.2.2 Why Do Our Lips Need Separate Care? (2)

As a result of the thin stratum corneum and poor barrier function, our lips are susceptible to a wide variety of external factors like wind, sun, smoke, etc., which play a major role in extrinsic aging or photoaging. Photoaging and intrinsic or chronological aging give rise to fine lines and wrinkles on the lips and perioral area. Our lips are also subjected to repeated trauma from chewing food and other habits. Thin lips and asymmetrical lips can also be genetic features. In order to prevent dryness, chapping, and dullness of lips, certain prophylactic and therapeutic measures can be undertaken, which are further discussed here.

21.2.3 Examination of the Lips

Any cutaneous condition affecting the lips requires a detailed history and complete evaluation of the lips, head, and neck area. An exhaustive history, including the use of topical and systemic medications, oral habits, and allergies, must be undertaken.

Examination of the lips included inspection and bi-digital palpation of the upper and lower borders.

Some of the dermatological disorders affecting lips, including developmental the anomalies are listed in Table 21.1 (3–6).

21.2.4 Lip-Licking Dermatitis (7)

Lip licking is the most common compensatory mechanism for dry and chapped lips, which temporarily reduces the symptoms but leads to chronic cheilitis, habit formation, secondary infections, and other complications. Some of the other common causes leading to lip licking include sunburn, anxiety, chronic nasal congestion, Sjogren's syndrome, lupus erythematosus, Crohn's disease, and sarcoidosis. The most effective method in the management of lip-licking dermatitis is the identification of the underlying condition, treatment of exacerbating factors, and following a regular and healthy routine which includes lip balms.

Cheilitis can be defined as an inflammatory process affecting the lips due to various causes. Patients with cheilitis present with dry, cracked, and eroded lips. Edema, exfoliation, and fissuring might occur in advanced cases.

Common causes of cheilitis are enumerated in Table 21.2 (4)

What Can Be done? (8)

- Avoid constant lip licking.
- Hydrate frequently and adequately.
- Usage of bland, non-flavored, non-irritating lip balms.
- Avoid products with fragrances, flavors, colors, and ingredients like camphor, lanolin, menthol, phenol, or salicylic acid.
- Photoprotection of lips is as equally important as any other part of our face. Bland lip balms with sunscreens are a great addition.

21.2.5 Lip Balms (9)

These are specific ingredients applied to our lips to prevent dryness and protect against various adverse environmental factors, including sunlight. They contain ingredients including ceramides, petrolatum, shea butter, dimethicone, and other excipients.

21.2.6 Recent Advances and Lip Fillers

Nowadays, products to increase lip fullness and give a more defined structure are available in the form of creams and lip fillers. Lip-lightening creams containing hydroquinone and

TABLE 21.1 Dermatological Disorders Affecting Lips

Developmental anomalies	• Fordyce spots • Cleft lip, cleft palate • Labial melanotic macules • Lentigines • Venous lakes • Infantile hemangioma
Traumatic	• Morsicatio labiorum • Mucoceles
Infectious	• Angular cheilitis • Herpes labialis • Molluscum contagiosum
Inflammatory	• Cheilitis • Sjogren disease • Xerostomia • Lichen planus • Psoriasis • Amyloidosis
Neoplastic	• Actinic cheilitis • SCC of lips

TABLE 21.2 Causes of Cheilitis

Chapped lips or cheilitis simplex
Eczematous cheilitis
Exfoliative cheilitis
Factitial cheilitis
Contact dermatitis
Actinic cheilitis
Infectious cheilitis

DOI: 10.1201/9780429243769-21

kojic acid, as well as chemical peels, are available for the management of dark lips.

Lip fillers are an important aspect of any anti-aging treatment. The most common indications for lip fillers are a deflating vermilion, drooping of angles of the mouth, and a thin upper lip. Commercially prepared hyaluronic acid-based injectable fillers like Restylane, Perlane, and Juvederm Ultra are used to achieve quick results with minimal downtime (10, 11).

In conclusion, our lips are the most visible and cosmetically relevant structures on our faces. Any physiological or pathological alterations could be physically and psychologically distressing to the patient. A careful evaluation, delineation between benign and pathological conditions, and lip care routine will ensure that our lips remain healthy and the most aesthetically pleasing structures on our faces.

21.3 Nail Care

Nail health is of utmost importance as a majority of us experience a nail disorder during our lifetime. The definition of a healthy nail includes one that is pink with a white free margin, a smooth and shiny surface, and attached cuticle and nail folds (12). Maintenance of healthy nails requires the knowledge of safe grooming practices.

Examination of nails forms an important aspect of a complete dermatological examination. Specific nail changes serve as important diagnostic clues for various dermatological disorders. These nail changes are listed in Table 21.3 (13).

Our nails can serve as a window to our body, sometimes as a manifestation of numerous systemic diseases. Some of them are enumerated in Table 21.4 (14).

Some important nail care practices include the following:

- Cut the nails frequently with a sterile clipper.
- Rounding the edges must be practiced cautiously and with expertise, as it can lead to the ingrowing of nails, especially on the toes.
- Avoid filing the nail plate as this can cause thinning and splitting of nails.
- Avoid cutting or pushing back the cuticle as it can lead to paronychia.
- Avoid nail biting or pulling off hangnails.
- Manicures and pedicures must be done with sterile instruments.

21.4 Nail Cosmetics

These include nail polish, gel polish, nail hardeners, and acrylic nails. Gel polish, which is otherwise known as UV-light-curable nail lacquer, contains photo-initiators that are photo-cured with UV light or a light-emitting diode. Complications of nail cosmetics include allergic contact dermatitis, pterygium formation, nail plate thinning and splitting, and eczema (15). Awareness of these complications is of utmost importance as they can be avoided or treated at an early stage.

21.5 Eye Care

More than two billion people around the world are affected by visual problems, out of which 50% suffer from vision impairment. Non-communicable eye diseases (NCED), including refractive errors, presbyopia, cataract, and glaucoma, are on the rise, resulting in a severe decrease in the quality of life.

21.5.1 Eye Health

The concept of eye health involves three important concepts: health education, reorientation, and advocacy. Some examples of ocular disorders which can be prevented by health education include night blindness and onchocerciasis due to the *Simulium* fly. These can be prevented by the formation of national programs for incorporating vitamin A, health education regarding vitamin A-rich foods, national programs for filariasis control, distribution of bed nets, and other similar measures.

21.5.2 Special Eye Care Measures

Periorbital skin is extremely thin and sensitive and among the first areas to manifest signs of aging, including fine lines, wrinkles, drooping of lids, hollowing, and crow's feet (16).

- Use regular moisturizer around the periorbital area.
- Regularly use an under-eye cream, preferably containing a low concentration of retinol.
- Hyaluronic acid, caffeine, vitamin K, and green tea extracts are some of the other ingredients that may be present in an under-eye cream.
- Use sunscreen regularly and frequently.
- Avoid smoking.
- Adequately sleep and hydrate.
- Follow a low-sodium diet, as increased salt consumption can lead to puffiness.

Some of the common dermatological conditions affecting the eye are described in Table 21.5 (17).

TABLE 21.3: Nail Changes and Dermatological Conditions

Onycholysis	• Psoriasis
	• Onychomycosis
	• Due to nail cosmetics
Pterygium	• Lichen planus
	• Cicatricial pemphigoid
	• Lupus erythematosus
	• Dyskeratosis congenita
	• Graft-versus-host disease
Pitting	• Psoriasis
	• SLE
	• Dermatomyositis
	• Pemphigus vulgaris
Melanonychia	• Racial
	• Melanocytic nevis
	• Malignant melanoma
	• Drug-induced

TABLE 21.4: Nail Changes and Systemic Diseases

Cardiovascular system	• Splinter haemorrhage
	• Koilonychia
	• Red lunula
Renal system	• Mees lines
	• Muehrcke's lines
	• Half and half nail
	• Terry's nail
Respiratory system	• Yellow nail syndrome
Gastrointestinal system	• Brittle nail
	• Azure lunula
	• Longitudinal striae
Endocrine system	• Periungual erythema
	• Longitudinal pigmented band
	• Brittle nail

TABLE 21.5 Skin Diseases Affecting the Eye

Infections	• Impetigo • External and internal hordeola • Orbital cellulitis, erysipelas • Herpes simplex, herpes zoster • Viral warts • Molluscum contagiosum
Infestations	• Pediculosis pubis • Démodé mite infestation
Inflammatory	• Atopic dermatitis • Psoriaiss • Seborrhoeic dermatitis • Contact dermatitis • Ocular rosasea
Erosive disorders	• SJS-TEN • Cicatricial pemphigoid • Pemphigus vulgaris
Benign nodules	• Seborrhoiec keratosis • Trichoepithelioma • Xanthelasma • Milia • Skin tags • Syringoma
Malignant lesions	• Actinic keratoses • SCC • BCC • Melanoma

21.6 Conclusion

The care of lips, eyes, and nails is important both from a clinical and aesthetic point of view. The inclusion of these in the general cutaneous examination cannot be stressed enough. The occurrence of skin cancers over our lips must be kept in mind, especially in Fitzpatrick types I–III. The use of eye, nail, and lip cosmetics must be done cautiously, as it can lead to a series of adverse effects. The use of Botox and fillers in and around the perioral and periorbital regions is gaining prominence and requires adequate counseling and deliberation before opting for these. To conclude, our lips, eyes, and nails require as much attention as our skin does, and one must not forget to include them in our daily skin care regimen.

Frequently Asked Questions

1. *Q: How to get rid of chapped lips and have smoother lips?*
   A: The key to having healthy lips is frequent moisturization. Regular use of a dermatologist-approved lip balm helps in restoring moisture. Drinking eight to ten glasses of water per day also keeps our lips soft and supple.
2. *Q: Can anything else be used in place of lip balm?*
   A: Other household ingredients, like coconut oil, almond oil, ghee, shea butter, milk cream, and petroleum jelly, can be used as alternatives to lip balm.
3. *Q: Is having a manicure or pedicure good for my nails?*
   A: One can opt for manicures and pedicures from a professional nail salon, keeping the following points

in mind: Make sure the salon uses clean and sterilized instruments. Do not go in very often; once every six to eight weeks should be sufficient. If you're opting for an artificial nail or other nail cosmetics, make sure you know about them and their care in detail first.
4. *Q: What about cuticle care?*
   A: Pushing back cuticles is the most common mistake made in nail salons and parlors. This exposes the underlying nail bed to external infections. So do not push back your cuticles. Moisturize them frequently to have healthy cuticles.
5. *Q: What causes dry eyes, and how do you treat them?*
   A: Dry eyes usually present with the blurring of vision and redness and itching in your eyes. Dry eyes can be due to a number of ocular and systemic conditions and warrant a visit to your ophthalmologist. It can be treated by the use of lubricating eye drops after ruling out any underlying condition.

References

1. Piccinin MA, Zito PM. Anatomy, Head and Neck, Lips. [Updated 2022 Jun 11]. In: StatPearls [Internet]. Treasure Island (FL): StatPearls Publishing; 2022 Jan.
2. Lévêque JL, Goubanova E. Influence of age on the lips and perioral skin. Dermatology. 2004;208(4):307–13. doi: 10.1159/000077838. PMID: 15178912.
3. Venkatesh R. Syndromes and anomalies associated with cleft. *Indian J Plast Surg.* 2009;42 Suppl(Suppl):S51-S55
4. Lugović-Mihić L, Pilipović K, Crnarić I, Šitum M, Duvančić T. Differential Diagnosis of Cheilitis - How to Classify Cheilitis?. *Acta Clin Croat.* 2018;57(2):342–351.
5. Hitz Lindenmüller I, Itin PH, Fistarol SK. Dermatology of the lips: inflammatory diseases. Quintessence Int. 2014 Nov-Dec;45(10):875–83.
6. Charly, M. M., Jean-PauI, S. I., Ngbolua, K.-T.-N., Hippolyte, S. N.-T., Erick, K. N., Alifi, P. B., Adelin, N. F., Mawunu, M., Mulongo, E. K., Anne, T. M. N., Mpiana, P. T., & Nestor, P. M. (2022). Review of the Literature on Oral Cancer: Epidemiology, Management and Evidence-based Traditional Medicine Treatment. *Annual Research & Review in Biology,* 37(6), 15–27.
7. Mini, P.N. & TM, Anoop. (2017). Lip–lick dermatitis. New Zealand Medical Journal. 130. 68–69.
8. Fonseca A, Jacob SE, Sindle A. Art of prevention: Practical interventions in lip-licking dermatitis. *Int J Womens Dermatol.* 2020;6(5):377–380.
9. Kokil, Suruchi & Kadu, Mayuri & Vishwasrao, Dr & Singh, Dr. (2014). Review on Natural Lip Balm. International Journal of Research in Cosmetic Science. 5.1
10. Luthra, Amit. Shaping Lips with Fillers. Journal of Cutaneous and Aesthetic Surgery 8(3):p 139–142, Jul–Sep 2015.
11. Keramidas E, Rodopoulou S, Gavala MI. A Safe and Effective Lip Augmentation Method: The Step-by-Step Φ (Phi) Technique. *Plast Reconstr Surg Glob Open.* 2021;9(2):e3332. Published 2021 Feb 2.
12. Johnson C, Sinkler MA, Schmieder GJ. Anatomy, Shoulder and Upper Limb, Nails. 2022 Jun 11. In: StatPearls [Internet]. Treasure Island (FL): StatPearls Publishing; 2022 Jan.
13. Lee DK, Lipner SR. Optimal diagnosis and management of common nail disorders. Ann Med. 2022 Dec;54(1):694–712.
14. Singal A, Arora R. Nail as a window of systemic diseases. Indian Dermatol Online J. 2015 Mar-Apr;6(2):67–74
15. Madnani NA, Khan KJ. Nail cosmetics. Indian J Dermatol Venereol Leprol 2012;78:309–317
16. Sarkar R, Ranjan R, Garg S, Garg VK, Sonthalia S, Bansal S. Periorbital Hyperpigmentation: A Comprehensive Review. *J Clin Aesthet Dermatol.* 2016;9(1):49–55.
17. Grzybowski A, Kels BD, Grant-Kels JM. Eye and skin disorders: part 1. Clin Dermatol. 2015 Mar-Apr;33(2):133–4.

CHAPTER 22: VITAMINS, ANTIOXIDANTS, AND PROTEINS

Shirin Lakhani

22.1 The Role of Nutrients in Skin Health

Nutritional status plays an important role in the maintenance of healthy skin, and changes in nutritional status that alter skin structure and function can also directly affect skin appearance.

22.2 Vitamins

Vitamins are nutrients required by the body in small amounts for a variety of essential processes. Most vitamins cannot be made by the body, so they need to be provided exogenously. They are essential for maintaining optimal levels of skin health, appearance, and function. Eating nutrient-dense foods, taking vitamin supplements, and using topical products containing vitamins can all be beneficial. In addition to aesthetic benefits, vitamins can also be used to manage a variety of skin conditions, such as acne, psoriasis, and the effects of photoaging. In many cases, vitamin deficiencies are associated with cutaneous effects. Many of the vitamins that are beneficial for skin health also exert an antioxidant effect.

22.2.1 Vitamin A

Vitamin A is a group of fat-soluble compounds that occur in two forms: retinoids (preformed vitamin A), which include retinol and its retinyl esters, and carotenoids (pro-vitamin A).

Retinol is found in foods such as liver, milk, and eggs and is the most biologically active form of the vitamin. Carotenoids are found in many fruits and vegetables and have strong antioxidant capabilities. Carotenoids need to be converted to retinoid forms to have a physiological effect. This occurs in the liver. Retinol is transported to the dermis bound to retinol-binding protein. Uptake into the cells occurs via receptor-mediated uptake or endocytosis. Keratinocytes and fibroblasts convert retinol first to retinaldehyde and then to all-trans-retinoic acid.

22.2.1.1 Actions of Retinoids
- Induce proliferation in keratinocytes resulting in epidermal hyperplasia.
- Modulate epidermal differentiation.
- Stimulate dermal fibroblasts to produce extracellular matrix proteins (especially when skin is damaged by wounding or UV radiation).
- Regulate pigmentation and can lighten hyperpigmented skin (reduce tyrosinase activity and increase exfoliation).
- Sebosuppression (isotretinoin).

22.2.1.2 Role of Retinoids in Aesthetic Dermatology
- *Photoprotection*
  Carotenoids exert an antioxidant effect and protect the skin against UV-light-mediated damage. The topical retinoid treatments inhibit the UV-induced, MMP-mediated breakdown of collagen and protect against UV-induced decreases in procollagen expression.
- *Photoaging*
  Clinical signs of photoaging include fine and coarse wrinkles, mottled hyperpigmentation, actinic lentigines, freckles, roughness, telangiectasia, and sallowness.

Topical retinoids lead to visible improvement in fine wrinkling, smoothness, and hyperpigmentation of photodamaged skin by inducing a number of histological changes in both the epidermis and dermis, which is reversible upon discontinuation. Therefore, a long-term maintenance regimen is necessary to sustain retinoid-induced improvements.
- *Skin lightening*
  Topical retinoids inhibit tyrosinase activity, thereby reducing the production of melanin. Furthermore, increased cell turnover leads to increase in the exfoliation of melanin-containing keratinocytes leading to a brighter complexion.
- *Wound healing*
  Vitamin A deficiency is associated with impaired immune function and delayed wound healing.
- *Acne*
  Topical tretinoin is considered a safe and effective treatment for mild to moderate acne, while oral isotretinoin is used to treat severe cases of acne that are resistant to topical therapies. Topical tretinoin influences the proliferation and differentiation of keratinocytes, thereby increasing follicular epithelial turnover, accelerating the shedding of corneocytes, and expelling mature comedones. Oral isotretinoin has unique inhibitory activity on sebaceous glands. It decreases the proliferation of basal sebocytes, suppresses sebum production, and inhibits sebocyte differentiation.

22.2.1.3 Limitations of Use
Side effects associated with topical tretinoin are local skin reactions, such as redness, peeling, dryness, itching, and burning. Although the use of topical retinoids is not associated with an increased incidence of birth defects in retrospective studies, it is still advised to abstain from their use during pregnancy. Oral isotretinoin, however, crosses the placenta and is teratogenic, meaning it causes developmental abnormalities. Therefore, oral isotretinoin is strictly contraindicated prior to and during pregnancy. Other side effects of oral retinoids resemble those associated with hypervitaminosis A and include mucocutaneous adverse effects, hyperostosis, and extraskeletal calcification.

When introducing topical retinoids to patients, it is imperative to educate them on the potential dryness and irritation; otherwise, they will not be compliant. There are two ways of initiating topical retinoids: start slow and increase gradually (e.g., twice a week), increase slowly to daily use, or start with daily application, omitting a day if the irritation is severe. The approach taken will depend on the patient, but the second approach results in faster tolerance and quicker results. An additional oat-based skin hydrator helps relieve the irritation in the first few weeks (1–5).

22.2.2 Vitamin C
Vitamin C (ascorbic acid) is the most abundant antioxidant in human skin, but as we lack the enzyme L-glucono-gamma lactone oxidase, we are unable to synthesize it and rely wholly on exogenous sources.

Vitamin C is found in citrus fruits and other fresh fruit and vegetables. It is also the most commonly taken supplement.

DOI: 10.1201/9780429243769-22

The absorption of vitamin C in the gut is limited by an active transport mechanism, and hence, a finite amount of the drug is absorbed despite high oral dosage[3]. Furthermore, the bioavailability of vitamin C in the skin is inadequate when it is administered orally.

L-Ascorbic acid is the most biologically active form of vitamin C. It is highly hydrophilic in nature, as well as unstable, especially on exposure to air, heat, and/or light. This provides challenges in the formulation of topical products.

22.2.2.1 Cutaneous Benefits of Vitamin C

- *Potent antioxidant effect*
  Vitamin C is the most plentiful antioxidant in human skin. When the skin is exposed to UV light, reactive oxygen species, such as the superoxide ion, peroxide, and singlet oxygen, are generated. Vitamin C protects the skin from oxidative stress by sequentially donating electrons to neutralize free radicals.
- *Collagen synthesis*
  Vitamin C is essential for collagen biosynthesis. It serves as a co-factor for the enzymes that are responsible for stabilizing and cross-linking the collagen molecules. Another mechanism by which vitamin C influences collagen synthesis is by stimulation of lipid peroxidation, which in turn stimulates collagen gene expression. It also directly activates the transcription of collagen synthesis and stabilizes procollagen mRNA, thereby regulating collagen synthesis. Clinical studies have shown that the topical use of vitamin C increases collagen production in young and aged human skin.
- *Prevention of skin aging*
  Studies have shown that the use of oral vitamin C is associated with improved skin appearance. Topical vitamin C use has also been shown to decrease wrinkles, improve skin texture, and increase collagen production.
- *Photoprotection from ultraviolet A and B*
  The antioxidant activity of vitamin C protects against UV-induced damage caused by free radicals. Topical application of vitamin C, alone or in combination with other compounds, may result in greater photoprotection than oral supplementation because of the more direct route of administration. It has been shown that topically applied combinations of vitamin C and vitamin E are more effective in preventing photodamage than either vitamin alone.
- *Lightening hyperpigmentation*
  Vitamin C interacts with copper ions at the tyrosinase-active site and inhibits action of the enzyme tyrosinase, thereby decreasing the melanin formation.
- *Improvement of a variety of inflammatory dermatoses*
  Vitamin C inhibits the activation of a number of pro-inflammatory cytokines such as TNF-α, IL1, IL6, and IL8. Vitamin C, therefore, has a potential anti-inflammatory activity and can be used in conditions like acne vulgaris and rosacea.
- *Wound healing*
  A notable feature of vitamin C deficiency (scurvy) is poor wound healing. Vitamin C has a multifactorial role in wound healing, limiting free radical damage and increasing collagen synthesis. It may also have a role in promoting keratinocyte differentiation, stimulating the formation of the epidermal barrier, and re-establishing the stratum corneum (1,4–10).

22.2.3 Vitamin E

Vitamin E is a group of compounds called tocopherols. It is a fat-soluble antioxidant that is essential for the maintenance of healthy skin. Dietary vitamin E is found in nuts, seeds, oils, dark green vegetables, and some seafood. Naturally occurring vitamin E is not a single compound; instead, vitamin E is a group of molecules with related structures, some of which may have unique properties in the skin.

Vitamin E is normally provided to the skin through the sebum. Topical application can also supply the skin with vitamin E and may provide specific vitamin E forms that are not available from the diet. Vitamin E is commonly used in creams and lotions for its moisturizing effect. As an antioxidant, vitamin E primarily reacts with reactive oxygen species. In addition, vitamin E can also absorb the energy from ultraviolet (UV) light. Thus, it plays an important role in photoprotection, preventing UV-induced free radical damage to the skin. It has been shown to have even more of a photoprotective effect when used in combination with vitamin C than either vitamin alone. Vitamin E may also have related anti-inflammatory roles in the skin (1, 4, 11).

22.2.4 Vitamin D

Vitamin D is synthesized in the epidermis in response to sunlight. It is actually a hormone rather than a vitamin. It is important to note that people with darker complexions synthesize less vitamin D on exposure to sunlight than those with lighter skin. Also, cultural or religious practices involving concealed clothing styles also play a factor in vitamin D deficiency.

Vitamin D has an important immune function, and deficiencies exacerbate eczema, psoriasis, and acne. Research has suggested that optimizing vitamin D can help these skin conditions.

Calcitriol (1,25-dihydroxy-vitamin D3) has been used topically to treat certain skin conditions, including psoriasis, a skin condition that involves a hyperproliferation of keratinocytes (1, 11–13).

22.2.5 The B Vitamins

B vitamins are a class of water-soluble vitamins that play important roles in cell metabolism. Though these vitamins share similar names, they are chemically distinct compounds that often coexist in the same foods. B vitamins are found in highest abundance in meat. They are also found in small quantities in whole, unprocessed carbohydrate-based foods. In addition to oral intake, B vitamins are included in topical preparations and are also commonly administered as mesotherapy to the dermis and epidermis (2).

22.2.5.1 Role in Dermatology

- *Thiamine* (B1) promotes collagen and elastin formation.
- *Riboflavin* (B2) maintains skin health and can help prevent acne breakouts.
- *Niacin* (B3) promotes skin hydration, reduces wrinkles and fine lines, and lightens skin by inhibiting the transfer of melanosomes to surrounding keratinocytes. Topical niacin can also exert antioxidant properties.
- *Pantothenic acid* (B5) has a strong anti-acne effect. It also promotes skin hydration and wound healing.
- *Pyridoxine* (B6) is useful in treating eczema, acne, dry skin, melanoma, and psoriasis.

22.2.6 Vitamin K

Vitamin K is a fat-soluble vitamin synthesized in the liver. Its role in blood coagulation is well documented, but in more recent years, its dermatological benefits have come to light. Research has shown the benefits of using vitamin K topically to help hyperpigmented areas and dark under-eye circles. Also, 5% vitamin K cream has been shown to diminish post-treatment bruising from cosmetic procedures (14,15).

22.3 Antioxidants

Skin cells, as all cells of the body, continuously produce highly reactive molecules called free radicals. Free radicals are waste substances produced by cells as the body processes food and reacts to the environment. If the body cannot process and remove free radicals efficiently, oxidative stress can result. This can harm cells and body function. Free radicals are also known as reactive oxygen species (ROS). Factors that increase the production of free radicals in the body can be internal, such as inflammation, or external, such as pollution, UV exposure, and cigarette smoke.

Antioxidants are substances that combine to neutralize reactive oxygen species, thus preventing oxidative damage to cells and tissues. The body produces some antioxidants, known as endogenous antioxidants. Antioxidants that come from outside the body are called exogenous. Many of the vitamins discussed have antioxidant properties.

Cosmeceuticals containing antioxidants are among the most popular anti-aging remedies. Topically applied antioxidants exert their benefits by offering protection from damaging free radicals produced when skin is exposed to ultraviolet light or allowed to age naturally.

Important Antioxidants in Skin Health

- Vitamin C
- Vitamin E
- Carotenoids (e.g., β-carotene, astaxanthin, lycopene)
- Polyphenols (flavonoids, resveratrol, green tea polyphenols)
- Curcumin
- Coenzyme Q10
- Glutathione

Glutathione and Skin Lightening

Glutathione is an important antioxidant and is indeed referred to as the "mother of antioxidants." It has multiple functions within the body.

There has been much interest in glutathione and its inhibitory effect on melanogenesis. It has therefore been used for skin lightening both as a topical agent as well as orally and parentally. IV glutathione has received poor publicity in recent years as people seek treatment to try and lighten the color of their skin. There is little evidence for the efficacy of glutathione used in this way, and there are inherent risks associated with IV therapy that should also be considered. Furthermore, any effects glutathione has on reducing pigmentation are reversed on discontinuation (12, 16).

22.4 Proteins and Amino Acids

Proteins are important for skin health, and studies have shown that women who consume less protein in their diet have more wrinkles. The main structural proteins in the skin are collagen and elastin. Collagen is the most abundant of animal proteins and can be found in all connective tissues. Collagen comprises one-third of the total protein in the body and three-quarters of the dry weight of the skin.

There has been much interest in oral collagen supplements and whether they have any effect on skin aging, with a particular interest in wrinkle depth, elasticity, and skin hydration. Oral supplementation for skin aging has generally been dismissed due to the breakdown of the constituents by stomach acid and gut enzymes. However, many recent studies have shown that hydrolyzed collagen does have an effect on upregulating collagen production in the dermis, particularly when combined with vitamins, minerals, and omegas. It must be noted that vitamin C is essential to promote the absorption of hydrolyzed collagen peptides from the gut and also that caffeine intake an hour before or after the collagen peptides inhibit their absorption.

Several amino acids have also been shown to play an important role in skin health.

Amino acids are the building blocks of peptides and proteins, and each amino acid performs a specific function in skin health. Amino acids help to strengthen the immune system and maintain the skin's hydration, resilience, and overall healthy appearance. They protect the skin from free-radical damage and reduce signs of aging.

All essential and non-essential amino acids play a role in getting beautiful skin, but there are some that have extra benefits:

- *Arginine* helps to restore visible skin damage.
- *Histidine* soothes the skin and has antioxidant properties.
- *Methionine* protects the skin from harmful substances.
- *Lysine* strengthens the skin's surface.
- *Proline, leucine, and glycine* make fine lines and wrinkles less deep (17, 18).

22.5 Oral Nutraceuticals

The term "nutraceutical" is used to describe nutrients within foods that have medicinal properties. They include vitamins, minerals, essential fatty acids, botanical extracts, prebiotics, and probiotics. Some nutrients have well-researched, proven benefits in skin health, such as vitamin A. Others, such as polyphenols, have limited evidence of benefit when taken as supplements over levels found in a healthy balanced diet rich in fresh fruit and

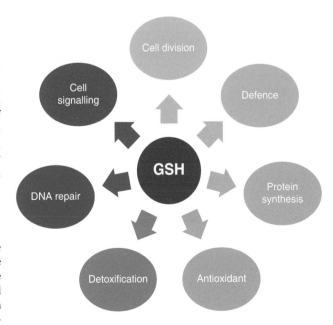

FIGURE 22.1 Role of glutathione in cell function.

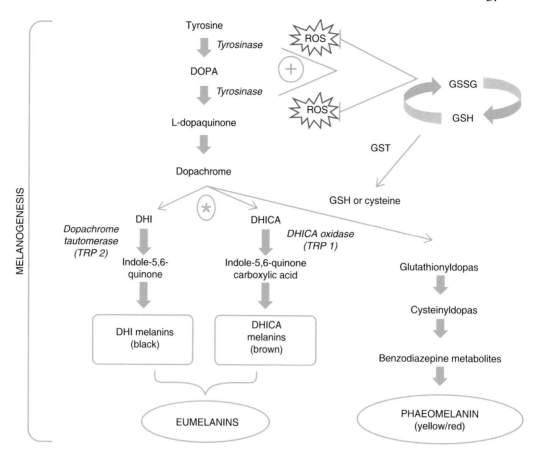

FIGURE 22.2   Effects of glutathione on skin lightening.

vegetables. However, there may be a benefit in dietary supplementation when these substances are not present in sufficient amounts in daily food intake. It is also worth noting that any systemically administered nutraceutical is distributed evenly throughout the body, and this needs to be considered when assessing dose requirements. Currently, there is a lack of good-quality randomized controlled trials in this area to draw any firm conclusions (19).

22.6 Conclusion

While there is plenty of evidence regarding the therapeutic benefits of certain vitamins and antioxidants, nutrition and skin aging remain controversial. Supplementation with nutraceuticals appears to show benefit in in vitro studies, but a lack of good quality human studies means that it is difficult to draw conclusions, and further study is required.

References

1. Park K. Role of micronutrients in skin health and function. Biomol Ther (Seoul). 2015;23(3):207–17
2. Dattola A, Silvestri M, Bennardo L, Passante M, Scali E, Patruno C, et al. Role of vitamins in skin health: A systematic review. Curr Nutr Rep. 2020;9(3):226–35
3. Boelsma E, Hendriks HF, Roza L. Nutritional skin care: health effects of micronutrients and fatty acids. Am J Clin Nutr. 2001;73(5):853–64.
4. Schagen SK, Zampeli VA, Makrantonaki E, Zouboulis CC. Discovering the link between nutrition and skin aging. Dermatoendocrinol. 2012;4(3):298–307.
5. Galimberti F, Mesinkovska NA. Skin findings associated with nutritional deficiencies. Cleve Clin J Med. 2016;83(10):731–9.
6. Farris PK. Topical vitamin C: A useful agent for treating photoaging and other dermatologic conditions. Dermatol Surg. 2005;31(7 Pt 2):814–7; discussion 818.
7. Cosgrove MC, Franco OH, Granger SP, Murray PG, Mayes AE. Dietary nutrient intakes and skin-aging appearance among middle-aged American women. Am J Clin Nutr. 2007;86(4):1225–31.
8. R DD, P B, P S, A G, D Y, C T, et al. Vitamin C prevents ultraviolet-induced pigmentation in healthy volunteers: Bayesian meta-analysis results from 31 randomized controlled versus vehicle clinical studies. J Clin Aesthet Dermatol. 2019;Feb;12(2):E53-E59
9. Al-Niaimi F, Chiang NYZ. Topical vitamin C and the skin: Mechanisms of action and clinical applications. J Clin Aesthet Dermatol. 2017;10(7):14–7.
10. Pullar JM, Carr AC, Vissers M. The roles of vitamin C in skin health. Nutrients. 2017;9(8):866.
11. Skin Health [Internet]. Oregonstate.edu. 2016 [cited 2021 Oct 28]. Available from: https://lpi.oregonstate.edu/mic/health-disease/skin-health
12. Lakdawala N, Babalola O III, Fedeles F, McCusker M, Ricketts J, Whitaker-Worth D, et al. The role of nutrition in dermatologic diseases: Facts and controversies. Clin Dermatol. 2013;31(6):677–700
13. Soliman YS, Hashim PW, Farberg AS, Goldenberg G. The role of diet in preventing photoaging and treating common skin conditions. Cutis. 2019;103(3):153–6.
14. Elson M, Nacht S. Treatment of periorbital hyperpigmentation with topical vitamin K/vitamin A. J Cosmetic Dermatol. 1999;12:323–5.
15. Leu S, Havey J, White LE, Martin N, Yoo SS, Rademaker AW, et al. Accelerated resolution of laser-induced bruising with topical 20% arnica: a rater-blinded randomized controlled trial: Topical treatments for bruising. Br J Dermatol. 2010;163(3):557–63.
16. Addor FAS. Antioxidants in dermatology. An Bras Dermatol. 2017;92(3):356–62.
17. Pérez-Sánchez A, Barrajón-Catalán E, Herranz-López M, Micol V. Nutraceuticals for Skin Care: A Comprehensive Review of Human Clinical Studies. Nutrients. 2018;10(4):3390 10040403.
18. Essential fatty acids and skin health [Internet]. Oregonstate.edu. 2016 [cited 2021 Oct 28]. Available from: https://lpi.oregonstate.edu/mic/health-disease/skin-health/essential-fatty-acids
19. Spiro A, Lockyer S. Nutraceuticals and skin appearance: Is there any evidence to support this growing trend? Nutr Bull. 2018;43(1):10–45.

CHAPTER 23: COSMECEUTICAL-RELATED DERMATITIS AND ALLERGIES

Sandeep Cliff, Abirami Pararajasingam, and Libin Mathew

23.1 Introduction

With the ever-increasing life expectancy of the population, there is a growing demand for youthful and healthy-looking skin, with consumers looking for non-invasive and economic aesthetic interventions. The term "cosmeceutical" was first coined by Kligman in 1984 and encompassed cosmetic products that are promoted as having "biologically active" ingredients with claims of improving skin health, rejuvenation, and healing. Cosmeceuticals are legally classified as cosmetics and not recognized as a distinct entity by the US Federal Food, Drug, and Cosmetic Act.[1] In the UK, the legal implications of this are that cosmetics are governed by the EU Cosmetics Directive. The fifth recital of the directive, the Cosmetic Directive, foresees cosmetic products having a secondary preventative (but not curative) purpose. Pharmaceuticals, on the other hand, are prescription-only medicines designed and rigorously proven to cure or treat a condition. As such, they must be prescribed for use and are governed by the Medicines and Healthcare Products Regulatory Agency regulating both medicines and medical devices nationally.[2] *Cosmeceutical* products therefore avoid the regulatory burden and costs associated with drug development.

It is therefore important that clinicians are vigilant of complications associated with cosmeceutical use and take appropriate steps to minimize risk to patients. In this chapter, we will describe the type of contact dermatitis commonly encountered in ethnic skin following the use of cosmeceuticals and approach to management.

23.2 Classification

Contact dermatitis is the most common complication associated with cosmeceutical use and can be categorized as allergic or irritant. **Allergic contact dermatitis** (ACD) occurs when contact with a particular substance elicits a delayed (type IV) hypersensitivity reaction. ACD usually presents as a well demarcated, intensely pruritic, eczematous eruption localized to skin that comes in direct contact with the allergen. **Irritant contact dermatitis** (ICD) results from exposure to substances that cause direct chemical irritation of the skin. Acute ICD presents with erythema, edema, vesicles or bullae, and oozing. In chronic ICD, lichenification, hyperkeratosis, and fissuring may predominate.[3] Mildly irritating cosmeceuticals can produce erythema, chapped skin, dryness, and fissuring. **Mild erythema may be masked in darker skins and be evident only as hyperpigmentation**. Pruritus and pain may be accompanying symptoms.

Of particular concern in ethnic skin is the development of dyschromias following the use of cosmeceuticals. *Pigmented contact dermatitis* (PCD) is a variant of contact dermatitis and is characterized by reddish-brown to slate-gray pigmentation in a reticulate pattern, usually without any active or preceding clinical dermatitis.[4, 5] Unlike most cases of contact dermatitis where the eczematous reaction resolves with the removal of the allergen, in PCD, pigmentation tends to persist for years, even after the withdrawal of the implicated allergen.[6] *Riehl's melanosis* is a subtype of PCD and is characterized by brown-gray pigmentation secondary to dermal melanin deposition. It is typically preceded by mild erythema and pruritus, followed by diffuse to reticuated hyperpigmentation.[7, 8]

Those with darker skin (Fitzpatrick III–VI) types are also predisposed to *post-inflammatory hyperpigmentation*, which is an acquired hypermelanosis occurring at the site of cutaneous inflammation, including contact dermatitis.[9] Another cause of pigmentation, although rare, is erythrose peribuccale pigmentaire de Brocq, thought to be caused by photodynamic substances in cosmetics.[10] It is characterized by diffuse, symmetrical red-brown pigmentation around the mouth with sparing of the vermillion border and may extend to the forehead, temples, and angles of the jaw.[11]

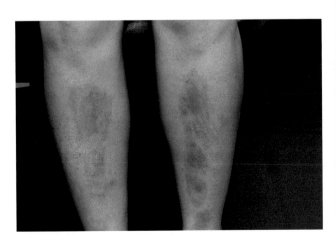

FIGURE 23.1 Allergic contact dermatitis to topical creams applied to the legs of an atopic individual.

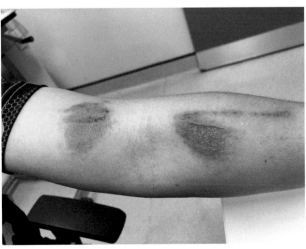

FIGURE 23.2 Irritant contact dermatitis following contact with the *Paederus* beetle.

DOI: 10.1201/9780429243769-23

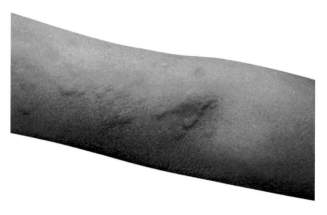

FIGURE 23.3 Urticaria.

Less commonly, individuals can also develop *contact urticaria* and *type 1 hypersensitivity* (or IgE-mediated) reactions. In the former condition, the reaction is limited to the site of cutaneous contact or present as generalized urticaria with concurrent involvement of internal organs. The four stages of the syndrome are as follows: stage 1: local symptoms ranging from non-specific symptoms, such as itching, tingling, and a burning sensation to a wheal-and-flare response restricted to the area of contact; stage 2: generalized urticaria following local cutaneous contact, which also includes angioedema; stage 3: extracutaneous manifestations, which may include the respiratory (bronchial asthma or rhinoconjunctivitis), orolaryngeal, or gastrointestinal tract; stage 4: anaphylactic reactions. IgE-mediated reactions occur in a previously sensitized individual and involve the coupling of percutaneously absorbed antigens with specific IgE molecules on the surfaces of mast cells, the symptoms resulting from the release of histamine. Pre-existing conditions, such as atopic dermatitis, may favor this condition.

23.3 Epidemiology

Contact dermatitis to cosmeceuticals is under-reported. This may in part be due to the difficulty in testing these products and the lack of standardized allergens. UK data reveals that as much as 23% of females and 13.8% of males experience adverse effects on personal care products.[12] Overall evidence suggests that the prevalence is equivalent between ethnicities.[13, 14]

23.4 Common Cosmeceutical Allergens

Cosmeceutical products contain a number of potential allergens, which will be discussed here.

23.4.1 Fragrance

Fragrances have been used in cosmetic products for centuries and are the most common cause of allergic contact dermatitis. Unfortunately, product labeling can be misleading as no specific information regarding fragrance components is usually listed on products, often being labeled as "fragrance" in the ingredient disclosure. To further complicate matters, there are several fragrance chemicals, such as benzyl alcohol, benzaldehydeyde, and ethylene brassylate, which that can have other functions in addition to being a fragrance. These chemicals can therefore be found in products labeled as "fragrance-free" Because of the prevalence of allergic reactions to fragrances, a fragrance mix is included in the standard series for patch testing.

23.4.2 Preservatives

Preservatives are used to prevent bacterial growth and oxidation and are found in all cosmeceutical products. They are the second most common cause of allergic contact dermatitis. Preservatives that have been reported as allergens include formaldehyde and formaldehyde releasers, parabens, and methylchloroisothiazolinone. At present, the latter is mainly used in rinse-off products to minimize the contact time and chance of allergic reaction.

23.4.3 Vitamins

A number of vitamins are incorporated into cosmeceutical products owing to their diverse properties, including anti-inflammatory, anti-aging, and skin-lightening effects. Contact dermatitis to vitamins, such as vitamin A (retinol), vitamin C (ascorbic acid), and vitamin E (tocopherol) have been reported in the literature.[15] Vitamin A is well recognised for improving signs of photoaging; however, its derivatives are commonly culpable for irritant contact dermatitis characterized by dryness and skin irritation. This is typically worse during the early phase of treatment and settles within four to six weeks.[16] Allergic contact dermatitis is rare but can be confirmed with patch testing. Vitamin C can be found in topical preparations and protects the skin from oxidative stress. With several reported benefits, vitamin C rarely causes irritant contact dermatitis due to low pH. ACD is also rare. Vitamin E is a common cause of both ICD and ACD.

23.4.4 Hydroxy Acids

Alpha-hydroxy acids (AHAs), beta-hydroxy acids (BHAs), and polyhydroxy acids (PHAs) are acids with exfoliating properties. Contact dermatitis is typically in the form of ICD. The larger size of the PHAs reduces skin penetration, which also lessens the opportunity for ICD to occur. More irritant reactions are seen with AHAs in the form of stinging and burning due to the low pH of these cosmeceuticals that rapidly penetrate the stratum corneum to reach the nerve endings in the dermis. AHAs that have been partially neutralized produce less contact dermatitis but also do not produce dramatic anti-aging effects. BHAs, such as salicylic acid, are oil-soluble and do not penetrate the stratum corneum well. For this reason, ICD is lessened but can still occur in individuals with compromised barrier function.[17, 18]

23.4.5 Botanicals

Botanicals are often considered by the consumer as natural and safer alternatives to their synthetic counterparts.[19] Aloe is commonly contained within cosmeceutical products, and there are reports of contact dermatitis following use. *Centella asiatica* has been purported to stimulate collagen production by fibroblasts, and numerous cases of contact allergy have been reported in the literature.

Peppermint, tea tree, and lavender oil, as well as causing contact dermatitis, have also been reported to cause stomatitis and burning mouth syndrome. Antigenic potential depends on the type of plant, the part used, and processing methods. Other botanicals with reported reactions are *Gingkgo biloba*, curcumin, and witch hazel.

23.5 Investigation

23.5.1 History and Physical Exam

Contact dermatitis is generally underdiagnosed on its first presentation. A detailed history is essential to establish the temporal correlation of exposure to the allergen and

TABLE 23.1: Common Causes of Contact Allergy Based on Anatomical Site

Site of involvement	Common source of allergen exposure
Face	Skin care products: moisturizers, sunscreens, makeup, cleansers, and perfumes
Eyelids	Eye cosmetics and nail cosmetics
Lips and mouth	Lipsticks, oral hygiene products (e.g., toothpaste, mouthwash, and dental floss), gum, and mints
Ears	Hair care products, perfumes, medicinal ear drops, and jewelry
Trunk	Moisturizers, sunscreens, cleansers, and perfumes
Hands	Moisturizers, cleansers, perfumes, and nailcare products
Scalp	Hair dyes, permanent waves, shampoos, hair sprays, and perfumes

Source: With permission from Ortitz and Yiannias. Contact dermatitis to cosmetics, fragrances and botanicals. Dermatologic Therapy. 2004, 264–271.[20]

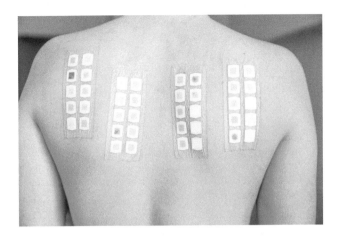

FIGURE 23.4 Patch test.

symptomology. Particular points to include are the list of products used by the patient (makeup, moisturizer, etc.), method of application, and removal. The importance of prompt recognition as a prerequisite for early treatment must be recognized, particularly in ethnic patients with darker skin types who may be predisposed to post-inflammatory hyperpigmentation. In addition, baseline pigmentation of the skin may mask clinical features of contact dermatitis, particularly if mild. One must also consider other causes for presentation, including primary dermatological disorders, including atopic dermatitis, contact urticaria, acneiform eruptions, rosacea, and seborrhoeic dermatitis.

Allergic contact dermatitis to cosmeceuticals can be found in any body area (Table 23.1). The physical exam can offer important clues to the cause of the eruption in most cases.

The face is a classic area of involvement as it is exposed to a multitude of potential allergens, including airborne allergens and irritants, as well as skin care products that are applied daily. A background of atopic eczema does not rule out allergic or irritant contact dermatitis as a cause for a flare of pre-existing dermatitis, and therefore, patch testing should be considered in these patients. The use of products on lips may cause perioral irritation. The scalp is affected by several hair cosmetics and, in particular, hair dyes.

The eyelids are particularly susceptible to contact dermatitis and may manifest the first signs of an allergic reaction to a product. The eyelids are most often affected by fragrances or preservatives. Infection should be considered in these patients as conjunctival injection and blepharitis can feature in both.

Truncal sites may be involved, typically secondary to the presence of preservatives and fragrances within products that have contact with wide body surface area (e.g., body lotion).

The history should also address the possibility of more passive allergic reactions to the cosmetics worn by the patient's partner or relatives. As such, it can sometimes be necessary to also review the cosmetics used by those they have an extended period of contact with.

23.5.2 Patch Testing

Patch testing is invaluable in the diagnosis of ACD. The process involves applying around 40 patches containing potential or suspected allergens, typically on the mid-upper back of the patient. The patches are removed and read after 48 hours and read again after 96 hours. Positive reactions and corresponding allergens are noted (Figure 23.4).

A sensible starting point would be testing for the standard series (for example, true test) and expanding the allergen series based on clinical suspicion. The whole product may be tested, but often, it is impossible to determine which of the many ingredients in the preparation is the culprit. Most large cosmeceutical companies can provide a sample of the raw material they use in their formulation for individual ingredient patch testing. As many of the cosmeceuticals are relatively new and standardized allergens are not available, testing the whole product may be helpful. If the product is a rinse-off product, then it should be diluted with water first to avoid irritant reactions.

23.6 Management

Dermatitis secondary to cosmetic use can be treated in the same way as allergic or irritant contact dermatitis secondary to other causes. The first step is to stop using the suspected product. Then follows the identification of the offending agent, as this is key in aiming to prevent future exposure to the agent. Once identified, the patient should be educated on avoiding the constituent and directed to alternative hypoallergenic products.[21] Patients should be encouraged to always read the labels of cosmetics to ensure it does not contain a component that they're allergic to. Patients should be given the INCI name of the ingredient they are allergic to, as this is how the ingredients are listed on labels. Generally, products with fewer ingredients will be a lower risk of causing a reaction. If tester samples are provided, patients can even patch test themselves by placing a small amount of product on an inconspicuous area, such as the inside of the elbow, and monitoring over the next 24–72 hours for a reaction.

In general, patients who have reacted to a fragrance should also avoid botanical products. Initially, patients are advised to avoid fragranced products for approximately six weeks. Once the dermatitis has cleared, patients can try one fragranced product at a time. New fragrances or fragranced products can be introduced every two weeks.

In the acute symptomatic setting, active treatment is used to bring about rapid symptom control. The aims are to reduce inflammation and to restore the epidermal barrier that has been disrupted by cosmeceutical dermatitis. The treatment usually overlaps whether it is an ACD or ICD reaction.

Emollients and moisturizers are recommended to all patients as they aid in reducing inflammation and restoring the epidermal barrier. They can also be soothing to irritated skin. Emollients and moisturizers can be applied repetitively during the day, and liberal application is advised as they can be easily wiped or washed off throughout the course of the day, which would reduce their effectiveness.[22] Oral antihistamines can be used to treat the pruritic or urticarial element that may be experienced.

Topical corticosteroids are considered first-line in managing ACD if not controlled with emollients alone.[23] Despite the lack of clinical evidence for their use in ICD, topical corticosteroids are also used empirically in ICD.

- For severe or milder reactions not involving the face or flexural areas, a super high-potency or high-potency corticosteroid can be used for up to four weeks.
- A medium- or low-potency corticosteroid is advised for reactions involving the face or flexural areas for up to two weeks.

The treatment between an ICD and ACD reaction diverges on topical calcineurin inhibitors. It can be used in ACD, where its effectiveness has been proven in clinical studies, although not directly in comparison with topical corticosteroids.[24] From clinical practice, it has been noted the onset of action is generally slower, with side effects including stinging. They have not been shown to be effective in ICD and are not recommended for use.

Oral corticosteroids are rarely used but can be considered for ACD when it covers a large body surface area (>20%). Phototherapy and oral systemic agents can be considered in chronic ACD that has been unresponsive to conventional treatment with corticosteroids.

23.6.1 Post-Inflammatory Hyperpigmentation

Following cosmeceutical dermatitis, post-inflammatory hyperpigmentation (PIH) is a common sequela that particularly affects ethnic skin (Fitzpatrick type III–VI). This often has a significant psychological impact on the patient. The PIH is typically isolated to the area of the inflammatory reaction. As well as treating the acute reaction, treatment should also be initiated early for the PIH. One of the most important steps is photoprotection to prevent any worsening. Patients should be advised to use at least a sun protection factor 30 sunscreen and carry out physical sun-protective measures, such as reducing exposure to the sun, using hats and umbrellas, or wearing appropriate clothing. They should be warned that UV irradiation makes hyperpigmentation darker and thus more noticeable. They also take longer to fade away after UV exposure.[25] The medical management of PIH can be challenging, and patients should be counseled that it tends to improve slowly over time. They should be warned that many of the treatments can in themselves irritate the skin as a side effect, worsening the hyperpigmentation. Figure 23.5 outlines the possible treatment algorithm that clinicians might consider when managing a patient with post-cosmeceutical-related dermatitis. Often combinations of treatments are required to attain a clinically significant improvement.

23.6.1.1 Hydroquinone

First-line treatment for PIH is topical hydroquinone, which can be used twice daily for 12–24 weeks.[26] The majority of evidence for hydroquinone arises from studies on its use in treating melasma,[27] with few studies looking at PIH alone. Backed by clinical experience, the treatment has translated to PIH. Hydroquinone can be bought over the counter in some countries at a 2% concentration and is usually prescribed at a 4% concentration. Patients should be advised it reduces pigmentation

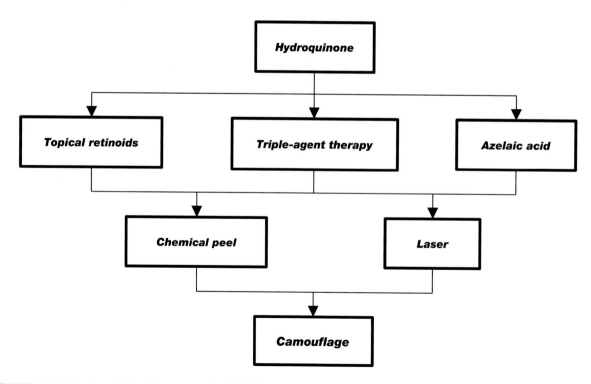

FIGURE 23.5 Treatment algorithm to consider for PIH.

of normal and hyperpigmented skin, and as such, care should be used when applying it. Over the face, it is advisable to treat the entire face to prevent irregularities in pigment.[26] Over the body, it can be used over the limited area of hyperpigmentation, but patients should be warned that a "halo" of hypopigmentation can appear at the periphery of treated areas which slowly resolves.

Hydroquinone should be used twice a day, then patients are assessed at week 12, at which point the treatment can be stopped if there is any considerable improvement or if there has been no response but can be continued for a further 12 weeks in those with some improvement. The side effects include a risk of ICD and ACD, which rises with higher concentrations. The most concerning side effects are exogenous ochronosis (blue-black pigment), which is associated with the use of hydroquinone for more than six months.[28] Treatment should be stopped if this occurs.

There are a wide variety of second-line therapies for PIH with limited evidence of their efficacy or comparison with hydroquinone.

23.6.1.2 Topical Retinoids

Retinoids increase the dispersion and removal of melanin.[29] There are three topical forms available for PIH: tretinoin, tazarotene, and adapalene. Data is limited to small trials; for example, in a study with 68 skin of color patients, tretinoin demonstrated greater improvement in PIH at 40 weeks.[30] The efficacy of tazarotene and adapalene has been demonstrated in similar small trials. These agents are applied once daily and typically at night.[31] Side effects include erythema and ICD (in the early treatment stages).

23.6.1.3 Triple-Agent Therapy

Triple-agent therapy consists of hydroquinone, topical tretinoin, and topical corticosteroid. It is postulated that tretinoin increases the penetration of hydroquinone, while corticosteroid decreases the risk of ICD.[32] Again, there is a lack of evidence regarding its efficacy. The treatment regimen is the same as for hydroquinone alone, with a maximum duration of treatment of 24 weeks. As with the aforementioned side effects of hydroquinone, there is the added potential side effect of corticosteroid-induced atrophy to be aware of.

23.6.1.4 Azelaic Acid

Azelaic acid is a naturally occurring agent derived from *Pityrosporum ovale*. It inhibits the actions of tyrosinase. There

are only small studies in patients with types IV–VI, where it has demonstrated significant improvement in PIH.[33] It is applied twice daily and may need a few months to attain a significant improvement. Side effects include stinging over the area of application.

23.6.1.5 Chemical Peels

Chemical peels are, in essence, targeted wounding of the skin surface with an exfoliating agent. There are different depths of skin to which the peel can induce injury, but this conversely increases the risk of PIH. Superficial peels reduce epidermal melanin and are used in the treatment of PIH. They are sometimes used in combination with the previously mentioned agents, improving their absorption.[34] Glycolic acid and salicylic acid are the most commonly used agents in superficial chemical peels. They are generally well tolerated in all skin types, with a series of multiple peels required for significant clinical improvement. The use of sunscreen is especially important both before and throughout the peel treatment until the skin has healed.

23.6.1.6 Lasers

There are several different laser and light devices that have been used in the treatment of PIH with variable success. The evidence is limited to small studies or case reports. It is important to note that laser therapy is associated with a potential adverse effect of PIH, and the risk increases with darker skin types. Longer-wavelength lasers are better in this regard, but the overall use of laser and light therapy should be limited to clinicians who are highly experienced in the area.

23.6.1.7 Camouflage

While not treating the PIH itself, camouflage products are useful for patients to minimize the visibility of the PIH while it slowly improves. The improvement of PIH can often take several months, and in those patients where this is especially slow or limited, camouflage products can be explored.[35]

Frequently Asked Questions

1. *Q: What to advise patients on hypoallergenic products?*
   A: Public perception of products that claim to be hypoallergenic can be that they are completely free of all allergens. In reality, companies simply use this term for products that they claim cause fewer allergic reactions. The products themselves may contain fewer ingredients or not contain the compounds that are commonly associated with allergic reactions. However, in many countries, including the United States, there are no legally set criteria that companies must meet to advertise their products as hypoallergenic. Patients should be made aware that while there may be a lower risk of developing dermatitis, there is no guarantee these products won't cause a reaction.

2. *Q: What should patients look for on product labels?*
   A: Firstly, as mentioned earlier in this chapter, patients should be made aware of the ingredient they are allergic to, and this is the first item to be looking for on the product label. The ingredients are displayed in the order of decreasing quantity in the product. As well as "hypoallergenic," companies often use expressions such as "pure," "natural," or "organic," among others, to describe their product. However, these terms often have very little in the way of scientific/medical relevance with regard

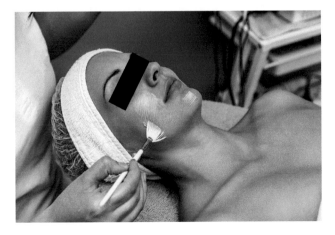

FIGURE 23.6 Application of a chemical peel.

to cosmetic dermatitis but describe products manufactured a certain way and are usually marketing terminology employed by companies to make their products appear more attractive.

On the other hand, products that are described as "fragrance-free" can be better tolerated by patients who are prone to reactions as fragrances are common causes of cosmetic-related dermatitis. It must be noted to patients that "unscented" products could contain fragrance chemicals to disguise any odor.

3. *Q: General advice on products that are marketed as skin lightening?*

A: Hydroquinone, which was mentioned earlier for use in PIH, is probably the most well-known agent for skin lightening and the gold standard of these agents. The lightening of skin is often sought by those with darker skin types, and there is a vast range of products targeted at them around the world. Hydroquinone interferes with melanogenesis and melanocytes. There are several concerns about the long-term use of this product, including dermatitis, vitiligo, and renal/hepatic toxicity. As such, there are limitations in several countries on the maximum concentration of hydroxyquinone in products, while countries such as Japan and Australia have banned it.

4. *Q: What is the prognosis, and how long will the reaction last?*

A: The reaction should begin to settle within a few days, provided the culprit cosmetic is not used again. Depending on the severity of the reaction, it can sometimes take six to eight weeks for the reaction to fully resolve, and patients should be made aware that it can be a lengthy reaction. Patients with Fitzpatrick types IV–VI have the propensity to experience post-inflammatory pigmentation and should be warned as such.

5. *Q: What else could the rash be?*

A: There are several skin conditions that are similar in appearance to cosmetic dermatitis. There are several subtypes of dermatitis, and differentials would also need to be considered for the potential precipitants of an irritant contact/allergic dermatitis reaction. The history will be key in diagnosing cosmetics as the cause and further investigations as outlined previously. An alternative cause for the rash should be considered for rashes that do not improve/resolve with abstinence from the suspected cosmetic product.

References

1. The Food and Drugs Administration, Federal Food, Drug and Cosmetic Act (FD&C Act) (US: The Food and Drugs Administration, 2010). www.fda.gov/RegulatoryInformation/Legislation/FederalFoodDrugandCosmeticActFDCAct.
2. Gov.uk, The Medicines and Healthcare Products Regulatory Agency. www.gov.uk/government/organisations/medicines-and-healthcare-products-regulatory-agency
3. Fisher AA. Contact dermatitis in black patients. Cutis. 1977;20:905–922.
4. Matsuo S, Nakayama H. A case of pigmented dermatitis induced by cinnamic derivatives (in Japanese). Hifu.1984;26:573–579.
5. Nakayama H, Matsuo S, Hayakawa K, Takhashi K, Shigematsu T, et al. Pigmented cosmetic dermatitis. Int J Dermatol.1984;23:299–305.
6. Nakayama H. Pigmented contact dermatitis and chemical depigmentation. Textbook of Contact Dermatitis, Springer, Berlin. 2001.
7. https://emedicine.medscape.com/article/1119818-clinical)
8. Khanna U, Khandpur S. Pigmented contact dermatitis. Pigment Disord. 2015;2:214.
9. Richards GM, Oresajo CO, Halder RM. Structure and function of ethnic skin and hair. Dermatol Clin. 2003;21:595–600.
10. Vashi NA, Kundu RV. Facial hyperpigmentation: Causes and treatment. Br J Dermatol. 2013 Oct;169 Suppl 3:41–56.
11. Khanna N, Rasool S. Facial melanoses: Indian perspective. Indian J Dermatol Venereol Leprol. 2011;77:552–563; quiz 564.
12. Orton DI, Wilkinson JD. Cosmetic allergy: Incidence, diagnosis, and management. Am J Clin Dermatol. 2004;5(5):327–337.
13. Deleo VA, Taylor SC, Belsito DV, Fowler JF Jr, Fransway AF, Maibach HI, Marks JG Jr, Mathias CG, Nethercott JR, Pratt MD, Reitschel RR, Sherertz EF, Storrs FJ, Taylor JS. The effect of race and ethnicity on patch test results. J Am Acad Dermatol. 2002 Feb;46(2 Suppl Understanding):S107–112.
14. Peters L, Marriott M, Mukerji B, Indra P, Iyer JV, Roy A, Rowson M, Ahmed S, Cooper K, Basketter D. The effect of population diversity on skin irritation. Contact Dermatitis. 2006 Dec;55(6):357–363.
15. Callender VD. Acne in ethnic skin: Special considerations for therapy. Dermatol Ther. 2004;17:184–195. See J-A, Goh CL, Hayashi N, Suh DH, Abad Casintahan F. Optimizing the use of topical retinoids in Asian acne patients. J Dermatol. 2018 May;45(5):522–528.
16. Kim WJ, Park JM, Ko HC, Kim BS, Kim MB, Song M. A split-faced, observer-blinded comparison study of topical adapalene/benzoyl peroxide and adapalene in the treatment of Asian acne patients. J Drugs Dermatol. 2013;12:149–151.
17. Monheit GD, Chastain MA. Chemical peels. Facial Plast Surg Clin North Am. 2001;9:239–255.
18. Zakopoulou N, Kontochristopoulos G. Superficial chemical peels. J Cosmet Dermatol. 2006;5:246–253.
19. Draelos ZD. Cosmeceuticals: What's real, what's not. Dermatol Clin. 2019 Jan;37(1):107–115. doi: 10.1016/j.det.2018.07.001. Epub 2018 Nov 1.
20. Ortitz KJ, Yiannias JA. Contact dermatitis to cosmetics, fragrances and botanicals. Dermatologic ther. 2004;264–271.
21. Mowad CM, Anderson B, Scheinman P, Pootongkam S, Nedorost S, Brod B. Allergic contact dermatitis: Patient management and education. J Am Acad Dermatol. 2016 Jun;74(6):1043–1054.
22. Yokota M, Maibach HI. Moisturizer effect on irritant dermatitis: An overview. Contact Dermatitis. 2006 Aug;55(2):65–72.
23. Bourke J, Coulson I, English J. Guidelines for the management of contact dermatitis: An update. British Association of Dermatologists Therapy Guidelines and Audit Subcommittee. Br J Dermatol. 2009;160(5):946.
24. Belsito D, Wilson DC, Warshaw E, Fowler J, Ehrlich A, Anderson B, Strober BE, Willetts J, Rutledge ES. A prospective randomized clinical trial of 0.1% tacrolimus ointment in a model of chronic allergic contact dermatitis. J Am Acad Dermatol. 2006;55(1):40.
25. Davis EC, Callender VD. Postinflammatory hyperpigmentation: A review of the epidemiology, clinical features, and treatment options in skin of color. J Clin Aesthet Dermatol. 2010;3(7):20–31.
26. Rossi AM, Perez MI. Treatment of hyperpigmentation. Facial Plast Surg Clin North Am. 2011;19(2):313.
27. Ennes SBP, Paschoalick RC, Mota de Avelar Alchorne M. A double-blind, comparative, placebo-controlled study of the efficacy and tolerability of 4% hydroquinone as a depigmenting agent in melisma. J Dermatolog Treat. 2000;11:173.
28. Levin CY, Maibach H. Exogenous ochronosis. An update on clinical features, causative agents and treatment options. Am J Clin Dermatol. 2001;2(4):213.
29. Kligman AM, Willis I. A new formula for depigmenting human skin. Arch Dermatol. 1975 Jan;111(1):40–48.
30. Bulengo-Ransby SM, Griffiths CE, Kimbrough-Green CK, Finkel LJ, Hamilton TA, Ellis CN, Voorhees JJ. Topical tretinoin (retinoic acid) therapy for hyperpigmented lesions caused by inflammation of the skin in black patients. N Engl J Med. 1993;328(20):1438.
31. Nighland M, Yusuf M, Wisniewski S, Huddleston K, Nyirady J. The effect of simulated solar UV irradiation on tretinoin in tretinoin gel microsphere 0.1% and tretinoin gel 0.025%. Cutis. 2006;77(5):313.
32. Ortonne JP, Passeron T. Melanin pigmentary disorders: Treatment update. Dermatol Clin. 2005 Apr;23(2):209–226.
33. Lowe NJ, Rizk D, Grimes P, Billips M, Pincus S. Azelaic acid 20% cream in the treatment of facial hyperpigmentation in darker-skinned patients. Clin Ther. 1998 Sep;20(5):945–959.
34. Grimes PE. Management of hyperpigmentation in darker racial ethnic groups. Semin Cutan Med Surg. 2009;28(2):77.
35. McMichael L. Skin camouflage. BMJ. 2012;344:d7921.

CHAPTER 24: EVALUATION AND ASSESSMENT FOR ETHNIC SKIN

Kavita Mariwalla

24.1 Introduction

The popularity of medical aesthetic procedures continues to grow, with a global market size valued at $86.2 billion in 2020 and an expected compounded annual growth rate of 9.8% until 2028.[1] What is fueling this drive? It is partly due to the entry of men into the cosmetic market but also the result of a generation of millennials who have grown up with words like "Botox" as part of their common vernacular. No longer taboo, the subject of aesthetic enhancement now permeates social media as well as magazines globally. While North America retains the largest share of the aesthetic market, the highest rates of growth in the market are expected to come from APAC countries due to expanding consumer knowledge, strong local economies, and a rise in medical tourism. As a result, it is important to understand the unique features of different ethnic groups and understand how to best evaluate and assess their skin. The problem we currently face is that the facial canon as it is taught and as it relates to aesthetics has mainly been based on the Euro-Caucasian model. This does not take into account racial and ethnic differences in appearance, nor does it keep in mind cultural cues that should be maintained in order to prevent racial morphing through the use of fillers and injectables. In this chapter, I will focus on the evaluation and assessment of ethnic skin in Asian, Southeast Asian, African, Hispanic, and Mediterranean skin.

24.2 What Are Consumers Looking For?

Before performing any facial assessment, it is important to have a general understanding of what patients are seeking. Allergan conducted a survey in 2019 of 14,584 aesthetically conscious consumers and 1,300 physicians in 18 countries, which demonstrated that while in many countries consumers look to celebrities to define beauty standards, in the US, Canada, and India, the definition of attractiveness is actually more derived from friends and family.[2] Top concerns worldwide are upper facial lines and wrinkles regardless of age, and 54% of women worldwide consider under-eye bags a top concern. Interestingly millennials (age 21–35) are more likely to seek preventative treatment compared to older cohorts and treatment as soon as they notice a concern. Globally speaking, of all consumers surveyed, 52% stated they would consider dermal filler treatments at some point in their life, and 82% feel the use of injectables is socially acceptable. As we no doubt witness in our daily practice, the most common questions, according to

those surveyed, during an initial appointment are cost, effectiveness of treatment, and safety, respectively.

In addition to facial injectables, body shape also ranked highly on the list for aesthetic improvement. Turkey, India, and Saudi Arabia exceeded the average score for caring about the shape of their body across genders, while Russia and South Korea scored well below the average across both men and women on this question. While body sculpting is beyond the scope of this chapter, the takeaway is that although we consider the assessment of the face, it may be important to discuss body contouring as well during aesthetic consultations, as many consumers are looking for these kinds of treatments.

The other notable data to come out of this global Allergan survey are the words consumers use to describe female beauty (Table 24.1). It is clear that our patients are looking for natural results and that the upper third of the face still predominates most aesthetic concerns.

TABLE 24.1: Words Used by Consumers in Varying Age Groups to Describe Beauty

AGES 21-35	AGES 36-55	AGES 56-65
Soft	Natural	Healthy
Smooth	Smooth	Natural
Curvy	Soft	Smooth
Natural	Healthy	Soft
Beautiful	Curvy	Clean
Strong	Beautiful	Glowing
Clean	Confident	Confident
Pretty	Glowing	Toned
Healthy	Pretty	Curvy
Confident	Toned	Fit
Fit	Fit	Beautiful
Glowing	Strong	Strong

Source: Alexiades M, Chantrey J, Chatrath V et al. Allergan 360° Aesthetics Report. Accessed online January 2021. https://www.allergan.com › Allergan-360-Report-Full

24.3 Differences in Intrinsic Aging across Ethnicities

We already understand that aging is a cumulative process occurring due to extrinsic and intrinsic factors. Intrinsically, the interplay between bony resorption changes and ligament

DOI: 10.1201/9780429243769-24

laxity and position, which can affect various fat compartments in the face, which lead to changes in skin folding and perceived volumetric changes. This, however, is not consistent among all ethnic groups.

In addition to an increase in melanin content and melanosomal dispersion in persons of color, we know that once transferred to keratinocytes, melanosomes are degraded more slowly in darker skin. Darker skin types may have more cornified cell layers and greater lipid content compared to white stratum corneum, which should inform recommendations for topicals to improve skin texture and skin quality. Black skin has been found to have more and larger fibroblasts, smaller collagen fiber bundles, and more macrophages compared to white skin. Asian skin tends to demonstrate greater collagen density than that of Caucasian skin. The collagen density manifests as a more vigorous fibroblastic response during wound healing which leads to more hyperemia during scar formation. It is important, therefore, to control any post-inflammatory erythema from procedures in Asian skin.

The density of the collagen across ethnic groups is likely also responsible for less solar damage among Africans and Asians compared to their North American and European counterparts, which may be why there is less wrinkling in areas like the upper chest. The dominance of fat ptosis is more noticeable in South Indians, Middle Easterners, and Asians compared to Africans and Hispanics, which is why one also notices a particular dominance of a desire to improve the jowls, nasolabial folds, and submental regions in these groups.

Among Asians, the lower face tends to have more of a pulling effect due to the thickness of the platysma muscle resulting in more visible sagging compared to just wrinkling. In the lower face, there is also a greater tendency toward masseter hypertrophy which compounds this downward-pulling effect on facial skin. And while wrinkling is more superficial among the Asian population in general, among Chinese patients frontal forehead lines do appear earlier than in Caucasian patients.

In Southeast Asians, depressor anguli oris hyperactivity leads to traction of skin at the oral commissures leading to early visibility of a downturned mouth. Similarly, mentalis hyperactivity occurs in both Asians and Southeast Asians. Marionette lines begin to appear earlier than nasolabial folds in Southeast Asians, and like Asians, Southeast Asians have more concerns regarding pigmented lesions. One notable difference, however, is that fine wrinkles are more evident in Southeast Asians, which does make this group a good candidate for toxin use.

Patients of African descent tend to age via folds and volume changes, particularly in the midface, compared to wrinkles in the upper third. The presence of dermatosis papulosa nigricans is common, as are pigmentary alterations, especially around the eyes and the upper lateral face. One area of aging that is evident in African patients is loss of lip volume. Unlike the typical ratio touted for Caucasian patients, lips in patients of African descent should be in a 1:1 ratio of upper to lower lip. Aging around the mouth is characterized by a loss of volume in this area and an increase in wrinkling of the lips, as well as a change in pigment.

The result of these anatomic differences in aging across ethnic groups should make the physician think not just about dynamic and static wrinkles in their assessment but also gravitational and structural wrinkles. These subtle differences in aging indicate that when thinking about treating ethnic skin, it is important to consider not only neuromodulators and fillers but also procedures.

24.3.1 Evaluation of Asian Skin

When we talk about "Asian" skin, we are really discussing a swath of countries ranging from China to Japan with quite distinct facial features and cultural expectations. Common among these countries is a desire by patients for skin tone evenness. While wrinkles are less evident in Asian skin compared to Caucasian skin, pigmentary changes occur earlier. These include a tendency toward post-inflammatory hyperpigmentation, melasma, lentigines and freckles, nevus of Ota, and Hori nevus. Skin phototype also ranges in this group from Fitzpatrick skin types II–IV, making the resolution of dyschromias something that must be nuanced. This is where chemical peels and lasers like picosecond devices are particularly useful. Ruby lasers are a traditional laser with excellent results in the Asian population.

In addition to aging, skin texture is also a primary concern. Ultraviolet radiation can increase oil production by the sebaceous gland leading to the worsening of skin texture and an increase in acne tropicana. Combined with an increase toward a sensitive skin type and a greater intolerance of retinoids, assessment of Asian patients should include modalities to improve not only dyschromia but also texture.

Based on cadaver dissections, East Asians have a thicker dermis, increased fat above and deep to the superficial muscular aponeurotic system, and dense fat and fibrous connections between the superficial muscular aponeurotic system and deep parotidomasseteric fascia.[2] In addition, muscle mass of the corrugators tends to be lower in East Asia than in Caucasians, and corrugators tend to be shorter, narrower, and less hyperdynamic. For this reason, it is very important to be cautious when using neuromodulators in the upper third of the face for Asian patients. Consider a three-point injection pattern with much lower units (e.g., eight units onabotulinumtoxinA or twelve units incobotulinumtoxinA) when injecting the glabellar region.

The East Asian aesthetic is typically based on data from Korea. For patients from China and Taiwan, the goal was traditionally a round "moon" face appearance, but in the last two decades, this has changed. Now the goal is to achieve a more pronounced taper from maxilla to mandible, giving a "V shape" to the overall frontal profile. Angles must be softened with both contouring, using modalities such as ultrasound and radiofrequency, and fillers and potentially threads. Neuromodulator injections to the masseter are quite popular for this reason.

Structurally, the Asian face is characterized by prominent malar eminences and a relative deficiency of the premaxillary region. Due to a wide mandibular angle, the face shape can appear square with a relative flattening of the midface region, and microgenia can contribute to the overall angled countenance. Ideally, for patients of Korean origin, fuller, oval-shaped cheeks and a small chin with a 0.8–0.9 length ratio of glabellar to nasolabial angle are ideal. Consideration should also be given to neuromodulators to thin out the masseter and filler in the chin and along the mandible to achieve a smooth contour and a narrower lower third.

Globally, we know that most women want improvement in the lower eye area, but in particular, it is important to understand beauty norms in Asian culture. For example, it is particularly important to understand the cultural implication of botulinumtoxinA injection for widening the palpebral aperture. Injections of neuromodulators can remove the pretarsal bulge and slightly lower the inferior ciliary margin to widen the palpebral aperture. However, in East Asians, the pretarsal muscular bulge is known as the "charming roll" and is considered a hallmark of female beauty. Fillers are used to re-establish it if it is lost. Trying to fill around it, if present naturally, will thus lead to an undesirable outcome for these patients. Similarly, the supratarsal crease in Asians is smaller compared to Caucasians, and there are more epicanthal folds in the eye area. A high lid crease and deep palpebral sulcus may give the appearance of a widened eye; however, it can make the Asian upper lid actually appear unnatural and aged. Brow position in the Asian patient tends to be flatter and lower in the lateral 2/3 than advocated for Caucasians, and lateral brow arching can give a "samurai eyebrow" appearance, which would not be considered an acceptable aesthetic result. Thus, if the frontalis is to be injected, consider two rows with six injection points using a microdroplet technique.

For the Asian patient, it is important to stress daily skin care and sun protection but also consider non-invasive skin tightening and lifting by RF energy or ultrasound energy. Fillers can be placed directly into folds, but caution should be used in reflating the midface as the outcome can sometimes be simply increasing face volume without improving contour. Finally, I recommend the assessment of the submental area as jowls and a thick platysmal band lead to gravitational wrinkles and sagging that can detract from the overall appearance of the face.

24.3.2 Evaluation of Southeast Asian Skin

Like Asians, Southeast Asians also suffer from dyschromias and issues with skin texture. The tendency to post-inflammatory hyperpigmentation is high, which does not in and of itself preclude laser procedures and peels but should be done by an experienced physician. The South Asian subcontinent represents a vast array of skin phototypes ranging from II–III in the north to V–VI in the south of India. Similarly, one notices a change in the process of aging, with early signs of aging appearing in north and east Indian ethnic groups first (around age 40) and at a later age in west and then south Indians, respectively.

Typically in South Asian patients, the aging parameters include the presence of forehead lines, brow position drop, and tear trough deformity.[3] Loss of cheek volume and increase in neck volume were higher in East Indians, while West Indians tend to show signs of dermatochalasis as early as 40–45 years of age.

Genetic predisposition to tear trough deformity and dyschromia around the eyes is very common in South Asian patients, and usually one of the top concerns of patients from this ethnic group. It may be worsened due to aging and chronic exposure to sunlight. Whereas in Caucasian populations, the severity of the tear trough deformity peaks in the 60s, South Asian patients present with medial hollowness as early as the thirties. A multimodal approach is important; assessment of the under-eye area should include remedies for volume loss but also improvement in pigment. This is where microneedling, radiofrequency, and also picosecond laser procedures can aid in periorbital rejuvenation and should always be considered before filler alone. A maintenance routine of topicals must also be discussed at any consultation for the eye area in South Asian patients. When evaluating the eye area, keep in mind brow position, as age-related brow drooping occurs more frequently in the south and east Indian ethnicities compared to the west and north Indian population.

When assessing South Asian patients, also keep in mind the extent to which pigment can enhance an aging process. This is particularly true in the marionette lines. This area becomes noticeable in most ethnic groups after their 50s, but in South Asians, women as young as their thirties have reported pigmented marionette lines. While this area can be prone to pigmentary demarcation lines, Singh et al. reported that 38% of Indian women over 30 showed moderate to severe pigmented marionette lines.[4] An approach to rejuvenation in this area

must, therefore, include not only fillers but also peels and frequent maintenance to control pigment in this area.

The approach to the South Asian patient should stress the use of sunscreen, including the use of chemical peels to improve skin clarity, as these are well tolerated in South Asian skin, and procedures for the under-eye area to improve pigment and hollows around the eyes. Fillers can be used in the mid-face but keep in mind that tightening procedures are more likely to be helpful in the 40s and 50s in this ethnic group since the volume changes are predominantly contributed to by ptosis of fat pockets. Lastly, the neck is a common concern in South Asian populations and should be addressed either with toxins for the necklace lines or skin-tightening procedures for neck fullness that is common in this demographic.

24.3.3 Evaluation of Middle Eastern Skin

For patients from the Middle East, the use of fillers and neuromodulators is quite high and well accepted. Body shape is of particular concern and should be discussed at any cosmetic consultation. Men and women in the Middle East belong to three distinct racial clusters: Bedouin (genetically closest to Europeans), Persian–South Asian (from which many Iranians are descendants), and African. Therefore, the approach to this ethnic group will be in some ways a combination of treatments from other ethnic groups, depending on the ancestry of the patient. In general, Middle Eastern beauty is characterized by striking eyes, defined cheeks, and full lips.[5]

When assessing Middle Eastern patients, one of the important things to keep in mind for any injection scheme is the cultural attire the patient wears on a regular basis. Rounder faces with fuller cheeks are preferred among women who wear a full hijab because it looks more attractive than a thinner, a narrower face enveloped by the scarf. For women who wear a niqab, large, wide, striking, almond-shaped eyes are considered the beauty ideal. A wide upper-lid margin area that further emphasizes the eye and eyebrows that are arched and elevated with a lateral eyebrow flare are favored.

For the submental area, sagging or submental fat is a top aesthetic concern, and facial contouring with liposuction in this area, cryolipolysis or ultrasound skin tightening is often sought after. As compared to Asians and Southeast Asians, the paradigm for the Middle East is a straight profile—in other words, an oval face, a straight nose, fuller lips, laterally full cheeks, a pointed chin, and elevated, thick, arched eyebrows.

To achieve this look, fillers are a key component of the consultation. Use of fillers should focus on the temple area, the lateral eyebrow, and potentially even into flat or convex areas of the forehead. It is important for patients in this ethnic subgroup to have a wide and high forehead and a smooth contour. Biostimulatory fillers are particularly useful for this application.

For eye shape, consider the injection of neuromodulators into the pretarsal orbicularis oculi and pretarsal palpebral muscles in the medial and lateral canthus to create wider-looking eyes. Fillers should be used to improve the tear trough area, and consider nonablative fractionated lasers for skin tone clarity. Due to the climate in this region, maintenance routines and frequent touch-ups to improve skin tone and brightness should be discussed during any comprehensive assessment to maintain results.

In general, an assessment of Middle Eastern patients should include sunscreen and the use of chemical peels to maintain skin tone. Fillers predominate the aesthetic toolbox for this subgroup as compared to many of the others, and body contouring for the submental region is a must.

24.3.4 Evaluation of African Skin

Like the other ethnic groups discussed so far, African patients can vary tremendously in skin phototype from IV to VI. On a cellular level, the pH of black skin is lower than that of white skin, and it is known that there is variable racial blood vessel reactivity across skin types. Dyschromia tends to be noted earlier and with greater intensity in this subgroup compared to Caucasian counterparts. There is also a tendency toward freckling, labial lentigos, and keloidal scarring. The latter is not affected by fillers but should be noted before attempting medium-depth peels or laser resurfacing.

For the African patient, volume loss in the midface is the predominant sign of aging, with flattening of the midface and prominence of the nasolabial folds. Jowls and neck fullness are secondary and appear much later in this ethnic group.

Benign growths of the skin, like dermatosis papulosa nigricans, are exceedingly common and can be cleared quickly and with little scarring risk via electrodesiccation. Dyschromias can be treated effectively with medium-depth peels, and while caution should be used with this type of chemical peel, African skin can tolerate them, and the results for dyschromia are quite impressive.

One of the key areas of aging that occurs in this ethnic group is around the mouth. Although African patients will have fewer perioral rhytids compared to Caucasians, black women will often seek augmentation not to increase the size of their lips but rather to restore their lip size to that of their youth. As such, it is usually not necessary to enhance the vermillion border. Rhytids that develop in this area occur predominantly in the body of the lip below the vermillion border. Typically, the lower lip will maintain its appearance while the upper lip loses volume and the philtral ridges flatten out. The ratio should approach more closely 1:1, and hyaluronic acid filler injections should be used to superiorly roll the lip. Minute doses of botulinumtoxinA can be used for relaxation of the periorbicularis oris musculature to resolve perioral rhytids, but this author tends to stay away from this technique in anyone over the age of 45 due to slight phonation changes that can occur.

In the midface, simple volume restoration ameliorates most nasolabial folds. Caution should be used to place filler at the apex of the cheek and in the medial midface as lateral placement can make the face look widened. The prominence of the zygomatic retaining ligament is amplified with time which can be softened and corrected with filler. A bolus of 0.1–0.2 ml of product is injected perpendicular to the periosteum to accurately place filler at the origin of the ligament and then create an elevation of the skin to soften the fat pad displacement.

In the tear trough area, medial hollowing occurs but usually not until the 50s for which filler is able to achieve the proper correction. Typically skin texture is not an issue, though pigmentary demarcation lines are common, like in the South Asian group.

Overall, the assessment of the African patient should pay attention to skin tone and post-inflammatory hyperpigmentation, followed by the appropriate use of fillers to volumize the lips, followed by the cheeks in order to soften the nasolabial folds.

24.3.5 Evaluation of Hispanic Skin

Outside of Caucasian patients, Hispanic/Latino patients represent the largest proportion of the growing aesthetic patient demographic. When surveyed, a majority were aware of facial treatments and procedures (over 75% for dermal fillers, under-chin fat reduction, neuromodulators, chemical peels, and skin-tightening procedures).[6] Fabi et al. reported results of a survey which showed that 69% of Hispanic and Latina women would consider neuromodulators in the next two years while 49% would consider laser skin resurfacing. The result is that when assessing a patient in this ethnic subgroup, be aware that you are most likely speaking with a very educated consumer who is aware of multiple modalities of treatment and also one who is willing to try procedures in the upper third of the face.

Dyschromia is a common concern for Hispanic patients and can be treated easily with chemical peels and intense pulsed light. The cautionary tale here is to remember that while this demographic can present as skin phototype II, the patient can hyperpigment after a procedure like a skin phototype IV. Thus it is important to pre-treat with retinoids or skin-lightening agents prior to any procedure for skin tone and to closely watch sun exposure afterward. Patients are compliant with maintenance routines, including topicals, and should be counseled on the regular use of sunscreen to help with pigment alterations.

As compared to the other patient groups discussed so far, Hispanic patients do often suffer the effects of solar damage that manifest as deeper lines and wrinkles in the forehead and in the crow's feet. An arched brow is desirable, so a neuromodulator injection scheme to address the forehead and glabellar lines should center around eyebrow elevation and lateral arch as well.

The other top area of concern is the submental region. Sagging of the neck and underneath the chin ranks as a relatively important area of concern for most patients in this group. While injectables for submental fat reduction are certainly an option, beware of lingering post-inflammatory hyperpigmentation that can result from bruising. The same goes for cryolipolysis.

Because the ethnic group contains such a truly diverse array of patients, assessment should be approached based on deficits commonly noted in that skin phototype. The assessment should also be informed by the fact that performing procedures carries very little taboo among Hispanic patients, and most are interested in trying procedures to ameliorate their cosmetic concerns.

24.4 Conclusion

Much of what we teach and are taught about facial aesthetics is based upon a Caucasian and Eurocentric viewpoint of ratios and angles. The facial canon for various ethnic groups has not been fully developed, and for this reason, it is important to learn from global thought leaders on the best techniques to respect facial architecture not across races but rather within ethnic groups. When performing an assessment, it is reassuring for patients to know that their treating physician understands their unique bony architecture and can create a paradigm that will help them to look their best.

References

1. Alexiades M, Chantrey J, Chatrath V et al. Allergan 360⁰ Aesthetics Report™. Accessed online January 2021: www.allergan.com/-/media/allergan/documents/us/Media-Resources/Allergan-360-Report-Full.pdf
2. Sundaram H, Huang PH, Hsu NJ et al. Aesthetic applications of botulinum toxin A in Asians: An international, multidisciplinary Pan-Asian consensus. Plast Reconstr Surg Glob Open. 2016;4:e872.
3. Shome D, Vadera S, Desai N et al. Aging and the Indian face: An analytical study of aging in the Asian Indian face. Plast Reconstr Surg Global Open. 2020 Mar;8(3):e2580.
4. Singh N, Thappa DM. Pigmentary demarcation lines. Pigment Int [serial online]. 2014;1:13–16.
5. Kashmar M, Alsufyani MA, Ghalamkarpour F. Consensus opinion on facial beauty and implications for aesthetic treatment in Middle Eastern Women. Plast Reconstr Glob Open. 2019;7:e2220.
6. Fabi S, Montes JR, Aguilerea SB. Understanding the female Hispanic and Latino American facial aesthetic patient. JDD. 2019;18(7):623–663

CHAPTER 25: AGING IN MIDDLE EASTERN SKIN

Sahar Ghannam

25.1 Introduction

People of color who identify as African American, Asian, Native American, Hispanic, and Arab are diverse both genotypically and phenotypically. Skin color and hair texture vary greatly among and within these groups. Appreciation of these differences, together with an understanding of their cultural habits, is crucial to be able to deliver the best care. Literature describing aging in the Middle Eastern region are scarce compared with those of Asians, African Americans, or Hispanics.[1-3] It is necessary for every physician dealing with Arab patients to be aware of the fact that the skin phenotype of people residing in the Middle East is generally between Fitzpatrick types III–VI, depending on their origins.[4] Egypt and the Arabian peninsula have seen waves of migrations over the past 50,000 years. Genotyping studies of Arabian peninsula populations reveal three distinct clusters that reflect their primary ancestry:[5]

1. Bedouin (genetically closest to Europeans)
2. Persian–South Asian (genetically between Bedouins and Asian and from which many Iranians are descended)
3. African (less closely related to the Middle Eastern cluster)

Residents of the Gulf area are usually a combination of these three types.[4, 6]

The physical characters of modern Egyptians are said to be derived from the originally indigenous African population (the pharaohs), Arabs, and Europeans (Greeks, British, and French).[4, 6, 7] The Lebanese, Syrians, and Palestinians have descended from the Phoenicians, who had their origins in the eastern Mediterranean but are also genetically influenced by the Islamic expansion from the Arabian peninsula and the Ottomans and European populations.[4, 8, 9]

The focus of this chapter will be on the Middle Eastern population and the biomechanics of aging in them. It is imperative to have a knowledge of these facts to understand the diversity among skin types and also appreciate why sometimes a person with Fitzpatrick type III might behave like a Fitzpatrick type V with procedures. It is not only the skin type that affects the aging process but also a wide range of extrinsic and intrinsic factors. Aging is inevitable and is a marker that reflects biological changes, as well as cultural and social conventions.[10, 11] More than 300 divergent theories have been put forward to explain why aging occurs.[10] While many are outdated and are only useful from a historical perspective, others have no experimental data to support or refute them. Overall the aging theories could be divided into three groups: causal, systemic, and evolutionary.[12, 13] A causal theory of particular interest is the theory of cellular damage, in which reactive oxygen species (ROS) are one of the factors that have been documented to contribute to cellular damage and aging.[14] Basically, the immune response produces an excess of ROS and matrix metalloproteinases which are enzymes that degrade the skin matrix and accelerate the external symptoms of aging.[15]

25.2 Stress and Aging Skin

Another contributing factor along the same lines is stress and telomere shortening. A great deal of literature has been described in relation to stress and aging wherein multiple studies have shown that stress impairs longevity.[16, 17] Internal, external, and emotional triggers contribute to aging skin as they create micro-inflammatory pathways that lead to cellular damage.[16, 18] Stress is majorly categorized into three types: acute stress, episodic acute stress, and chronic stress. A recent category added due to technological advancements, global events, and the rapid rate of communication by social media is termed cultural stress, to accurately reflect the changing events in human history. Cultural stress is pervasive and constant.[10]

Although we all know the effects of stress on our bodies, little is spoken about it in the context of facial rejuvenation. Why do some patients get dramatic results with energy-based devices or injectables, and why do others not? The answer may be related to their stress levels and how various individuals deal with it.

25.3 Cutaneous Anatomical Features and Aging Skin

The diversity of skin type plays a large role in skin response and facial structure differences.

A large anthropometric study comparing different ethnic groups of North American Caucasians revealed that the most significant differences in facial proportions were in the orbital region, nasal heights, and nasal widths.[19] Caucasian intercanthal widths were identical to the African ethnic group, in contrast with the Middle Eastern and Asian groups that showed greater intercanthal widths with smaller eye openings. A narrower nasal base and larger tip projection were noted in Caucasians compared to Asians and African Americans.[19] Skin aging is also associated with progressive atrophy of the dermis and changes in the architectural organization leading to folds and wrinkles.[20] Asian and black skin has a relatively thicker and more compact dermis, a thicker stratum corneum, and a greater lipid content, compared to fairer skin types, with the thickness being proportional to the degree of pigmentation.[21-23] This likely contributes to the lower incidence of facial rhytides in them.

Akin to Asians and Hispanics, there is a wide variety of skin types and ethnicities comprising the term Arabs and/or Middle Easterners. In general, they tend to have more sebaceous glands, which explains the typical concern about open pores. They also have rounder heavy faces, especially in the midface, sometimes similar to Hispanics, which could lead to an increased predisposition to develop marionette lines, deep nasolabial grooves, and unsightly jowls.[24, 25]

They also have a greater tendency to develop periorbital changes like periocular hyperpigmentation, accentuation of tear trough, and perioral changes in the form of deep marionette lines.[1, 23]

25.4 Pigmentary Disorders

Melanin is the major determinant of skin color, and the concentration of epidermal melanin in darker skin is much higher compared to lightly pigmented skin types.[26] In addition, melanosome degradation within the keratinocyte is slower in dark-pigmented people. Overall, darker skin has singly dispersed,

DOI: 10.1201/9780429243769-25

large melanosomes that contain more melanin compared with the smaller, aggregated, less melanin-containing melanosomes that occur in lighter-skinned persons. The melanin content and melanosomal dispersion pattern are thought to confer protection from accelerated aging induced by ultraviolet (UV) radiation.[27, 28] In fact, Kaidbey et al. demonstrated that a greater epidermal melanin content provided greater photoprotection (SPF of 13.40).[27] Although the increased melanin provides protection from many harmful effects of UV radiation, including photodamage and skin cancers, it also makes darkly pigmented skin more vulnerable to dyspigmentation. Therefore, inconsistent pigmentation with both hypo- and hyperpigmentation is a sign of photoaging in people with skin of color.

Dyschromia and hyperpigmentation are two of the primary complaints in Middle Eastern patients. In fact, El-Essawi et al. reported that uneven skin tone and skin discoloration are two of the most concerning skin problems among Arab Americans, with more than 50% of the survey participants expressing such concerns.[29] This has also been repeatedly reported in other ethnic groups.[30]

These hyperpigmentation disorders are usually in the form of melasma, post-acne eruptive hyperpigmentation, pigmented contact dermatitis (Riehl's melanosis), and lichen planus pigmentosus, which are usually exaggerated with aging.[30] It is very crucial, when addressing problems of pigmentation in Middle Eastern patients, to achieve a balance between tolerability and efficacy without causing additional inflammation or damage that could trigger even more post-inflammatory hyperpigmentation (PIH).

25.5 Consultation for the Aging Face

The first consultation is long and extensive, usually lasting for 45–60 minutes. The patient is given a full detailed explanation of the aging process together with all the rejuvenating options available, including surgery. If the patient opts for a nonsurgical method, the need for multiple treatment sessions must be explained to them. Sessions could be with injectables alone or injectables together with energy-based devices. The interval between any two sessions is not less than three weeks.

A detailed history of their home care cosmeceutical regimen, including sun protection, is noted.

Although almost all patients acknowledge having sunblocks and applying them, they either apply very little or do not reapply after a couple of hours. The importance of sunscreens is explained to the patients, not only to guard against further pigmentation but also because it was shown that the daily use of a facial broad-spectrum photostable sunscreen might visibly reverse signs of existing photodamage.[31] In calculating the sun protection factor (SPF), the FDA uses a dose of 2.2 mg/cm² of exposed skin.[32] In reality, individuals apply as little as or less than a quarter of this recommended dose which reduces the effect of the sunscreen by almost four times.[33]

Educating people to apply a quantity that they feel is too much or too greasy will simply not work! To add to this dilemma, we now know that visible light (VL) may have a role in increasing pigmentation in conditions aggravated by sun exposure, such as PIH and melasma, especially in dark-skinned individuals.[34]

Patients are educated that everything they apply in the morning should contain photoprotection; the moisturizer or the primer should have an SPF, and a tinted or non-tinted sunblock with an SPF of 50 topped with a tinted blemish balm (BB) cream, or another tinted sunblock with an SPF of 50 must be used. The goal is applying as much as two fingers' worth of product. This will give approximately 9%, which is one area of the body in accordance with the rule of nine. This will provide a dose that approximates the required 2 mg/cm². The importance of tinted sunscreens is also emphasized over clear ones, as tinted sunscreens, especially those containing iron oxide, are capable of absorbing visible light.[30, 35] All patients should be put on a home-based rejuvenating topical regimen. For patient compliance, it is best to change home care creams every few months. The most commonly prescribed cosmeceuticals are retinol, L-ascorbic acid, exfoliators, hydroquinone, or non-hydroquinone products.[30]

A detailed history of diseases and medications, if any, should be noted and explained, as chronic diseases such as diabetes mellitus, which is an aging disease on its own, can make the rejuvenating process difficult. Stress is another major issue, and its effect on aging is explained to the patient.

The author typically tells patients to consider aging as a chronic disease, and like any other chronic disease, this, too, needs lifelong treatment. A pre-procedure photograph of the patient is taken after obtaining consent. During the procedure, a diagram of the procedure is inserted in the patient chart for ease of follow-up (Figure 25.1).

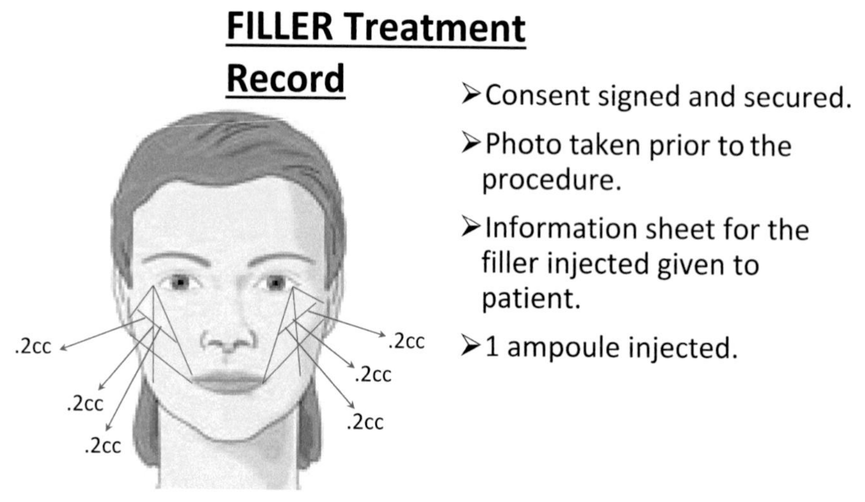

FILLER Treatment Record

> Consent signed and secured.

> Photo taken prior to the procedure.

> Information sheet for the filler injected given to patient.

> 1 ampoule injected.

.2cc .2cc .2cc .2cc .2cc .2cc

FIGURE 25.1   Dermatology and cosmetology clinic.

25.6 Case 1

A female aged 50 years presented with the typical features of aging like deep nasolabial folds, marionette lines, blotchy pigmentation, and open pores. She began her treatment in 2011. The pre- and post-photographs are listed eight years apart (Figure 25.2).

Through the years, she was injected with 7.5 mL of calcium hydroxyl apatite and 16 mL of hyaluronic acid fillers. The repair of deep nasolabial and marionette lines in elderly females should be performed in stages. Injection points were typically placed on the zygoma at two points, where the maximum lift occurs. The jawline was addressed with two or three points 5 mm apart. Injections at any given point were not more than 0.01–0.02 mL. Sessions were spaced three to four months apart.

The injectable sessions were coupled with superficial chemical peels for her dyschromia and home care in the form of sun protection and retinol, L-ascorbic acid, and non-hydroquinone-based night cream, along with occasional use of hydroquinone.

This was a case successfully demonstrating the process of rejuvenation with non-invasive procedures.

25.7 Cases 2 and 3

Two female patients aged around 50 years, with skin type III, presented with typical features of aging, like deep nasolabial grooves and deep marionette lines. Both of them declined doing any kind of energy-based devices (EBD), although they agreed on the session treatments with injectables and home care.

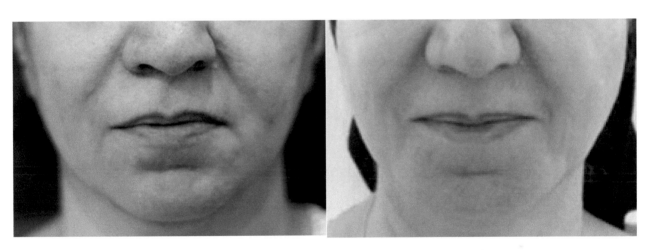

Pre   Post 8 years

FIGURE 25.2A   Case 1 (A).

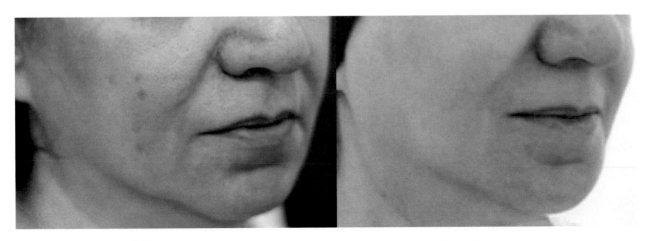

pre   Post 8 years

FIGURE 25.2B   Case 1 (B).

Case #2 achieved improvement after five sessions, three to four months apart, injecting not more than 2 mL of hyaluronic acid at any given time (Figure 25.3).

Case #3 could not achieve a satisfying improvement even after eight sessions, three to four months apart, again injecting anywhere between 2–3 mL of hyaluronic acid at any given time. This patient had other comorbidities in the form of diabetes mellitus and inflammatory bowel disease, increasing the burden of inflammatory mediators and ROS, which could be one of the contributory factors in the failure of her treatment (Figure 25.4).

In both cases, to repair the nasolabial and the marionette grooves, injections were first placed on the zygomatic bone as a rule. The home care regimen was sunscreens in the morning and a vitamin C serum at night topped with a retinol cream. Topical brands were changed every few months for compliance.

25.8 Case 4

A 45-year-old female with an inherent heavy midface began treatment in 2009. Through the years, she was injected with 30 mL of hyaluronic acid. Heavy-faced patients require a lot of hyaluronic acid, which should be done in stages to achieve the desired appearance. Injection points should be deep on the bone, totally avoiding the already inherent heavy midface. It must be noted here that the patient's left marionette fold was not totally ameliorated, the main reason being that the patient had lost a tooth and did not replace it. Dentition is of clinical significance as it affects the outcome of the procedure and should be outlined to the patient. She also had eight sessions of bipolar radiofrequency, four sessions of platelet-rich plasma (PRP) therapy through the years. The patient was also put on home care in the form of exfoliators, retinol, and L-ascorbic acid together, with sun protection (Figures 25.5 and 25.6).

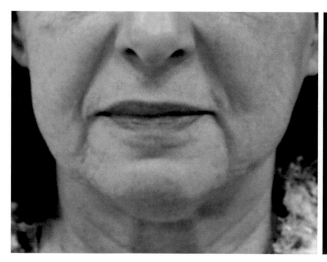
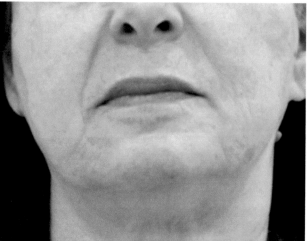

FIGURE 25.3　Case 2.

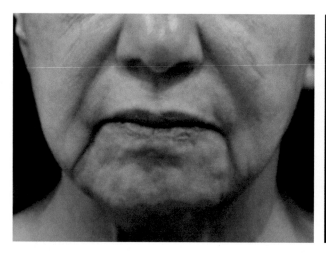
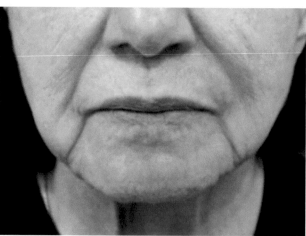

FIGURE 25.4　Case 3.

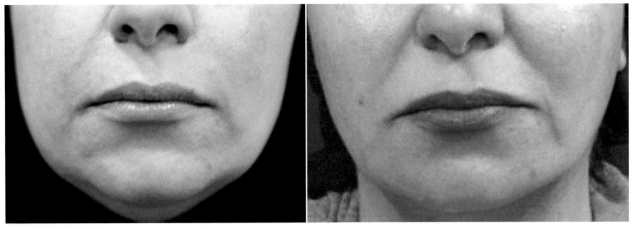

pre   Post 9 years

FIGURE 25.5 Case 4.

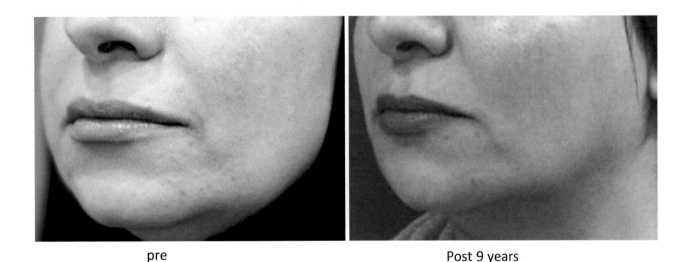

pre   Post 9 years

FIGURE 25.6 Case 4.

25.9 Case 5

A 55-year-old female presented to us with long-standing melasma. Her treatment regimen was in the form of various forms of triple combination creams omitting the steroids and adding L-ascorbic acid together at times with azelaic acid and superficial chemical peels. For patients of melasma with a greater tendency toward post-inflammatory hyperpigmentation, like our current patient, the author prefers retinol-based chemical peels. The course of treatment was complicated with remissions and flares. Patients with melasma should be informed about the chronic nature of the condition and that relapses are common whenever there is unprotected sun exposure. Attempts to repair her marionette fold with injectables failed until the patient fixed her teeth which emphasizes the importance of dentition as the backbone supporting soft tissue structures (Figures 25.7 and 25.8).

25.10 Case 6

A 50-year-old female patient presented with severe nasolabial and melolabial folds. She was initiated on a home-care regimen initially and later started on injections of 8 ml hyaluronic acid for 13 consecutive months (Figure 25.9).

25.11 Cases 7, 8, and 9

Three elderly female patients, all in their 50s, presented with various forms of dyschromia, blotchy hyperpigmentation, and melasma. After a thorough explanation of their condition, a conservative approach was considered best to begin with, in the form of sun protection and local home care, starting with a combination cream of hydroquinone, retinol, and L-ascorbic acid on alternate days at night. The patients were followed up after two weeks to observe for signs of irritation and later

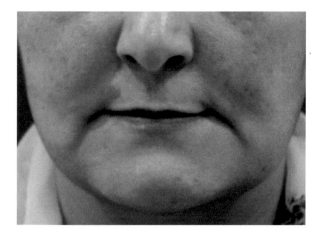

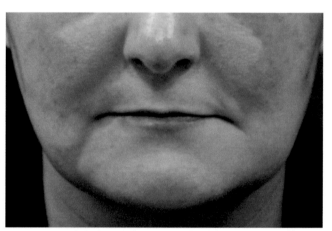

pre

Improvement of melasma

FIGURE 25.7 Case 5.

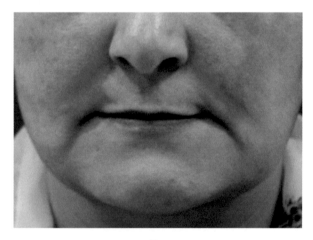

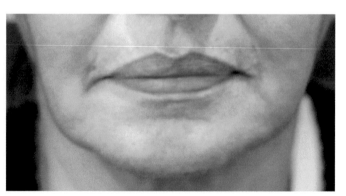

Pre

Relapse of melasma
Improved melobial fold

FIGURE 25.8 Case 5.

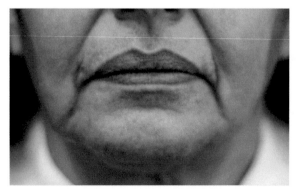

pre

post

FIGURE 25.9 Case 6.

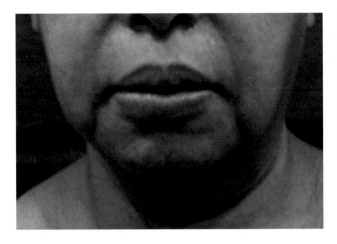

FIGURE 25.10 Case 7.

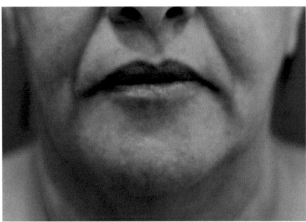

FIGURE 25.11 Case 8.

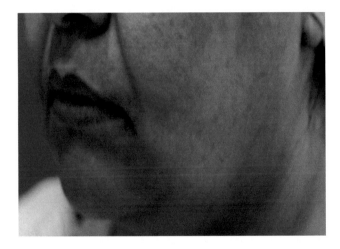

FIGURE 25.12 Case 9.

advised to switch to daily application. A step-wise treatment is a way to ensure efficacy avoiding the risk of more PIH. Superficial chemical peels were only introduced later on once the compliance of the patient was established (Figures 25.10, 25.11, and 25.12).

References

1. Vashi N, Buainain M, Kundu RV. Aging differences in ethnic skin. J Clin Aesthet Dermatol. 2016;9(1):31–38.
2. Halder R, Richards G. Photoaging in patients of skin colour. In: Rigel D, Weiss R, Lim H, Dover J, editors. Photoaging. New York: Marcel Dekker; 2004: 55–63.
3. de Rigal J, Des Mazis I, Diridollou S, et al. The effect of age on skin color and color heterogeneity in four ethnic groups. Skin Res Technol. 2010;16(2):168–178.
4. Kashmar M, Ghannam S, Ghalamkarpour F, et al. Consensus opinions on facial beauty and implications for aesthetic treatment in Middle Eastern women. PRS Global Open. 2019;1–11.
5. Omberg L, Salit J, Hackett N, et al. Inferring genome-wide patterns of admixture in Qataris using fifty-five ancestral populations. BMC Genet. 2012;13:49.
6. National Geographic. Genographic project/reference populations-geno 2.0 next generation 2018. Available at https://genographic.nationalgeographic.com/reference-populations-next-gen/. Accessed 19 January 2018.
7. National Geographic. Genetic Study Reveals Ancient Legacies in Lebanon. Genographic Project. 2008. Available at https://genographic.nationalgeographic.com/genetic-study-reveals-ancientlegacies-in-lebanon/ Accessed 18 January 2018.
8. Zalloua PA, Platt DE, El Sibai M, et al. Identifying genetic traces of historical expansions: Phoenician footprints in the Mediterranean. Am J Hum Genet. 2008;83:633–691.
9. Zalloua PA, Xue Y, Khalife J, et al. Y-chromosomal diversity in Lebanon is structured by recent historical events. AM J Hum Genet. 2008;82:873–882.
10. Murad H. Thoughts on the process of aging. Cosmetic Dermatol. 2009 February; 22(2):74–78.
11. Kirkwood TB. The origins of human ageing. Philos Trans R Soc Lond B Biol Sci. 1997;352:1765–1772.
12. Zs-Nagy I. The Membrane Hypothesis of Aging. Sark, Great Britain: International Antiaging Systems; 2003.
13. Kyriazis M. The Cross-Linking Theory of Aging. Sark, Great Britain: International Antiaging Systems; 2003.
14. Murad H. Skin immunity-the new anti-aging frontier. Les Nouvelles Esthetiques Spa. 2008;7:130–136.
15. Ferguson MW, O'Kane S. Scar-free healing: From embryonic mechanisms to adult therapeutic intervention. Phil Trans R Soc Land B Biol Sci. 2004;359:839–850.
16. Sapolsky RM. Organismal stress and telomeric aging: An unexpected connection. Proc Natl Acad Sci U S A. 2004;101:17323–17324.
17. Riddle CC, Liu D, Aires DJ. Antiaging: Where are the data? Cosmet Dermatol. 2007;20:313–320.
18. Jiang H, Ju Z, Rudolph KL. Telomere shortening and ageing. Z Gerontol Geriatr. 2007;40:314–324.
19. Farkas LG, Katic MJ, Forrest CR, et al. International anthropometric study of facial morphology in various ethnic groups/races. J Craniofac Surg. 2005;16(4):615–646.
20. Lapiere CM. The ageing dermis: The main cause for the appearance of "old" skin. Br J Dermatol. 1990;122(Suppl 35):5–11.
21. Montagna W, Prota G, Kenney J. The structure of black skin. In: Montagna W, Prota G, Kenney J, editors. Black Skin Structure and Function. Gulf Professional Publishing; 1993.
22. Sugino K, Imokawa G, Maibach H. Ethnic differences in stratum corneum lipid in relation to stratum corneum function (abstr). J Invest Dermatol. 1993;100:594.
23. de Rigal J, Des Mazis I, Diridollou S, et al. The effect of age on 22. Skin color and color heterogeneity in four ethnic groups. Skin Res Technol. 2010;16(2):168–178.
24. Alexis AF, Alam M. Racial and ethnic differences in skin aging: Implications for treatment with soft tissue fillers. J Drugs Dermatol. 2012;11(8):s30–s32; discussion s2.
25. Cobo R, Garcia CA. Aesthetic surgery for the Mestizo/Hispanic patient: Special considerations. Facial Plastic Surg. 2010;26(2):164–173.
26. Iozumi K, Hoganson GE, Pennella R, et al. Role of tyrosinase as the determinant of pigmentation in cultured human melanocytes. J Invest Dermatol. 1993;100(6):806–811.
27. Kaidbey KH, Agin PP, Sayre RM, Kligman AM. Photoprotection by melanin—a comparison of black and Caucasian skin. J Am Acad Dermatol. 1979;1(3):249–260.
28. Taylor SC. Skin of color: Biology, structure, function, and implications for dermatologic disease. J Am Acad Dermatol. 2002;46(2 Suppl Understanding):S41–S62.
29. El-Esaawi D, Musial JL, Hammad A, et al. A survey of skin disease and skin related issues in Arab Americans. J Am Acad Dermatol. 2007;56:913–938.

30. Silpa-archa N, Kohli I, Chaowattanapanit S, et al. Postinflammatory hyperpigmentation: A comprehensive overview. J Am Acad Dermatol. 2017;77;591–605.

31. Randhawa M, Wang S, Leyden JJ, et al. Daily use of a facial broad spectrum sunscreen over one year significantly improves clinical evaluation of photoaging. Derm Surg. 2016;42:1135–1361.

32. Maslin D. Do sunscreens protect us? Int J Dermatol. 2014;1319–1323.

33. Reich A, Harupa M, Bury M, et al. Application of sunscreen preparation: A need to change the regulations. Photodermatol Photoimmunol Photomed. 2009;25:242–244.

34. Mahmoud BH, et al. Impact of long-wavelength and visible light on melanocompetent skin. J Invest Dermatol. 2010;130:2092.

35. Castanedo-Cazares JP, Hernandez-Blanco D, Carlos-Ortega B, et al. Near visible light and UV photoprotection in the treatment of melasma: A double-blind randomized trial. Photodermatol Photoimmunol Photomed.2014;30:35–42.

CHAPTER 26: MINIMIZING COMPLICATIONS IN SKIN OF COLOR

Jaishree Sharad

Aesthetic procedures in Fitzpatrick skin types IV–VI have always been challenging in the past due to the impending complications. However, in the recent past, better technologies, research, and studies have been helpful in reducing the complications with procedures such as peels, lasers, injectables, and so on, for skin of color.

Ethnic skin, or skin of color, is characterized by increased epidermal melanin, larger melanosomes that are more singly dispersed and widely distributed within epidermal keratinocytes, labile melanocytes, and reactive fibroblast responses (1). These characteristics pose bigger challenges while treating skin of color with laser and light-based devices.

Careful patient selection and setting realistic expectations prior to starting treatment are the most important preliminary steps to ensure a favorable outcome.

The following is the protocol while doing aesthetic procedures on skin of color:

- *History*: In order to prevent or reduce the chances of complications with any procedure, a careful history is extremely essential. History of herpes simplex infections, keloids, hypertrophic scarring, contact dermatitis, atopic dermatitis, photosensitivity, use of photosensitive drugs, and most importantly, post-inflammatory hyperpigmentation (PIH) should be asked (2). Also, ask the patient about his/her habits, such as exposure to sunlight, occupation of the patient, picking the skin, outdoor activities (be it for work or sport), regular scrubbing, swimming, and smoking—all of which can aggravate the chances of PIH post-procedure. History of any side effects with any treatments in the past must not be missed.
- *Examination*: Careful examination under good lighting is mandatory. Look for any signs of infection, eczema, scaling, keloids, and PIH. Sometimes, habitual pickers will not give you their history, but upon examination, you can identify them.
  The treatment site should be examined again on the day of the treatment to rule out any active infection or hotspots (erythema, dryness, flaking of skin) (3).
- *Counseling*: Pre-treatment counseling about pre- and post-care, immediate reaction of the skin to treatment, downtime, and what to expect will go a long way in obtaining better results. Do not forget to ask if the patient has any events that require public appearances (e.g., marriage, parties, conference) within two weeks of any treatment to avoid unpleasant surprises. Time your treatments well before such events.

26.1 General Pre-Treatment Care for Chemical Peels, Microneedling, Microneedling Radiofrequency (MNRF), Platelet-Rich Plasma, and Laser and Light Devices

Complications can be avoided or minimized with proper pre-treatment care.

26.1.1 Pre-Treatment Priming (4)

Priming the skin reduces wound healing time. It also enforces the concept of a maintenance regimen. In the case of chemical peels, priming also helps in uniform penetration of the peeling agent, thereby decreasing PIH.

Three to four weeks prior to the treatment:

- Start the patient on broad-spectrum sunscreen.
- A skin-lightening cream containing kojic acid, hydroquinone, azelaic acid, lactic acid, and vitamin C can be added.
- Topical retinoids, salicylic-acid-based creams, or 6% glycolic acid cream are other options that help in mild exfoliation and make the stratum corneum more compact.

One week prior to treatment:

- Stop salicylic acid or glycolic-acid-based face wash.
- Avoid scrubs, loofahs, facials, and microdermabrasion.
- Avoid bleaching, waxing, electrolysis, and laser hair removal.
- Avoid hair dyeing and permanent hair straightening.

Four to five days prior to treatment:

- Stop all priming creams.

On the day of treatment:

- Avoid scrubbing and use of colognes and cosmetics. In the case of peels, avoid shaving too.

General post-treatment care:

- Immediate post-treatment cooling using ice is mandatory in case of chemical peels (except leave-on peels) and laser and light treatments.
- In the case of treatments like microneedling or MNRF, a topical antibiotic may be given (5, 6).
- In case of erythema more than expected or if a patient complains of a burning sensation, icing followed by the application of a mild corticosteroid can help prevent further damage.
- Patients should be strongly encouraged to use all means of sun protection. A broad-spectrum sunscreen, umbrellas, wide-rimmed hats wherever possible, and of course, avoiding outdoor activities for a week after the peel or laser will minimize risks of prolonged erythema, PIH, and scarring.
- A soap-free cleanser should be used to wash the face.
- Irritant cleansers such as Dettol and abrasive scrubs should be strictly avoided for a week.
- The importance of letting the skin heal on its own and not picking at the skin should be emphasized thoroughly.
- The patient should also be advised against getting into chlorinated water for at least 72 hours to prevent PIH.
- Avoid retinoids and AHA creams for a week or until the skin peels.

- Facial procedures like steaming, scrubbing, waxing, bleaching, or facials should not be allowed for at least ten days to two weeks after the treatment.
- Use of emollients can be advocated.
- The patient must be advised to immediately inform the doctor if there is excessive burning/pain, redness, swelling, crusting, oozing, or blister formation after any procedure.

26.2 Special Considerations While Doing Chemical Peels: Step-by-Step, Shehnaz in Aesthetic Derm

- *Agent used and its concentration*: Select a peel according to patient characteristics, desired depth, and indication. Always start with low peel concentration and titrate to tolerability. Both the strength of the peel and the time to neutralization can be increased with each subsequent peel. Also decide on the volume of peel to be used. Overusing a product will not give better results (7).
- *Pre-peel preparation*: Remove all makeup. Tie a hair band so that the peel doesn't get spilled onto the hair and trickle onto the face. Proper degreasing with chlorhexidine, acetone, and spirit is important for better penetration of the peel. Apply occlusive ointment to under eyes, lips, and ala corners, and also protect the ear canal.
  - Keep a neutralizer at hand in case hot spots develop.
  - Never hold a peel bottle over a patient's head.
  - Keep a syringe with cold water ready in case of any spillage of peel solution into the patient's eyes (8).
- *Method of application*: Sequential application over the entire surface that needs to be peeled can prevent overlap. Decide on the number of coats and adhere to them. Avoid rubbing the peel on the skin. If you notice any erythema or flaking in any area, avoid applying a peel in that area. Time your peels and neutralize accordingly, in order to prevent a longer duration of contact than desired. In the case of some peels like Trichloroacetic acid (TCA), do not apply more peel solution in areas where you begin to see frosting. Apply ice if there is undesired frosting or a severe burning sensation.
  - Use clean cotton buds and brushes to apply the peel to prevent any infection.
  - Avoid causing demarcation lines by feathering the peel into the surrounding normal skin.
- *Special post-care advice*
  Advise the patient not to use hot water to wash the face or take steam.

  Patients should be informed that after a peel, erythema and desquamation may occur for one to seven days. Ask the patient not to remove the skin, which starts peeling in a day or two, however tempting it may be. Tell them the significance of not picking at the skin.

  If there is severe crusting, a topical antibacterial ointment should be used to prevent infection.

  Space peels should be two to four weeks apart.

  Bleaching, waxing, or any other form of hair removal should only be done two weeks after a peel.

  One must also avoid any laser treatments after a peel for at least three weeks in dark-skinned patients.

  Do not prescribe any new topical agent during the maintenance period after a peel.

Ask the patient to avoid any home remedies for quicker peeling or healing of the skin in order to prevent irritant contact dermatitis or allergic contact dermatitis.

- *Gel peels*: In case of dark-skinned patients with a history of PIH or sensitive skin, or even atopic skin, gel peels may be considered to avoid complications. Gel peels allow slow penetration of the peeling agent and ensure maximum acid delivery to the target area without causing irritation.

  They minimize pooling and runoff of the solution.

Immediate care in case of a suspected complication:

- *Pain, burning, or persistent erythema*: Prolonged sun exposure, inadequate application of sunscreen, and using a topical retinoid or glycolic acid immediately after peels can lead to these complications (9). Paradoxically, in some patients, sunscreens can cause contact sensitization or irritant dermatitis (10).
- *Pruritus*: It may be a normal occurence following re-epithelialization. In such cases, an emollient will help. Pruritis may also occur due to contact dermatitis to a topical agent (retinoid or citric acid or any chemical in their cosmetics or home remedies used by them for quicker healing). If papules, pustules, and erythema occur along with pruritus, it is suspected to be contact dermatitis, and treatment should start as early as possible to prevent PIH (9).
- *Infection*: Both topical and systemic antibiotics should be given immediately in case of any pustules or bacterial infection. Oral acyclovir should be started a day before a peel in case of patients with history of herpes simplex infection. However, sometimes patients may forget to give such a history, and there may be a flare-up of herpes post-peel. A proper course of acyclovir or valacyclovir should be given immediately in such cases.
- *PIH*: If you suspect PIH, give a mild corticosteroid topically. Ask the patient to avoid sun exposure and slather sunscreen even indoors. Topical tacrolimus also helps in reducing PIH. Do not attempt any treatment to reduce the PIH for at least a month to six weeks. You may do mild peels, or a Q-switched Nd:YAG laser after four to six weeks to treat the PIH.

26.3 Special Considerations While Doing Laser Treatments

Complications largely depend on laser settings which are further determined by the indication and the skin type of the patient.

Since responses vary widely among patients, a test spot is vital to determine the optimal parameters for the lesion in that patient. It also allows the patient to become familiar with and understand the procedure.

26.4 Points to Remember before Any Laser Treatment (1, 11)

1. The importance of the history of keloids has already been mentioned. It is equally important to examine existing scars, if any, to mark any keloidal tendency.
2. Reactivation of the herpes simplex virus may occur after any laser treatment. Widespread facial lesions, delayed

epithelialization, and scarring are seen especially after fractional laser resurfacing. All at-risk patients must be administered antiviral prophylaxis (valacyclovir or famciclovir 500 mg twice daily in patients) starting a day before the procedure and continued ten days thereafter to prevent herpes simplex virus reactivation (11, 12).

3. Hypersensitivity to topical anesthetic has been well documented. If itching or erythema develops after the application of topical anesthetic cream, the procedure must be postponed, and other options, such as nerve blocks or infiltration anesthesia, may be considered in the subsequent sessions.

4. Ocular injury can be prevented by adhering to laser protection guidelines strictly (13). Laser glasses are mandatory and are rated by optical density at various wavelengths. An optical density of >4 for a particular wavelength is considered safe. Ocular injury depends upon the wavelength of the laser used, duration of exposure, beam size, and incidence of the laser beam (1).

5. Treatment parameters—employ settings that minimize the extent of epidermal and dermal injury (typically more conservative than in SPT I–III, often requiring a greater number of sessions), such as lower fluences and longer pulse durations for laser hair removal; lower treatment densities (microthermal zones cm²) for fractional laser resurfacing

6. Judicious epidermal cooling must be done, such as slower treatment speeds when using lasers with contact cooling, pausing between passes of resurfacing lasers to reduce bulk heating, and ice packs post-procedure.

7. Consider topical corticosteroids post-treatment (to reduce inflammation), especially when significant post-procedure erythema or edema noted

26.5 Points to Remember Pertaining to Specific Lasers

Q-switched lasers (pigment lasers): Devices with a Gaussian beam profile are more prone to adverse effects as compared to those with a top hat beam. Picosecond lasers are supposed to be superior to nanosecond devices in dark skin though a skilled laser specialist can deliver equally good results without complications in dark skin, even with nanolasers.

Selecting the treatment parameters while treating with Q-switched lasers:

1. Fluence: Always use the lowest fluence which can produce an immediate whitening on the treated skin. Increase the fluence gradually if you do not see whitening. If there is a significant debris or if there is bleeding, lower the fluence (14).

2. Spot size: For epidermal conditions, opt for a spot size just enough to cover the lesion. Larger spot will damage the normal skin and may lead to dyschromia. Use a larger spot size for conditions with dermal component such that you see immediate whitening on the lasered area. As with all lasers, the larger the spot size deeper the penetration and lesser is the splatter (15).

3. Endpoint: Immediate whitening (pseudo frosting) of the treated lesion is considered to be the endpoint of the treatment. Avoid overtreating in order to prevent complications.

4. Never stack pulses while treating pigmented lesions in order to prevent PIH (16).

Fractional lasers: Ablative full-face resurfacing is best avoided on Indian skin owing to a significant risk of hyperpigmentation and scarring.

1. Energy and density are key parameters that determine the efficacy and safety of both ablative as well as nonablative fractional lasers. The higher the treatment density, the higher the risk of PIH (17).

2. The fewer the number of passes, the lesser the chances of PIH, burns, and scarring (18).

3. Interval between two treatment sessions can be increased in case PIH occurs.

4. Pre- and post-treatment cooling, as well as additional cooling between passes to reduce bulk heating, will reduce the risk of pain, edema, crusting, PIH, burns, and scarring (10, 19).

26.6 Hair Removal Lasers

While treating patients with skin of color, keep the following points in mind to avoid complications (1).

1. Always do a test spot laser. Test spots should be chosen in an area with similar skin color, sun exposure, and hair density as the site to be treated. In general, two to four different fluence settings are recommended for testing, and at least four overlapping spots should be administered for each fluence and pulse duration. The best and safest parameters can be selected according to the results (20).

2. Wavelength: Opt for lasers with longer wavelengths in order to allow deeper penetration. This prevents the chances of epidermal melanin from competing as a target chromophore. It increases the ratio of the temperature of the hair bulb to the temperature of the epidermis, allowing follicular destruction with relative sparing of the epidermis. This reduces the chances of PIH, burns, and scarring.

3. Treatment parameters: Use conservative settings such as lower fluences and longer pulse durations to minimize the extent of the epidermal and dermal injury and facilitate epidermal cooling, although these parameters may require a greater number of sessions

4. For areas with higher hair density, such as the beard and upper back, the initial fluence must be even lower due to the increased risk of thermal damage that results from heat diffusion of closely adjacent hairs (21).

5. Fluence should be decreased in case of prolonged erythema or edema. Avoid blistering and crusting as endpoints, as these will surely lead to discoloration and scarring in dark skin. Reduce the fluence if the patient complains of severe pain.

6. Pre-treatment cooling with ice, cooling during treatment with a built-in chill tip or external modalities, and post-treatment cooling with ice reduce chances of adverse effects.

7. Pre- and post-treatment sun protection is mandatory.

8. Use of exfoliants, scrubs, and creams that cause exfoliation should be stopped a week before laser hair removal.

9. Laser hair removal should not be done within two weeks of bleaching and chemical peels.

10. Topical anesthetic preparations have a high potential of causing irritant reactions and, subsequently, burns with

laser. Hence, it is better to avoid topical anesthesia, especially on dark or sensitive skin.

11. Thin long hair, which develops after a few treatment sessions, needs to be treated with a different wavelength, such as 755 nm alexandrite laser or higher fluences with extensive cooling may be used.

12. Paradoxical hypertrichosis: Appropriate delivery of energy using optimal laser settings may reduce the incidence of paradoxical hypertrichosis. Subtherapeutic thermal injury to the surrounding vellus hair stimulates conversion into terminal follicles. Inflammatory mediators and upregulatory cytokines may also play a role. Protecting the peripheral nontreatment area with cold packs during the procedure may help prevent this complication (22).

26.7 Special Considerations While Doing Injectables

While the complications seen in Fitzpatrick skin types III–VI are not any different than those seen in skin types I and II when it comes to injectables, dyschromias can occur in dark skin. There are no reports of keloids and scarring with injectables in skin of color (23).

One must abstain from or minimize the use of multiple puncture techniques to prevent hyperpigmentation. Taylor et al. reported hyperpigmentation in 13% of patients with Fitzpatrick skin types IV, V, and VI treated with hyaluronic acid fillers using multiple puncture techniques as opposed to hyperpigmentation in only 2% of patients who were injected by linear threading techniques. Patients in whom the injection times were slightly longer also showed an increased PIH. Hence, it was concluded that slower injection rates decrease the incidence of PIH and clinical bruising with occasional subsequent hemosiderin deposition in black patients (24).

In case of PIH or dyschromia due to trauma, advise patients to protect themselves from sun exposure and use sunscreen and a topical lightening agent. Chemical peels, such as salicylic acid or glycolic acid, will help in this regard (25).

If the dyschromia is related to the hyaluronic acid filler, it is better to dissolve the filler with hyaluronidase. Persistent dyschromia may be the result of hemosiderin deposition in which case a neodymium-YAG laser would help to clear the discoloration (26).

In conclusion, careful selection of patients, strict pre- and post-treatment care, and the right procedural parameters and protocols will help minimize any complication in skin of color.

References

1. Alexis AF. Lasers and light-based therapies in ethnic skin: Treatment options and recommendations for Fitzpatrick skin types V and VI. *Br J Dermatol*. 2013;169(suppl 3):91–97.

2. Savant SS. Superficial and medium depth chemical peeling. In: Savant SS (Ed), *Text book of dermatosurgery and cosmetology*. 2nd ed. ASCAD; 2005. P. 177–195.

3. Grimes PE. The safety and efficacy of salicylic acid chemical peels in darker racial-ethnic groups. *Dermatol Surg*. 1999;25:18–22.

4. Khunger N. Standard guidelines of care for chemical peels. *Indian J Dermatol Venereol Leprol*. 2008;74(suppl 1):5–12.

5. Sharad J. Combination of microneedling and glycolic acid peels for the treatment of acne scar in dark skin. *J Cosmet Dermatol*. 2011;10:317–323.

6. Sharad J. Microneedling. In: Khunger N (Ed), *Step by step treatment of acne scars*. Jaypee Brothers Medical Publishers; 2014. P. 102–113.

7. Sharad J. Glycolic acid peel therapy—a current review. *Clin Cosmet Investig Dermatol*. 2013;6:281–288. Published 2013 Nov 11. Doi:10.2147/CCID.S34029.

8. Khunger N. Chemical peeling in dark skin. In Khunger N (Ed), *Step by step chemical peels*. Jaypee Brothers Medical Publishers; 2014. P. 210–219.

9. Nikalji N, Godse K, Sakhiya J, Patil S, Nadkarni N. Complications of medium depth and deep chemical peels. *J Cutan Aesthet Surg*. 2012;5:254–260.

10. Uday K, Sushil P, Nischal K. Sunscreens. In: *Handbook of dermatological drug therapy*. 1st ed. Elsevier; 2007. P. 299–304.

11. Chandrashekar BS, Shenoy C, Madura C. Complications of laser and light-based devices therapy in patients with skin of color. *Indian J Dermatol Venereol Leprol*. 2019;85:24–31.

12. Gilbert S. Improving the outcome of facial resurfacing—Prevention of herpes simplex virus type 1 reactivation. *J Antimicrob Chemother*. 2001;47(suppl T1):29–34.

13. Lolis M, Dunbar SW, Goldberg DJ, Hansen TJ, MacFarlane DF. Patient safety in procedural dermatology: part II. Safety related to cosmetic procedures. *J Am Acad Dermatol*. 2015;73:15–24.

14. Goldberg DJ. Pigmented lesions, tattoos, and disorders of hypopigmentation. In: Goldberg DJ (Ed), *Laser dermatology pearls and problems*. 1st ed. Blackwell Publishing; 2008. P. 71–114.

15. Kilmer SL, Farinelli WF, Tearney G, Anderson RR. Use of a larger spot size for the treatment of tattoos increases clinical efficacy and decreases potential side effects. *Lasers Surg Med*. 1994;6:S51.

16. Tiwari A. Lasers for pigmentation. In: Sharad J (Ed), *Aesthetic dermatology: Current perspectives*. Jaypee Brothers Medical Publishers; 2019. P. 326–334.

17. Treatment of acne scarring in Fitzpatrick skin types v to vi: Practical approaches to maximizing safety. *Cutis*. 2013;92(6):272–273.

18. Chan HH, Manstein D, Yu CS, Shek S, Kono T, Wei WI. The prevalence and risk factors of post-inflammatory hyperpigmentation after fractional resurfacing in Asians. *Lasers Surg Med*. 2007 Jun;39(5):381–385.

19. Mysore V, Pall A. Fractional lasers. In: Sharad J (Ed), *Aesthetic dermatology: Current perspectives*. Jaypee Brothers Medical Publishers; 2019. P. 307–317.

20. Nouri K, Tiwari A. Laser hair removal in ethnic skin. In: Sharad J (Ed), *Aesthetic dermatology: Current perspectives*. Jaypee Brothers Medical Publishers; 2019. P. 318–325.

21. Battle EF, Jr., Hobbs LM. Laser-assisted hair removal for darker skin types. *Dermatol Ther*. 2004;17:177–183.

22. Radmanesh M. Paradoxical hypertrichosis and terminal hair change after intense pulsed light hair removal therapy. *J Dermatolog Treat*. 2009;20:52–54.

23. Burgess C et al. Ethnic and gender considerations in the use of facial injectables: African-American patients. *Plast Reconstr Surg*. Nov 2015;136(5S):28S–31S.

24. Taylor SC, Burgess CM, Callender VD. Safety of nonanimal stabilized hyaluronic acid dermal fillers in patients with skin of color: A randomized, evaluator-blinded comparative trial. *Dermatol Surg*. 2009;35(suppl 2):1653–1660.

25. Talakoub L, Wesley NO. Differences in perceptions of beauty and cosmetic procedures performed in ethnic patients. *Semin Cutan Med Surg*. 2009;28:115–129.

26. Burgess CM. Special considerations in African American skin. In: Alam M, Bhatia A, Kundu R et al. (Eds), *Cosmetic dermatology for skin of color*. McGraw-Hill Companies; 2008. P. 163–167.

CHAPTER 27: SOP FOR AN AESTHETIC DERMATOLOGY CLINIC

Sahana P. Raju and Mukta Sachdev

27.1 Introduction

The fascination to keep one's skin beautiful dates all the way back to ancient times, be it Queen Cleopatra's renowned rituals or the Indian practice involving the use of many natural ingredients. Thousands of years later, in the present era, the inclination to "stay young forever" is at its zenith.

Aesthetic dermatology and surgery have gained increasing acclaim worldwide owing to their safety and wide availability. What was once considered a minor subspeciality has now grown into a thriving and independent market. In addition to being performed in hospital settings or an outpatient clinic, aesthetic procedures are also being done in nonmedical locales, which call for a standard guideline describing the do's and don'ts of setting up an Aesthetic practice.

This chapter briefly describes the general requirements and protocols to be followed while establishing an aesthetic dermatology clinic.

27.2 What Does Aesthetic Dermatology Comprise?

The word "aesthetic" is derived from the Greek word "aisthëtikos," meaning "perception by the senses." The American Board of Cosmetic Surgery has defined cosmetic surgery as a subspeciality of medicine and surgery that exclusively confines itself to the betterment of appearance through surgical and medical techniques. Medical aesthetics is best defined as the harmonious fusion of cosmetic procedures as treatment options for various dermatological indications.[1]

27.3 The State of Aesthetic Healthcare Practice

Aesthetic dermatology has only recently risen to popularity as an informal subspecialty of dermatology. The surging problems related to body image, the desire to "look perfect," and a rise in cosmetic-related dermatological problems have compelled many dermatologists and non-dermatologists to look into a career in aesthetics. However, the present scenario entails that a dermatologist, during his/her residency, doesn't receive a formal training in aesthetics, which forms the very foundation of their education. Development and incorporation of a systematic and exclusive curriculum for aesthetic and cosmetic dermatology, with a futuristic and translational approach, is the need of the day.

In this chapter, the basic framework of an aesthetic dermatology clinic—including the infrastructure, qualifications of the treating physician and other staff required, equipment required, and the principles of ethical aesthetic practice—are outlined.

Before we dive into it, there are three key points that must be kept in mind for any aesthetic healthcare practitioner.[3]

- *Knowledge, skill, and performance*: Take part in activities that increase one's competence and upgrade one's knowledge.

- *Safety and quality*: Follow good clinical practice guidelines, monitor patient outcomes, and ensure that your setup is suitable, equipped, and staffed.
- *Communication, partnership, and teamwork*: Form a credible relationship with the patient and build a support system with seasoned colleagues.

27.4 Infrastructure

• *Office facility*

- An environment with a soothing ambiance is vital to make the patient feel at ease.
- The individual room and overall building design must adhere to the state and local fire, safety, and sanitation guidelines for physicians' offices.
- A waiting area or reception with the front desk and billing counter, consultation rooms, procedure rooms (including a separate laser room if applicable), a photography room, and hygienic washrooms form the mainstay of any clinic.
- Proper hand washing amenities must be available with measures to decrease contamination.
- An air-conditioning system is a must as it makes the environment remain relatively dust free and is useful for machine longevity.
- Inside the procedure room, a dental chair/cosmetic chair/ophthalmic chair that can be operated manually or electrically, with a movable task light fitted to it, is preferred. A rotatable surgeon's chair with an adequate backrest must be in position.
- Electrical requirements: A three-phase electric connection is advised if multiple machines, lasers, and cooling devices are being used. Online and offline uninterrupted power supplies (UPS) are recommended, with each socket board stabilized by proper earthing or grounding. In case of a general power failure, a backup lighting system must be in place to avoid disruption of any procedure underway.[4]
- Ventilation: Adequate windows that are screened or closed must be present in each room. All outside air openings to the surgical area must be sealed against the entrance of insects.

• *Specific designing of a laser procedure room*[5]

- The ideal dimensions should be 12 feet by 12 feet with ample space to accommodate a patient chair, a trolley with a laser machine, a cooling device and other required equipment, a laser operator, and at least one assistant.
- The door should be made up of opaque material to prevent transmission of laser light, and reflective surfaces must be avoided.
- A smoke evacuator with specific features must be present to reduce damage due to laser plumes.
- A fire extinguisher with an ISI mark should be available nearby.

27.5 Physician Qualifications and Staff Requirements

- A qualified dermatologist (MD/DNB/diploma in dermatology), with at least six months of training from a recognized center if the specialized training was not imparted during post-graduation, can perform aesthetic and cosmetic procedures.
- However, this was the previous norm, and of late, medical and surgical specialists, including non-dermatologists, plastic surgeons, and general practitioners, are also dabbing their hands in aesthetic procedures.
- Plastic surgeons are more well-versed in performing procedures like blepharoplasty (it can also be performed by an ophthalmologist), breast implants, abdominoplasty, brow lift, rhytidectomy, rhinoplasty, and phlebectomy.[6]
- Other essential members of the team must include a receptionist, registered nurses, laser technicians, helping staff, security, a biomedical waste management team, and a technical manager.
- All staff members must be trained to follow the standard operating guidelines and understand the importance of maintaining a clean and professional environment.

Workplace safety

- The staff must be aware of workplace hazards and the means to minimize risk.
- Universal precautions must be practiced prior to any procedure.
- The physician and appropriate staff must be familiar with basic life support methods.
- A plan of action must be preformulated for all anticipated emergencies.
- Specific measures for laser procedures, like smoke evacuation, eye protection, fire avoidance, and methods to minimize plume, must be followed aptly.

27.6 Equipment[7]

- In the past, the only instrument dermatologists were familiar with was the magnifying glass, which then broadened to involve basic equipment, such as a Wood's lamp, cautery machine, cryotherapy, and radiofrequency. In today's practice, hundreds of specialized pieces of equipment are available to carry out a multitude of basic and complicated aesthetic procedures.
- The awareness about the maintenance and management needs of these instruments is equally important. Poor maintenance compromises efficacy and safety, not to mention the possibility of financial losses.
- The annual maintenance contract (AMC), which is procured from the supplier of the particular equipment with details about the warranty period, has to be kept available, along with the updated insurance documents.[5]
- The managing staff have to organize regular visits by a service engineer as per the manufacturer's recommendations.
- Earthing of the equipment is a must to avoid damage to the machines, not to mention electrical shocks to the operator.

- A low ambient temperature, dust-free environment, and well-grounded power supply without voltage fluctuation are described as the crucial elements for lasting and safe maintenance of equipment.[8]
- In the procedure room, stainless steel surgical instruments of appropriate quality and quantity must be kept in place before each procedure, wherever required.
- A sphygmomanometer must be available in the vicinity of the instrument trolley.
- An electrosurgical device (cautery or radiofrequency device) as a means of hemostasis must be available.
- Emergency drugs and additional equipment which must be available in the premises but not limited to are outlined in Table 27.1.

Sterilization, disinfection, and biomedical waste management

- In outpatient clinics, alcohols like ethanol or isopropanol are sufficient for hand disinfection.
- Medical and surgical devices can be divided into *critical* (e.g., surgical instruments required for scar revisions, acne surgery, or liposuction) *semi-critical* (instruments that come in contact with an intact mucous membrane), and *non-critical* (laser probes, microdermabrasion tips, laser and phototherapy glasses) depending on the potential risk of infection involved.
- Critical items require complete sterility by means of autoclaving, semi-critical items can be chemically sterilized by glutaraldehyde, and non-critical items can be managed by simply washing with a detergent.[9]
- Disinfection of the procedure room is to be done by fogging by using agents like 8–10% hydrogen peroxide, glutaraldehyde, and quaternary ammonium compounds, though the conventional use of formaldehyde gas still prevails. The contact time should be 60 minutes, after which the room can be used immediately.[10]
- Periodic cleaning of lasers and other machines must be carried out by authorized personnel, with the help of acetone or betadine.
- Proper waste disposal methods are an important part of healthcare, and strict laws have been sanctioned for waste disposal and environmental safety.
- Biomedical waste management involves segregation and safe disposal.
- The different types of waste generated in dermatology clinics and their methods of safe disposal are described in Table 27.2.

TABLE 27.1: Outline of Essential Emergency Drugs and Equipment

Emergency Drugs	Emergency Equipment
• Adrenaline	• Pulse oximeter
• Antihistamine	• Cardiac monitor
• IV fluids	• Laryngoscope with an
• Sodium bicarbonate	endotracheal tube
• Vasopressor	• Ambubag with a mask
• Corticosteroids	
• Vasodilator	
• IV lidocaine	
• Anticonvulsants	

TABLE 27.2: Summary of Biomedical Waste Management

Category	Type of Waste Generated	Methods of Disposal	Color and Type of Container
6	Solid waste contaminated with blood and bodily fluids	Incineration or microwaving	Yellow plastic bag
7	Solid waste from disposable items like tubings, IV sets, etc.	Chemical disinfection with 1% sodium hypochlorite solution or others	Red plastic bag
4	Sharps	Chemical disinfection followed by shredding/mutilation	Sealed puncture-proof container in blue/white translucent plastic bag

TABLE 27.3: Classification of Procedures According to the Risk Involved

Low Risk	Moderate Risk	High Risk
PRP—scalp, hands	PRP—face, without mask	Fillers—lips
Cryolipolysis	RF—face, without mask	QS lasers, PDL, KTP—face
Laser hair removal—non-facial areas	Laser hair removal—face	Fractional and non-fractionals lasers—face
RF—body	Nonablative lasers	

Specific precautionary measures due to the COVID-19 pandemic

- Training of staff and front desk regarding the basic preventive measures must be undertaken.
- Patients coming in for aesthetic procedures must be screened for fever, cough, and breathlessness by means of an infrared thermometer and relevant history.
- Frequent hand sanitization and social distancing must be encouraged.
- Use of personal protective equipment (PPE), which includes a head cap, face shield, N95 respirator, disposable gown, and shoe covers, must be worn by the consulting doctor.
- The procedures performed can be divided into low-, moderate-, and high-risk according to the degree of exposure involved (Table 27.3). Low-risk procedures require only the use of an N95 respirator, while moderate- and high-risk procedures require other measures as well, along with a smoke evacuation device.
- Disinfection of all surfaces must be undertaken using 1% sodium hypochlorite solution or alcohol-based solutions like 70% isopropyl alcohol. The procedure rooms must be fumigated every night.
- Wearing appropriate PPE, sanitization measures, and other general protective measures go a long way in decreasing the risk of contracting COVID-19.

27.7 Pre-Procedure Checklist

Selection of patients

- Before any procedure is undertaken, the practitioner must ensure that the patient
  - Is medically and psychologically fit to undergo the procedure,
  - Understands the risks and complications involved, and
  - Has no life-threatening medical conditions or, if there are any, must have them managed appropriately.
- Although most people are satisfied with the outcomes of cosmetic surgery, the main cause of disputes arises from a small subsection of people with unrealistic expectations who tend to be dissatisfied, which was clearly defined as a predictor of poor outcomes.[11]

- A 19-item ASPECT scale was developed for determining internal and external expectations for cosmetic treatment outcome, which can assist physicians in identifying patients who may require further psychological assessment.[12] This, however, is not widely implemented due to its time-consuming nature.

Counseling, including the cost of the procedure

- The diagnosis, management options available and the one chosen, the anesthesia planned, nature of the procedure to be performed, downtime and pain involved, postoperative care including the necessity of dressing, need of antibiotics, and possible complications that could occur must be discussed in detail with the patient.[5]
- Patients must be made aware of the complete financial implications of the procedure involved, including the consultation fee and follow-up charges. The fact that the results of some procedures are not permanent must be clearly explained to the patient so that they are aware of the need for repeat procedures.[13]

Informed consent

The following points must be clearly written in the consent form, in a language that the patient understands:[5]

- Name of the institute/clinic where the treatment is planned.
- Name of the patient and doctor.
- Diagnosis of the condition.
- Name of the procedure to be done.
- Most common complications of the procedure involved. If and when required, the entire list available in the literature may be explained.
- Consent for photography can be taken in the same form—it must include points protection of the patient's identity and consent for the use of the images for academic purposes in journals with all efforts made to maintain anonymity.

Recordkeeping and documentation

A complete clinical history, routine general examination, and cutaneous examination findings must be noted down in the patient's file. Procedure registers for each category must be maintained and updated on a daily basis.

Pre-procedure workup

- Relevant investigations like S.HbsAg, S.HIV, and VDRL must be done before invasive procedures and ablative skin resurfacing.
- A complete hemogram and bleeding and clotting profile may be advised if coagulation disorders are suspected.

Photography[14]

- Clinical photography plays a vital role in a dermatologist's armamentarium.
- It is essential for serial evaluation of the condition, documentation purposes, and academics and also in further formulating a treatment strategy.
- Professional and high-quality images are a must.
- After taking consent, the patient must be properly positioned against a non-reflective background (plain light blue, black, or green).
- Identifying features like hats, jewelry, and glasses must be avoided.
- DSLR/SLR cameras, a tripod, and photographic frames are some of the essential prerequisites.
- A resolution of $768 \times 512 \times 24$—around 0.4 megapixels—is considered suitable for photography in dermatology.[15]

27.8 Procedures That Can Be Performed

According to the Cosmetic Surgical Practice Working Party,[16] cosmetic treatments can be divided as follows:

- *Level 1a*: Invasive; medium to high risk; may require general anesthesia and overnight stay
- *Level 1b*: Invasive; low to medium risk; usually performed as an outpatient procedure and only requires local anesthesia
- *Level 2*: Minimally invasive; lower risk; usually reversible; daycare; local anesthetic if any

Procedures performed in an aesthetic clinic are usually noninvasive or minimally invasive. Some of them are listed in Table 27.4.

TABLE 27.4: Non-Invasive and Minimally Invasive Aesthetic Procedures

Chemical peels
Microdermabrasion
Microneedling
Mesotherapy
Botox
Fillers
Platelet-rich plasma therapy (PRP)
Aesthetic cryotherapy
Radiofrequency skin rejuvenation
Intense pulsed light (IPL)
Nonablative lasers
Photodynamic therapy (PDT)
Sclerotherapy

- Some of the invasive procedures, other than the various surgical modalities performed for a wide variety of indications, are enumerated in Table 27.5.

27.9 Post-Procedure Care

- Precise instructions must be given regarding the products to be used after a facial cosmetic procedure; the type of cleanser and moisturizer to be used must be explained in detail to the patient.
- Photoprotection must be greatly emphasized after any facial aesthetic procedure.
- Any other post-procedural instructions relevant to the specific procedure must be given.
- Medication instructions and prescriptions (pain medications and antibiotics) must be given.
- Details about the next visit and protocol to be followed at home must be explained.
- Here, the patient must also be counseled regarding postprocedural erythema, swelling, bruising, and so on and that these will only be temporary.
- The optimum time to see visible results must be explained, which depends on each individual procedure.

27.10 Pharmacy and Dispensing

- Some dermatologists prefer to have a pharmacy in affiliation with their clinics or an in-house dispensing facility.
- The three As, which are often practical and must be followed while treating any patient, are as follows:
  1. *Assess*: Diagnose the patient
  2. *Advise*: Either a medical or a procedural modality as required
  3. *Assist*: Offer the patient the security and accessibility of purchasing the right kind of products.
- Various studies have shown that in-house dispensing leads to better outcomes and is more convenient for patients, and the chance of the wrong products ending up in the patients' hands is almost nil.
- Informational displays, including brochures, testers, and prices of the products, can be placed.

27.11 Telemedicine and Virtual Consultation

- Keeping the legal aspects in mind, telemedicine is highly relevant for improved delivery of dermatological care, including aesthetic care in the periphery and remote regions.
- The patients can have the advantage of deciding the choice of therapy without wasting money on travel.
- The suitability of a particular lesion for treatment by procedures and pre-surgery counseling can be easily done through teleconsultations.

TABLE 27.5: Invasive Aesthetic Procedures

Liposuction
Fat transplantation
Fractional lasers
Scar revision methods

27.12 Publicity and Promotion[17]

- With 80% of people searching the internet for health information, there is a liability for practitioners to maintain a presence on social media to allay misinformation and communicate evidence-based knowledge.
- Newsletters, personal blogs, webinars, and personalized websites can be used to broadcast useful information, interact with the general public and let them know what's new in your practice.
- However, the best way to build up a practice is to offer an unmatched patient experience by respecting their time, working to decrease the waiting period, and making sure that the whole team comes together to take good care of the patient.

27.13 The Ethical Issues of Cosmetic Procedures

- The difficulty in drawing accurate and consistent distinctions between therapeutic procedures, cosmetic procedures, medical aesthetics, and beauty practices has given rise to a number of ethical issues.
- The tremendously commercial environment and the basis of cosmetic procedures being undertaken for appearance-related reasons are major troubling factors.
- Social media platforms act as a double-ended sword, with rising levels of body dissatisfaction among teenagers, the general public wanting to match "celebrity culture," air-brushed images, and setting high and unnecessary beauty standards.
- There are no clear-cut requirements for practitioners to have particular qualifications and competence in the field.
- These are some of the issues that need to be identified and rapidly addressed by the concerned authorities.

27.14 Conclusion

Thanks to an economic boom and the desire to look better, an increasing number of surgical and non-surgical cosmetic procedures are being performed globally. The concept of cosmetic medical tourism is also on the rise, with increasing numbers of people going out of their countries seeking aesthetic procedures. To visualize and fulfill the needs of patients, it is necessary to ensure that the technologies being invested in are foolproof and dependable. Providing an unbiased and ethical view and doing what is best for the patient should be our ultimate goal.

Elegance is when the inside is as beautiful as the outside.
—*Chanel*

References

1. Arora S, Arora G. Recognizing "medical aesthetics" in dermatology: The need of the hour. *Indian J Dermatol Venereol Leprol* 2021;87:1–2.
2. Dogra S. Fate of medical dermatology in the era of cosmetic dermatology and dermatosurgery. *Indian J Dermatol Venereol Leprol* 2009;75:4–7.
3. Guidance for doctors who offer cosmetic interventions www.gmc-uk.org.
4. Olson R. Continuous power to the OR and other critical care areas. *Dimensions Health Serv* 1975;52:29–30.
5. Dhepe N. Minimum standard guidelines of care on requirements for setting up a laser room. *Indian J Dermatol Venereol Leprol* 2009;75:101–110.
6. Malaysian medical council guidelines on aesthetic medical practice. https://www.moh.gov.my/moh/images/gallery/Garispanduan/GUIDELINES.
7. Drake et al. Guidelines of care for office surgical facilities. Part II. Self-assessment checklist. *J Am Acad Dermatol* 1995;33:265–270.
8. Kerr DR. Electrical design and safety in the operating room and intensive care unit. *Int Anaesthesiol Clin* 1981;19:27–48.
9. Favero MS. Chemical disinfection of medical and surgical materials. In: Block SS, editor. *Disinfection, sterilization and preservation.* 3rd ed. Philadelphia: Lea and Febiger; 1983. P. 469–492.
10. Patwardhan N, Kelkar U. Disinfection, sterilization and operation theater guidelines for dermatosurgical practitioners in India. *Indian J Dermatol Venereol Leprol* 2011;77:83–93.
11. Honigman RJ, Phillips KA, Castle DJ. A review of psychosocial outcomes for patients seeking cosmetic surgery. *Plast Reconstr Surg* 2004;113(4):1229.
12. Pikoos TD, Rossell SL, Tzimas N, Buzwell S. Assessing unrealistic expectations in clients undertaking minor cosmetic procedures: The development of the aesthetic procedure expectations scale. *Facial Plast Surg Aesthet Med* 2021 Jul–Aug;23(4):263–269.
13. *Professional standards for cosmetic practice.* Cosmetic Surgical Practice Working Party.
14. Muraco L. Improved medical photography: Key tips for creating images of lasting value. *JAMA Dermatol* s 2020;156(2):121–123.
15. Bittorf A, Fastasch M, Schuler G, Diepgen TL. Resolution requirements for digital images in dermatology. *J Am Acad Dermatol* 1997;37:195–198.
16. *Professional standards for cosmetic practice.* Cosmetic Surgical Practice Working Party.
17. Laughter MR, Zangara T, Maymone MB, Rundle CW, Dunnick CA, Hugh JM, Sadeghpour M, Dellavalle RP. Social media use in dermatology. *Dermatol Sin* 2020;38:28–34.

Part V
Procedures

CHAPTER 28: CHEMICAL PEELS

Niti Khunger and Charvi Chanana

28.1 Introduction

Chemical peels, also referred to as chemexfoliation, is a method of controlled destruction of all or part of the epidermis and dermis using chemical agents.[1–4] It is a frequently practiced procedure and is witnessing a resurge in recent times. A wide array of conditions like acne, pigmentary disorders like melasma, and scars are being treated with chemical peels. The use has been extended to facial rejuvenation and to reverse the effect of photoaging. They can be used alone or in combination with other aesthetic procedures.

Chemical peels have been classified according to their depth of penetration into superficial, medium, and deep types (Table 28.1). The depth of the peel is determined by the concentration, pH, nature of the peeling agent, priming agents, and mode of application.[5, 6]

Very superficial peels exfoliate the stratum corneum. Superficial peels exfoliate the skin from the stratum corneum to the papillary dermis. They cause reduced corneocyte adhesion and epidermolysis and increased dermal collagen deposition.[7–10]

Examples of superficial peels include 10–30% salicylic acid (SA), 20–70% glycolic acid (GA), Jessner solution (JS), solid carbon dioxide slush, and 20% or lower concentrations of trichloroacetic acid (TCA).

TABLE 28.1: Classification of Chemical Peels

Type	Depth	Indication
Very superficial	Stratum corneum	Texture improvement (Party Peel) Skin brightening Comedonal acne
Superficial	Part or entire epidermis upto the papillary dermis	Melasma PIH Freckles Mild superficial acne scars Mild photoaging
Medium-depth	Upto the upper reticular dermis	Melasma PIH Superficial acne scars Moderate photoaging Fine lines
Deep	Upto the mid-reticular dermis	Deep acne scars Static wrinkles

Medium-depth peels penetrate deeper than superficial peels. They penetrate the papillary dermis to the upper reticular dermis.[4, 5] They result in extensive protein precipitation, resulting in coagulative necrosis of cells.

Examples of medium-depth peels include 35–50% TCA peel. TCA 35% may be combined with glycolic acid 70% or Jessner's solution or solid carbon dioxide to form a combination medium-depth peel.[11]

Deep peels penetrate the mid-reticular dermis. They denature the epidermal keratin and dermal proteins, causing complete epidermolysis and mid-dermal injury. Phenol peel formulas cause deep peels.

28.2 Indications[8]

The indications of chemical peels are given in Table 28.2.

Acne: Superficial chemical peels are effective for mild to moderate acne.[12–16] They can improve comedonal and inflammatory papular and pustular acne, as well as pigmentation associated with acne (Figure 28.1). SA 30% and GA 30% were similarly effective in a split-face randomized control trial.[12]

Melasma: Chemical peels are effective for pigmentary disorders like melasma and post-inflammatory hyperpigmentation. A study comparing JS plus 20% TCA versus 20% TCA alone in individuals with higher Fitzpatrick skin phototypes found that JS plus 20% TCA was more effective in treating melasma but with greater immediate discomfort. There was no significant difference in PIH.[17, 18] Sarkar et al. compared hydroquinone 2%, tretinoin 0.05% cream, and hydrocortisone 1% cream to 30% GA peels performed every three weeks for six sessions. The GA group showed significant improvement compared to bleaching cream only.[19]

Post-inflammatory pigmentation: Grimes et al. treated patients with SA 20% to 30% peels every two weeks for five sessions. Eighty percent had 75% improvement, and 20% had 51% to 75% improvement in PIH.[20] Chemical peels are a useful adjunct to the management of PIH and can hasten response (Figure 28.2).

Photo-rejuvenation: Medium-depth peel is particularly effective in treating lentigines and fine wrinkles. They can be applied as spot peels to the localized lesions and superficial peels for overall rejuvenation.

Infraorbital melanosis: Four-weekly 3.75% TCA and 15% lactic acid peels resulted in excellent improvement in 90% of patients at six months of follow-up.[21] GA 20% and lactic acid 15% showed 73% and 56% improvement in periorbital melanosis.[22]

DOI: 10.1201/9780429243769-28

TABLE 28.2: Indications of Chemical Peels

Pigmentary disorders	Ephelides
	Lentigines
	Melasma
	Post-inflammatory pigmentation
Inflammatory	Acne vulgaris
	Comedones
	Rosacea
Scarring	Acne scarring
	Traumatic scarring
Epidermal proliferations and tumors	Actinic keratoses
	Dermatosis papulosa nigra
	Milia
	Seborrhoeic keratoses
	Sebaceous hyperplasia
	Warts
Aesthetic procedures	Photoaging
	Superficial fine rhytides
	Superficial scars

28.2.1 Contraindications

Earlier chemical peels were performed rarely in darker skins due to the risk of PIH. However, with the advent of newer peels and combination peels that are safer, they are now commonly performed in dark skin types. Use of isotretinoin within six months was a contraindication, but recent evidence shows that superficial peels are safe, medium-depth peels should be used with caution, and deep peels should be avoided. Precaution should be taken with high-strength glycolic acid peels.[23] The contraindications are summarized in Table 28.3.

28.3 Patient Workup and Counseling

Chemical peels should be advised to patients who are motivated. Patients should have a realistic expectation about the results. Informed consent has to be taken before the procedure and all risks to be explained.

A thorough history and examination should be done for all the patients.

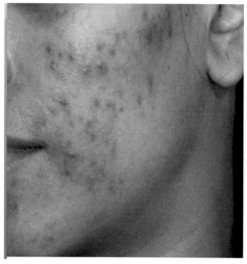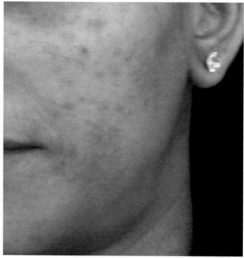

FIGURE 28.1   Improvement of acne and PIH following three sessions of salicylic acid–mandelic acid combination peel at two-week intervals and one session of combination peel containing glycolic acid, kojic acid, and citric acid.

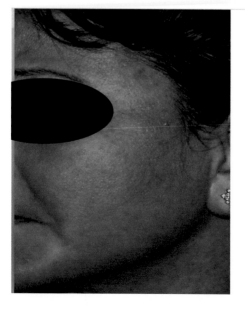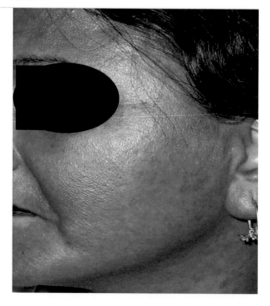

FIGURE 28.2   Improvement of PIH following lichen planus pigmentosus in sensitive skin. Mandelic acid gel peel 40% after eight peels at two-weekly intervals.

TABLE 28.3: Contraindications of Chemical Peels

Absolute	• Active infection (bacterial, viral, or fungal) • History of allergy to peeling ingredient • Isotretinoin therapy within the previous six months (for medium-depth and deep chemical peels) • Open wounds • Pregnancy
Relative	• Inflammatory dermatosis (e.g., rosacea, atopic dermatitis, and psoriasis) • Radiation exposure • Recent facial rejuvenation surgery

28.3.1 History

Any history regarding cardiac, renal, or hepatic disease, diabetes mellitus, and immunosuppression has to be asked, as these patients are more prone to side effects and delayed wound healing.[24, 25]

Past or current episodes of herpes simplex, photosensitivity, keloid, or hypertrophic scarring have to be assessed.[26] Any prior radiotherapy also increases the risk of delayed healing.

Any concurrent dermatological disease like psoriasis, eczema, vitiligo, rosacea, and connective tissue disease might get worsened by chemical peels.[3–11]

Current or past medication with isotretinoin in the last 6–12 months increases the risk of scarring, especially with medium-depth and deep peels.[27]

The patient's occupation is asked in order to assess the degree of sunlight exposure.

Smoking cessation is advised for at least six months during the peeling period, particularly for medium-depth and deep peels, which can delay healing and increase the chances of complications. Pregnancy and lactation status has to be assessed before initiation of peels and before every peel.[26]

28.3.2 Examination

Physical examination involves assessing the patient's skin type, severity and extent of the condition being treated, and any dermatological skin disease.

Skin type is assessed using the Fitzpatrick skin phototype scale.[2, 11]

Intact pilosebaceous glands, skin thickness, and presence of any hypertrophic scar or keloid are evaluated.

28.3.3 Photographic Documents

Baseline photographs must be taken before and after treatment, for comparison.

28.3.4 Patient Selection

Superficial peels can be applied on all skin types,[27] while for medium-depth and deep peels, the ideal candidates are fair-skinned and blue-eyed patients.[28, 29] Patients with Fitzpatrick III–VI phototypes are at higher risk of scarring and post-inflammatory pigmentation.[30] Men have thick, coarse skin; hence, penetration of peeling agents is unpredictable.

28.3.5 Test Spot Testing

Test spot testing is basically done for medium-depth and deep peels. It involves the application of the peeling agent to a small area of skin. Common sites for test-spot testing are the lateral temple, anterior hairline, and pre-auricular region.[31, 32]

Test spot testing helps us to predict the course of healing and any post-peel complication that might develop. It makes the doctor more confident about the procedure.

28.4 Pre-Procedure Care

Pre-procedure care involves the application of agents that makes the stratum corneum thin in order to enhance the penetration of peels and accelerate healing. They also help in identifying the patients who are non-adherent with treatment regimens, making them less suitable candidates for chemical peeling.

Priming is the term given to all the pre-treatment and preparation activities that are performed on the skin prior to chemical peeling. Priming enhances patients' compliance and reduces the risk of complications such as post-inflammatory hyperpigmentation and scarring.[5, 9, 33]

Pre-treatment should begin at least two to four weeks before the chemical peel and cease three to five days prior. Patients are instructed to apply a broad-spectrum sunscreen with a sun protection factor of 50+ that blocks both UVA and UVB. Patients are also advised to limit sun exposure Sunscreen ideally started three months prior to the procedure and continued thereafter.

Other agents for priming are tretinoin, hydroquinone, glycolic acid, 5–10% salicylic acid, 5–10% kojic acid, 1–4%, azelaic acid, and topical corticosteroids.[34, 35]

Tretinoin decreases the epidermal adhesion resulting in thinning of the stratum corneum. It is available in 0.025–0.05% cream, which is applied for a minimum of two weeks before the chemical peel. Tretinoin also enhances epithelial differentiation and proliferation.[36] Retinoid dermatitis is a possible complication that can be avoided by initial application for a short duration and gradually increasing application time. The peeling procedure should not be initiated and discontinued if retinoid dermatitis develops. Hydroquinone 2–4% cream reduces the risk of post-inflammatory hyperpigmentation.

In patients who are at increased risk of post-inflammatory hyperpigmentation, hydroquinone is initiated at least two weeks before a chemical peel and reintroduced one to two weeks post-peel. Hydroquinone reversibly inhibits the enzyme tyrosinase. Patients are instructed to avoid waxing for a minimum of three to four weeks prior to chemical peeling. Individuals with a history of recurrent herpes simplex virus infection should be commenced on systemic antiviral treatment prior to medium-depth and deep chemical peeling.

28.5 Procedure

Prior to peeling, the patient should wash their face and should not use moisturizers and makeup. On the day of the procedure, the patient should wash their skin with a non-residue cleanser. Before applying the peeling agent the skin should be degreased with acetone, triclosan, or isopropyl alcohol to remove residual cosmetics, oils, loose keratin, and other debris.

28.5.1 Peeling Technique

Chemical peeling should be done in a room with appropriate lighting, adequate ventilation, and access to resuscitation equipment. Personnel should be present to make the patient comfortable and position properly, manage equipment, and blot tears from the medial canthal regions to prevent the backtracking of the peeling agent into the eye. The patient should not be left alone during the procedure.

The peeling agent should be checked and poured into a small, clearly labeled glass receptacle or prepared according to the product specification. Any crystals that have formed in the solution should be removed as these may increase the concentration of the solution that is applied. The peeling agent should be securely stored and never passed across the patient in case of inadvertent spillage. Neutralizing agents and eye irrigation solutions, such as water, saline, or glycerine, must be readily available. Local occupational health and safety practices and infection control guidelines must be followed. This includes wearing gloves throughout the procedure.

28.5.2 Reagents

Choosing the right peeling agent is the most important factor leading to success. The indication for the peel, the depth of the pathology, and the type of patient's skin are factors that guide the choice of the peeling agent (Table 28.4). Generally, alcohol-based agents are preferred for oily skin and gel-based peels for dry and sensitive skin. Combination peels are safer for darker skins as they combine lower concentrations of peeling agents.

28.5.2a Tretinoin Peel

Tretinoin peels are used for rejuvenation and to treat melasma and acne. Tretinoin 5% to 10% peels is left on for six hours as a facial mask.[36, 37] It causes mild erythema and desquamation on post-peel day 2.[37]

28.5.2b Salicylic Acid (SA)

SA is a beta-hydroxy acid and a phenolic compound. It is lipophilic and comedolytic; hence, it is useful in comedonal acne. SA 20% to 30% in ethanol crystallizes as the ethanol evaporates, yielding a pseudofrost, which can be easily removed from the skin with water. The crystals cannot penetrate the skin, hence making it self-limiting and safe for all

skin types. SA is also present in polyethylene glycol (PEG) base, which makes it safer. PEG vehicle causes slow delivery and increases penetration into follicles. It is particularly used for acne, comedones.[38, 39]

28.5.2c Trichloroacetic Acid

TCA is a highly water-soluble peel. Depth of penetration correlates directly to concentration. It is available in varying concentrations. TCA penetrates slowly, and frosting occurs at the endpoint. The currently accepted standard preparation of TCA is weight to volume. Other preparation methods are weight-to-weight grams of TCA per 100 ml of water.[40]

28.5.2d Glycolic Peel

GA is a water-soluble alpha-hydroxy acid. The endpoint for glycolic peel is erythema, and it has to be neutralized with 10% sodium bicarbonate and water. It is available in varying concentrations. At lower concentrations, it is safe; however, side effects increase with increasing concentration. Sometimes erythema quickly progresses to frosting. This is associated with scarring or PIH.

28.5.2e Jessner's and Modified Jessner's Solution

JS consists of 14% resorcinol, 14% SA, and 14% lactic acid (LA) in 95% ethanol. It is used for treating melasma and post-inflammatory hyperpigmentation.[41] Modified JS solution contains 17% lactic acid, 17% salicylic acid, and 8% citric acid (all in weight to volume) and ethanol anhydrous.

28.5.2f Phenol Peel

Phenol 88% is a medium-depth peel and is associated with cardiotoxicity and hypopigmentation.[10, 42] Phenol immediately coagulates epidermal and superficial dermal proteins with increased collagen and elastic fibers histologically.

28.5.3 Procedure

The patient is positioned supine with the head elevated on a pillow at 45° and a towel placed around the neck. Their eyes should remain closed for the procedure. A surgical cap is used to keep the hair off the treatment site. Petrolatum or zinc oxide paste may be applied to the lateral canthi, nasal alar grooves, nasolabial folds, lips, and oral commissures to prevent the pooling of the peeling agent in these areas.

Before applying the peeling agent, the skin should be degreased with acetone, triclosan, or isopropyl alcohol to remove residual cosmetics, oils, loose keratin, and other debris.

The chemical peel is applied using a brush or a cotton tip and is started from areas of thick skin. The forehead, cheeks, nose, and chin are treated first, followed by the perioral and periorbital skin. The agent is applied in an upward direction with firm, even strokes. Care should be taken to avoid overlapping brush strokes and skipping areas. A feathering technique is employed at the edge of the treatment field to avoid sharp demarcation lines. In areas of deep wrinkling, skin is stretched to prevent the pooling of the peeling agent.

Pain control must be adequately taken care of. This is done by physical agents like ice packs and fans and oral agents like paracetamol, non-steroidal anti-inflammatory agents, regional nerve blocks, and general anesthesia for deep peels. Superficial peels generally do not require anesthesia, while phenol peeling requires sedation and regional or general anesthesia.[43]

TABLE 28.4: Choice of Peeling Agents

Indication	Peeling Agent
Active acne	• Salicylic acid 20–30%
	• Mandelic acid 20–50%
	• Glycolic acid 20–35%
	• Tretinoin peel 1–5%
	• Retinol peel 1–5%
	• Jessner's solution
	• Pyruvic acid 40–50%
	• Combination peels
Melasma and other pigmentary disorders	Salicylic acid 20–30%
	Mandelic acid 20–50%
	Glycolic acid 20–70%
	Tretinoin peel 1–5%
	Retinol peel 1–5%
	Jessner's solution
	TCA 15–25%
Photoaging	Salicylic acid 20–30%
	Glycolic acid 35–70%
	Pyruvic acid 40–50%
	TCA 25–35%
	Tretinoin peel 1–5%
	Retinol peel 1–5%
	Jessner's solution
	Mandelic acid 20–50%
	Monheit's peel—Jessner's followed by TCA 35%
	Coleman's peel—glycolic acid 70% followed by TCA 35%
Skin brightening (Party Peel)	Lactic acid 92%
	Ferulic acid
	Phytic acid

28.6 Post-Procedure Care

Patients are explained about the care that needs to be taken after the chemical peel procedure.

They are instructed to wash their face with a non-soap cleanser and to avoid rubbing, scrubbing, scratching, or picking. A bland emollient and sunscreen should be applied regularly to the skin till healing is complete. If there is crusting, a topical antibacterial agent is applied. Makeup can be applied once re-epithelization is complete. Sun avoidance is advised.

28.7 Side Effects and Their Management

Chemical peeling is a relatively safe procedure. Appropriate patient selection and pre-procedure care minimize the risk. However, there are side effects, which can be mild or severe (Table 28.5).

Excessive irritation and burning are managed with topical steroids. A short course of oral steroids can also be given. Bacterial infections are managed with topical and oral antibiotics. Prolonged erythema may be treated with pulsed-dye or dual-wavelength vascular lasers.[44] PIH is more common in skin of color but is usually temporary and can be managed with skin-lightening agents like kojic acid, azelaic acid, arbutin, or hydroquinone (Figure 28.3).

28.8 Clinical Pearls in Treating Ethnic Skin/Skin of Color

* Skin of color is prone to post-inflammatory hyperpigmentation. Priming with skin-lightening agents and tretinoin for at least four to six weeks prior to peeling, along with strict sun protection, reduces risks.
* Start with lower-strength peels and gradually build up. Combination peels are safer.

28.9 Conclusion

Chemical peels are versatile office procedures useful in the treatment of acne, pigmentation, and photoaging. Choosing the right peeling agent with the right strength, careful technique, and regular post-procedure care are the key factors in achieving success.

TABLE 28.5: Adverse Effects of Chemical Peels

Mild	Moderate	Severe
• Irritation	• Infection (bacterial, fungal, and viral)	• Scarring (atrophic, hypertrophic, and keloid)
• Burning	• Persistent erythema	• Allergic reactions
• Erythema	• Demarcation lines	• Laryngeal edema
• Pruritus	• Milia	• Toxic shock syndrome
• Scaling	• Pigmentary changes (hyperpigmentation and hypopigmentation)	• Cardiotoxicity
• Edema	• Textural changes	• Acute kidney injury
• Acneiform eruptions	• Increased pigmentation of naevi	• Lower-lid ectropion
	• Salicylism	• Corneal damage
		• Significant scarring
		• Dyspigmentation

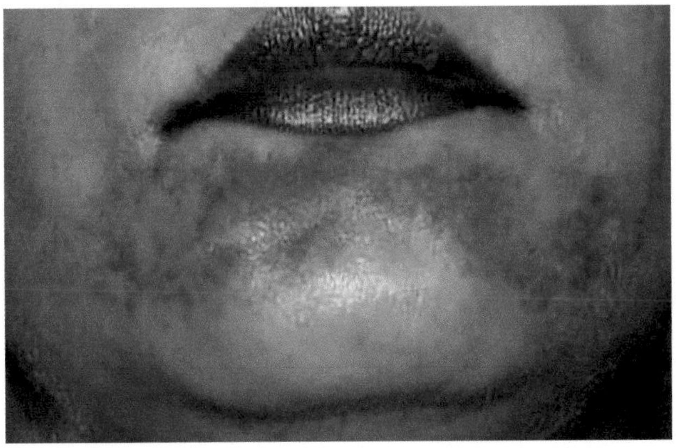

SCHEMATIC APPROACH

Patient assessment

▼

Good candidate for chemical peel

▼

Start priming regimen for 2-4 weeks

▼

Counselling, consent, photographs

▼

Skin preparation

▼

Select and apply peeling agent

▼

Terminate the peel after achieving endpoint

▼

Home care instructions

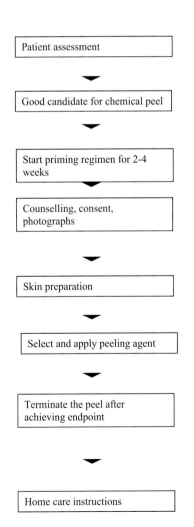

FIGURE 28.3 Complication with PIH in the perioral region following glycolic acid peeling 70%.

Frequently Asked Questions

1. *Q: Is chemical peeling indicated?*

   A: Chemical peeling can now be safely done on skin of color, using the appropriate peeling agent, with due care. Superficial and medium-depth peels are safe, whereas deep peels have a higher risk for pigmentary changes. Acne, pigmentary disorders, photoaging, and skin rejuvenation are the main indications.

2. *Q: Are there any contraindications?*

   A: Recent suntan, infection, delayed healing, prolonged sun exposure, and uncooperative patients with non-adherence to home care regimens are relative contraindications to chemical peels.

3. *Q: Which peel should be choosen and at what strength?*

   A: The peeling agent and strength depend on the condition to be treated, the type of patient's skin (dry, oily, mature, or sensitive), and the degree of photodamage.

4. *Q: How often are they repeated?*

   A: Very superficial peels can be repeated every one to two weeks, superficial peels every two to four weeks, and medium-depth peels once in six months.

5. *Q: What side effects are expected, and how are they avoided?*

   A: The commonest side effects are excessive irritation, dryness, burning, and edema, which can be avoided by initially selecting peeling agents of lower strength and gradually building up. PIH can be avoided by sun protection and strictly following pre- and post-peel care regimens.

References

1. O'Connor AA, Lowe PM, Shumack S, Lim AC. Chemical peels: A review of current practice. *Australas. J. Dermatol.* 2018; 59: 171–181.
2. Drake LA, Dinehart SM, Goltz RW et al. Guidelines of care for chemical peeling. Guidelines/outcomes committee: American academy of dermatology. *J. Am. Acad. Dermatol.* 1995; 33: 497–503.
3. Landau M. Chemical peels. *Clin. Dermatol.* 2008; 26: 200–208.
4. Khunger N, Force IT. Standard guidelines of care for chemical peels. *Indian J. Dermatol. Venereol. Leprol.* 2008; 74: S5–12.
5. Zakopoulou N, Kontochristopoulos G. Superficial chemical peels. *J. Cosmet. Dermatol.* 2006; 5: 246–253.
6. Langsdon PR, Rodwell DW 3rd, Velargo PA et al. Latest chemical peel innovations. *Facial Plast. Surg. Clin. North Am.* 2012; 20: 119–123.
7. Rendon MI, Berson DS, Cohen JL et al. Evidence and considerations in the application of chemical peels in skin disorders and aesthetic resurfacing. *J. Clin. Aesthet. Dermatol.* 2010; 3: 32–43.
8. Berson DS, Cohen JL, Rendon MI et al. Clinical role and application of superficial chemical peels in today's practice. *J. Drugs Dermatol.* 2009; 8: 803–811.
9. Matarasso SL, Glogau RG, Markey AC. Wood's lamp for superficial chemical peels. *J. Am. Acad. Dermatol.* 1994; 30: 988–992.
10. Camacho FM. Medium-depth and deep chemical peels. *J. Cosmet. Dermatol.* 2005; 4: 117–128.
11. Jackson A. Chemical peels. *Facial Plast. Surg.* 2014; 30: 26–34.
12. Kessler E, Flanagan K, Chia C, Rogers C, Glaser DA. Comparison of alpha- and beta-hydroxy acid chemical peels in the treatment of mild to moderately severe facial acne vulgaris. *Dermatol. Surg.* 2008; 34: 45–50.
13. Al-Talib H, Al-Khateeb A, Hameed A, Murugaiah C. Efficacy and safety of superficial chemical peeling in treatment of active acne vulgaris. *An Bras Dermatol.* 2017; 92: 212–216.
14. Dayal S, Amrani A, Sahu P, Jain VK. Jessner's solution vs. 30% salicylic acid peels: A comparative study of the efficacy and safety in mild-to-moderate acne vulgaris. *J. Cosmet. Dermatol.* 2017; 16: 43–51.
15. Kligman DE, Draelos ZD. Combination superficial peels with salicylic acid and post-peel retinoids. *J. Drugs. Dermatol.* 2016; 15: 442–450.
16. Vemula S, Maymone MBC, Secemsky EA et al. Assessing the safety of superficial chemical peels in darker skin: A retrospective study. *J. Am. Acad. Dermatol.* 2018; 79: 508–513.
17. Abdel-Meguid AM, Taha EA, Ismail SA. Combined Jessner solution and trichloroacetic acid versus trichloroacetic acid alone in the treatment of melasma in dark-skinned patients. *Dermatol. Surg.* 2017; 43: 651–656.
18. Brody HJ. Commentary on combined Jessner solution and trichloroacetic acid versus trichloroacetic acid alone in the treatment of melasma in dark-skinned patients. *Dermatol. Surg.* 2017; 43: 657.
19. Sarkar R, Kaur C, Bhalla M, Kanwar AJ. The combination of glycolic acid peels with a topical regimen in the treatment of melasma in dark-skinned patients: A comparative study. *Dermatol. Surg.* 2002; 28: 828–832.
20. Grimes PE. The safety and efficacy of salicylic acid chemical peels in darker racial ethnic groups. *Dermatol. Surg.* 1999; 25: 18–22.
21. Vavouli C, Katsambas A, Gregoriou S et al. Chemical peeling with trichloroacetic acid and lactic acid for infraorbital dark circles. *J. Cosmet. Dermatol.* 2013; 12: 204–209.
22. Dayal S, Sahu P, Jain VK, Khetri S. Clinical efficacy and safety of 20% glycolic peel, 15% lactic peel, and topical 20% vitamin C in constitutional type of periorbital melanosis: A comparative study. *J. Cosmet. Dermatol.* 2016; 15: 367–373.
23. Mysore V, Omprakash HM, Khatri GN. Isotretinoin and dermatosurgical procedures. *Indian J. Dermatol. Venereol. Leprol.* 2019; 85: 18–22.
24. Peters W. The chemical peel. *Ann. Plast. Surg.* 1991; 26: 564–571.
25. Mangat DS, Tansavatdi K, Garlich P. Current chemical peels and other resurfacing techniques. *Facial Plast. Surg.* 2011; 27: 35–49.
26. Anitha B. Prevention of complications in chemical peeling. *J. Cutan. Aesthet. Surg.* 2010; 3: 186–188.
27. Fabbrocini GDP, De Padova MP, Tosti A. Chemical peels: What's new and what isn't new but still works well. *Facial Plast. Surg.* 2009; 25: 329–336.
28. Cortez EA. Chemical face peeling. *Otolaryngol. Clin. North Am.* 1990; 23: 947–961.
29. Stough DB 3rd. The chemical face peel. *Cutis.* 1976; 18: 239–240.
30. Monheit GD. Chemical peels. *Skin Ther. Lett.* 2004; 9: 6–11.
31. Cortez EA, Fedok FG, Mangat DS. Chemical peels: Panel discussion. *Facial Plast. Surg. Clin. North Am.* 2014; 22: 1–23.
32. Swinehart JM. Test spots in dermabrasion and chemical peeling. *J. Dermatol. Surg. Oncol.* 1990; 16: 557–563.
33. Khunger N. *Step by Step Chemical Peels.* New Delhi: Jaypee, 2014.
34. Langsdon PR, Rodwell DW 3rd, Velargo PA et al. Latest chemical peel innovations. *Facial Plast. Surg. Clin. North Am.* 2012; 20: 119–123.
35. Peters W. The chemical peel. *Ann. Plast. Surg.* 1991; 26: 564–571.
36. Magalhaees G, Borges M, Queiroz A, Capp A, Pedrosa S, Diniz M. Double-blind randomized study of 5% and 10% retinoic acid peels in the treatment of melasma: Clinical evaluation and impact on the quality of life. *Surg. Cosmet. Dermatol.* 2011; 3: 17–22.
37. Khunger N, Sarkar R, Jain RK. Tretinoin peels versus glycolic acid peels in the treatment of Melasma in dark-skinned patients. *Dermatol. Surg.* 2004 May; 30(5): 756–760; discussion 760.
38. Dainichi T, Ueda S, Imayama S, Furue M. Excellent clinical results with a new preparation for chemical peeling in acne: 30% salicylic acid in polyethylene glycol vehicle. *Dermatol. Surg.* 2008; 34: 891–899.
39. Dainichi T, Amano S, Matsunaga Y et al. Chemical peeling by SA-PEG remodels photo-damaged skin: Suppressing p53 expression and normalizing keratinocyte differentiation. *J. Invest. Dermatol.* 2006; 126: 416–421.
40. Bridenstine JB, Dolezal JF. Standardizing chemical peel solution formulations to avoid mishaps. Great fluctuations in actual concentrations of trichloroacetic acid. *J. Dermatol. Surg. Oncol.* 1994; 20: 813–816.
41. Wambier C, Brody H. Classification of chemical peels. In: da Costa A, ed. *MinimallyInvasive Aesthetic Procedures for Dermatologists and Plastic Surgeons.* Atlanta, GA: Springer Nature, 2019:1–12.
42. de Mendonca MCC, Segheto NN, Aarestrup FM, Aarestrup BJV. Punctuated 88% phenol peeling for the treatment of facial photoaging: A clinical and histopathological study. *Dermatol. Surg.* 2018; 44: 241–247.
43. Rubin MG, Wiest LG, Gout U. *IllustratedGuide to Chemical Peels.* New Malden: Quintessence, 2014.
44. Maloney BP, Millman B, Monheit G, McCollough EG. The etiology of prolonged erythema after chemical peel. *Dermatol. Surg.* 1998; 24: 337–341.

CHAPTER 29: MICRODERMABRASION

Atchima Suwanchinda and Natthachat Jurairattanaporn

29.1 Introduction

Microdermabrasion (MDA) is one of the most performed minimally invasive aesthetic procedures for skin rejuvenation that physically removes the superficial part of the epidermis, including the stratum corneum (SC), to the upper dermis by mechanical abrasion (1–3). The wound-healing process then occurs, resulting in an increase in epidermal thickness, neocollagenesis, and neo-elastogenesis (4). Due to exfoliation, it also acts as a delivery system with an increase in the absorption of active ingredients. Studies have shown improved skin permeability and enhanced delivery of transdermal medications and cosmeceuticals (5–8). MDA is used to treat mild photoaging skin, uneven texture, scars, seborrhea, stretch marks, acne, acne scars, and superficial hyperpigmentation (9). Recently, there are various indications using the combination with other modalities to increase its efficacy. MDA technique is considered safe for all Fitzpatrick skin types. The downtime is acceptable with minimal side effects (10, 11). It has been considered as initial skin rejuvenation suitable for both female and male patients (12–14).

29.2 Type of Devices

Basically, this procedure relies on an abrasive component and a vacuum component. The original foundation of the system consisted of the headpiece and the operating machine. This MDA uses a closed-loop negative pressure system. There are various MDA systems that differ based on the source of the abrasive component. Mostly used devices include crystal-containing and non-crystal-containing systems (15, 16). Regardless of the abrasive stimulus, MDA devices are basically a closed-loop system (15, 16).

29.2.1 Crystal-Containing MDA

This device requires aluminum oxide (Al_2O_3) or sodium chloride (NaCl) as a major abrasive material. The other crystals, such as magnesium oxide and sodium bicarbonate, are less commonly employed (12). The headpiece is basically composed of a tip and a small chamber that deliver abrasive elements on the skin (15). The crystal has a diameter of 100 microns and shows excellent abrasive properties due to multiple sharp edges on its structure with water insolubility. The abrasive crystals are gradually propelled on the skin surface, creating superficial abrasion and exfoliating the outermost layer of the SC. The crystals are suctioned back as a closed-loop system (15). Some devices can create aerosolized crystals, but it has a concerning disadvantage because both patient and operator can accidentally inhale the aerosol during the procedure. The crystals may also cause ocular injury to the patient if proper eye protection is not performed. Normally, the crystal cannot be reused and should be disposed of after a single application (15, 16). Figure 29.1 shows corundum MDA.

29.2.2 Non-Crystal-Containing MDA

The headpiece has a special tip with an abrasive property, such as diamond or bristle, that is embedded on the distal part of the treatment tip. It has various grit patterns that create different aggressiveness of abrasion across the skin. These systems rely on the abrasiveness of the handpiece, much like a diamond fraise in mechanical dermabrasion, to disrupt the skin surface and promote exfoliation (16). The treatment tip can be used again after proper sterilization. This device has been increasingly performed as it lowers the risk of ocular injury or inhalation of abrasive elements to the respiratory system. Figure 29.2 shows non-crystal-containing corundum MDA.

Various MDA systems that differ based on the source of the abrasive component have been developed.

29.2.3 Oxygen MDA (Oxybrasion)

Current MDA uses other substances as abrasive material. This novel method involves the application of a stream of saline solution (0.9% NaCl) and compressed air on the skin surface (9). Application of the NSS stream causes skin cooling, which reduces discomfort during exfoliation. It is considered safe and gentle for the skin as the physiological saline used is neutral to the skin, and the whole procedure is carried out without any contact with the skin. It minimizes the risk of bleeding or

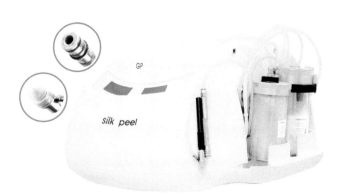

FIGURE 29.1 Crystal microdermabrasion device.

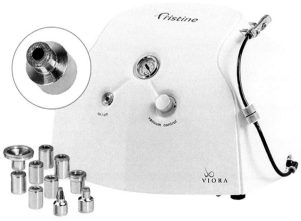

FIGURE 29.2 Non-crystal-containing microdermabrasion device.

DOI: 10.1201/9780429243769-29

exudation and carries a minimal risk of complications (9). It helps to increase skin hydration and significantly decrease skin hydrolipid coat and pH (9).

29.3 Mechanism of Action

MDA detaches the SC, which is the outermost layer of the skin (1–3). It creates a superficial depth of exfoliation with the repetitive application of shearing force of either crystal element or diamond tip on the epidermis (10, 11). After the wound-healing process, the skin texture gradually improves. Even though the depth of penetration of MDA is mainly in the uppermost part of the epidermis, which is the SC, it also influences the deeper layers of the epidermis and dermis. Basically, the penetration depth depends on the type of abrasive elements used in MDA and the number of passes. An increased number of passes of MDA may enhance penetration to the stratum granulosum or even the superficial part of the papillary dermis or full epidermis. The optimization of MDA for controlled depth of the injury strongly depends on the crystal flow rate and exposure time and only weakly on the pressure or static/dynamic mode operation (2). However, a more aggressive depth of penetration to the reticular dermis cannot be achieved by conservative MDA. To achieve that level of penetration, aggressive dermabrasion and medium-depth to deep chemical peeling or ablative resurfacing laser should be employed. Besides the operator's technique, the differences between crystal and non-crystal MDA offers different results, as summarized in Table 29.1.

29.4 Histological Evaluation

Histological evaluation of the skin after the immediate application of this procedure shows thinning of the SC. There is a thickening of the epidermis and dermis, a flattening of rete ridges at the dermal-epidermal junction, increased collagen fiber density at the dermal-epidermal junction, vascular ectasia in the reticular dermis, perivascular inflammation, and hyalinization of the papillary dermis with newly deposited collagen and elastic fibers (4, 17). MDA also demonstrates upregulation of wound-healing transcription factors and matrix metalloproteinases in the dermis (18). Few comparative histological studies after chemical peeling and MDA have shown interesting findings. Abdel-Motaleb et al. compared

dermal morphological changes following salicylic acid (30%) application and MDA, which demonstrated that both salicylic acid and MDA were associated with a thickened epidermal layer, thin dermal papillae, dense collagen, and elastic fiber formation (19). Another study found that the histological change after MDA showed more microvessel formation than chemical peeling (20). El-Domyati M. et al. histological analysis of different cutaneous conditions such as melasma, acne scars, striae distensae, and photoaging revealed that after the eighth week of weekly treatment of MDA, the histological section had decreased melanization and more regular distribution of melanosomes in the epidermis in melasma group. Moreover, there was an increase in collagen fibers with the more organized arrangement in acne scars, striae, and photoaging groups (1).

29.5 Transdermal Drug Delivery

MDA has been shown to improve transdermal drug delivery by removing the SC as it is the main barrier which limits the percutaneous diffusion of drugs and other molecules(6). One study demonstrated that a viable epidermis offers a significant permeability barrier that becomes rate limiting upon sufficient permeabilization of SC. The removal of SC dramatically increased skin permeability to all compounds tested. Furthermore, removal of full epidermis increases skin permeability and facilitates drug delivery (8, 21). A previous study demonstrated that full epidermal removal with MDA can increase skin permeability to insulin at a level sufficient to reduce blood glucose level similar to subcutaneous insulin injection (8). In addition, MDA has been employed to improve drug delivery using vitamin C, lidocaine, and 5 FU, and cosmeceuticals (8, 22, 23). Even though, ongoing research shows promising results, the feasibility of using MDA in clinical practice for this purpose is still unknown (6, 8, 22). An advanced form of dermabrasion combines microdermabrasion with simultaneous infusion of a combination of natural extracts, hyaluronic acid and a complex of peptide to the treatment area (Figure 29.3).

29.6 The Effect of Skin Barrier Function

29.6.1 Sebum
Several studies showed the significant sedum reduction of a series of 5 to 6 biweekly corundum MDA on different areas of the face (forehead, nose, right and left cheek, chin) (17, 24, 25). Another recent study also demonstrated sebum reduction immediately after MDA irrespective of skin type and face area. In addition, the sebum value was found to return to baseline one hour after the procedure (26).

29.6.2 Skin Hydration
A statistically significant difference in SC hydration 30 minutes after treatment on the cheek and immediately after the procedure on the T-zone area has been demonstrated (26). The observed changes in epidermal barrier function may be responsible for the clinical improvement (26).

29.6.3 Transepidermal Water Loss (TEWL)
Several studies reported a significant increase in TEWL immediately after a single diamond MDA on the forehead and cheek, which remained for 24 hours (27). Similar results for NaCl and AL_2O_3 MDA showed that TEWL values decreased to levels below the baseline level (28).

TABLE. 29.1: The Differences between Microdermabrasion Devices

	Crystal MDAs	Non-Crystal MDAs
Abrasive element	Disposable crystals • Aluminum oxide (AL_2O_3) • Sodium chloride (NaCl)	Non-disposable abrasive tip • Diamond • Bristle
Depth of penetration	Deep penetration (More with multiple passes)	Moderate penetration
Suitable candidate	Thick skin	Thin skin
Pain	Mild	Low
Risk	Inhalation of aerosolized particles	Contamination risk from inadequate sterilization of the tip

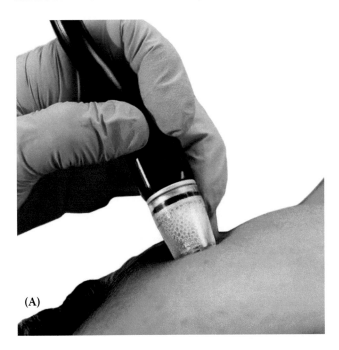

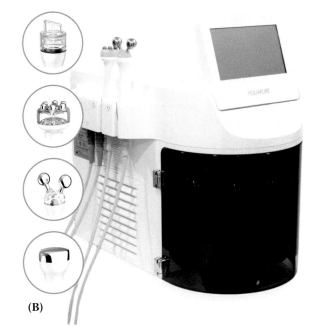

FIGURE 29.3 Microdermabrasion with concurrent multiple solution infusion. A) Advanced technology of dermabrasion combines microdermabrasion with simultaneous infusion of a combination of natural extracts, hyaluronic acid, and a complex of peptides to the treatment area. B) Electroporation, microcurrent and cooling are also available for combination treatment in one treatment session.

29.6.4 Skin pH

There is a significant decrease in skin pH, which may be associated with an increase in hydrogen ions in the treatment area (9, 29). The pH of the skin is between 4.1 and 5.8 (30). There are several benefits of having acidic skin pH. An acidic skin pH may inhibit tyrosinase activity, which could be one of the responsible factors in pigmentation reduction. In addition, it may also decrease susceptibility to infection that may have therapeutic effects and prevent bacterial colonization, such as in acne vulgaris and dry and sensitive skin conditions, since pathogenic bacteria grow better in an alkaline environment (31–33).

29.6.5 The Effect of Skin Pigmentation

MDA alone also showed lower epidermal melanization and more regular distribution of melanosomes with Fontana-Masson staining after a series of six MDA treatments on the forearms (9). MDA causes a rearrangement of melanosomes in the basal layer of the epidermis (17). In addition, an acidic pH environment inhibits tyrosinase activity, which could result in a reduction in pigmentation (9, 31).

29.6.6 Indications

- *Improving skin texture*: Irregular skin texture includes surface roughness, fine lines, enlarged pores, and superficial scars. After a single MDA session, Karimipour DJ et al. found that there is a significant increase in pro-inflammatory transcription factors (AP-1 and nuclear factor-kappa binding; NF-kB) and cytokines (interleukin-1 beta and tumor necrosis factor-alpha). These factors and cytokines play a potential role as matrix metalloproteinases (MMP) regulators. Moreover, around 20% of the subjects showed the elevation of type I collagen after the treatment (18). MDA also enhances hydration and helps in sebum reduction, which leads to better skin texture.
- *Abnormal pigmentation*: Dyspigmentation includes solar-damaged skin or superficial hyperpigmentary disorders.

Shim et al. reported histological change of mottled skin hyperpigmentation associated with photoaging with more regular distribution of melanosomes and decreased melanization of epidermis (34). Combination treatment study of MDA followed by low-fluence Q-switch Nd:YAG laser in female patients with mixed type melasma demonstrated more than 95% melasma clearance after three to four treatment sessions in more than 60% of patients with minimal adverse effects. Only mild erythema was observed, with no long-term hypopigmentation or guttate leukoderma (35).

- *Acne with mild to moderate severity*: Weekly treatment of MDA in acne patients as an adjunctive treatment for a total of eight weeks showed excellent to good results in 72% of the subjects in one study. However, the improvement may not be fully from MDA alone since subjects still use their acne medication (36). Wang et al. using MDA in combination with 1,450 nm diode laser in comparison with 1,450 diode laser alone demonstrated no significant additional benefit in terms of clinical efficacy. However, both the combination and laser groups showed significant improvement in inflammatory acne lesion count (37).
- *Transdermal drug delivery*: MDA exhibits an enhanced delivery of cosmeceuticals and the degree of penetration, which depends on lipophilicity. Hydrophilic compounds may penetrate into the skin more than lipophilic ones after application (7). MDA has been shown to improve 5-aminolevulinic acid (ALA) absorption, shortening the incubation time to minutes. Moreover, it can enhance the absorption of hydrophilic substances through the lipophilic epidermal barrier as well. Abdel-Motaleb et al. demonstrated significantly greater MASI reduction in combination with MDA before 70% glycolic acid than 70% GA alone in dark-skinned patients (7, 38). Moreover, MDA has been used as an adjunctive modality for vitiligo patients in combination with standard topical treatments. Farajzadeh S et al. conducted a single-blind, randomized study in nonsegmental

TABLE 29.2: Microdermabrasion Indications

Indications

- Acne with mild to moderate severity
- Uneven skin texture (surface roughness, fine lines, enlarged pores, or superficial scars)
- Pigmentary disorders (melasma or post-inflammatory hyperpigmentation)
- Photoaging
- Seborrheic skin
- Fine wrinkles
- Enlarged pores
- Scar, including acne scar
- Striae distensae
- Drug delivery
  — 5% aminolevulinic acid (ALA)
  — Glycolic acid
  — Tacrolimus and pimecrolimus
  — Insulin

* Including the case study and report in the literature.

TABLE 29.3: Microdermabrasion and Combination Treatment

Combination Treatment	Indication
MDA + 70% glycolic peeling (48)	Melasma
MDA + low-fluence Q-switched Nd: YAG (35)	Melasma
MDA + topical tranexamic acid 5%(49)	Hyperpigmentation
MDA + topical tacrolimus (40)	Vitiligo
MDA + topical pimecrolimus 1%(39)	Vitiligo
MDA + 5% retinoic acid (45)	Photoaging
MDA + 5-FU (47)	Vitiligo
MDA + 20% aminolaevulinic acid (44)	Photodynamic therapy
MDA + 595 nm pulsed dye laser, long-pulsed 755 nm alexandrite laser (42)	Keratosis pilaris
MDA+ 1,450 nm diode laser (50)	Acne
MDA+ sonophoresis (46)	Striae distensae

* Including the case study and report in the literature.

childhood vitiligo by performing MDA followed by the application of topical pimecrolimus (1%) compared with the topical application alone and placebo. Of the patches, 60.5% showed a clinical response in the combination group, followed by 32.1% and 1.7% in the topical treatment and the placebo group, respectively (39). In addition, a single-blind, randomized placebo-controlled study compared clinical response between the daily treatment of topical tacrolimus (0.03%) with or without monthly MDA. By the end of three months, the combination group demonstrated moderate to excellent response in 65.7% and the topical treatment group in 25.8% of the vitiliginous patches. Only 12% of the subjects experienced the mild adverse effect of a burning sensation during MDA (40). Andrews et al. reported that MDA could facilitate the delivery of insulin embedded as a transdermal reservoir patch by full epidermal that which can increase skin permeability to insulin at a level sufficient to reduce blood glucose level (8).

Reported indications of MDA are summarized in Table 29.2 and Table 29.3 (6, 16, 35, 39, 41–47).

29.7 Patient Workup/Counseling

- A thorough patient history is necessary, with a review of underlying medical conditions focusing on some

TABLE 29.4: Microdermabrasion Contraindications

Contraindication (12, 51)

- Impaired skin integrity, open wounds, or cutaneous erosions over the treatment area
- Active skin infections within the treatment area, including other bacterial, viral, or fungal infections, or inflammatory lesions, such as active inflammatory acne or rosacea and telangiectasias, eczema, psoriasis herpes simplex virus, varicella zoster virus, human papillomavirus, and impetigo
- Cutaneous disorders with active Koebner phenomena, such as psoriasis, lichen planus, or vitiligo
- Underlying medical conditions that may impair the wound healing process, such as bleeding disorders, diabetes mellitus, and immunosuppression
- Contact allergies to the abrasive crystals (e.g., aluminum allergy)
- Concurrent medications that may affect proper wound healing, such as bleeding tendencies from anticoagulants, isotretinoin use within the last six months, or current use of immunosuppressive agents
- Known history of bleeding disorders or taking anticoagulant (blood thinner) therapies, such as warfarin, heparin, or low-dose aspirin
- Autoimmune diseases or immunosuppression due to medical conditions or medications
- Pregnancy and lactation
- Keloid or hypertrophic scarring predisposition
- Sunburn or tan or sun exposure in the next two weeks after treatment
- MDA immediately after injections or laser/IPL in the area to be treated
- After waxing
- Patients with uncontrolled diabetes
- Patients with unidentified or suspicious lesions, undiagnosed skin cancer
- Unrealistic expectations and body dysmorphic disorder
- Patients who cannot adhere to appropriate post-treatment care and sun avoidance

diseases that may interfere with proper wound healing, such as diabetes mellitus, hematological conditions that affect coagulopathy, or previous history of herpes simplex virus infection. The contraindication of this procedure are mentioned in Table 29.4
- Evaluate the Fitzpatrick skin type.
- A full discussion with the patients regarding their main concerns and a detailed explanation of MDA indications, expected results, and alternative treatments is important. Counseling is also required about possible clinical results from MDA to meet the patient's realistic expectations, pre- and post-treatment care, possible side effects, and expected downtime after the procedure.

29.8 Pre-Procedure Care

- Patients should be instructed to avoid the application of any chemical peels or irritating substances before the procedure for a few weeks.
- Patients should avoid direct sun exposure for a few weeks prior to treatment sessions.
- In patients with a previous history of herpetic infection, prophylactic antiviral therapy should be initiated 48 hours before the procedure to prevent a herpetic attack afterward.
- Advise the patient to avoid wearing contact lenses before the procedure, especially when crystal MDA is performed.
- No local anesthesia is needed since the pain during the procedure is tolerable.

29.9 Procedure

29.9.1 Patient Preparation

- Clean the treatment area with a gentle cleanser and later with alcohol. Wait at least two minutes for the alcohol to dry before starting the procedure.
- The patient should be lying in a supine position, and cover the patient's eyes with a gauze pad or proper eye protection, especially when an aerosolized crystal MDA system is being used.

29.9.2 Device and Equipment Preparation

- Choose an appropriate sterilized abrasive treatment tip for a non-crystal-containing system and check the crystal delivery system for the crystal-containing system.
- Set vacuum pressure and recheck the system circuit by occluding the treatment tip with the operator's thumb.

29.9.3 Operator Preparation

- Wear protective eyewear and appropriate surgical attire since MDA is considered a high-risk procedure that may create aerosolized particles. Appropriate face mask, face shield, or protective clothing should be employed, especially in the era of SARS-CoV-2 infection (52).

29.9.4 Steps of Treatment

- Areas that should be avoided during MDA are periocular and perioral areas since the skin is fragile and may cause unwanted side effects, such as petechiae or purpura.
- The device uses negative pressure, and it pulls the skin into the handpiece. Firmly stretching the area with the operator's fingers helps to fully expand the treatment site.
- The device releases the abrasive crystals at a controlled flow rate. Gently press the headpiece on the skin and move slowly and gently across the skin and parallel to skin tension lines. The pattern of the treatment technique is shown in Figure 29.4. Short strokes can also be applied if there is any discomfort. It is imperative to avoid uneven pressure or pressing the headpiece with too much pressure, particularly on bony prominences.
- Move the headpiece in the same fashion to cover all the treatment zone, such as the forehead, glabella, lateral eyes, nose, cheeks, and chin.
- Surface debris and the stratum corneum layer of cells are removed. The particles will be collected in a reservoir to be later discarded (6).
- Multiple passes of MDA can be achieved by moving the headpiece in a diagonal direction against the previous round.
- A single treatment usually requires three passes over the treated are. The operator should be aware that the degree of SC removal is dependent on the crystal flow rate and exposure time (6).
- The desirable clinical endpoint is mild erythema of the treatment area. Intense petechiae, purpura, or intolerable pain should be avoided.
- The entire procedure typically takes 30–60 minutes (6).
- The remaining crystal and debris are wiped away with NS-soaked gauze and pat-dried with dry gauze.

29.10 Post-Procedure Care

- For the first few days after the procedure, the patient may develop mild erythema or dryness. A bland moisturizer with or without anti-inflammatory ingredients may be applied during this period to hasten recovery. If there is a scale-crust formation, local wet dressing with normal saline or topical petrolatum ointment should be employed to facilitate wound healing. Patients should be instructed to avoid skin picking to prevent scar formation.
- Irritating topical medications such as retinoids, benzoyl peroxide, and chemical peels should be avoided for at least two weeks after the procedure to prevent further skin irritation.
- Broad-spectrum sunscreen should be applied daily (SPF more than 30 with high UVA protection) with proper avoidance of UV exposure and other physical protection as needed.
- Four to six weekly treatments are normally required to achieve desired results (6).

29.11 Side Effects and Their Management

- Erythema is a frequent side effect that can be expected, which is usually mild and subsides in hours to days. However, some patients with a dark skin complexion may have a longer duration of erythema of about a week.
  Management: If erythema occurs immediately after the procedure, an ice pack or single application of high-potency topical corticosteroid should be employed. In some patients where erythema persists, mild-potency topical corticosteroids can be used for a short period of time until erythema subsides.
- Abrasion can occur in patients with multiple passes of treatment or treated with excessive pressure during the procedure of MDA. After creating a deeper level of penetration, the abrasion later turns to scale crust formation.
  Management: Petrolatum ointment can be applied to facilitate wound healing. Avoid picking and sun exposure to prevent PIH or scar formation.
- Petechiae or purpura can occur in a high-vacuum setting or in elderly patients with fragile, thin epidermis or taking anticoagulants. When petechiae or purpura occurs, it takes longer time to heal than erythema (up to two to three weeks). To prevent this complication, a low-vacuum setting and fewer passes should be employed.
- Urticaria is the most serious adverse effect, especially in patients who have a previous history of allergic reaction to latex or a history of chronic inducible urticaria, especially symptomatic dermographism.
- Post-inflammatory hyperpigmentation (PIH) can occur in dark-skinned patients (Fitzpatrick skin types IV–VI) who underwent multiple passes of MDA with an aggressive depth of penetration.
  Management: Avoid aggressive MDA in dark-skinned patients. If PIH occurs, sun avoidance and sun protection should be encouraged. Topical whitening and bleaching agents should be prescribed to fasten PIH recovery.
- Ocular injury can occur with aerosolized crystal systems. Appropriate eye protection for both patient and operator should be strictly adhered to.
- Flaring of erythema in rosacea patients, especially with multiple passes and high vacuum setting.
- Eruptive keratoacanthoma has been reported in a patient that underwent MDA and photodynamic therapy with aminolevulinic acid for the treatment of actinic keratosis. A 70-year-old patient developed multiple eruptive monomorphic dome-shaped papules on his bilateral cheeks. Histopathology was done, and the diagnosis of keratoacanthoma was confirmed. However, all lesions completely subsided within five weeks without any treatments (53).

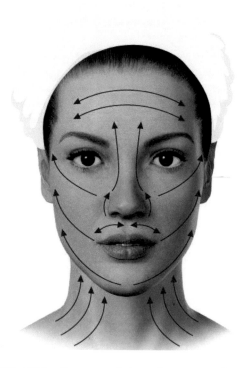

FIGURE 29.4 Recommended stroke pattern for microdermabrasion.

29.12 Clinical Pearls in Treating Ethnic Skin (14)

Patients with a dark complexion may have a higher risk of developing PIH or hypopigmentation. Even MDA is considered a minimally invasive procedure and a safe option for skin rejuvenation for ethnic skin types. Aggressive or multiple passes of MDA that cause deep exfoliation may induce substantial damage to the dermo-epidermal junction and later cause melanophages or melanocyte stimulation. In addition, dyspigmentation may occur if an inappropriate technique is used or if there is inadequate local wound care after the procedure.

29.13 Special Precautions—Do's and Don'ts

Do's

- Choose MDA for patients who expect only superficial exfoliation; the expectation of deep exfoliation should be counseled prior to the procedure.
- Appropriate choice of the MDA system, number of passes, and vacuum setting should be considered according to the patient's Fitzpatrick skin type, indication, and underlying medical conditions or preexisting skin conditions in the treatment area.
- Clinical endpoint for MDA is mild erythema.
- Perform the treatment with caution in dark-skinned patients since dyspigmentation may occur exclusively.

Don'ts

- Avoid too aggressive depth of treatment.
- Avoid treatment on periorbital skin or lip areas.
- Avoid endpoints of purpura or petechiae.

Frequently Asked Questions

1. *Q: Even though MDA is considered a high-safety aesthetic treatment, post-inflammatory hyperpigmentation (PIH) can occur in dark-skinned patients (Fitzpatrick skin types IV–VI). How can it be prevented?*
   A: To prevent this, multiple passes, too-aggressive depth of penetration, irritating active ingredients of cosmeceuticals and medication, and heat and sun exposure should be avoided.
2. *Q: What factors should be taken into consideration to do the MDA procedure effectively?*
   A: It is important to choose an appropriate MDA system, number of passes, crystal flow rate, vacuum setting, and abrasion elements to determine the abrasive level according to the patient's problem, Fitzpatrick skin type, and underlying medical conditions.
3. *Q: What is the precaution for the MDA procedure?*
   A: Greater attention should be addressed when the procedure is performed in dark-skinned patients, especially in sensitive areas, such as the periorbital or perioral areas and newly scarred or healed areas.
4. *Q: Can MDA be a good alternative for scar treatment?*
   A: It can be an alternative for scar treatment. However, for newly formed scars, care has to be taken to adjust the abrasive level and also make sure the vacuum setting is not too aggressive. For old scars, deeper exfoliation can also be done with extra precautions. The combination of other aesthetic treatments, such as chemical peeling, laser treatment, sonophoresis, and drug delivery systems, is very helpful.
5. *Q: How is the penetration depth in MDA increased?*
   A: The penetration depth of the abrasive level can be increased by using crystal MDA, increasing crystal flow rate, vacuum setting, exposure time, and the number of passes.

References

1. El-Domyati M, Hosam W, Abdel-Azim E, Abdel-Wahab H, Mohamed E. Microdermabrasion: A clinical, histometric, and histopathologic study. *J Cosmet Dermatol.* 2016;15(4):503–513.
2. Andrews SN, Zarnitsyn V, Bondy B, Prausnitz MR. Optimization of microdermabrasion for controlled removal of stratum corneum. *Int J Pharm.* 2011;407(1–2):95–104.
3. Gill HS, Andrews SN, Sakthivel SK, Fedanov A, Williams IR, Garber DA, et al. Selective removal of stratum corneum by microdermabrasion to increase skin permeability. *Eur J Pharm Sci.* 2009;38(2):95–103.
4. Freedman BM, Rueda-Pedraza E, Waddell SP. The epidermal and dermal changes associated with microdermabrasion. *Dermatol Surg.* 2001;27(12):1031–1033; discussion 3–4.
5. Zhou Y, Banga AK. Enhanced delivery of cosmeceuticals by microdermabrasion. *J Cosmet Dermatol.* 2011;10(3):179–184.
6. Shah M, Crane JS. *Microdermabrasion.* StatPearls. Treasure Island (FL) 2021.
7. Zhou Y, Banga AK. Enhanced delivery of cosmeceuticals by microdermabrasion. *J Cosmet Dermatol.* 2011;10(3):179–184.
8. Andrews S, Lee JW, Choi SO, Prausnitz MR. Transdermal insulin delivery using microdermabrasion. *Pharm Res.* 2011;28(9):2110–2118.
9. Jarząbek S, Rotsztejn H. Effect of oxybrasion on selected skin parameters. *J Cosmet Dermatol.* 2021;20(2):657–663.
10. Fernandes M, Pinheiro NM, Crema VO, Mendonça AC. Effects of microdermabrasion on skin rejuvenation. *J Cosmet Laser Ther.* 2014;16(1):26–31.
11. Spencer JM. Microdermabrasion. *Am J Clin Dermatol.* 2005;6(2):89–92.
12. Grimes PE. Microdermabrasion. *Dermatol Surg.* 2005;31(9 Pt 2):1160–1165; discussion 5.
13. Cohen BE, Bashey S, Wysong A. Literature review of cosmetic procedures in men: Approaches and techniques are gender specific. *Am J Clin Dermatol.* 2017;18(1):87–96.

14. Davis EC, Callender VD. Aesthetic dermatology for aging ethnic skin. *Dermatol Surg.* 2011;37(7):901–917.

15. Bhalla M, Thami GP. Microdermabrasion: Reappraisal and brief review of literature. *Dermatol Surg.* 2006;32(6):809–814.

16. Karimipour DJ, Karimipour G, Orringer JS. Microdermabrasion: An evidence-based review. *Plast Reconstr Surg.* 2010;125(1):372–377.

17. Tan MH, Spencer JM, Pires LM, Ajmeri J, Skover G. The evaluation of aluminum oxide crystal microdermabrasion for photodamage. *Dermatol Surg.* 2001;27(11):943–949.

18. Karimipour DJ, Kang S, Johnson TM, Orringer JS, Hamilton T, Hammerberg C, et al. Microdermabrasion: A molecular analysis following a single treatment. *J Am Acad Dermatol.* 2005;52(2):215–223.

19. Abdel-Motaleb AA, Abu-Dief EE, Hussein MR. Dermal morphological changes following salicylic acid peeling and microdermabrasion. *J Cosmet Dermatol.* 2017;16(4):e9–e14.

20. Hussein MR, Ab-Deif EE, Abdel-Motaleb AA, Zedan H, Abdel-Meguid AM. Chemical peeling and microdermabrasion of the skin: Comparative immunohistological and ultrastructural studies. *J Dermatol Sci.* 2008;52(3):205–209.

21. Andrews SN, Jeong E, Prausnitz MR. Transdermal delivery of molecules is limited by full epidermis, not just stratum corneum. *Pharm Res.* 2013;30(4):1099–1109.

22. Lee WR, Shen SC, Kuo-Hsien W, Hu CH, Fang JY. Lasers and microdermabrasion enhance and control topical delivery of vitamin C. *J Invest Dermatol.* 2003;121(5):1118–1125.

23. Prausnitz MR, Langer R. Transdermal drug delivery. *Nat Biotechnol.* 2008;26(11):1261–1268.

24. Davari P, Gorouhi F, Jafarian S, Dowlati Y, Firooz A. A randomized investigator-blind trial of different passes of microdermabrasion therapy and their effects on skin biophysical characteristics. *Int J Dermatol.* 2008;47(5):508–513.

25. Kolodziejczak A, Wieczorek AM, Rotsztejn HP. The assessment of the effects of the combination of microdermabrasion and cavitation peeling in the therapy of seborrhoeic skin with visible symptoms of acne punctata. *J Cosmet Laser Ther.* 2019;21(5):286–290.

26. Fak M, Rotsztejn H, Erkiert-Polguj A. The early effect of microdermabrasion on hydration and sebum level. *Skin Res Technol.* 2018;24(4):650–655.

27. Kim HS, Lim SH, Song JY, Kim MY, Lee JH, Park JG, et al. Skin barrier function recovery after diamond microdermabrasion. *J Dermatol.* 2009;36(10):529–533.

28. Rajan P, Grimes PE. Skin barrier changes induced by aluminum oxide and sodium chloride microdermabrasion. *Dermatol Surg.* 2002;28(5):390–393.

29. Mauro T, Grayson S, Gao WN, Man M-Q, Kriehuber E, Behne M, et al. Barrier recovery is impeded at neutral pH, independent of ionic effects: Implications for extracellular lipid processing. *Arch Dermatol Res.* 1998;290(4):215–222.

30. Lambers H, Piessens S, Bloem A, Pronk H, Finkel P. Natural skin surface pH is on average below 5, which is beneficial for its resident flora. *Int J Cosmet Sci.* 2006;28(5):359–370.

31. Segger D, Aßmus U, Brock M, Erasmy J, Finkel P, Fitzner A, et al. Multicenter study on measurement of the natural pH of the skin surface. *Int J Cosmet Sci.* 2008;30(1):75.

32. Marrakchi S, Maibach HI. Biophysical parameters of skin: Map of human face, regional, and age-related differences. *Contact Derm.* 2007;57(1):28–34.

33. Percival SL, McCarty S, Hunt JA, Woods EJ. The effects of pH on wound healing, biofilms, and antimicrobial efficacy. *Wound Repair Regen.* 2014;22(2):174–186.

34. Shim EK, Barnette D, Hughes K, Greenway HT. Microdermabrasion: A clinical and histopathologic study. *Dermatol Surg.* 2001;27(6):524–530.

35. Kauvar AN. Successful treatment of melasma using a combination of microdermabrasion and Q-switched Nd:YAG lasers. *Lasers Surg Med.* 2012;44(2):117–124.

36. Lloyd JR. The use of microdermabrasion for acne: A pilot study. *Dermatol Surg.* 2001;27(4):329–331.

37. Wang SQ, Counters JT, Flor ME, Zelickson BD. Treatment of inflammatory facial acne with the 1,450 nm diode laser alone versus microdermabrasion plus the 1,450 nm laser: A randomized, split-face trial. *Dermatol Surg.* 2006;32(2):249–255; discussion 55.

38. Abdel-Motaleb AA, Bakr RM. Microdermabrasion assisted delivery of glycolic acid 70% peel for the treatment of melasma in dark-skinned patients. *Dermatol Ther.* 2021:e15025.

39. Farajzadeh S, Daraei Z, Esfandiarpour I, Hosseini SH. The efficacy of pimecrolimus 1% cream combined with microdermabrasion in the treatment of nonsegmental childhood vitiligo: A randomized placebo-controlled study. *Pediatr Dermatol.* 2009;26(3):286–291.

40. Abd-Elazim NE, Yassa HA, Mahran AM. Microdermabrasion and topical tacrolimus: A novel combination therapy of vitiligo. *J Cosmet Dermatol.* 2020;19(6):1447–1455.

41. Abdel-Latif A, Elbendary A. Treatment of striae distensae with microdermabrasion: A clinical and molecular study. *JEWDS.* 2008;5:24–30.

42. Lee SJ, Chung WS, Kim J, Cho SB. Combination of 595-nm pulsed dye laser, long-pulsed 755-nm alexandrite laser and microdermabrasion treatment for keratosis pilaris. *J Dermatol.* 2012;39(5):479–480.

43. Lee SJ, Choi MJ, Zheng Z, Chung WS, Kim YK, Cho SB. Combination of 595-nm pulsed dye laser, long-pulsed 755-nm alexandrite laser, and microdermabrasion treatment for keratosis pilaris: Retrospective analysis of 26 Korean patients. *J Cosmet Laser Ther.* 2013;15(3):150–154.

44. Linkner RV, Jim On S, Haddican M, Singer G, Shim-Chang H. Evaluating the efficacy of photodynamic therapy with 20% aminolevulinic acid and microdermabrasion as a combination treatment regimen for acne scarring: A split-face, randomized, double-blind pilot study. *J Clin Aesthet Dermatol.* 2014;7(5):32–35.

45. Faghihi G, Fatemi-Tabaei S, Abtahi-Naeini B, Siadat AH, Sadeghian G, Ali Nilforoushzadeh M, et al. The effectiveness of a 5% retinoic acid peel combined with microdermabrasion for facial photoaging: A randomized, double-blind, placebo-controlled clinical trial. *Dermatol Res Pract.* 2017;2017:8516527.

46. Nassar A, Ghomey S, El Gohary Y, El-Desoky F. Treatment of striae distensae with needling therapy versus microdermabrasion with sonophoresis. *J Cosmet Laser Ther.* 2016;18(6):330–334.

47. Garg T, Chander R, Jain A. Combination of microdermabrasion and 5-fluorouracil to induce repigmentation in vitiligo: An observational study. *Dermatol Surg.* 2011;37(12):1763–1766.

48. Abdel-Motaleb AA, Bakr RM. Microdermabrasion assisted delivery of glycolic acid 70% peel for the treatment of melasma in dark-skinned patients. *Dermatol Ther.* 2021:e15025.

49. Batory M, Wolowiec-Korecka E, Rotsztejn H. The influence of topical 5% tranexamic acid at pH 2.38 with and without corundum microdermabrasion on pigmentation and skin surface lipids. *Dermatol Ther.* 2020;33(6):e14391.

50. Wang SQ, Counters JT, Flor ME, Zelickson BD. Treatment of inflammatory facial acne with the 1,450 nm diode laser alone versus microdermabrasion plus the 1,450 nm laser: A randomized, split-face trial. *Dermatol Surg.* 2006;32(2):249–255.

51. Nguyen T. Dermatology procedures: Microdermabrasion and chemical peels. *FP Essent.* 2014;426:16–23.

52. Kandhari R, Kohli M, Trasi S, Vedamurthy M, Chhabra C, Shetty K, et al. The changing paradigm of an aesthetic practice during the COVID-19 pandemic: An expert consensus. *Dermatol Ther.* 2021;34(1):e14382.

53. Gogia R, Grekin RC, Shinkai K. Eruptive self-resolving keratoacanthomas developing after treatment with photodynamic therapy and microdermabrasion. *Dermatol Surg.* 2013;39(11):1717–1720.

CHAPTER 30: MICRONEEDLING

Atchima Suwanchinda

30.1 Introduction

Microneedling (MN) or percutaneous collagen induction (PCI) therapy is a minimally invasive procedure in which fine needles are used to repetitively puncture the epidermis and/or dermis creating microwounds in a controlled injury without causing any significant damaged to the epidermis (1–3). These multiple microwounds stimulate the release of growth factors, inducing the production of new collagen, elastin, capillaries, and dermal substance (4). MN was initially utilized as collagen induction therapy for facial rejuvenation and scar treatment, but now it is widely used for multiple indications, which include dyschromia, melasma, vitiligo, enlarged pores, and surgical scar (5). (Table 30.1) These also include a transdermal delivery system for therapeutic drugs and in combination therapy. Various topical agents and other technologies are frequently used in combination to increase therapeutic efficacy. MN procedure uses an instrument that contains up to 540 needles (2). The needle size varies from 0.1–0.25 mm in diameter and 0.2–3 mm in length (4). MN has increasing popularity due to its high efficacy, safety, and minimal post-treatment recovery rates. It is considered relatively safe, particularly in skin of color. However, untoward side effects can occur.

30.2 Mechanisms of Action

Microwounds are created by MN with controlled skin injury and minimal epidermal damage, and thereby, they stimulate the dermal wound healing cascade (inflammation, proliferation, and remodeling) to take place. This leads to the release of various growth factors, such as platelet-derived growth factor (PDF), transforming growth factor alpha and beta (TGF-α and TGF-β), connective tissue activating protein, connective tissue growth factor, and fibroblast growth factor (FGF) (6, 7). This, in turn, causes neovascularization and neocollagenesis secondary to the fibroblast proliferation and migration. Fibronectin, which is created after five days of the skin injury, provides a matrix for collagen type III deposition, resulting in skin tightening and rhytid reduction over weeks to months and persisting for five to seven years in the form of collagen III (8, 9). There is an increase in gene and protein expression of type I collagen with upregulation of glycosaminoglycans and various growth factors including vascular endothelial growth factors, FGF-7, and epidermal growth factor (9, 10). In addition, there is upregulation of TGF-β3, which promotes regeneration and scarless wound healing (10). The depth of neocollagenesis has been found to be 5–600 μm with the use of 1.5 mm long needle. There is up to 400% increase in collagen and elastin deposition at six months postoperatively, with a thickened stratum spinosum and normal rete ridges at one year postoperatively after four MN sessions one month apart (11). In addition, MN has an action of enhancing the delivery of various drugs by bypassing the stratum corneum (SC) barrier and depositing the drug directly up to the vascularized dermis (12). These drugs include peptides, DNA, and other molecules. It has also been shown to cause a significant widening of the follicular infundibulum by 47%, which may contribute to the increased penetration of the medication across the skin barrier (13).

30.3 Devices

MN devices have evolved over the past decade. There are multiple devices with different needle lengths, needle quantities, needle diameters, configurations, materials, drum sizes, and automation types (14, 15). These allow physicians to select and customize the chosen devices according to each patient's condition. Modern MN devices consist of stamps, rollers, and pens.

30.4 Roller MN

Roller MN devices are among the commonly used devices (2). (Figures 30.1 and 30.3) Rollers can pierce the skin deeper when treating at a 90-degree angle perpendicular to the skin. The quality of rollers is crucial. The most important factor is the needle length. A high ratio of tip length to diameter (13:1) is an important property of good needles (1). Needle length is generally 0.2–3.0 mm with a diameter of 0.25 mm. The proper length is selected depending on the indication and skin thickness of the treated area. There are several needle materials, such as stainless steel, which is the most common type, titanium, which usually stays sharper for a longer time, or silver and gold, which offer antimicrobial properties and less risk of allergic reactions (1). At-home devices are also available, but the quality of the needle is crucial.

30.5 Stamp MN

Stamps have different needle lengths (0.2–3 mm) and a diameter of 0.12 mm. It is useful to treat scars and a small surfaces where great control is beneficial, such as periorbital, perioral, and nasal regions. It is also helpful for use on isolated scars and wrinkles (14, 16). (Figure 30.2). Recently, an MN stamp and MN roller with a fixed needle length and customizable vial for needling infusion have been made available to directly administer as a form of mesotherapy.

30.6 Pen MN

Currently, sophisticated automated pen MN devices with adjustable needle length, depth, and speed for customized treatment options are increasingly popular among physicians. Most pens utilize sterile single-use cartridges and sterile needle cartridges with a range of different needle configurations. (Figure 30.4) The pen itself is reusable, and most of them have a protective disposable sleeve. The needle tips are disposable. Most devices can be operated in high-speed mode (700 cycles/minute) and low-speed mode (412 cycles/minute) in a vibrating stamp-like manner (17, 18). The automated pen device allows the operator to define the penetration depth and frequency of the needle penetration and control the treatment area and coverage. The valuable current automated MN devices contain multiple fine, sterile needles, typically 0.5–3.0 mm in length (18). Its advantage is the ability to work on curved and small areas, such as nasal ala and periocular and perioral areas, because of the smaller size of the tips.

DOI: 10.1201/9780429243769-30

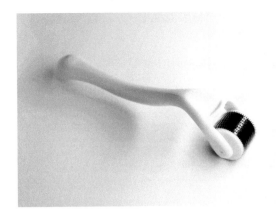

FIGURE 30.1 Derma roller.

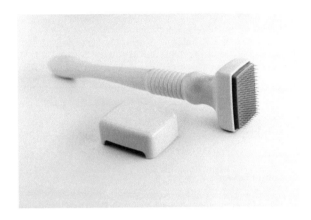

FIGURE 30.2 Stamp microneedling.

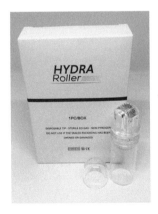 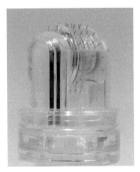

FIGURE 30.3 Roller microneedling attached with microchamber.

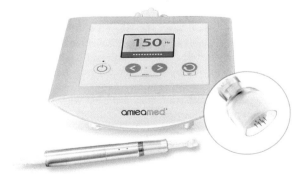

FIGURE 30.4 Automatic pen microneedling.

30.7 Other Variations in MN Devices

1. Fractional radiofrequency MN (3, 14)
2. Devices combining MN and vacuum-assisted infusion (3)
3. Devices combining MN, microdermabrasion simultaneous deep tissue serum infusion, and light-emitting diode (LED) therapy, Dermafrac (3, 14)
4. LED MN rollers (3)
5. Stamps and roller MN, which have attached microchamber (14, 19) (Figure 30.4)
6. Home care roller MN: this device contains a needle of about 0.1 mm in length and is used for transcutaneous delivery of anti-aging agents (14)

30.8 Patient Considerations and Clinical Assessment

- A meticulous visual assessment of the overall skin quality and texture, including the evaluation of the treatment areas, should be done.
- Risks, benefits, and alternative treatment options should be thoroughly discussed with the patients.
- A consent form should be completed.
- Photography should be performed before each treatment session to compare the baseline and post-treatment.
- Patient realistic expectation is important and must be discussed, including compliance with postoperative care.
- The downtime period must be informed. Minimal downtime with an average of 3.7 days was reported after MN procedure (95).
- MN should be avoided or delayed in patients with obvious signs of sun exposure to reduce the risk of PIH (7, 95).
- Patients with a history of bleeding disorders, coagulopathies, taking anticoagulants, or antiplatelet aggregation have an increased risk of prolonged erythema, ecchymosis, and bleeding. This must be informed and discussed before the treatment (2). However, oral anticoagulants need not be discontinued as the risk of uncontrolled bleeding during the procedure is insignificant (7).
- Absolute and relative contraindications should be carefully analyzed by the operator (Table 30.2).

Pre-procedure care recommendations (7, 15, 46):

- Photoprotection is advised for at least a week prior to MN. The treatment is not recommended in patients with a history of recent sun exposure to avoid the risk of PIH.
- Any home skin care regimen (antioxidants, growth factor, moisturizer) can be used up until the time of the procedure (7).
- Even though preoperative skin preparation with vitamin A formulations is recommended for at least a month, in order to maximize dermal collagen formation, in skin-of-color patients, any possible irritating drug or cosmetics should be stopped, at least three to seven days to avoid the higher risk of PIH (19, 49).
- MN is often used in combination with other modalities; the order of treatments can be applied from deep to superficial (15).

TABLE.30.1: Dermatological Indications

Dermatological indications that have been reported

- Skin rejuvenation (10, 19, 28–34)
- Rhytid reduction (11, 24, 35)
- Acne vulgaris (36–41)
- Acne scar (25, 42–54)
- Acne-related post-inflammatory erythema (55)
- Varicella scar (54, 56)
- Rosacea (57, 58)
- Burn scar (49, 59–63)
- Traumatic scar (17, 64)
- Surgical scar (17, 64)
- Periorbital melanosis (19)
- Infraorbital hyperpigmentation (65)
- Melasma and hyperpigmentation (19, 66–68)
- Senescence-induced aging hyperpigmentation (69)
- Vitiligo (70–81)
- Drug delivery (82)
- Striae distensae (83, 84)
- Androgenic alopecia (85–90)
- Alopecia areata (61)
- Primary axillary hyperhidrosis (27)
- Warts (91, 92)
- Actinic keratosis (93, 94)

Sources: From (1, 2, 19–27).

TABLE 30.2: Microneedling Contraindications

Contraindications

- Active infection within the treatment area, active herpes simplex, including bacterial, viral, or fungal infection, or inflammatory lesions, such as active inflammatory acne, eczema, psoriasis, vitiligo, or autoimmune disease
- Hepatitis or human immunodeficiency virus (HIV) infection
- Keloid or hypertrophic scarring predisposition
- Immunosuppression due to medical conditions or medications
- History of clotting or bleeding disorders, such as hemophilia
- Anticoagulant (blood thinner) therapies, such as warfarin, heparin, or low-dose aspirin
- Uncontrolled diabetes
- Currently taking acne medication with the ingredient isotretinoin (Accutane) or has taken isotretinoin in the past six months
- Patients who are tan or planning to be in the sun in the two weeks following the procedure
- Malignancy or current or imminent treatments using chemotherapy, radiotherapy, or steroids
- Pregnancy or breastfeeding
- Patients who are allergic to stainless steel or to topical or local anesthetics or have a history of contact dermatitis to these products

Source: According to the US FDA (www.fda.gov/medical-devices/aesthetic-cosmetic-devices/microneedling-devices) (7).

TABLE 30.3: Recommended Needle Length According to the Dermatologic Indication

Dermatologic Indication	Needle Length Recommendation
Acne and other scars	1.5–2 mm
Scars and sun-damaged skin	1.5–3.0 mm
Skin aging and wrinkle treatment	0.5–1.0 mm
Melasma and hyperpigmentation	0.5–1.5 mm
Androgenic alopecia	1.5 mm *One study showed a greater result with 0.6 than 1.2 mm (61).
Alopecia areata	1.5 mm
Striae	1.5–2.5 mm

Sources: From (14, 19, 46, 61, 97).

TABLE 30.4: Recommended Needle Length According to the Treatment Location

Treatment Location	Needle Length Recommendation
Forehead, lower eyelids, and nasal bridge	0.5–1.0 mm
Cheeks, perioral regions	1.5–3.0 mm
Scars	1.5–2.5 mm
Body	1.5–3.0 mm
Scalp	1.5 mm

Source: From (15, 61).

- Prophylactic one-week course of oral antiviral therapy is recommended in patients with a history of herpes simplex (7).
- MN should be avoided in patients with active acne or other inflammatory lesions because treatment of the lesions may lead to the development of bacterial micro-abscesses or granuloma (7).

30.9 Operative Techniques (7)

- Preparing the device used by selecting the appropriate devices, needle length, and needle material to match the clinical indication is important for a successful outcome (96).
- Needle length must be selected according to the dermatologic indication, epidermal and dermal thickness, and skin characteristics (3, 14). (Tables 30.3 and 30.4). The thicker or more fibrotic skin should be treated with deeper needle depths (15).
- Generally, a needle length of 1.5–2 mm is preferred when treating acne and other scars, 0.5–1.0 mm is recommended for skin aging and wrinkle treatment, while 1.5–3.0 mm is favored for the use of scars and sun-damaged skin (14, 46).

- When using the automated pen device, the power speed, sterile disposable cartridge with different array counts, needle lengths, and sizes of the needle gauge must be carefully chosen to tailor the therapy based on specific treatment indications and locations (15).
- Meticulous skin preparation is important to decrease the risk of superficial skin infections and granuloma.
- A gentle skin cleanser is used to remove makeup and debris from the skin's surface.
- Locally numb the treatment area with topical anesthetic cream or gel, leave it for 30–45 minutes, and wash the treatment area with the NSS-soaked gauze.
- Prepare the skin with the treated site with preferred antiseptics, alcohol, or chlorhexidine in alcohol or in water immediately before the procedure (19).
- Treatment techniques will depend on specific devices and the special location of the treatment area. Basic rules are precisely and uniformly followed with the clinical endpoint of uniform pinpoint bleeding.
- Treatment area is divided into small regions or quadrants to create more precise and uniform coverage.
- Sufficient gliding gels, such as hyaluronic acid or other active ingredients solution for skin rejuvenation (pharmaceutical grade is strongly recommended), are typically applied to the treatment area to facilitate gliding and to prevent injury to the overlying epidermis. An additional amount can be added if needed.

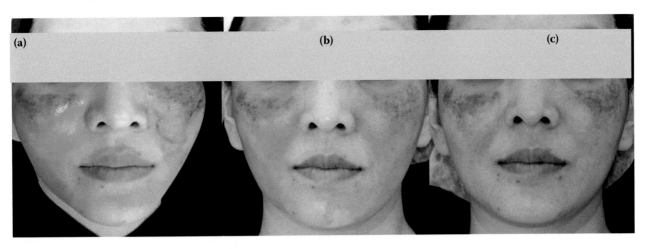

FIGURE. 30.5a Uniform pinpoint bleeding and erythema were demonstrated after three passes, which is the visual endpoint of the skin needling treatments. Excess bleeding and serum can be removed using the cold saline-soaked sterile gauze and pat-dried with gentle pressure to stop the bleeding using a dry sterile gauze.

FIGURE. 30.5b Immediate erythema after MN treatment.

FIGURE. 30.5c After 24 hours, the degree of erythema subsided. Area of pinpoint bleeding became dark red. Mild desquamation was seen.

TABLE 30.5: Combinations of Therapeutic Drugs and Active Ingredients Used with MN

Substance used during and/or after MN procedures

(0.05% tretinoin + 4% hydroquinone + 1% fluocinolone acetonide) (103)
Hydroquinone (104)
Tranexamic acid (TA) (105–107)
Topical vitamin C (105, 108): magnesium lascorbyl-2-phosphate
  (VC-PMG), L-ascorbic acid
Bimatoprost (109)
Vitamin A (99)
Bleomycin (110)
Indocyanine green (111)
Corticosteroid (112)
Minoxidil (113)
5-aminolaevulninic acid (114)
5-fluouracil (78, 92)
Tacrolimus (74)
Jessner's solution (115)
Autologous PRP (19, 116, 117)
Cultured or extracted bone marrow-derived mesenchymal cells (19, 117)
Stem cell-conditioned medium (19, 117)
Non-cultured autologous skin cell (62)
Peptides (99)

- Gentle manual skin traction is done with the non-dominant hand and firmly hold the device and smoothly move or roll MN devices perpendicular over the skin surface in a circular motion over the treatment area in a multidirectional or cross-hatching pattern, involving the combination of different directions of horizontal, vertical, and oblique passes over the treatment area back and forth to homogeneously treat the areas repeatedly. Approximately three to ten passes are needed until the effacement of the lesion is seen or until reaching the therapeutic endpoint of fine pinpoint bleeding (19, 97, 98). (Figure 30.5).

- Special technique is applied when treating deep rhytids or scars by using the "rocking" or "stamping" technique to increase the density of the microwounds.

- Be careful of too much pressure or increased speed, particularly on bony prominences, which can increase the risk of epidermal tear.

- Cold saline-soak sterile gauze is used to remove excess blood and achieve hemostasis. The coolness helps to comfort the skin. Avoid tap water as the possible contamination with pathogenic organisms leads to an increased risk of infection. Dry sterile gauze can be applied with gentle pressure for several minutes to stop further bleeding, if any.

- Icepack can also be applied to reduce discomfort.

- A thin layer of healing-aid ointment, topical hydrocortisone-containing balm, antioxidants, therapeutic drugs, or biologicals is immediately applied according to preferences (19). There are many substances reported to be used to combine with MN. (Table 30.5) Thin layer of active ingredients, such as hyaluronic acid, vitamin C, vitamin A, and other depigmenting agents, can be immediately applied when finished (3, 99). Serum-containing vitamins A and C are recommended as the best chemicals to be used by some experts (99). They enhance the regenerative process of MN, inducing greater wound healing clinically and histologically (49, 99). Please be conscious that immediate use of topical medications or cosmetics skin care after MN treatment may induce a local or systemic hypersensitivity reaction through microchannels that act as a gateway stimulating immune response, which leads to PIH afterward (100).

30.10 Post-Procedure Care

- In the first few hours, the transient feeling of mild sunburn can occur. It can be treated with analgesics or HA-based hydrating serum (101).

- Product selection for concurrent use is crucial. There are multiple concurrent drugs reported to be used. (See Table 30.5.)

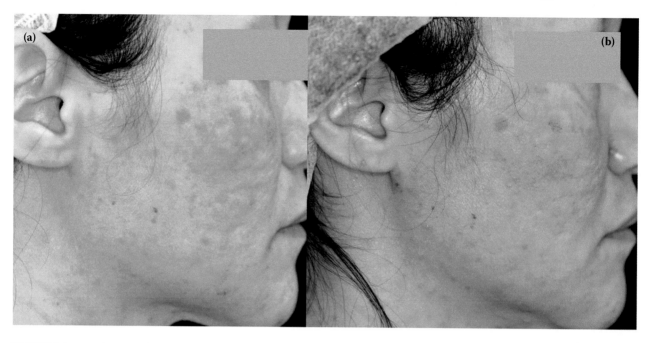

FIGURE 30.6 Photograph of patients with acne scar before treatment (a) and after four MN treatment sessions at monthly intervals (b).

- After four hours, non-allergenic moisturizing cream or healing ointment and mild corticosteroid are applied two times a day for three days.
- Erythema usually subsided after 24 hours, with some areas of pinpoint bleeding becoming darker. Erythema and mild desquamation may be seen for about two to three days or, in some patients, may last up to five days (102). (see Figure 30.6.).
- Limit skin inflammation by avoidance of exposure to chemical-based irritant skin care, makeup, facial cleanser, and sunscreen.
- In the first few weeks after the MN procedure, prescribed skin care products and mild non-allergic cleansers are recommended.
- Nonirritating makeup and routine skin care application can be introduced at least seven days after procedures depending on individual wound healing completion (19).
- Avoidance of sun exposure and strict use of sun-protective measures with physical (mineral) sunblock, at least SPF 50, are suggested even at home.
- Advise patients that a final result could take over three to six months period due to the process of neocollagenesis (3, 49).

30.11 Number and Frequency of Treatments

- Multiple session of MN is recommended.
- MN is generally recommended at biweekly or monthly intervals until the desired clinical outcome is met (7, 103). Some recommendations are after a minimum of three weeks (3, 49, 118–120).

- A study showed 3 mm MN done once a month for a total of four sessions, with 1 mm MN done once a week for a total of four sessions. This weekly needling gave superior results.
- The number and interval of treatments also depend on the indication for which it is being done and the needle length used, as well as the severity of the problems (14). In the case of deep acne scars, the number of treatments can be frequent and numerous.
- For rejuvenation purposes or maintenance sessions, every three to six months or once a year to enhance the aesthetic outcome is recommended (19, 121).

30.12 Side Effects and Their Management

Even though MN carries a decreased risk of many cutaneous adverse effects, patients with darker skin types can continue to be at risk for dyspigmentation (15). Whereas histological analysis of skin melanocytes 24 hours after MN demonstrated neither change in melanocyte number nor any epidermal disruption, PIH can occur after MN, particularly in skin of color, possibly because melanocytes are vulnerable to any kind of injury (122). (Figure 30.7). The severity and duration of the adverse reactions are variable depending on different devices and techniques (123). The selection of MN devices and tailored meticulous technique is crucial to lessen the adverse effects. The few seen with pen-type devices may be attributed to the automated features of these electric devices that allow for varying speeds of penetration, while the pressure and depth are controlled and uniform. This may ultimately reduce the likelihood of operator-related side effects. Additionally, disposable needles confer the advantage of reducing infection and

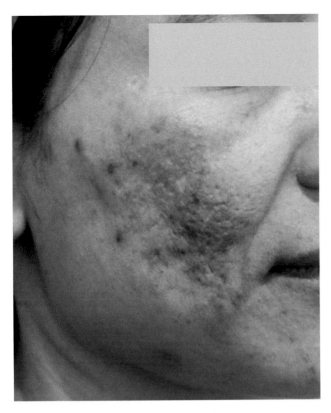

FIGURE 30.7 Unusual tram-tracking linear scar and post-inflammatory hyperpigmentation after MN treatment in Asian patients.

cross-contamination after use (2). Common side effects and other reported side effects are shown in Table 30.6 (19, 28, 33, 40, 45, 82, 123–130).

30.13 Special Precautions

Physicians should take extra precautions when combining MN with other procedures to prevent the risk of side effects.

The product used during and after MN procedures should only be the products that are approved by the FDA for mesotherapy to avoid granuloma infection.

MN procedure should be done with an aseptic technique.

30.14 Conclusion

MN is a minimally invasive procedure widely used in dermatology, plastic surgery, and other aesthetic practices. It is a simple procedure with relatively short downtime. The procedure itself is well tolerable with minimal risk, particularly for skin of color. It was originally used for skin rejuvenation and scar treatment. Currently, novel uses include transcutaneous medication delivery with many ingredients, including cell therapy. It can also be combined with other treatment modalities, such as chemical peeling, subcision, microdermabrasion, LED, and fractional laser resurfacing. Even though there is a limited number of large, well-controlled studies, there are many anecdotal reports and small case series that have demonstrated significant improvement when used for several dermatologic conditions.

Frequently Asked Questions

1. *Q: Which products can be used safely with MN?*
   A: Only FDA-approved drugs are recommended. Please refer to Table 30.1 for reported substances that are used during, before, and after an MN procedure. Avoidance of non-approved substances for intradermal use is strongly suggested due to a higher risk of dermatitis and granuloma formation because the microchannel created by microneedling, which have been reported to remain open for several hours after treatment.

2. *Q: Is it necessary to pre-treat the skin with bleaching cream before MN treatment in skin of color?*
   A: The pre-treatment regimen is not mandatory. The risk of dyspigmentation after MN is minimal with proper techniques when compared to other cutaneous resurfacing procedures, even in skin of color. There are recommendations from experts to use vitamin A formulations, such as retinoic acid 0.1%, to pre-treat the skin to hasten healing, normalize skin cells, and promote normal collagen in a lattice pattern (99). But one should be cautious when using this in skin-of-color patients as it might increase the risk of dermatitis, which leads to PIH.

3. *Q: Are there any special precautions for MN treatment in ethnic skin/skin of color?*
   A: Patients with darker skin types can be at risk for dyspigmentation. The risk of PIH is between 0 and 17% (141). Most of the adverse effects occur in scar, hyperhidrosis, and skin rejuvenation treatment. The application of MN and drug delivery systems for melasma or melanosis showed no reported side effects. Significant PIH was observed in patients with inadequate sun protection (141). Strict use of sunscreen and sun protection measures are strongly advocated. The risk is higher with improper technique, concomitant agent use, improper postoperative care, and the patient's skin condition (19).

4. *Q: How are the combination treatment of MN and other rejuvenation modalities managed?*
   A: When MN is used in combination with other modalities, the order of treatments should be from deep to superficial (15). When fillers are combined with MN, fillers are done before MN (143). When combined with laser, as laser targets deeper tissues, it will be used first, followed by MN (144). MN will go after to maintain visual landmarks and prevent diffusion of injectables caused by tissue edema or bleeding.

5. *Q: What are the factors that make each device different?*
   A: The quality of the needle is critical. It should be evaluated before its use for sharpness, the strong attachment of the needle to the drum, material used, needle length, needle diameter, and total number of needles. The differences in roller, stamps, pen automation, and radiofrequency MN affect the resultant efficacy with different applications and anatomical areas. Each device has some advantages and disadvantages. An appropriate selection to tailor to the patient's condition is crucial.

Essentials for Aesthetic Dermatology in Ethnic Skin

TABLE 30.6: Adverse Effects after Microneedling

Side Effects	Description	Management
Erythema*	The post-procedure transient erythema is expected (131, 132). Normally, it will last for a day; if prolonged, it can last from three to seven days (34, 132–136). Irritation and mild edema may be seen. Erythema was more likely to occur with the stamp, pen, roller, and RF energy, respectively (2).	Often self-remission within three to seven days
Pain*	The pain during the procedure is usually mild and tolerable (3).Topical anesthetics are helpful if used appropriately. Increasing pain with each successive roller MN treatment was reported in one study (137). Pain is found more with pen MN than the roller and RF (2).	No specific treatment is needed
Edema*	Edema was reported in many studies, which often resolves spontaneously within 24 hours (54, 137, 138). Some cases can prolong to couple of days (2). Edema is found most with roller MN and less with pen and RF MN (2).	Generally subsides in hours to days. No specific treatment is needed. Arnica can be used
Post-inflammatory hyperpigmentation (PIH)*	The overall risk is significantly lower than when using energy-based devices (lasers) (3). In multiple MN sessions, PIH may occur (19, 52, 83, 139, 140). PIH was more likely to occur with the roller and RF energy than with the stamp (2). Significant PIH is also related to inadequate sun protection (141). The use of topical medications or cosmetics skin care immediately after MN may also increase the incidence of adverse effect as MN creates a microchannel within the epidermis and dermis as a gateway to potentially stimulate the immune response inducing a local or systemic hypersensitivity reaction which leads to PIH afterward (100).	Spontaneously resolves or with the aid of topical bleaching cream (52, 124)
Ecchymosis	Ecchymosis can be observed over bony prominences in some patients even without a history of bleeding disorder without residual hyperpigmentation (43, 138, 142).	Spontaneously resolves
Bleeding	The therapeutic endpoint is the presence of pinpoint bleeding in the treatment areas. Bleeding was more likely to occur with the roller than with RF energy (2).	Apply gentle pressure during the procedure for prevention
Epidermal tear	There are many factors, such as low-quality products, dull or loose needles, or incorrect techniques because of too much pressure or increased speed (14, 19).	Healing ointment
Tram-tracking scarring	Tram-tracking was more likely to occur with the roller than with the stamp (2). The risk is primarily related to improper technique, such as inappropriate use of a large needle or excessive pressure over a bony prominence (19, 54, 141). It was shown as discrete papular scars in a linear pattern in the horizontal and vertical direction, similar to a tram track.	Topical corticosteroid, silicone gel
Granuloma	Allergic granulomatous reactions have been noted. It was reported after the application of serums in patients with hypersensitivity to serum ingredients. Three patients were reported after the use of high doses of topical lipophilic vitamin C during an MN session (100).	Topical corticosteroid, topical calcineurin inhibitor, oral prednisolone, oral doxycycline (33) Fumaderm* (off-label use) (127)
Infection	Localized superficial infections, such as impetigo and reactivation of herpes simplex. There was a report of unintended widespread facial autoinoculation of varicella by a home microneedling roller device (123).	Antibiotics and antiviral treatment
Contact dermatitis	The concomitant use of MN with topical agents can occur, particularly allergic and irritant dermatitis. The risk is higher when using unapproved products for intradermal application (128). Contact dermatitis from topical arnica cream was also reported (82). Allergic contact dermatitis to needle materials was reported (129, 138).	Topical and/or systemic corticosteroid
Lymphadenopathy	The painful swollen retroauricular lymph nodes were reported shortly after MN treatment (130).	Oral antibiotics
Peeling, discomfort, burning, milia, pruritus, dryness, rough skin, tight pustules, scabbing and crusting, recurrence, flare0up of acne, dysesthesia	Others reported side effects from publication and warnings from the US FDA (www.fda.gov/medical-devices/aesthetic-cosmetic-devices/microneedling-devices).	Symptomatic treatment

* Common side effects.

References

1. Houshmand EB. *Microneedling: Global Perspectives in Aesthetic Medicine*. Wiley Online Library; 2021.

2. Gowda A, Healey B, Ezaldein H, Merati M. A systematic review examining the potential adverse effects of microneedling. *Journal of Clinical and Aesthetic Dermatology.* 2021;14(1):45–54.

3. Litchman G, Nair PA, Badri T, Kelly SE. *Microneedling.* StatPearls. Treasure Island (FL); 2021.

4. Yadav S, Dogra S. A cutaneous reaction to microneedling for postacne scarring caused by nickel hypersensitivity. *Aesthetic Surgery Journal.* 2016;36(4):NP168–NP170.

5. Cercal Fucci-da-Costa AP, Reich Camasmie H. Drug delivery after microneedling: Report of an adverse reaction. *Dermatologic Surgery.* 2018;44(4):593–594.

6. Kloth LC. Electrical stimulation for wound healing: A review of evidence from in vitro studies, animal experiments, and clinical trials. *The International Journal of Lower Extremity Wounds.* 2005;4(1):23–44.

7. Alster TS, Graham PM. Microneedling: A review and practical guide. *Dermatologic Surgery.* 2018;44(3):397–404.

8. Fernandes D. Minimally invasive percutaneous collagen induction. *Oral and Maxillofacial Surgery Clinics.* 2005;17(1):51–63.

9. Aust M, Reimers K, Kaplan H, Stahl F, Repenning C, Scheper T, et al. Percutaneous collagen induction–regeneration in place of cicatrisation? *Journal of Plastic, Reconstructive & Aesthetic Surgery.* 2011;64(1):97–107.

10. Aust M, Reimers K, Gohritz A, Jahn S, Stahl F, Repenning C, et al. Percutaneous collagen induction. Scarless skin rejuvenation: Fact or fiction? *Clinical and Experimental Dermatology: Clinical Dermatology.* 2010;35(4):437–439.

11. Aust MC, Fernandes D, Kolokythas P, Kaplan HM, Vogt PM. Percutaneous collagen induction therapy: An alternative treatment for scars, wrinkles, and skin laxity. *Plastic and Reconstructive Surgery.* 2008;121(4):1421–1429.

12. Bernadete Riemma Pierre M, Cristina Rossetti F. Microneedle-based drug delivery systems for transdermal route. *Current Drug Targets.* 2014;15(3):281–291.

13. Serrano G, Almudéver P, Serrano JM, Cortijo J, Faus C, Reyes M, et al. Microneedling dilates the follicular infundibulum and increases transfollicular absorption of liposomal sepia melanin. *Clinical, Cosmetic and Investigational Dermatology.* 2015;8:313.

14. Houshmand EB. Introduction to microneedling. *Microneedling: Global Perspectives in Aesthetic Medicine.* 2021:1–9.

15. Alster TS, Graham PM. Microneedling: A review and practical guide. *Dermatologic Surgery.* 2018;44(3):397–404.

16. McCrudden MT, McAlister E, Courtenay AJ, González-Vázquez P, Raj Singh TR, Donnelly RF. Microneedle applications in improving skin appearance. *Experimental Dermatology.* 2015;24(8):561–566.

17. Arora S, Gupta PB. Automated microneedling device-a new tool in dermatologist's kit-a review. *Journal of Pakistan Association of Dermatologists.* 2012;22(4).

18. Ablon G. Safety and effectiveness of an automated microneedling device in improving the signs of aging skin. *Journal of Clinical and Aesthetic Dermatology.* 2018;11(8):29.

19. Suwanchinda A. Treatment of hyperpigmentation with microneedling. *Microneedling: Global Perspectives in Aesthetic Medicine.* 2021:52–80.

20. Iriarte C, Awosika O, Rengifo-Pardo M, Ehrlich A. Review of applications of microneedling in dermatology. *Clinical, Cosmetic and Investigational Dermatology.* 2017;10:289–298.

21. El-Domyati M, Abdel-Wahab H, Hossam A. Combining microneedling with other minimally invasive procedures for facial rejuvenation: A split-face comparative study. *International Journal of Dermatology.* 2018;57(11):1324–1334.

22. West L, He B, Vandergriff T, Goff HW. The use of microneedling to treat striae distensae. *Dermatologic Surgery.* 2021 Oct 1;47(10):1407–1408.

23. Sitohang IBS, Sirait SAP, Suryanegara J. Microneedling in the treatment of atrophic scars: A systematic review of randomised controlled trials. *International Wound Journal.* 2021 Oct;18(5):577–585.

24. Wamsley CE, Kislevitz M, Barillas J, Basci D, Kandagatla V, Hitchcock T, et al. A single-center trial to evaluate the efficacy and tolerability of four microneedling treatments on fine lines and wrinkles of facial and neck skin in subjects with Fitzpatrick skin types I-IV: An objective assessment using non-invasive devices and 0.33mm microbiopsies. *Aesthetic Surgery Journal.* 2021 Oct 15;41(11):NP1603–NP1618.

25. Gupta M, Barman KD, Sarkar R. A comparative study of microneedling alone versus along with platelet-rich plasma in acne scars. *Journal of Cutaneous and Aesthetic Surgery.* 2021;14(1):64–71.

26. Faghihi G, Nabavinejad S, Mokhtari F, Fatemi Naeini F, Iraji F. Microneedling in androgenetic alopecia: Comparing two different depths of microneedles. *Journal of Cosmetic Dermatology.* 2021;20(4):1241–1247.

27. Kim M, Shin JY, Lee J, Kim JY, Oh SH. Efficacy of fractional microneedle radiofrequency device in the treatment of primary axillary hyperhidrosis: A pilot study. *Dermatology.* 2013;227(3):243–249.

28. Kaplan H, Kaplan L. Combination of microneedle radiofrequency (RF), fractional RF skin resurfacing and multi-source non-ablative skin tightening for minimal-downtime, full-face skin rejuvenation. *Journal of Cosmetic and Laser Therapy.* 2016;18(8):438–441.

29. Merati M, Woods C, Reznik N, Parker L. An assessment of microneedling with topical growth factors for facial skin rejuvenation: A randomized controlled trial. *Journal of Clinical and Aesthetic Dermatology.* 2020;13(11):22–27.

30. Alessa D, Bloom JD. Microneedling options for skin rejuvenation, including non-temperature-controlled fractional microneedle radiofrequency treatments. *Facial Plastic Surgery Clinics of North America.* 2020;28(1):1–7.

31. Chun S. Fractional microneedling radiofrequency and fractional 1927 nm thulium laser Treatment offer synergistic skin rejuvenation: A pilot case series. *Laser Therapy.* 2018;27(4):283–291.

32. Badran KW, Nabili V. Lasers, microneedling, and platelet-rich plasma for skin rejuvenation and repair. *Facial Plastic Surgery Clinics of North America.* 2018;26(4):455–468.

33. Soltani-Arabshahi R, Wong JW, Duffy KL, Powell DL. Facial allergic granulomatous reaction and systemic hypersensitivity associated with microneedle therapy for skin rejuvenation. *JAMA Dermatology.* 2014;150(1):68–72.

34. Lee HJ, Lee EG, Kang S, Sung JH, Chung HM, Kim DH. Efficacy of microneedling plus human stem cell conditioned medium for skin rejuvenation: A randomized, controlled, blinded split-face study. *Annals of Dermatology.* 2014;26(5):584–591.

35. Haimovic A, Ibrahim O, Lee NY, Dover JS. Ensuring consistent results when microneedling perioral rhytides. *Dermatologic Surgery.* 2018;44(4):595–597.

36. Bhargava S, Kumar U, Varma K. Subcision and microneedling as an inexpensive and safe combination to treat atrophic acne scars in dark skin: A prospective study of 45 patients at a tertiary care center. *Journal of Clinical and Aesthetic Dermatology.* 2019;12(8):18.

37. Mehran G, Sepasgozar S, Rohaninasab M, Goodarzi A, Ghassemi M, Fotooei M, et al. Comparison between the therapeutic effect of microneedling versus tretinoin in patients with comedonal acne: A randomized clinical trial. *Iranian Journal of Dermatology.* 2019;22(3):87–91.

38. Ramaut L, Hoeksema H, Pirayesh A, Stillaert F, Monstrey S. Microneedling: Where do we stand now? A systematic review of the literature. *Journal of Plastic, Reconstructive & Aesthetic Surgery.* 2018;71(1):1–14.

39. Kim ST, Lee KH, Sim HJ, Suh KS, Jang MS. Treatment of acne vulgaris with fractional radiofrequency microneedling. *Journal of Dermatology.* 2014;41(7):586–591.

40. Kim ST, Lee KH, Sim HJ, Suh KS, Jang MS. Treatment of acne vulgaris with fractional radiofrequency microneedling. *Journal of Dermatology.* 2014;41(7):586–591.

41. Kwon HH, Park HY, Choi SC, Bae Y, Jung JY, Park GH. Novel device-based acne treatments: Comparison of a 1450-nm diode laser and microneedling radiofrequency on mild-to-moderate acne vulgaris and seborrhoea in Korean patients through a 20-week prospective, randomized, split-face study. *Journal of the European Academy of Dermatology and Venereology.* 2018;32(4):639–644.

42. Leheta TM, Abdel Hay RM, Hegazy RA, El Garem YF. Do combined alternating sessions of 1540 nm nonablative fractional laser and percutaneous collagen induction with trichloroacetic acid 20% show better results than each individual modality in the treatment of atrophic acne scars? A randomized controlled trial. *Journal of Dermatological Treatment.* 2014;25(2):137–141.

43. Dogra S, Yadav S, Sarangal R. Microneedling for acne scars in A sian skin type: An effective low cost treatment modality. *Journal of Cosmetic Dermatology.* 2014;13(3):180–187.

44. Minh PPT, Bich DD, Van Nguyen Thi Hai TN, Van VTC, Khang TH, Gandolfi M, et al. Microneedling therapy for atrophic acne scar: Effectiveness and safety in Vietnamese patients. *Open Access Macedonian Journal of Medical Sciences.* 2019;7(2):293.

45. Min S, Park SY, Yoon JY, Suh DH. Comparison of fractional microneedling radiofrequency and bipolar radiofrequency on acne and acne scar and investigation of mechanism: Comparative randomized controlled clinical trial. *Archives of Dermatological Research.* 2015;307(10):897–904.

46. Doddaballapur S. Microneedling with dermaroller. *Journal of Cutaneous and Aesthetic Surgery.* 2009;2(2):110.

47. Chandrashekar BS, Sriram R, Mysore R, Bhaskar S, Shetty A. Evaluation of microneedling fractional radiofrequency device for treatment of acne scars. *Journal of Cutaneous and Aesthetic Surgery.* 2014;7(2):93.

48. Mujahid N, Shareef F, Maymone MB, Vashi NA. Microneedling as a treatment for acne scarring: A systematic review. *Dermatologic Surgery.* 2020;46(1):86–92.

49. Singh A, Yadav S. Microneedling: Advances and widening horizons. *Indian Dermatology Online Journal.* 2016;7(4):244.

50. Chawla S. Split face comparative study of microneedling with PRP versus microneedling with vitamin C in treating atrophic post acne scars. *Journal of Cutaneous and Aesthetic Surgery.* 2014;7(2):209.

51. Asif M, Kanodia S, Singh K. Combined autologous platelet-rich plasma with microneedling verses microneedling with distilled water in the treatment of atrophic acne scars: A concurrent split-face study. *Journal of Cosmetic Dermatology.* 2016;15(4):434–443.

52. Sharad J. Combination of microneedling and glycolic acid peels for the treatment of acne scars in dark skin. *Journal of Cosmetic Dermatology.* 2011;10(4):317–323.

53. Schoenberg E, O'Connor M, Wang JV, Yang S, Saedi N. Microneedling and PRP for acne scars: A new tool in our arsenal. *Journal of Cosmetic Dermatology.* 2020;19(1):112–114.

54. Pahwa M, Pahwa P, Zaheer A. "Tram track effect" after treatment of acne scars using a microneedling device. *Dermatologic Surgery.* 2012;38(7 pt1):1107–1108.

55. Min S, Park SY, Yoon JY, Kwon HH, Suh DH. Fractional microneedling radiofrequency treatment for acne-related post-inflammatory erythema. *Acta Dermato-Venereologica.* 2016;96(1):87–91.

56. Costa IM, Costa MC. Microneedling for varicella scars in a dark-skinned teenager. *Dermatologic Surgery.* 2014;40(3):333–334.

57. Wang B, Deng Y-X, Li P-Y, Yan S, Xie H-F, Li J, et al. Efficacy and safety of non-insulated fractional microneedle radiofrequency for treating difficult-to-treat rosacea: A 48-week, prospective, observational study. *Archives of Dermatological Research.* 2021:1–8.

58. Ledon JA, Bennett RG. *Miscellaneous Procedures: Intense Pulsed Light, Photodynamic Therapy, Cryotherapy, Cryolipolysis, Microdermabrasion, Salabrasion, Dermabrasion, Microneedling, Radiofrequency, and Ultrasound.* Practical Dermatologic Surgery: CRC Press; 2021. P. 207–214.

59. Zeitter S, Sikora Z, Jahn S, Stahl F, Strauß S, Lazaridis A, et al. Microneedling: Matching the results of medical needling and repetitive treatments to maximize potential for skin regeneration. *Burns.* 2014;40(5):966–973.

60. Aust M, Fernandes D, Bender R. The value of medical needling in burn scars. *Microneedling: Global Perspectives in Aesthetic Medicine.* 2021:22–40.

61. Chandrashekar B, Yepuri V, Mysore V. Alopecia areata-successful outcome with microneedling and triamcinolone acetonide. *Journal of Cutaneous and Aesthetic Surgery.* 2014;7(1):63.

62. Busch K, Bender R, Walezko N, Aziz H, Altintas M, Aust M. Combination of medical needling and non-cultured autologous skin cell transplantation (ReNovaCell) for repigmentation of hypopigmented burn scars. *Burns.* 2016;42(7):1556–1566.

63. Aust MC, Knobloch K, Reimers K, Redeker J, Ipaktchi R, Altintas MA, et al. Percutaneous collagen induction therapy: An alternative treatment for burn scars. *Burns.* 2010;36(6):836–843.

64. Bandral MR, Padgavankar PH, Japatti SR, Gir PJ, Siddegowda CY, Gir RJ. Clinical evaluation of microneedling therapy in the management of facial scar: A prospective randomized study. *Journal of Maxillofacial and Oral Surgery.* 2019;18(4):572–578.

65. Ghandehari R, Robati RM, Niknezhad N, Hajizadeh N, Tehranchinia Z. Efficacy and safety of fractional CO2 laser and tranexamic acid versus microneedling and tranexamic acid in the treatment of infraorbital hyperpigmentation. *Journal of Dermatological Treatment.* 2020:1–6.

66. Korobko IV, Lomonosov KM. A pilot comparative study of topical latanoprost and tacrolimus in combination with narrow-band ultraviolet B phototherapy and microneedling for the treatment of nonsegmental vitiligo. *Dermatologic Therapy.* 2016;29(6):437–441.

67. Tahoun AI, Mostafa WZ, Amer MA. Dermoscopic evaluation of tranexamic acid versus vitamin C, with microneedling in the treatment of melasma: A comparative, split-face, single-blinded study. *Journal of Dermatological Treatment.* 2021:1–7.

68. Bailey AJM, Li HO-Y, Tan MG, Cheng W, Dover JS. Microneedling as an adjuvant to topical therapies for melasma: A systematic review and meta-analysis. *Journal of the American Academy of Dermatology.* 2022 Apr;86(4):797–810.

69. Lee YI, Kim E, Lee DW, Kim J, Kim J, Lee WJ, et al. Synergistic effect of 300 μm needle-depth fractional microneedling radiofrequency on the treatment of senescence-induced aging hyperpigmentation of the skin. *International Journal of Molecular Sciences.* 2021;22(14):7480.

70. Marasca C, Fabbrocini G, D'Andrea M, Luciano MA, De Maio G, Ruggiero A. Low dose oral corticosteroids, microneedling, and topical 5-fluorouracil: A novel treatment for recalcitrant pediatric vitiligo. *Pediatric Dermatology.* 2021;38(1):322–323.

71. Joseph-Michel Bailey A, Oi-Yee Li H, Zheng D, Glassman SJ, Tan MG. Microneedling as an adjuvant to local therapies for vitiligo: A systematic review and meta-analysis. *Dermatologic Surgery.* 2021 Sep 1;47(9):1314–1316.

72. Salloum A, Bazzi N, Maalouf D, Habre M. Microneedling in vitiligo: A systematic review. *Dermatologic Therapy.* 2020;33(6):e14297.

73. Neinaa YME, Lotfy SS, Ghaly NR, Doghaim NN. A comparative study of combined microneedling and narrowband ultraviolet B phototherapy versus their combination with topical latanoprost in the treatment of vitiligo. *Dermatologic Therapy.* 2021;34(2):e14813.

74. Ebrahim HM, Elkot R, Albalate W. Combined microneedling with tacrolimus vs tacrolimus monotherapy for vitiligo treatment. *J Dermatolog Treat.* 2020:1–6.

75. Andrade Lima EV, Aandrade Lima MMD, Miot HA. Induction of pigmentation through microneedling in stable localized vitiligo patients. *Dermatologic Surgery.* 2020;46(3):434–435.

76. Jha AK, Sonthalia S. 5-Fluorouracil as an adjuvant therapy along with microneedling in vitiligo. *Journal of the American Academy of Dermatology.* 2019;80(4):e75–e76.

77. Giorgio CM, Caccavale S, Fulgione E, Moscarella E, Babino G, Argenziano G. Efficacy of microneedling and photodynamic therapy in vitiligo. *Dermatologic Surgery.* 2019;45(11):1424–1426.

78. Mina M, Elgarhy L, Al-Saeid H, Ibrahim Z. Comparison between the efficacy of microneedling combined with 5-fluorouracil vs microneedling with tacrolimus in the treatment of vitiligo. *Journal of Cosmetic Dermatology.* 2018;17(5):744–751.

79. Kumar A, Bharti R, Agarwal S. Microneedling with Dermaroller 192 needles along with 5-fluorouracil solution in the treatment of stable vitiligo. *Journal of the American Academy of Dermatology.* 2019;81(3):e67–e69.

80. Ebrahim HM, Albalate W. Efficacy of microneedling combined with tacrolimus versus either one alone for vitiligo treatment. *Journal of Cosmetic Dermatology.* 2020;19(4):855–862.

81. Stanimirovic A, Kovacevic M, Korobko I, Situm M, Lotti T. Combined therapy for resistant vitiligo lesions: NB-UVB, microneedling, and topical latanoprost, showed no enhanced efficacy compared to topical latanoprost and NB-UVB. *Dermatologic Therapy.* 2016;29(5): 312–316.

82. Fucci-da-Costa APC, Camasmie HR. Drug delivery after microneedling: Report of an adverse reaction. *Dermatologic Surgery.* 2018;44(4):593–594.

83. Khater MH, Khattab FM, Abdelhaleem MR. Treatment of striae distensae with needling therapy versus CO_2 fractional laser. *Journal of Cosmetic and Laser Therapy.* 2016;18(2):75–79.

84. Nassar A, Ghomey S, El Gohary Y, El-Desoky F. Treatment of striae distensae with needling therapy versus microdermabrasion with sonophoresis. *Journal of Cosmetic and Laser Therapy.* 2016;18(6):330–334.

85. Yu AJ, Luo YJ, Xu XG, Bao LL, Tian T, Li ZX, et al. A pilot split-scalp study of combined fractional radiofrequency microneedling and 5% topical minoxidil in treating male pattern hair loss. *Clinical and Experimental Dermatology.* 2018;43(7):775–781.

86. Jha AK, Udayan UK, Roy PK, Amar AKJ, Chaudhary R. Platelet-rich plasma with microneedling in androgenetic alopecia along with dermoscopic pre-and post-treatment evaluation. *Journal of Cosmetic Dermatology.* 2018;17(3):313–318.

87. Dhurat R, Mathapati S. Response to microneedling treatment in men with androgenetic alopecia who failed to respond to conventional therapy. *Indian Journal of Dermatology.* 2015;60(3):260.

88. Jha AK, Vinay K, Zeeshan M, Roy PK, Chaudhary R, Priya A. Platelet-rich plasma and microneedling improves hair growth in patients of androgenetic alopecia when used as an adjuvant to minoxidil. *Journal of Cosmetic Dermatology.* 2019;18(5):1330–1335.

89. Dhurat R, Sukesh M, Avhad G, Dandale A, Pal A, Pund P. A randomized evaluator blinded study of effect of microneedling in androgenetic alopecia: A pilot study. *International Journal of Trichology.* 2013;5(1):6.

90. Gentile P, Dionisi L, Pizzicannella J, De Angelis B, de Fazio D, Garcovich S. A randomized blinded retrospective study: The combined use of micro-needling technique, low-level laser therapy and autologous non-activated platelet-rich plasma improves hair re-growth in patients with androgenic alopecia. *Expert Opinion on Biological Therapy.* 2020;20(9):1099–1109.

91. Gamil HD, Nasr MM, Khattab FM, Ibrahim AM. Combined therapy of plantar warts with topical bleomycin and microneedling: A comparative controlled study. *Journal of Dermatological Treatment.* 2020 May;31(3):235240.

92. Ghonemy S, Ibrahim Ali M, Ebrahim HM. The efficacy of microneedling alone vs its combination with 5-fluorouracil solution vs 5-fluorouracil intralesional injection in the treatment of plantar warts. *Dermatologic Therapy.* 2020;33(6):e14179.

93. Steeb T, Niesert AC, French LE, Berking C, Heppt MV. Microneedling-assisted photodynamic therapy for the treatment of actinic keratosis: Results from a systematic review and meta-analysis. *Journal of the American Academy of Dermatology.* 2020;82(2):515–519.

94. Bencini PL, Galimberti MG, Pellacani G, Longo C. Application of photodynamic therapy combined with pre-illumination microneedling in the treatment of actinic keratosis in organ transplant recipients. *British Journal of Dermatology.* 2012;167(5):1193–1194.

95. Leheta T, El Tawdy A, Abdel Hay R, Farid S. Percutaneous collagen induction versus full-concentration trichloroacetic acid in the treatment of atrophic acne scars. *Dermatologic Surgery.* 2011;37(2):207–216.

96. Nair PA, Arora TH. Microneedling using dermaroller: A means of collagen induction therapy. *GMJ.* 2014;69(1):24–27.

97. Lima EdA. Microneedling in facial recalcitrant melasma: Report of a series of 22 cases. *Anais brasileiros de dermatologia.* 2015;90:919–921.

98. Sasaki GH. Micro-needling depth penetration, presence of pigment particles, and fluorescein-stained platelets: Clinical usage for aesthetic concerns. *Aesthetic Surgery Journal.* 2016;37(1):71–83.

99. Fernandes D. A short history of skin needling. *Microneedling: Global Perspectives in Aesthetic Medicine.* 2021:10–21.

100. Kontochristopoulos G, Kouris A, Platsidaki E, Markantoni V, Gerodimou M, Antoniou C. Combination of microneedling and 10% trichloroacetic acid peels in the management of infraorbital dark circles. *Journal of Cosmetic and Laser Therapy.* 2016;18(5):289–292.

101. Lee JC, Daniels MA, Roth MZ. Mesotherapy, microneedling, and chemical peels. *Clinics in Plastic Surgery.* 2016;43(3):583–595.

102. Aust MC, Fernandes D, Kolokythas P, Kaplan HM, Vogt PM. Percutaneous collagen induction therapy: An alternative treatment for scars, wrinkles, and skin laxity. *Plastic and Reconstructive Surgery.* 2008;121(4):1421–1429.

103. Fabbrocini G, De Vita V, Fardella N, Pastore F, Annunziata M, Mauriello M, et al. Skin needling to enhance depigmenting serum penetration in the treatment of melasma. *Plastic Surgery International.* 2011;2011.

104. Ramirez-Oliveros JF, de Abreu L, Tamler C, Vilhena P, de Barros MH. Microneedling with drug delivery (hydroquinone 4% serum) as an adjuvant therapy for recalcitrant melasma. *Skinmed.* 2020;18(1):38–40.

105. Budamakuntla L, Loganathan E, Suresh DH, Shanmugam S, Suryanarayan S, Dongare A, et al. A randomised, open-label, comparative study of tranexamic acid microinjections and tranexamic acid with microneedling in patients with melasma. *Journal of Cutaneous and Aesthetic Surgery.* 2013;6(3):139.

106. Menon A, Eram H, Kamath PR, Goel S, Babu AM. A split face comparative study of safety and efficacy of microneedling with tranexamic acid versus microneedling with vitamin C in the treatment of melasma. *Indian Dermatology Online Journal.* 2020;11(1):41–45.

107. Kaur A, Bhalla M, Pal Thami G, Sandhu J. Clinical efficacy of topical tranexamic acid with microneedling in melasma. *Dermatologic Surgery.* 2020;46(11):e96–e101.

108. Ismail ESA, Patsatsi A, Abd el-Maged WM, Nada EEDAeA. Efficacy of microneedling with topical vitamin C in the treatment of melasma. *Journal of Cosmetic Dermatology.* 2019;18(5):1342–1347.

109. Wilson BN, Aleisa A, Menzer C, Rossi AM. Bimatoprost drug delivery with laser and microneedling for the management of COVID-19 prone positioning-induced atrophy and hypopigmentation. *JAAD Case Reports.* 2021 Sep;15:26–29.

110. Kaul S, Caldito EG, Jakhar D, Kaur I, Kwatra SG, Mehta S. Comparative efficacy and safety of intralesional bleomycin relative to topical bleomycin with microneedling in the treatment of warts: A systematic review. *Journal of the American Academy of Dermatology.* 2021;84(3):816–819.

111. Nieboer MJ, Meesters AA, Almasian M, Georgiou G, de Rie MA, Verdaasdonk RM, et al. Enhanced topical cutaneous delivery of indocyanine green after various pretreatment regimens: Comparison of fractional CO2 laser, fractional Er: YAG laser, microneedling, and radiofrequency. *Lasers in Medical Science.* 2020;35(6):1357–1365.

112. Juhasz M, Fackler N, Pham C, Mesinkovska NA. Combination therapy using radiofrequency microneedling and corticosteroids for hypertrophic scars: A case report. *Journal of Clinical and Aesthetic Dermatology.* 2020;13(12):27–28.

113. Hong JY, Kwon TR, Kim JH, Lee BC, Kim BJ. Prospective, preclinical comparison of the performance between radiofrequency microneedling and microneedling alone in reversing photoaged skin. *Journal of Cosmetic Dermatology.* 2020;19(5):1105–1109.

114. Giorgio CM, Babino G, Caccavale S, Russo T, De Rosa AB, Alfano R, et al. Combination of photodynamic therapy with 5-aminolaevulinic acid and microneedling in the treatment of alopecia areata resistant to conventional therapies: Our experience with 41 patients. *Clinical and Experimental Dermatology.* 2020;45(3):323–326.

115. Ali B, ElMahdy N, Elfar NN. Microneedling (Dermapen) and Jessner's solution peeling in treatment of atrophic acne scars: A comparative randomized clinical study. *Journal of Cosmetic and Laser Therapy.* 2019;21(6):357–363.

116. Duncan DI. Microneedling with biologicals: Advantages and limitations. *Facial Plastic Surgery Clinics of North America.* 2018;26(4):447–454.

117. Duncan DI. Microneedling with biologicals: Advantages and limitations. *Facial Plastic Surgery Clinics.* 2018;26(4):447–454.

118. Jha AK, Vinay K. Androgenetic alopecia and microneedling: Every needling is not microneedling. *Journal of the American Academy of Dermatology.* 2019;81(2):e43–e44.

119. Boen M, Jacob C. A review and update of treatment options using the acne scar classification system. *Dermatologic Surgery.* 2019;45(3):411–422.

120. Almohanna HM, Perper M, Tosti A. Safety concerns when using novel medications to treat alopecia. *Expert Opinion on Drug Safety.* 2018;17(11):1115–1128.

121. El-Domyati M, Barakat M, Awad S, Medhat W, El-Fakahany H, Farag H. Multiple microneedling sessions for minimally invasive facial rejuvenation: An objective assessment. *International Journal of Dermatology.* 2015;54(12):1361–1369.

122. Aust MC, Reimers K, Repenning C, Stahl F, Jahn S, Guggenheim M, et al. Percutaneous collagen induction: Minimally invasive skin rejuvenation without risk of hyperpigmentation—fact or fiction? *Plastic and Reconstructive Surgery.* 2008;122(5):1553–1563.

123. Leatham H, Guan L, Chang ALS. Unintended widespread facial autoinoculation of varicella by home microneedling roller device. *JAAD Case Reports.* 2018;4(6):546.

124. Osman MAR, Shokeir HA, Fawzy MM. Fractional erbium-doped yttrium aluminum garnet laser versus microneedling in treatment of atrophic acne scars: A randomized split-face clinical study. *Dermatologic Surgery.* 2017;43:S47–S56.

125. Chae WS, Seong JY, Jung HN, Kong SH, Kim MH, Suh HS, et al. Comparative study on efficacy and safety of 1550 nm Er: Glass fractional laser and fractional radiofrequency microneedle device for facial atrophic acne scar. *Journal of Cosmetic Dermatology.* 2015;14(2):100–106.

126. Kwon H, Park H, Choi S, Bae Y, Jung J, Park GH. Novel device-based acne treatments: Comparison of a 1450-nm diode laser and microneedling radiofrequency on mild-to-moderate acne vulgaris and seborrhoea in Korean patients through a 20-week prospective, randomized, split-face study. *Journal of the European Academy of Dermatology and Venereology.* 2018;32(4):639–644.

127. Eisert L, Zidane M, Waigandt I, Vogt PM, Nast A. Granulomatous reaction following microneedling of striae distensae. *JDDG: Journal der Deutschen Dermatologischen Gesellschaft.* 2019;17(4):443–445.

128. Cary JH, Li BS, Maibach HI. Dermatotoxicology of microneedles (MNs) in man. *Biomedical Microdevices.* 2019;21(3):1–8.

129. Yadav S, Dogra S. A cutaneous reaction to microneedling for postacne scarring caused by nickel hypersensitivity. *Aesthetic Surgery Journal.* 2016;36(4):NP168–NP170.

130. Elghblawi E. Intense retroauricular lymphadenopathy postmicroneedling. *Journal of Cosmetic Dermatology.* 2019;18(6):2048–2049.

131. Al Qarqaz F, Al-Yousef A. Skin microneedling for acne scars associated with pigmentation in patients with dark skin. *Journal of Cosmetic Dermatology.* 2018;17(3):390–395.

132. Majid I. Microneedling therapy in atrophic facial scars: An objective assessment. *Journal of Cutaneous and Aesthetic Surgery.* 2009;2(1):26–30.

133. Sharad J. Combination of microneedling and glycolic acid peels for the treatment of acne scars in dark skin. *Journal of Cosmetic Dermatology.* 2011;10(4):317–323.

134. Chawla S. Split face comparative study of microneedling with PRP versus microneedling with vitamin C in treating atrophic post acne scars. *Journal of Cutaneous and Aesthetic Surgery.* 2014;7(4):209–212.

135. Budamakuntla L, Loganathan E, Suresh DH, Shanmugam S, Suryanarayan S, Dongare A, et al. A randomised, open-label, comparative study of tranexamic acid microinjections and tranexamic acid with microneedling in patients with melasma. *Journal of Cutaneous and Aesthetic Surgery.* 2013;6(3):139–143.

136. Park KY, Kim HK, Kim SE, Kim BJ, Kim MN. Treatment of striae distensae using needling therapy: A pilot study. *Dermatologic Surgery.* 2012;38(11):1823–1828.

137. Alam M, Han S, Pongprutthipan M, Disphanurat W, Kakar R, Nodzenski M, et al. Efficacy of a needling device for the treatment of acne scars: A randomized clinical trial. *JAMA Dermatology.* 2014;150(8):844–849.

138. Torezan L, Chaves Y, Niwa A, Sanches Jr JA, Festa-Neto C, Szeimies RM. A pilot split-face study comparing conventional methyl aminolevulinate-photodynamic therapy (PDT) with microneedling-assisted PDT on actinically damaged skin. *Dermatologic Surgery.* 2013;39(8):1197–1201.

139. Garg S, Baveja S. Combination therapy in the management of atrophic acne scars. *Journal of Cutaneous and Aesthetic Surgery.* 2014;7(1):18.

140. Majid I. Microneedling therapy in atrophic facial scars: An objective assessment. *Journal of Cutaneous and Aesthetic Surgery.* 2009;2(1):26.

141. Cohen BE, Elbuluk N. Microneedling in skin of color: A review of uses and efficacy. *Journal of the American Academy of Dermatology.* 2016;74(2):348–355.

142. Fabbrocini G, De Vita V, Monfrecola A, De Padova MP, Brazzini B, Teixeira F, et al. Percutaneous collagen induction: An effective and safe treatment for post-acne scarring in different skin phototypes. *Journal of Dermatological Treatment.* 2014;25(2):147–152.

143. Casabona G, Marchese P. Calcium hydroxylapatite combined with microneedling and ascorbic acid is effective for treating stretch marks. *Plastic and Reconstructive Surgery Global Open.* 2017;5(9).

144. Karadağ Köse Ö, Borlu M. Efficacy of the combination of Q-switched Nd: YAG laser and microneedling for melasma. *Journal of Cosmetic Dermatology.* 2021;20(3):769–775.

CHAPTER 31: LASERS AND LIGHTS

Kimberly A. Huerth, Nordeep Panesar, Ginette Okoye, and Eliot Battle

31.1 Introduction

Individuals with skin of color (SOC) comprise 80% of the world's population and represent a wide range of racial and ethnic groups, as well as those with blended ancestry.[1] Historically (and paradoxically), the literature on laser and light-based therapies has focused on lightly pigmented individuals of European ancestry. The dearth of studies involving those with darker skin types has been attributed to demographic, cultural, and socioeconomic factors, as well as safety limitations of first-generation energy-based technologies.[2] Available studies on the use of these technologies in SOC have, in large part, involved patients of South or East Asian descent. As a result, there remains a paucity of data on the safety and efficacy of laser and light-based devices for individuals with more richly pigmented skin. This gap in the literature can be compensated for by a practitioner's knowledge of the unique biological characteristics of SOC, how these characteristics bear upon cutaneous reactions to energy-based treatments, and the consequent nuances that must be considered when delivering these treatments.

31.2 Biological Characteristics and Classification of Skin of Color

There are a number of key biological characteristics unique to richly pigmented skin that the clinician must be cognizant of when administering laser or light-based therapies. Larger, non-aggregated melanosomes that are more slowly degraded are more widely and densely dispersed in the keratinocytes of heavily pigmented skin and serve to increase the overall amount of epidermal melanin.[3] Melanocytes themselves tend to evince more labile responses to cutaneous injury and inflammation, engendering increases or decreases in melanin production, which clinically manifest as hyper- or hypopigmentation, respectively.[2, 4] Dermal structural differences also exist between racial groups. In contrast to those with European ancestry, individuals of African descent have been found to possess more numerous fibroblasts, which tend to be larger and multinucleated and contain more biosynthetically active organelles.[5] Dermal fibroblasts have also been shown to increase both epidermal melanin and melanogenic gene expression in vitro.[6] Broadly speaking, race-related differences in skin characteristics can account for the tendency for individuals of African descent to develop keloids and post-inflammatory hyperpigmentation, for East and Southeast Asians to present with melasma, lentigines, and dermal melanocytosis, and for South Asians and Pacific Islanders to develop acne scars and trauma-induced dyspigmentation.[7]

While bearing significantly upon treatment choices and outcomes, racial identity is often more complex than a patient's physical features would suggest and is not always easily determined or classified. Perhaps the most commonly utilized framework for classifying skin is one devised by Fitzpatrick. Originally developed to guide the selection of initial doses of oral psoralen with ultraviolet A for the treatment of psoriasis in white patients, the Fitzpatrick skin type scale did not at its inception include skin phototypes (SPT) V and VI, which were added later.[8, 9] Although this classification system can be used as a starting point to anticipate how a patient will respond to laser and light treatment, assignment of SPT should not be based solely upon the provider's visual perception of a patient's ethnicity and clinical phenotype, as studies have identified high rates of discordance between self-perceived race and that which has been recorded by providers in clinical records.[10, 11] Mixed race individuals add an additional layer of complexity to the challenge of classifying an individual based on clinical phenotype alone.

Classification of skin phototypes based on incorrect assumptions about race can have potentially disastrous consequences for patients. Obtaining a detailed history that elicits details on both a patient's ancestry and on their historical responses to UV exposure and cutaneous injury may reveal considerations that are critical to optimizing a patient's chances of a successful outcome with laser procedures.

31.3 Lasers in Skin of Color: General Considerations and Precautions

All lasers exert cutaneous effects by targeting specific endogenous chromophores—namely, water, hemoglobin, and melanin. Melanin must be fastidiously considered when it is targeted as a chromophore in heavily pigmented skin. By virtue of melanin's broad absorption spectrum of 250–1200 nm, laser light intended for dermal melanin or hemoglobin may be errantly absorbed by epidermal melanin and converted to heat that may cause thermal injury to the epidermis. Whereas mild and transient erythema, edema, or desquamation are permissible reactions to laser treatment, excessive pain, erythema, graying of the skin, and blistering that evolves to pigmentary changes and scarring indicates that the epidermis has been thermally damaged by heating to temperatures in excess of 45°C.[7] Although it is prudent to perform a test spot in the pre-auricular or submental area with the intended laser and settings, manifestations of thermal damage may be delayed by at least 48 hours, which is the minimum amount of time that should elapse before declaring the tested device and parameters safe.[7] Occasionally, pre-treatment testing may not predict the occurrence of adverse events, regardless of which laser or light system is employed.[12]

In addition to thermal injury caused by energy absorption by epidermal melanin, laser-induced effects on melanin production or melanocytes themselves can cause hyper- or hypopigmentation. Although possible with any energy-based treatment, there is a greater risk of undesired pigmentary alterations in SOC with laser resurfacing procedures. Post-inflammatory hyperpigmentation (PIH) has been reported to occur in up to 36% of SPT III–VI patients undergoing laser resurfacing and correlates with injury extending to the papillary dermis.[13] Deeper injury may cause hypopigmentation, which may be actual and apparent six to twelve months after treatment, or relative when treated areas are inadequately blended with adjacent untreated areas. Overall, iatrogenic dyschromias can be very distressing to patients, who in many

DOI: 10.1201/9780429243769-31

cases may have originally sought treatment for endogenous dyschromias.

PIH can be addressed with a combination of sunscreen, topical lightening agents, light chemical peels, and microdermabrasion.[14] Attempts to improve hypopigmentation can be made with topical tacrolimus, which has been shown to promote tyrosinase activity and melanocyte migration,[15] or topical bimatoprost, which has been shown to increase melanogenesis histologically.[16] Bimatoprost has also improved laser-induced hypopigmentation when used in conjunction with fractional resurfacing devices,[17] which on their own have been reported to improve iatrogenic hypopigmentation through the creation of microthermal injury zones that stimulate melanocyte migration from adjacent intact skin during the healing process.[18, 19]

Epidermal melanin can additionally be protected by carefully controlling device settings, delivery technique, and skin care in the periprocedural period. Longer wavelengths that allow for deeper skin penetration and longer pulse durations with lower fluences than those utilized for SPT I–III mitigate excessive heating of epidermal melanin. Limiting the number of pulses in a given treatment area, minimizing stacking and overlap, and holding the laser handpiece perpendicular to the skin surface to avoid overlapping during pulses confer additional epidermal protection. When employing fractionated technology, utilizing a lower density of microthermal zones per unit area, and pausing between passes, may further attenuate the risks associated with excessive tissue heating.[2]

Delivery of efficient precooling, parallel cooling, and postcooling affords additional protection against thermal damage to the epidermis without compromising laser intensity. The application of refrigerated gels or ice packs prior to treatment can lower epidermal temperature, while cold air and the inherent cooling of the laser system are administered during treatment. Examples of inherent cooling techniques include chilled copper plates or sapphire windows, whose effects are enhanced when pulses are delivered at a lower speed, and cryogen spray that is applied 20–100 milliseconds (ms) prior to the pulse of laser energy. Following treatment, inherent cooling devices can be reapplied to the treated area, as can ice packs. It is of import to note that while epidermal cooling is essential to protect the epidermis from excessive heating, improper cooling technique can itself induce pigmentary abnormalities in darker skin types. Resultant hypopigmentation may be attributable to melanocyte destruction at temperatures of around −5°C,[20] while it has been proposed that cold-induced hyperpigmentation results from reactive melanocyte and keratinocyte hyperactivity.[21]

Additional ancillary precautions to minimize the risk of scarring and pigment-related complications include screening patients for a history of keloids or hypertrophic scarring, hyperpigmentation due to trauma, photosensitivity disorders, photosensitizing medications, and prophylaxis for viral and bacterial infections. Excessive sun exposure prior to laser treatment should be minimized, as increased epidermal melanin promotes its behavior as a competing chromophore and predisposes it to thermal epidermal injury. Post-treatment sun exposure should similarly be avoided. Topical lightening agents can be used for at least six weeks prior to treatment to prime the skin and decrease the chance of post-procedure hyperpigmentation, and they are continued as needed for maintenance afterward. Topical steroids may be considered for patients with significant post-treatment edema or erythema, as this may be a harbinger of PIH.

31.4 Laser Hair Removal

When utilized for hair removal, laser and light sources target both melanin in the hair shaft and pigmented cells of the follicular matrix. Epidermal melanin's presence as a competing chromophore in more heavily pigmented skin necessitates the use of longer red or near-infrared (IR) wavelengths that combine an adequate depth of penetration with follicular melanin absorption. Capable devices include long-pulsed ruby (694 nm), alexandrite (755 nm), diode (800 to 810 nm), and Nd:YAG (1,064 nm) lasers, and intense pulsed light (590–1,200 nm).[12]

The 1,064 nm neodymium-doped yttrium aluminum garnet (Nd:YAG) laser has been shown to have the lowest risk of adverse events when utilized for laser hair removal (LHR) in SPT V–VI.[2, 12] While lower fluences of 30–40 J/cm^2 have been recommended by practitioners who perform high volumes of LHR on SPT V–VI patients,[12] others have found the highest tolerable fluences to be up to 100 J/cm^2 in SPT V[22] and 50 J/cm^2 in SPT VI.[22, 23] Recommended pulse durations when employing the 1,064 nm Nd:YAG for LHR in darker SPT range from 3–40 ms, with at least 30 ms favored for SPT V–VI. Both Nd:YAG and diode lasers usually require more treatments than would be required in lighter SPT due to the need for lower fluences with longer pulse durations intended to shield epidermal melanin from thermal injury. The diode can cautiously be used in SPT V–VI; however, adverse events such as erythema, blistering, and pigmentary complications are more common.[24, 25] Though there have been reports of successful hair reduction with the diode at fluences of 10–40 J/cm^2 at pulse widths of 30–40 ms in SPT V–VI, others have recommended at least 100 ms in SPT V and 400 ms in SPT VI in order to heat follicular melanin slowly enough to minimize the aforementioned complications.[26] Some of these complications may be related to the type of hair being treated. Thick terminal hairs retain more heat[27] and may warrant additional decreases in fluence and/or increases in pulse width when treating pseudofolliculitis barbae, acne keloidalis nuchae, folliculitis decalvans, and dissecting cellulitis of the scalp.[2]

Thermal relaxation time (TRT) is the time required for a target tissue to dissipate half of the energy with which it was heated and is around 100 milliseconds for terminal hair follicles and 700 microseconds for skin tissue.[28] A 650-microsecond 1,064 nm Nd:YAG has shown good efficacy in LHR with a favorable side effect profile in higher SPT.[29, 30] In a study of SPT V patients undergoing axillary LHR, around a 75% reduction in hair was observed after four treatments spaced one month apart with fluences ranging from 21 to 36 J/cm^2.[30] The 650-microsecond device confers protection against collateral thermal damage to surrounding tissue by heating the therapeutic target more rapidly than the rate at which heat can be conducted to the surrounding skin, and by allowing pulses to travel through the epidermis 30–50 times faster than millisecond lasers.[31] In the authors' experience, this device is also capable of safely treating active acne, hidradenitis suppurativa, hyperpigmentation, and rejuvenating skin in SPT V–VI.

The long-pulsed 755 nm alexandrite laser and intense pulsed light (IPL) can both be utilized with caution for LHR in SPT I–IV. For example, in a study comparing the use of Nd:YAG, diode, and alexandrite for photoepilation in SPT IV–VI, the alexandrite laser was found to have the highest incidence of adverse events, with 90% of patients reporting redness, 60.6% reporting superficial burns, and 40% reporting hyperpigmentation.[25] IPL has been reported to be as effective as 1,064 nm Nd:YAG in SPT V after five monthly sessions, with a low incidence of post-treatment burning and hyperpigmentation, when administered with a wavelength range of 650–950 nm, 25–45 ms pulse duration, and 3.5–4.5 J/cm^2.[31] Despite such reports of its safety and efficacy in higher SPT patients, it is the authors' opinion that LHR with IPL in SPT V–VI should be avoided when possible due to the risk of hyperpigmentation.

31.5 Skin Rejuvenation and Resurfacing

Energy-based skin rejuvenation aims to improve the appearance of rhytids, scars, enlarged pores, benign epidermal lesions, photoaging, and laxity. For the purpose of fully ablative resurfacing, the 10,600 nm CO_2, 2,940 nm erbium-doped:yttrium-aluminum-garnet (Er:YAG), and 2,790 nm erbium-doped:yttrium-scandium-gallium-garnet (Er:YSGG) target water as a chromophore to both vaporize the epidermis and create controlled partial-thickness damage to the level of the dermis, which denatures, shrinks, and stimulates collagen. Though these lasers yield the most significant outcomes, they are also associated with a higher risk of adverse events such as infections, permanent hypopigmentation, temporary hyperpigmentation, lingering erythema, and scarring.[2, 4, 32] These devices are frequently contraindicated in SPT V–VI, and must be used with extreme caution in SPT III–IV.[4, 33]

In contrast to fully ablative resurfacing, fractionated ablative resurfacing with CO_2, Er:YAG, and Er:YSGG creates microscopic columns of controlled dermal tissue ablation and vaporization encased in thermally denatured collagen, which is surrounded by areas of intact skin that serve as a nidus for wound healing. Fractionally ablative lasers allow for complete reepithelialization within one week, rather than two to three weeks with fully ablative lasers, but may require more than one treatment to achieve desired results. Though they are less aggressive than fully ablative devices, they nevertheless pose a risk for infection, scarring, and dyspigmentation, which requires caution and careful consideration when treating SPT V–VI, in whom their use has not been well studied.[2, 4] There are reports of fractional ablative CO_2 being used in SPT III–IV Asian and Hispanic patients that yielded 25–50% improvement in acne scars and photoaging, with adverse effects such as transient hyperpigmentation and erythema that persisted several weeks.[34, 35]

The emergence of nonablative resurfacing lasers has afforded those with more heavily pigmented skin a safer means of skin rejuvenation. These devices heat water in the papillary and midreticular dermis to stimulate collagen remodeling while causing subclinical injury to an intact epidermis.[36] Nonablative lasers offer faster recovery time and a lower risk of scarring and dyspigmentation compared to ablative lasers, but in exchange, they yield less impressive results and can require four to six treatments to achieve maximal improvement. Nonablative nonfractionated lasers include the 1,319 nm pulsed energy, 1,320 nm Nd:YAG, and the 1,450 nm diode and have been demonstrated to reduce wrinkles and improve scarring in type III–V Asian skin.[37, 38] The microsecond 1,064 nm Nd:YAG has also been utilized in a nonablative fashion for acne scarring in SPT III–VI, showing improvement in skin texture and minimal side effects.[39, 40]

Nonablative fractionated lasers combine a more aggressive pulse with the safety of fractionation to create microthermal zones (MTZ) of tissue injury to the epidermis and upper dermis, thereby inducing dermal collagen remodeling while leaving the stratum corneum intact. They include the 1,410 nm and 1,440 nm Nd:YAG, the 1,540 nm and 1,550 nm erbium glass, and the 1927 nm thulium fiber lasers. As is the case with other nonablative technology, moderate improvements in skin tone and texture are produced over the course of several treatments, with less downtime and fewer adverse effects compared to ablative lasers. Though the majority of studies have been performed in SPT I–IV, these devices can be utilized with caution to treat regional disorders such as acne scarring in more deeply pigmented skin.[27] Parameters must be adjusted to ensure safety in SOC. For example, lower treatment densities and fewer passes administered over several treatment sessions have been shown to decrease the risk of PIH without compromising treatment efficacy.[41, 42]

31.6 Endogenous Epidermal and Dermal Pigmented Lesions

Treatment of dyschromia due to melasma, ephelides, lentigines, and dermal melanocytoses, such as nevus of Ota and Hori nevus, is one of the most frequent indications for which individuals with SOC seek the care of dermatologists.[43, 44] Given the prevalence of congenital and acquired pigmentary disorders in East Asian populations (who are often SPT III–IV), the use of lasers and IPL for these conditions has been well studied.[14, 45] Despite these concerns being shared by SPT V–VI patients, there is a relative dearth of studies to guide the use of lasers and light sources for their treatment. Complicating this matter is the fact that, in many cases, the treatment itself can induce or exacerbate dyschromia and that there is no laser that is universally effective for complexion blending in more heavily pigmented skin.[7]

31.6.1 Melasma

Laser toning with a Q-switched 1,064 nm Nd:YAG delivered in a multi-pass technique with low fluences (less than 5 J/cm^2), high repetition rate (5–10 Hz), and large spot sizes (6–10 mm) at weekly intervals for five to ten sessions, is not only used for skin rejuvenation, but has also gained popularity in Asia and elsewhere for the treatment of melasma.[32, 46, 47] This technique is based on the theory of subcellular selective photothermolysis (SSP), in which high peak power from fluence delivered over an ultrashort pulse width causes selective photothermolysis of stage IV melanosomes while permitting melanocyte survival.[48] In contrast, traditional laser treatment is based on selective photothermolysis that results in the death of pigment-containing cells.[49] By preventing cell death, SSP is thought to minimize inflammation that may contribute to disease recurrence. It is this very mechanism, however, that is accountable for mottled hypopigmentation that can be observed with laser toning, in which a preserved number of melanocytes severely lack melanosomes.[46, 50] Treating once every two weeks instead of weekly, applying tacrolimus ointment, and administering excimer laser, have been recommended as ways to circumvent this adverse effect.[51] Conversely, monthly maintenance treatments are recommended to prevent rebound hyperpigmentation.[32]

In addition to laser toning with 1,064 nm Nd:YAG, Q-switched 694 nm ruby and 755 nm alexandrite have also been used to treat melasma, with varied results. In one split-face study, laser toning with 755 nm alexandrite and 1,064 nm Nd:YAG were equally effective at improving moderate to severe melasma in a group of mostly SPT III–IV patients, though varying degrees of relapse were common by week 12.[52]

Recurrence and PIH have also been associated with attempts to treat melasma with Q-switched 694 nm ruby.[53, 54] Low-power fractional CO_2 laser has been compared with Q-switched 1,064 nm Nd:YAG laser toning, with the former demonstrating more significant improvements than the latter.[55] It is thought that fractional CO_2 improves melasma when transepidermal elimination of MTZs engenders the removal of dermal melanophages.[56] The fractional nonablative 1,550 nm laser is the only laser treatment that has been approved by the US Food and Drug Administration for melasma. Initial pilot studies on SPT III–V patients reported 75–100% clearing of melasma in 60%.[57] However, as with many other treatments that have been attempted, relapse is common, and there is a risk of adverse effects with increasing skin phototype. For this reason, patients should first be medically optimized with topical lightening agents and conscientious sun protection and extensively counseled on the high risk of recurrence before any laser or light-based therapies directed at melasma are attempted.

31.6.2 Ephelides, Lentigines, and Dermal Melanocytosis

The treatment of ephelides, lentigines, and congenital and acquired dermal melanocytoses, such as nevus of Ota and Hori nevus, are of particular concern to Asian patients, who tend to manifest these lesions more commonly than other races.[14] There is a paucity of studies that examine the use of laser and light treatments for these conditions in SPT V–VI. Q-switched lasers, such as the 694 nm ruby, the 755 nm alexandrite, and the 532 nm frequency-doubled or 1064 nm Nd:YAG have long been used to treat these lesions in SPT III–IV patients in a manner similar to laser toning employed for the treatment of melasma.[58] Though these devices can be used to treat epidermal melanin, they carry a higher risk of PIH when doing so and are thus preferred for dermal lesions.[7] More recently, a 755 nm picosecond alexandrite laser has been used to treat both endogenous dermal and epidermal pigmented lesions in SPT III–IV, with comparable efficacy to Q-switched 532 nm frequency-doubled and 1,064 nm Nd:YAG and 694 nm ruby lasers.[59] Similarly, a 532 nm picosecond laser demonstrated good to excellent results in treating epidermal pigmented lesions in SPT III–IV, with a low risk of PIH.[60] These studies offer mounting evidence that visible light and near-infrared picosecond lasers possess clinical applications beyond tattoo removal. Some studies have suggested that longer pulsed devices (microseconds) and IPL may confer a lower risk of PIH when treating pigmented lesions, as the microsecond domain more closely approximates the thermal relaxation time of the epidermis. In a study of SPT III women with ephelides and lentigines, IPL was found to provide a better therapeutic effect than Q-switched 755 nm alexandrite laser.[61] Anecdotally, PIH following the treatment of lentigines may be mitigated by compressing the skin with the handpiece. This helps to remove hemoglobin as a competing chromophore by emptying dermal blood vessels.[14]

31.7 Conclusion

Technological advances continue to give rise to devices with improved safety profiles in more richly pigmented skin, but this is not a substitute for the practitioner's crucial understanding of how racial ancestry and resultant skin phototype guide the selection of technology and treatment settings. Minimizing the risks of post-procedural pigmentary alterations and scarring, while concurrently achieving a desired therapeutic outcome, requires a thorough understanding of the parameters that influence selective photothermolysis. How these parameters are expressed in the context of the specific device being employed, methods of laser delivery that provide an increased level of protection to a more melanin-rich epidermis, and the unique biological characteristics of SOC. More studies determining safety, tolerability, and outcomes of existing and new laser technologies, especially in SPT V–VI patients are needed to ameliorate longstanding gaps in research.

Frequently Asked Questions

1. *Q: What are the biological characteristics of skin of color that create a heightened risk of adverse outcomes with laser and light-based treatments?*

   A: Increased amounts of epidermal melanin are attributable to the presence of larger, widely dispersed, and more degradation-resistant melanosomes. Melanocytes tend to react in a more labile manner to cutaneous injury and inflammation. Dermal fibroblasts are more numerous, larger, biosynthetically active, and capable of increasing epidermal melanin and melanogenic gene expression.

2. *Q: What interval of time should be permitted to elapse before evaluating the response to a laser test spot in SOC?*

   A: It is recommended that test spots be re-evaluated no sooner than 48 hours after they were placed, as manifestations of thermal damage may take this long (and in the authors' experience, sometimes as long as one to two weeks) to appear.

3. *Q: Why has the 1064 nm 650-microsecond Nd:YAG been purported to offer an enhanced safety profile in SPT V–VI?*

   A: Thermal relaxation time is around 100 milliseconds for terminal hair follicles and 700 microseconds for skin tissue. By heating therapeutic targets more rapidly than the rate at which heat dissipates to the surrounding skin and by allowing pulses to travel through the epidermis 30–50 times faster than millisecond lasers, the 650-microsecond Nd:YAG minimizes collateral thermal damage to surrounding tissue.

4. *Q: What is the purported mechanism that underlies laser toning, as well as a potential related untoward consequence?*

   A: Subcellular selective photothermolysis (SSP) occurs when high peak power from fluence delivered over an ultrashort pulse width causes selective photothermolysis of stage IV melanosomes while permitting melanocyte survival. A potential consequence of SSP is mottled hypopigmentation that is thought to be attributable to melanosome destruction in preserved melanocytes.

5. *Q: What are some strategies that can be employed to mitigate hypopigmentation that is induced by laser toning?*

   A: Treating once every two weeks instead of weekly, applying tacrolimus ointment, and utilizing an excimer laser have been recommended as ways to mitigate laser toning-induced hypopigmentation.

References

1. Talakoub L, Wesley NO. Differences in perceptions of beauty and cosmetic procedures performed in ethnic patients. *Semin Cutan Med Surg.* 2009;28(2):115–129.

2. Alexis AF. Lasers and light-based therapies in ethnic skin: Treatment options and recommendations for Fitzpatrick skin types V and VI. *Br J Dermatol.* 2013;169 Suppl 3:91–97.

3. Smit NP, Kolb RM, Lentjes EG, Noz KC, van der Meulen H, Koerten HK, Vermeer BJ, Pavel S. Variations in melanin formation by cultured melanocytes from different skin types. *Arch Dermatol Res.* 1998;290(6):342–349.

4. Richter AL, Barrera J, Markus RF, Brissett A. Laser skin treatment in non-Caucasian patients. *Facial Plast Surg Clin North Am.* 2014;22(3):439–446.

5. Montagna W, Carlisle K. The architecture of black and white facial skin. *J Amer Acad Dermatol.* 1991;24(6 Pt. 1):929–937.

6. Duval C, Cohen C, Chagnoleau C, Flouret V, Bourreau E, Bernerd F. Key regulatory role of dermal fibroblasts in pigmentation as demonstrated using a reconstructed skin model: Impact of photo-aging. *PloS One.* 2014;9(12):e114182.

7. Battle EF. Cosmetic laser treatments for skin of color: A focus on safety and efficacy. *J Drugs Dermatol.* 2011;10(1):35–38.

8. Fitzpatrick TB. Soleil et peau. *J Med Esthet.* 1975;2:33–34.

9. Fitzpatrick TB. Ultraviolet-induced pigmentary changes: Benefits and hazards. *Curr Probl Dermatol.* 1986;15:25–38.

10. Boehmer U, Kressin NR, Berlowitz DR, Christiansen CL, Kazis LE, Jones JA. Self-reported vs administrative race/ethnicity data and study results. *Am J Public Health.* 2002;92(9):1471–1472.

11. Harwell TS, Hansen D, Moore KR, Jeanotte D, Gohdes D, Helgerson SD. Accuracy of race coding on American Indian death certificates, Montana 1996–1998. *Public Health Rep.* 2002;117(1):44–49.

12. Breadon JY, Barnes CA. Comparison of adverse events of laser and light assisted hair removal systems in skin types IV–VI. *J Drugs Dermatol.* 2007;6(1):40–46.

13. Alexiades-Armenakas M, Dover JS, Arndt KA. The spectrum of laser skin resurfacing: Nonablative, fractional, and ablative laser resurfacing. *J Am Acad Dermatol.* 2008;58(5):719–737.

14. Chan HL. Effective and safe use of lasers, light sources, and radiofrequency devices in the clinical management of Asian patients with selected dermatoses. *Lasers Surg Med.* 2005;37(3):179–185.

15. Kang HY, Choi YM. FK506 increases pigmentation and migration of human melanocytes. *Br J Dermatol.* 2006;155(5):1037–1040.

16. Kapur R, Osmanovic S, Toyran S, Edward DP. Bimatoprost-induced periocular skin hyperpigmentation: Histopathological study. *Arch Ophthalmol.* 2005;123(11):1541–1546.

17. Regis A, MacGregor J, Chapas A. Fractional resurfacing and topical bimatoprost for the treatment of laser induced postinflammatory hypopigmentation on the lower extremities. *Dermatol Surg.* 2018;44(6):883–886.

18. Glaich AS, Rahman Z, Goldberg LH, Friedman PM. Fractional resurfacing for the treatment of hypopigmented scars: A pilot study. *Dermatol Surg.* 2007;33(3):289–294.

19. Gan SD, Bae-Harboe YC, Graber EM. Nonablative fractional resurfacing for the treatment of iatrogenic hypopigmentation. *Dermatol Surg.* 2014;40(1):87–89.

20. Gage AA, Meenaghan MA, Natiella JR, Greene GW. Sensitivity of pigmented mucosa and skin to freezing injury. *Cryobiology.* 1979;16(4):348–361.

21. Manuskiatti W, Eimpunth S, Wanitphakdeedecha R. Effect of cold air cooling on the incidence of postinflammatory hyperpigmentation after Q-switched Nd: YAG laser treatment of acquired bilateral nevus of Ota–like macules. *Arch Dermatol.* 2007;143(9):1139–1143.

22. Ross EV, Cooke LM, Timko AL, Overstreet KA, Graham BS, Barnette DJ. Treatment of pseudofolliculitis barbae in skin types IV, V, and VI with a long-pulsed neodymium: Yttrium aluminum garnet laser. *J Am Acad Dermatol.* 2002;47(2):263–270.

23. Alster TS, Bryan H, Williams CM. Long-pulsed Nd: YAG laser-assisted hair removal in pigmented skin: A clinical and histological evaluation. *Arch Dermatol.* 2001;137(7):885–889.

24. Greppi I, Ross EV. Diode laser hair removal of the black patient. *Lasers Surg Med.* 2001;28(2):150–155.

25. Galadari I. Comparative evaluation of different hair removal lasers in skin types IV, V, and VI. *Int J Dermatol.* 2003;42(1):68–70.

26. Battle EF, Hobbs LM. Laser-assisted hair removal for darker skin types. *Dermatol Ther.* 2004;17(2):177–183.

27. Rossi AM, Perez MI. Laser therapy in Latino skin. *Facial Plast Surg Clin North Am.* 2011;19(2):389–403.

28. Walsh JT, Flotte TJ, Anderson RR, Deutsch TF. Pulsed CO_2 laser tissue ablation: Effect of tissue type and pulse duration on thermal damage. *Lasers Surg Med.* 1988;8(2):108–118.

29. Burgess C, Chilukuri S, Campbell-Chambers DA, Henry M, Saedi N, Roberts WE. Practical applications for medical and aesthetic treatment of skin of color with a new 650-microsecond laser. *J Drugs Dermatol.* 2019;18(4):s138–s143.

30. Khatri KA, Lee RA, Goldberg LJ, Khatri B, Garcia V. Efficacy and safety of a 0.65 millisecond pulsed portable Nd: YAG laser for hair removal. *J Cosmet Laser Ther.* 2009;11(1):19–24.

31. Bs B, Chittoria RK, Thappa DM, Mohapatra DP, Mt F, Dineshkumar S, Pandey S. Are lasers superior to lights in the photoepilation of Fitzpatrick V and VI skin types?—A comparison between Nd: YAG laser and intense pulsed light. *J Cosmet Laser Ther.* 2017;19(5):252–255.

32. Jalalat S, Weiss E. Cosmetic laser procedures in Latin skin. *J Drugs Dermatol.* 2019;18(3 Suppl):127–131.

33. Battle EF, Soden CE. The use of lasers in darker skin types. *Sem Cutan Med Surg.* 2009;28(2):130–140.

34. Ho C, Nguyen Q, Lowe NJ, Griffin ME, Lask G. Laser resurfacing in pigmented skin. *Dermatol Surg.* 1995;21(12):1035–1037.

35. Manuskiatti W, Triwongwaranat D, Varothai S, Eimpunth S, Wanitphakdeedecha R. Efficacy and safety of a carbon-dioxide ablative fractional resurfacing device for treatment of atrophic acne scars in Asians. *J Am Acad Dermatol.* 2010;63(2):274–283.

36. Fatemi A, Weiss MA, Weiss RA. Short-Term histologic effects of nonablative resurfacing: Results with a dynamically cooled millisecond-domain 1320-nm Nd: YAG laser. *Dermatol Surg.* 2002;28(2):172–176.

37. Chua S, Ang P, Khoo LSW, Goh C. Nonablative 1450-nm diode laser in the treatment of facial atrophic acne scars in type IV to V Asian skin: A prospective clinical study. *Dermatol Surg.* 2004;30(10):1287–1291.

38. Chan HH, Lam L, Wong DSY, Kono T, Trendell-Smith N. Use of 1320 nm Nd: YAG laser for wrinkle reduction and the treatment of atrophic acne scarring in Asians. *Lasers Surg Med.* 2004;34(2):98–103.

39. Badawi A, Tome MA, Atteya A, Sami N, Morsy IAL. Retrospective analysis of non-ablative scar treatment in dark skin types using the sub-millisecond Nd: YAG 1064-nm laser. *Lasers Surg Med.* 2011;43(2):130–136.

40. Lipper GM, Perez M. Nonablative acne scar reduction after a series of treatments with a short-pulsed 1064-nm neodymium: YAG laser. *Dermatol Surg.* 2006;32(8):998–1006.

41. Alexis AF. Fractional laser resurfacing of acne scarring in patients with Fitzpatrick skin types IV–VI. *J Drugs Dermatol.* 2011;10(12 Suppl):s6–s7.

42. Chan HH, Manstein D, Yu CS, Shek S, Kono T, Wei WI. The prevalence and risk factors of post-inflammatory hyperpigmentation after fractional resurfacing in Asians. *Lasers Surg Med.* 2007;39(5):381–385.

43. Alexis AF, Sergay AB, Taylor SC. Common dermatologic disorders in skin of color: A comparative practice survey. *Cutis.* 2007;80(5):387–394.

44. Halder RM, Grimes PE, McLaurin CI, Kress MA, Kenney JA. Incidence of common dermatoses in a predominantly black dermatologic practice. *Cutis.* 1983;32(4):388–390.

45. Ho SGY, Chan NPY, Yeung CK, Shek SY, Kono T, Chan HH. A retrospective analysis of the management of freckles and lentigines using four different pigment lasers on Asian skin. *J Cosmet Laser Ther.* 2012;14(2):74–80.

46. Chan NPY, Ho SGY, Shek SYN, Yeung CK, Chan HH. A case series of facial depigmentation associated with low fluence Q-switched 1064-nm Nd: YAG laser for skin rejuvenation and melasma. *Lasers Surg Med.* 2010;42(8):712–719.

47. Parra CAH, Careta MF, Valente NYS, De SO, Torezan LAR. Clinical and histopathologic assessment of facial melasma after low-fluence Q-switched neodymium-doped yttrium aluminium garnet laser. *Dermatol Surg.* 2016;42(4):507–512.

48. Mun JY, Jeong SY, Kim JH, Han SS, Kim I. A low fluence Q-switched Nd: YAG laser modifies the 3D structure of melanocyte and ultrastructure of melanosome by subcellular-selective photothermolysis. *J Electron Microsc.* 2011;60(1):11–18.

49. Anderson RR, Parrish JA. Selective photothermolysis: Precise microsurgery by selective absorption of pulsed radiation. *Science.* 1983;220(4596):524–527.

50. Jang YH, Park J, Park YJ, Kang HY. Changes in melanin and melanocytes in mottled hypopigmentation after low-fluence 1064-nm Q-switched Nd: YAG laser treatment for melasma. *Ann Dermatol.* 2015;27(3):340–342.

51. Aurangabadkar S. Optimizing Q-switched lasers for melasma and acquired dermal melanoses. *Indian J Dermatol Venereol Leprol.* 2019;85(1):10–17.

52. Fabi SG, Friedmann DP, Niwa Massaki AB, Goldman MP. A randomized, split-face clinical trial of low-fluence Q-switched neodymium-doped yttrium aluminum garnet (1064-nm) laser versus low-fluence Q-switched alexandrite laser (755-nm) for the treatment of facial melasma. *Lasers Surg Med.* 2014;46(7):531–537.

53. Kopera D, Hohenleutner U. Ruby laser treatment of melasma and postinflammatory hyperpigmentation. *Dermatol Surg.* 1995;21(11):994.

54. Taylor CR, Anderson RR. Ineffective treatment of refractory melasma and postinflammatory hyperpigmentation by Q-switched ruby laser. *J Dermatol Surg Oncol.* 1994;20(9):592–597.

55. Jalaly NY, Valizadeh N, Barikbin B, Yousefi M. Low-power fractional CO_2 laser versus low-fluence Q-switch 1064-nm Nd: YAG laser for treatment of melasma: A randomized, controlled, split-face study. *Am J Clin Dermatol.* 2014;15(4):357–363.

56. Hantash BM, Bedi VP, Sudireddy V, Struck SK, Herron GS, Chan KF. Laser-induced transepidermal elimination of dermal content by fractional photothermolysis. *J Biomed Opt.* 2006;11(4):041115.

57. Rokhsar CK, Fitzpatrick RE. The treatment of melasma with fractional photothermolysis: A pilot study. *Dermatol Surg.* 2005;31(12): 1645–1650.

58. Seo HM, Choi CW, Kim WS. Beneficial effects of early treatment of nevus of Ota with low-fluence 1064-nm Q-switched Nd: YAG laser. *Dermatol Surg.* 2015;41(1):142–148.

59. Levin MK, Ng E, Bae YC, Brauer JA, Geronemus RG. Treatment of pigmentary disorders in patients with skin of color with a novel 755-nm picosecond, Q-switched ruby, and Q-switched Nd: YAG nanosecond lasers: A retrospective photographic review. *Lasers Surg Med.* 2016;48(2):181–187.

60. Kung KY, Shek SY, Yeung CK, Chan HH. Evaluation of the safety and efficacy of the dual wavelength picosecond laser for the treatment of benign pigmented lesions in Asians. *Lasers Surg Med.* 2019;51(1): 14–22.

61. Wang C, Sue Y, Yang C, Chen C. A comparison of Q-switched alexandrite laser and intense pulsed light for the treatment of freckles and lentigines in Asian persons: A randomized, physician-blinded, split-face comparative trial. *J Am Acad Dermatol.* 2006;54(5): 804–810.

CHAPTER 32: NON-LIGHT ENERGY-BASED DEVICES

Vivek Mehta

32.1 Introduction

The two most frequently utilized devices in any aesthetic practice are lasers and non-light energy-based devices. Lasers are devices that use light as an energy source to modify the skin. Examples are hair removal lasers (GentleLase), tattoo removal lasers (RevLite), and lasers for remodeling the skin by removing a layer of skin (resurfacing lasers such as Fraxel, CO2RE, and eMatrix). The rest of the devices that use alternative means, such as electricity, ultrasound, and cold, are known as non-light energy-based devices. Energy-based devices have become safer and more effective over the years, much like other technology in our lives.

Radiofrequency is not based on light but is based on electricity. An energy is developed that has a positive and negative pole, and the heat generated is due to the resistance of the skin as the energy travels through it. This can cause general "bulk" heating in the case of monopolar radiofrequency, where the heating causes the cells that make new collagen to be very active, as well as change the way the collagen sits in the skin in an advantageous way that makes the skin firmer or tighter. We can also use radiofrequency to resurface the skin, which, by means of tiny electrodes (positive and negative poles), causes heating just under the skin surface, which is helpful in treating wrinkles, scars, and pores. The advantage of radiofrequency is that it is color-blind, in that the color and type of skin do not matter. Excessive heating of the skin can affect people of different colors differently, leading to hyperpigmentation or darkening of the skin.

Most recently a new energy source—cold—has been utilized for various purposes. Cryo-lipolysis removes heat from the fat, causing many of the cells to undergo apoptosis and be reabsorbed by the body. This takes advantage of the fact that fat has a higher melting point compared to skin so that we can selectively damage the fat without damaging the skin.

Finally, another new energy modality is ultrasound. Mainly known for being a diagnostic test, ultrasound energy is used as the basis for high-intensity focused ultrasound, a lifting and tightening device for the face and neck. The high-intensity focused ultrasound uses sound waves to find the proper plane of treatment in the skin and then can deliver a focused beam of sound to a very exact spot in the skin to cause an invisible wound that makes remodeling faster and more effective. We can focus ultrasound on three different depths of the skin very precisely and make multiple tiny unseen wounds that cause a massive amount of new collagen to be built by our own bodies, resulting in the lifting of the skin and smoothing out of creases, wrinkles, and folds of the neck, jowls, cheeks, and forehead.

32.2 Classification

Non-light energy-based devices are divided into the following types:

1. Radiofrequency
2. Ultrasound
3. Cryolipolysis

32.3 Indications

1. Skin rejuvenation
2. Skin tightening
3. Treatment of scars
4. Body contouring
5. Treatment of acne
6. Vaginal rejuvenation

32.4 Radiofrequency

Radiofrequency (RF) current is formed when charged particles flow through a closed circuit. As the energy meets resistance in the tissue, heat is produced. The amount of heat will vary depending on the amount of current, the resistance levels in the targeted tissue, and the characteristics of the electrodes. Human tissues, including the skin, are rich in electrolytes and an array of compounds that allow current conductance with varying degrees of impedance and resultant heat formation. The amount of RF energy applied can be configured to target specific tissues. In addition, the water content of the skin varies between different areas of the body with the time of the day, environmental humidity, internal hydration, and the use of topical moisturizing agents. Thus, the flow of RF through the skin depends on multiple factors that may not be uniform from one treatment to the next. This reaction is dictated by the following formula: energy (J) = I2 × R × T (where I = current, R = tissue impedance, and T = time of application). High-impedance tissues, such as subcutaneous fat, generate greater heat and account for deeper thermal effects of RF devices (1, 2).

32.5 Nonablative Radiofrequency Skin Tightening

Nonablative RF is one of the commonly performed procedures, especially for the treatment of skin laxity. This is a therapeutic modality that produces a selective and controlled rise in tissue temperature from a high-frequency alternating current (0.3 to 10 MHz). The rising temperature and the depth of heating depends on the level of energy used and on the impedance of biological tissues. The final goal is to induce thermal damage to stimulate changes in collagen conformation and produce neocollagenesis in deep layers of the skin and subcutaneous tissue (3, 4).

Electromagnetic fields (EMF) can act on tissues in several ways, causing thermal and/or non-thermal effects. Most of the authors cite thermal effects caused by the increase in local tissue temperature, the contraction of collagen, and the stimulus to the synthesis of collagen fibers. The literature also cites some non-thermal effects, where EMF could induce biological changes through interaction with cellular membrane receptors or channels. According to Bachl et al., EMFs are able to stimulate the synthesis of a cytoprotective growth factor. Goodman et al. mentioned an increase in enzyme activity, level of transcription of specific genes, and mRNA expression. Tokalov et al. reported, in their experiments with human cell cultures, that EMFs lead to a significant induction of heat shock genes (5, 6).

DOI: 10.1201/9780429243769-32

Alvares et al. also mentioned the effects on the synthesis of mucopolysaccharides and elastic fibers, which leads to dermal thickening, thus improving the firmness and elasticity of the skin (7).

RF for the treatment of skin laxity and wrinkles is based on the use of a source of heat for the denaturation of collagen (which occurs at temperatures ranging from 50°C to 75°C in the dermis) and the consequent contraction of the connective tissue. These processes lead to tissue repair response, establishing long-term dermal remodeling. Zelickson et al. demonstrated, through abdominal skin biopsies, that eight weeks after the denaturation of collagen, there is an induction of new collagen synthesis (neocollagenesis) (8).

The process of thermal contraction of collagen begins with denaturing the triple helix, where the intramolecular cross-links are broken, and collagen undergoes a transition from a highly organized crystalline structure to a gel-like state (denaturation). The collagen contraction occurs by the cumulative effect of the "unwinding" of the triple helix due to the destruction of intermolecular cross-links and the residual stress of such links (9, 10).

The frequencies used in the reviewed studies ranged from 1 MHz to 6 MHz, with the highest percentage of studies reporting a frequency of 6 MHz. According to Abraham and Mashkevich, during the treatment cycle with an EMF at 6 MHz, it is determined that polarity alternates at a rate of six million cycles per second, which stimulates the movement of charged particles and creates an electrical current within the tissue, treated by attracting and repelling electrons and ions. The literature reports that the penetration depth of RF is an inverse function of its frequency—that is, in lower frequencies (0.8 MHz) occurs a greater penetration and in higher frequencies (2.45 MHz), a lower penetration (11). Zelickson et al. mentioned, however, that it is possible to change the depth of penetration of the treatment by changing the electrode geometry, the amount of power supplied, and the duration of treatment (10).

In all the analyzed studies, the authors mention the need to reach high temperatures in the dermis in order to achieve therapeutic goals. In this review, however, none of the authors measured the temperature of the therapeutic target, the dermis. On measuring the temperature of the epidermis, it remained around 40°C and 42°C, and that of the dermis, around 65°C.

Most pieces of equipment use capacitive methods (bipolar, tripolar, or multipolar electrodes) for transmitting energy to the skin. According to Montesi et al., the main difference between the inductive and the capacitive method is the configuration of the electrodes to be applied to the skin, which will result in the way energy is transmitted to the tissues. The inductive method (monopolar electrode) uses an active and a passive electrode, the latter acting as a grounding electrode. Power is transmitted to the tissue via a single point of contact, which increases the penetration of the generated current. In the capacitive method (bipolar, tripolar, or multipolar electrode), energy alternates between two electrodes situated a short distance from one another. In the tripolar and multipolar devices, bipolar energy switches between different poles at every moment. The energy is concentrated at the site of treatment, and the achieved depth is half of the distance between the two electrodes (12).

32.6 Classification of Radiofrequency

1. Monopolar RF
2. Bipolar RF
3. Unipolar RF
4. Multipolar RF

1. *Monopolar RF*: Monopolar means that the patient is grounded, and the RF is delivered through the skin, into the body, and ultimately to the grounding electrode. Typically, RF travels through structures with the highest water content and the greatest resistance. Monopolar devices are further divided into the following:
   a. Stamping or static monopolar devices: Short cycles of one to two seconds are delivered while the handpiece is held in place. A single pulse is delivered; the handpiece is then moved to an adjacent marked area and fired again. This is performed for hundreds of pulses until the pre-marked area is treated. Each pulse is measured for temperature while spray cooling is applied so the skin temperature does not exceed 45°C.
   b. Dynamic monopolar RF devices: RF is delivered in a continuous pulse with a constant rotation of the handpiece. The handpiece is continuously moved, and specific areas of laxity can be targeted in a relatively short time to reach a final temperature. The surface temperature measurements are continuously monitored, and the measurement tool is often built into the handpiece.
2. *Bipolar RF*: When using the bipolar method of RF delivery, the RF travels to and from the positive and negative poles, which are usually built into the handpiece. With a specific distance between the electrodes, the depth of penetration and heating is predetermined by the spacing of the electrodes and typically confined to within 1–4 mm of the skin surface. Multiple variations of the bipolar RF concept include the following:
   a. Fractional or fractionated RF constructed of mini-bipolar electrodes
   b. Bipolar-insulated needle electrodes mechanically inserted into the dermis
3. *Unipolar RF*: Another form of delivery is unipolar, in which there is one electrode, no grounding pad, and a large field of RF is emitted in an omnidirectional field around a single electrode. This is analogous to a radio tower broadcasting signals in all directions.

32.7 Fractional Sublative Radiofrequency

Fractional bipolar RF addresses some of the limitations of both ablative and nonablative skin rejuvenation. Also known as sublative rejuvenation, treatment is delivered via a hand-held applicator. Sublative rejuvenation causes limited epidermal disruption-less than 5% of the surface is treated with one pass, which translates to minimal downtime for patients. The bulk of the effect is coagulative and occurs mainly in the mid-dermis and, therefore, has the most effect on wrinkles and scars.

Mechanism of action: RF modality in bipolar electrode scheme applies the configured energy in a pyramid shape, which creates a predetermined controlled wound with a small epidermal component and large volume in deeper tissues. Epidermal ablation takes place within the first 10 ms of the pulse and up to another 100 ms of controlled RF travels between the electrode array to further heat the dermal tissue for optimal remodeling of both collagen and elastin. The tip of the sublative rejuvenation applicator contains an array of 64 electrode pins, each 200 microns wide, which directly contact the dry stratum corneum of the epidermis. The RF energy flows between the positively and negatively charged electrode pins to form a closed circuit of bipolar RF current within the tissue that passes through the epidermis deep into the dermis, delivering 1 MHz of conducted RF current into the tissue. The electric field produces a pyramid-shaped thermal injury zone with the tip of the pyramid at the epidermal surface branching out to the wider area deeper into the dermis. The RF energy penetrates the dermis with a coagulative effect up to 450 microns depth, with only 200 microns epidermal width of the effect.

The variable energy of RF current can create different spatial and depth impacts with a larger relative area and volume of dermal tissue affected than epidermal tissue, thereby promoting neocollagenesis, providing rhytid reduction, and minimizing dermal atrophic scarring. The healing process is focused mainly on fibroblast stimulation and ECM dermal remodeling.

32.8 Nano-Fractional Radiofrequency

Nano-fractional radiofrequency is the next-generation fractional RF that allows increased penetration of RF. The increased efficacy, due to its improved control of both power and pulse duration, results in improved control of tissue ablation or coagulation ratio. This allows for more aggressive treatments, which helps result in fewer treatments to reach cosmetic goals. The smaller pin footprint allows for the creation of micro-wounds in the targeted skin, resulting in decreased side effects and shorter downtime. The energy is delivered to each micro pin individually, not only maximizing patient comfort but also helping to ensure that the tissue is treated uniformly, resulting in homogenous, consistent, and reproducible clinical outcomes. The patented tip technology with a depth of penetration of up to 500 microns allows for varying energy densities to be used during treatment, enabling complete precision control over the ablation of the epidermis and coagulation of the underlying dermis for enhanced treatment efficacy. This technique minimizes the post-treatment recovery time and the potential risk for infection, scarring, and hyperpigmentation. For acne scar treatments, the 80 pins/tip is predominantly used as it forms a bigger loop of RF, can go deeper to target the deep-seated scars, and also results in minimizing the downtime associated with treatment.

Goel et al. conducted a study on 20 healthy male and female Indian patients aged 16 to 60 years, with Fitzpatrick skin types ranging from IV to V and acne scar lesions ranging from moderate to severe, who received one to three treatments with a nano-fractional RF aesthetic device. Results showed that the vast majority of study patients achieved improvement in the appearance of their acne scar lesions; the majority of patients mostly demonstrated improvement in a box and rolling type scars, with less impact on ice pick scar type. Patients responded very well to the nano-fractional RF treatment, and overall patient satisfaction from treatment at the six-month follow-up visit was very high (13).

In one recent study conducted by Hongcharu et al., 12 female patients received a single treatment with a nano-fractional RF device for the treatment and improvement of different aesthetic indications such as varying degrees of rhytids, hyperpigmentation, and acne redness. Results showed the treatment to be effective in improving all of these indications, particularly skin texture and pigmentation (14).

32.9 Fractional Microneedling Radiofrequency

The concept of using needles as the electrodes allowing the RF energy to be delivered into the dermis was proposed in a pilot study by Hantash and colleagues in 2009, and that was the genesis of microneedling RF. The fractional RF system is one of the novel fractional resurfacing techniques. It creates controlled thermal damage in the dermis and stimulates wound healing response, initiating the collagen remodeling process by using thermal production from tissue impedance and subsequent heat diffusion to deeper tissue. An advantage of fractional RF is that it causes less epidermal disruption by only 5%, compared with 10–70% of that of fractional ablative laser systems

When the shafts of the needles are not insulated, the needles, as electrodes, are active all the way from the epidermis to the needle tips. This necessitates epidermal cooling to protect the epidermis from electrothermal damage and leads to designs incorporating insulation of the needle shaft, restricting RF energy delivery to the very tip of the needle, but simple physical needling damage to the epidermis occurs, thereby stimulating regeneration of a young epidermis over the restructured dermis.

The mechanisms involved are neocollagenesis by needle penetration stimulating the release of growth factors and relative sparing of epidermis and adnexal structures, which contribute to rapid healing.

Manuskiatti et al. conducted a study to investigate the histological response after FRMS treatment with varying energy settings and pulse stacking techniques in dark-skinned individuals by using histopathology and immunohistochemistry to identify zones of denatured collagen, inflammatory infiltration, neoelastogenesis, and neocollagenesis, as well as any side effects to pigmentation and textural alteration, throughout the three-month study. The study demonstrated the potential application of FRMS to induce neocollagenesis by creating multiple microscopic zones of denatured collagen or RF thermal zone (RFTZ) intervening with normal tissue in the dermis as the result of the fractional thermal response. In addition, the study showed that the depth of RFTZ could be controlled by the radio wave duration and time of electrodes existing in the skin. The formation of denatured collagen zones was not detectable at the site treated with electrode insertion alone and at the site treated with low energy level (energy level 1). However, the zone of collagen denaturation was initially observed at energy level 2 (50 watts, wave duration of 50 ms, and electrode insertion duration of 300 ms). This observation implies that an induction of neocollagenesis requires an optimum level of dermal heating, and physical insertion of the electrode only without a sufficient thermal influence may not be able to stimulate a process of new collagen formation. Zones of denatured collagen had been replaced by newly formed collagen fiber by three months after a single FRMS treatment. This corresponds with the presence of an increasing amount of mucin deposition surrounding RFTZs from one- to three-month follow-up visits (15).

Gold et al. conducted a study wherein 13 patients with mild to moderate acne scars were treated with bipolar fractional RF and concluded that fractional bipolar RF is a safe and effective treatment for acne scars, with 67–92% of patients satisfied with the results (16).

Cho et al. evaluated the efficacy of fractional RF in the treatment of 30 patients with mild to moderate acne scars and large facial pores. The grade of acne scars and global investigator assessment of large pores improved in more than 70% of the patients (17).

32.10 High-Intensity Focused Ultrasound

High-intensity focused ultrasound (HIFU) acoustic energy, known to propagate much deeper through tissue than laser or RF energy, has been previously investigated for use in bulk heating for the treatments of solid organ tumors and recently adapted for the treatment of subcutaneous lipolysis. The ultrasound waves penetrate into tissue, leading to vibration in molecules at the site of beam focus. The friction between tissue molecules produces heat and thermal injury at the focal site of the beam. Penetration depth is determined by frequency in which higher frequency waves produce a shallow focal injury zone and lower frequency waves have a greater depth of penetration to produce focal thermal injury zones (TIZs) at deeper layers (18, 19).

For transcutaneous treatment, modifications of short pulse durations coupled with higher-frequency transducers allow MFUS to deliver precise zones of coagulative necrosis, so-called TIZs. Each TIZ is tightly focused at a given depth and heated precisely using shorter pulses (150 ms) to produce small zones (1 mm³) of coagulative necrosis at the site with surrounding tissue and superficial layers essentially unaffected. The epidermal surface remains unaffected as long as the energy delivered is not excessive for the given focal depth and frequency emitted by a given transducer, eliminating the need for superficial cooling and speeding the recovery process, as healing occurs rapidly from untreated adjacent tissue (20, 21).

The MFUS device is able to penetrate deeper into the tissue to affect superior tissue tightening and longevity of results by selectively targeting the superficial musculoaponeurotic system (SMAS). The SMAS lies deep in the subcutaneous fat, envelops the muscles of facial expression, and extends superficially to connect with the dermis (22).

Alam et al. conducted the first clinical study of full-face and neck MFUS treatment in 35 patients, looking at safety and efficacy. In standardized photographs, 86% of the patients achieved significant improvement as measured by blinded physician assessment. Photographic measurements demonstrated a mean brow lift of 1.7 mm (23).

Chan et al. evaluated the safety of MFUS skin tightening in 49 Chinese patients using an advanced protocol. All patients underwent full facial and neck treatment without significant or persistent adverse effects (24).

Alster and Tanzi established the first report of clinical efficacy in non-facial areas. Paired sites in 18 women were evaluated on the arms, knees, or medial thighs, where dual plane treatment with the 4-MHz 4.5-mm-depth and 7-MHz 3-mm-depth transducer was compared with single-plane treatment with the 4-MHz 4.5-mm-depth transducer alone. Global assessment scores of skin tightening and lifting were determined by two blinded physician raters and graded using a quartile grading scale. At the six-month follow-up visit, statistically significant improvement was seen at all three body sites, with the arms and knees demonstrating more noticeable improvement than the thighs (25).

For fat reduction, high-frequency acoustic energy (2 MHz, >1,000 W/cm) was used to ablate focal areas of SAT (subcutaneous adipose tissue), sparing any damage to surrounding connective tissues, blood vessels, nerves, and overlying skin.

Thermal effects of HIFU rapidly raise the adipose temperature above 55°C, producing coagulative necrosis, whereas the mechanical (cavitational) effects of this technology lead to adipocyte membrane disruption secondary to negative acoustic pressure (26).

Post-treatment adverse events with HIFU are transient and limited to tenderness, edema, focal induration, and ecchymosis. Bony areas, such as the lateral margin of the lower abdomen overlying the anterior superior iliac spine, are best avoided to prevent wave reflection and subsequent cutaneous injury.

Body HIFU device functions by using a mechanical scanner that moves the ultrasound transducer over a square area that measures 9 cm² (3 × 3 cm), heating the SAT (at focal point 1.3 cm below the skin) with the thermo-acoustic energy generated to promote adipocyte apoptosis. The entirety of a scan performed over a square is called a stack; the device can be programmed to repeat several scans over the same square site. This is done by modifying the stacking time. For example, if the stacking time is set to two, the device will complete two stacks in the same square (27–30).

In a study done by Silva et al., 30 subjects with a mean age of 35.4 years underwent one or two HIFU treatments with contact cooling. The mean total energy dose was 509.4 J/cm², 495 J/cm², and 374 J/cm² for groups A, B, and C, respectively; the whole study mean total fluence was 459.47 J/cm². Mean waist circumference reduction was 2.95 cm, 2.4 cm, and 3.8 cm for groups A, B, and C, respectively. A significant mean waist circumference reduction of 3.05 cm from baseline was observed. Most subjects (63.3%) reported being satisfied or very satisfied with the results; 80% of the investigators reported satisfactory results (31). It is speculated that contact cooling of the system used for this study contributes to the high fluence tolerability while maintaining the incidence of adverse events low, comparable to the incidence of adverse events reported by several authors using lower fluence in devices without surface cooling.

32.11 Cryolipolysis

Cryolipolysis has emerged as a new non-invasive body contouring method using controlled cooling to selectively destroy fat cells without damaging the skin and other surrounding tissues. Precise application of cold temperatures triggers the death of adipocytes that are subsequently engulfed and digested by macrophages. No changes in subcutaneous fat are noticeable immediately after treatment. An inflammatory process stimulated by apoptosis of adipocytes, as reflected by an influx of inflammatory cells, can be seen within three days after treatment and peaks at approximately 14 days thereafter as the adipocytes become surrounded by histiocytes, neutrophils, lymphocytes, and other mononuclear cells. At 14–30 days after treatment, macrophages and other phagocytes surround, envelope, and digest the lipid cells as part of the body's natural response to injury. Four weeks after treatment, the inflammation lessens, and the adipocyte volume is decreased. Two to three months after treatment, the interlobular septa are distinctly thickened, and the inflammatory process further decreases. By this time, the fat volume in the treated area is apparently decreased, and the septae account for the majority of the tissue volume (32–35).

The cryolipolysis device consists of a cup-shaped applicator with two cooling panels that is applied to the treatment area. The tissue is drawn into the handpiece under a moderate vacuum, and the selected temperature is modulated by thermoelectric elements and controlled by sensors that monitor the heat flux out of the tissue. Each area is treated for approximately 45 minutes and should be massaged for two minutes upon completion to improve the clinical outcome. The patient is then discharged home and is free to resume normal activities immediately after treatment. The number of treatment cycles needed depends on the treatment area. While good results at the flanks can usually be achieved with only one treatment, the back and the inner and outer thighs often require more than two treatments. Repeated treatment sessions should be spaced eight weeks apart to allow the inflammatory process to resolve. Studies have shown that multiple additional pre-/post-treatment options, such as massage, can enhance the efficacy of the outcome (36–38).

Several studies in humans have shown comparable results. One study published in 2009 involving ten subjects reported a 20.4% and 25.5% reduction in the fat layer two months and six months after treatment, respectively (39). More recently, a retrospective multicenter study using patient surveys, photographic documentation, and caliper measurements was published by Dierickx et al. These investigators reported that 86% of 518 subjects showed improvement. The body sites at which cryolipolysis was most effective were the abdomen, back, and flank. The majority described minimal to tolerable discomfort during the procedure (40).

In a report on the clinical and commercial experience with cryolipolysis in a private plastic surgery practice, only six of 528 patients were dissatisfied with the clinical outcome; four of these six patients were satisfied when treated a second time. A study by Garibyan et al. used a three-dimensional camera to evaluate the amount of fat loss after cryolipolysis. Mean fat loss between baseline and the two-month follow-up visit was 56.2 ± 25.6 cc on the treated side and 16.6 ± 17.6 cc on the control side (P < 0.0001). Two months post-treatment, the mean difference in fat loss between the treated and untreated sides was 39.6 cc (41). In an uncontrolled study by Ferraro et al., cryolipolysis was combined with acoustic waves to achieve possible synergistic effects. These authors reported significant reductions of up to 6.7 cm in circumference and up to 4.5 cm in thickness of the fat layer 12 weeks after three to four treatments (42).

Expected side effects are temporary erythema, bruising, and transient numbness that usually resolves within 14 days after treatment. With more than 850,000 procedures performed worldwide, only around 850 adverse events have been reported. The most common complaint is late-onset pain, occurring two weeks post-procedure, that resolves without intervention. Paradoxical adipocyte hyperplasia, a condition where additional fat grows at the treatment site and occurs approximately six months postoperatively, has been reported in 33 cases (43, 44).

32.12 Conclusion

Although the indications for these devices are cosmetic in nature, many of them were developed for medical indications. This does not mitigate the inherent risks of the procedure itself, as the adverse events can be disfiguring and debilitating. Only adequately trained professionals can partake in the safe and effective use of cosmetic lasers and other energy-based devices. The rapid advances in laser-based, light-based, and other energy-based devices are evidence of the increased consumer demand, the zeal for technology, and new paradigms of aesthetic medicine.

References

1. Capurro S, Fiallo P. Epidermal deepithelialization by programmed diathermosurgery. *Dermatol Surg.* 1997;23:600–601.
2. Belenky I, Margulis A, Elman M, Bar-Yosef U, Paun SD. Exploring channeling optimized radiofrequency energy: A review of radiofrequency history and applications in esthetic fields. *Adv Ther.* 2012;29:249–26611.
3. Alster T S, Jason R L. Nonablative cutaneous remodeling using radiofrequency devices. *Clin Dermatol.* 2007;25:487–491.
4. Bachl N, Ruoff G, Wessner B, Tschan H. Electromagnetic interventions in musculoskeletal disorders. *Clin Sports Med.* 2008;27:87–105. Viii–viii.
5. Goodman R, Blank M. Insights into electromagnetic interaction mechanisms. *J Cell Physiol.* 2002;192:16–22.
6. Tokalov SV, Gutzeit HO. Weak electromagnetic fields (50 Hz) elicit a stress response in human cells. *Environ Res.* 2004;94:145–151.
7. Alvarez N, Ortiz L, Vicente V, Alcaraz M, Sánchez-Pedreño P. The effects of radiofrequency on skin: Experimental study. *Lasers Surg Med.* 2008;40:76–82.
8. Anolik R, Chapas AM, Brightman LA, Geronemus RG. Radiofrequency devices for bodyshaping: A review and study of 12 patients. *Semin Cutan Med Surg.* 2009;28:236–243.
9. Arnoczky SP, Aksan A. Thermal modification of connective tissues: Basic science considerations and clinical implications. *J Am Acad Orthop Surg.* 2000;8:305–313.
10. Zelickson BD, Kist D, Bernstein E, Brown DB, Ksenzenko S, Burns J, et al. Histological and ultrastructural evaluation of the effects of a radiofrequency-based nonablative dermal remodeling device. *Arch Dermatol.* 2004;140:204–209.
11. Abraham MT, Mashkevich G. Monopolar radiofrequency skin tightening. *Facial Plast Surg Clin North Am.* 2007;15:169–177.
12. Montesi G, Calvieri S, Balzani A, Gold MH. Bipolar radiofrequency in the treatment of dermatologic imperfections: Clinicopathological and immunohistochemical aspects. *J Drugs Dermatol.* 2007;6:890–896.
13. Goel A, Gatne V. Use of nanofractional radiofrequency for the treatment of acne scars in Indian skin. *J Cosmet Dermatol.* 2017 Jun;16(2):186–192.
14. Hongcharu W, Gold M. Expanding the clinical application of fractional radiofrequency treatment: Findings on Rhytides, hyperpigmentation, rosacea, and acne redness. *J Drugs Dermatol.* 2015 Nov;14(11):1298–304.
15. Manuskiatti W, Pattanaprichakul P, Inthasotti S, Sitthinamsuwan P, Hanamornroongruang S, Wanitphakdeedecha R, Chuongsakol S. Thermal response of in vivo human skin to fractional radiofrequency microneedle device. *BioMed Res Int.* 2016, Article ID 6939018.
16. Gold M, Biron J. Treatment of acne scars by fractional bipolar radiofrequency energy. *J Cosmet Laser Ther.* 2012;14:172–178.
17. Cho SI, Chung BY, Choi MG, Baek JH, Cho HJ, Park CW, et al. Evaluation of the clinical efficacy of fractional radiofrequency microneedle treatment. In acne scars and large facial pores. *Dermatol Surg.* 2012;38:1017–1024.
18. MacGregor JL and Tanzi EL. Microfocused ultrasound for skin tightening. *Semin Cutan Med Surg.* 32:18–25.
19. White WM, Makin IR, Slayton MH, et al. Selective transcutaneous delivery of energy to porcine soft tissues using intense ultrasound (IUS). *Lasers Surg Med.* 2008;40:67–75.
20. White WM, Makin IR, Barthe PG, et al. Selective creation of thermal injury zones in the superficial musculoaponeurotic system using intense ultrasound therapy: A new target for noninvasive facial rejuvenation. *Arch Facial Plast Surg.* 2007;9:22–29.
21. Laubach HJ, Makin IR, Barthe PG, et al. Intense focused ultrasound: Evaluation of a new treatment modality for precise microcoagulation within the skin. *Dermatol Surg.* 2008;34:727–734.
22. Har-Shai Y, Bodner SR, Egozy-Golan D, et al. Mechanical properties and microstructure of the superficial musculoaponeurotic system. *Plast Reconstr Surg.* 1996;98:59–70.
23. Alam M, White LE, Martin N, et al. Ultrasound tightening of facial and neck skin: A rater-blinded prospective cohort study. *J Am Acad Dermatol.* 2010;62:262–269.
24. Chan NP, Shek SY, Yu CS, et al. Safety study of transcutaneous focused ultrasound for non-invasive skin tightening in Asians. *Lasers Surg Med.* 2011;43:366–375.
25. Alster TS, Tanzi EL. Noninvasive lifting of arm, thigh, and knee skin with transcutaneous intense focused ultrasound. *Dermatol Surg.* 2012;38:754–759.
26. Fatemi A. High-intensity focused ultrasound effectively reduces adipose tissue. *SeminCutan Med Surg.* 2009 Dec;28(4):257–262.
27. Haar GT, Coussios C. High intensity focused ultrasound: Physical principles and devices. *Int J Hyperthermia.* 2007;23:89–104.
28. Solish N, Lin X, Gatley RA. A randomized, single-blind, postmarketing study of multiple energy levels of highintensity focused ultrasound for noninvasive body sculpting. *DermatolSurg.* 2012;38:58–67.

29. Jewell ML, Desilets C, Smoller BR. Evaluation of a novel high-intensity focused ultrasound device: Preclinical studies in a porcine model. *Aesthet Surg J.* 2011;31(4):429–434.

30. Robinson DM, Kaminer MS, Baumann L, Burns AJ, Brauer JA, Jewell M, Lupin M, Narurkar VA, Struck SK, Hledik J, Dover JS. High-intensity focused ultrasound for the reduction of subcutaneous adipose tissue using multiple treatment techniques. *Dermatol Surg.* 2014 Jun;40(6):641–651.

31. Silva HL, Hernandez EC, Blanco AP, Vazquez MG, Lee S, Delgado SL. High-intensity focused ultrasound with surface cooling non-invasive abdominal subcutaneous adipose tissue reduction. *Int J Current Res;*8(8).

32. Manstein D, Laubach H, Watanabe K, Farinelli W, Zurakowski D, Anderson RR. Selective cryolysis: A novel method of non-invasive fat removal. *Lasers Surg Med.* 2008;40(9):595–604.

33. Zelickson B, Egbert BM, Preciado J, et al. Cryolipolysis for noninvasive fat cell destruction: Initial results from a pig model. *Dermatol Surg.* 2009;35(10):1462–1470.

34. Nelson AA, Wasserman D, Avram MM. Cryolipolysis for reduction of excess adipose tissue. *Semin Cutan Med Surg.* 2009;28(4):244–249.

35. Avram MM, Harry RS. Cryolipolysis for subcutaneous fat layer reduction. *Lasers Surg Med.* 2009;41(10):703–708.

36. US Food and Drug Administration 510(k) clearance K133212. 2014. [Accessed May 17, 2014]. Available from: www.accessdata.fda.gov/cdrh_docs/pdf13/K133212.pdf.

37. 17. Jalian HR, Avram MM. Cryolipolysis: A historical perspective and current clinical practice. *Semin Cutan Med Surg.* 2013;32(1):31–34. [PubMed] [Google Scholar].

38. 18. Stevens WG, Pietrzak LK, Spring MA. Broad overview of a clinical and commercial experience with CoolSculpting. *Aesthetic Surg J.* 2013;33(6):835–846. [PubMed] [Google Scholar].

39. Coleman SR, Sachdeva K, Egbert BM, Preciado J, Allison J. Clinical efficacy of noninvasive cryolipolysis and its effects on peripheral nerves. *Aesthetic Plast Surg.* 2009;33(4):482–448.

40. Dierickx CC, Mazer JM, Sand M, Koenig S, Arigon V. Safety, tolerance, and patient satisfaction with noninvasive cryolipolysis. *Dermatol Surg.* 2013;39(8):1209–1216.

41. Garibyan L, Sipprell WH, Jalian HR, Sakamoto FH, Avram M, Anderson RR. Three-dimensional volumetric quantification of fat loss following cryolipolysis. *Lasers Surg Med.* 2014;46(2):75–80.

42. Ferraro GA, De Francesco F, Cataldo C, Rossano F, Nicoletti G, D'Andrea F. Synergistic effects of cryolipolysis and shock waves for noninvasive body contouring. *Aesthetic Plast Surg.* 2012;36(3):666–679.

43. Bernstein EF. Longitudinal evaluation of cryolipolysis efficacy: Two case studies. *J Cosmet Dermatol.* 2013;12(2):149–152.

44. Jalian HR, Avram MM, Garibyan L, Mihm MC, Anderson RR. Paradoxical adipose hyperplasia after cryolipolysis. *JAMA Dermatol.* 2014;150(3):317–319.

CHAPTER 33: INJECTABLES
Toxins—Intrinsic Aspects and Special Precautions

Vandana Chatrath

33.1 Introduction

Botulinum toxin treatment was among the top five minimally invasive procedures performed in 2020, as per the American Society of Plastic Surgeons Survey. According to the ASPS statistics, 4.4 million of the 13.2 million cosmetic procedures performed were toxin injections [1]. However, this data has the limitation of being indicative only of the procedures performed in the United States. Extrapolating this number to the rest of the world would make botulinum toxin injection the most commonly performed minimally invasive procedure worldwide. As with statistics, clinical evidence and recommendations for toxin treatments in ethnic skin are scarce in the literature. This chapter attempts to highlight the nuances of botulinum toxin treatment in ethnic skin types. The differences among ethnicities in terms of dosing, injection technique, and side effect profile have been elucidated in keeping with the essence of the book.

The types of botulinum toxin and their dilutions are mentioned in Table 33.1 [2].

- Xeomin is the same as Bocouture.
- Dysport is also marketed as Azzalure.
- Nabota (Daewoong Pharmaceuticals) is the same as Jeuveau.
- Letybo is also letibotulinumtoxin A marketed by Croma.
- Alluzience (abobotulinum toxin A) is the first liquid toxin developed by Ipsen.

33.2 Botulinum Toxin for Glabella and Forehead

Glabella and the forehead region are typically injected with the same technique in Asians and Indians as described in Caucasians. The difference lies in the doses of toxin used, which is usually lower than what is used to treat Caucasians (Table 33.2) and for good reason. As is true for all facial rhytides in Asians, the presence of a thicker dermis provides a sort of cushion, allowing the skin to crease less despite repetitive muscle action. Additionally, as a cultural preference, Indians in particular, prefer a more "natural look," wanting effacement of only a few lines with toxin treatment, as long as it maintains some facial expression. Using a smaller dose of toxin has shown to have a shorter-lasting effect, but this seems to be acceptable to patients as long as it avoids the "frozen look." Lastly, like Asians, Indians tend to have a heavier upper eyelid which gets compounded by skin laxity secondary to aging [4] (Figure 33.1) Frontalis being the sole brow elevator, if treated aggressively with botulinum toxin A, can cause inadvertent brow ptosis, adding to the heaviness of upper eyelid (Figure 33.2). Women who experience this often complain of difficulty in applying eye make-up.

TABLE 33.1: Types of Botulinum Toxin and Dilution

Type of Botulinum Toxin	Brand Name/Company	Vial Size	Dilution	Units/0.1 mL
Onabotulinumtoxin A	Botox/Vistabel (Abbvie)	100 IU	2.5 mL	4 U
Abobotulinumtoxin A	Dysport (Ipsen)	500 U	1.5 mL	20 U
Incobotulinumtoxin A	Xeomin (Merz)	100 IU	2.5 mL	4 U
Prabotulinumtoxin A	Jeuveau (Evolus)	100 IU	2.5 mL	4 U
Letibotulinumtoxin A	Botulax (Hugel)/Letybo	100 IU	2.5 mL	4 U
Rimabotulinumtoxin B	Myobloc (Solstice	2500 IU	2.1 mL	
Daxibotulinumtoxin A	Neurosciences)	5000 IU	(2500 IU)	200 U
	Daxxify (Revance)	10,000 IU	0.6/1.2 mL	8 U
		50 U/100 U		

TABLE 33.2: Consensus Dose Recommendations of Onabotulinum Toxin A for Various Ethnic Groups [3, 4, 5]

	Indians	Caucasians	Asians
Glabellar complex	16–20 U	12–40 U	12–20 U
Lateral canthal lines	8–12 U per side	6–15 U per side	6–12 U per side
Forehead	6–12 U (higher dose in men)	8–25 U	5–12 U
Masseter	15–30 U per side	15–40 U per side	20–100 U per side
Mentalis	6–8 U	4–10 U	2–20 U
Depressor anguli oris (DAO)	2–3 U per side	2–4 U per side	2–8 U per side
Platysma	8–10 U per band	6–12 U per band	10–80 U total

Sources: From [2, 9, 10].

DOI: 10.1201/9780429243769-33

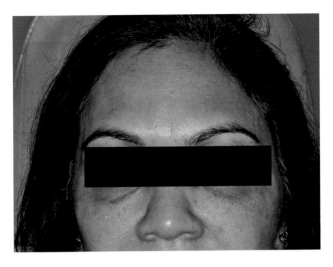

FIGURE 33.1 A 61-year-old Indian woman shows heavy upper eyelids with skin laxity secondary to aging.

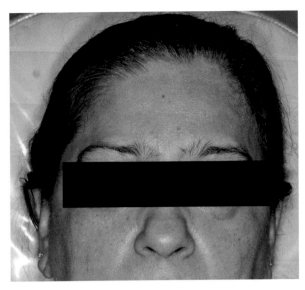

FIGURE 33.2 Brow ptosis, flat brows, and heaviness of the upper eyelids in a 58-year-old Indian woman. If the forehead needs to be treated with botulinum toxin A in such a case, the toxin must be injected high on the forehead, and the minimal dose must be used to avoid exaggeration of the pre-existing brow ptosis.

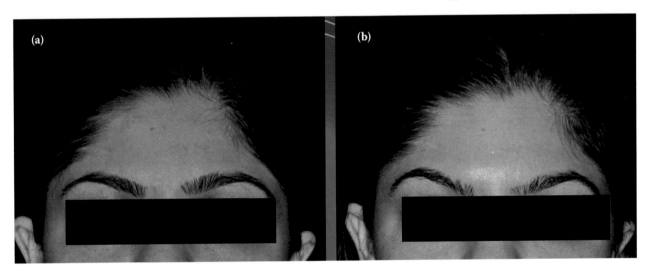

FIGURE 33.3 A 32-year-old Indian woman before (a) and after (b) botulinum toxin A treatment. 20 U of onabotulinum toxin A was injected into the glabella in five injection points and 10 U of onabotulinum toxin A in the forehead for brow shaping. There is brow elevation with arching of the brows post-treatment, as desired by the patient.

The interplay of brow depressors in the glabella and the brow elevator in the forehead can be utilized for brow shaping with botulinum toxin treatment. Although ideal brow aesthetics for men and women have been clearly defined [6], cultural preferences need to be considered when toxin is used for brow shaping. Indians, for example, prefer an arched brow over a horizontal brow with a lateral flare that is a more popular trend in the west. Strategic placement of botulinum toxin A in the glabella and forehead will allow the preferred brow shape (Figure 33.3). As mentioned previously, a hooded upper eyelid with skin excess that worsens with age in Asians makes brow elevation a much-desired aesthetic goal (Figure 33.4). In order to achieve this, the frontalis muscle must retain some of its action over the brow depressors. Thus, the dose of botulinum toxin A used in the frontalis should always be either the same or less than the dose used in the glabellar region for the brow depressors. Another

good technique is to place the toxin injections higher up in the forehead (above the C-line) [7] (Figures 33.5 and 33.6) so that the lower part of the frontalis muscle is able to retain its brow elevation function. This will ensure that there is no brow ptosis with the desired brow shape (Figure 33.7). If injections are to be placed below the C-line to address the lines in the lower third of the forehead, they must be very superficial (intradermal) to allow some residual frontalis action to avoid brow ptosis.

33.3 Treating Lateral Canthal Lines with Botulinum Toxin

Aging is a complex process and is influenced by both intrinsic and extrinsic factors. The cutaneous effects of aging are greatly influenced by the structural and functional differences

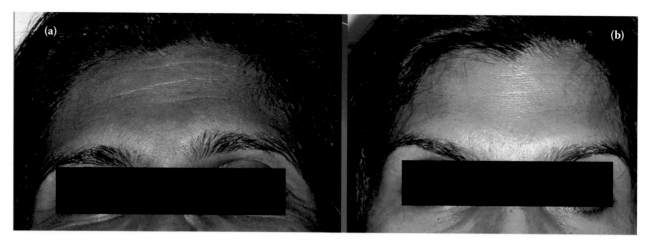

FIGURE 33.4 Hooded upper eyelid with low set brows is seen pre-treatment (a). Effacement of the forehead lines, brow elevation, and a natural arched brow are apparent post-treatment with onabotulinum toxin A (b).

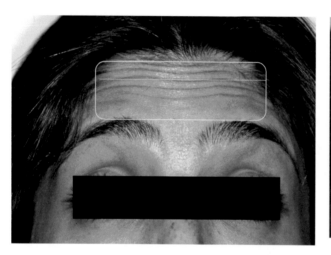

FIGURE 33.5 Horizontal forehead lines on raising eyebrows (surprised look). The forehead is divided into the upper one-third and lower two-thirds (yellow line) based on the bidirectional muscle action of the frontalis where the upper third of the muscle is responsible for moving the skin of the scalp down and the lower two-thirds causes brow elevation.

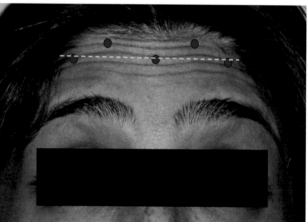

FIGURE 33.6 C-line (yellow line) divides the forehead into upper third and lower two-thirds and roughly corresponds to the second forehead rhytid from the hairline. All injection points for botulinum toxin (blue circles) should be placed at and above this line to allow the lower part of the frontalis muscle to retain its brow elevator action. This will reduce the incidence of brow ptosis.

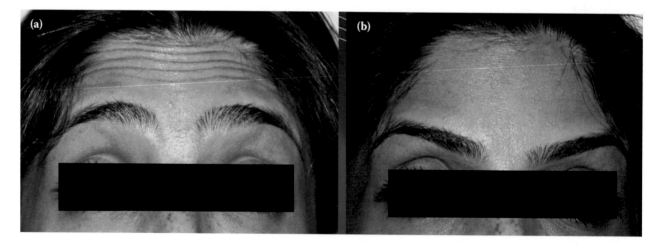

FIGURE 33.7 Before (a) and after (b) treatment of the glabella (20 U) and forehead (10 U) with onabotulinum toxin A keeping the C-line in consideration for the forehead injection. There is good brow elevation with no apparent forehead lines on animation.

in skin among ethnicities. Therefore, manifestations of cutaneous signs of aging are an interplay of internal and external influences based on ethnicity. Periorbital rhytides are a perfect example of this interplay. There are two factors in ethnic skin that positively influence the aging process in this anatomical area particularly. One of them is melanin. The concentration of melanin in ethnic skin provides protection from accelerated aging induced by ultraviolet radiation [8]. The consequence is a less severe manifestation of photoaging in the form of wrinkles in darker skin types. Therefore, people with skin of color are likely to exhibit fewer periorbital rhytides (crow's feet) than their age-matched white counterparts [9]. The other protective factor in ethnic skin is the thickness of the dermis. Asian skin has a thicker and more compact dermis than Caucasians, with the thickness being directly proportional to the degree of melanin in the skin [10]. As skin aging is associated with atrophy of the dermis leading to lines and folds, ethnic skin tends to have fewer facial rhytides (Figure 33.8). Keeping these two factors in mind, it is obvious that lateral canthal lines are less likely to be a cause of concern in ethnic skin types [11]. This means that the dose of botulinum toxin A needed to address these lines is usually lesser than that needed for Caucasians (Table 33.2).

There is one important anatomic feature that needs to be considered while treating Asians and Indians with botulinum toxin in the periorbital area. Indians have a narrow midface with a retruded maxilla causing early periorbital aging due to a lack of structural support [11]. A manifestation of this accelerated aging is hollowness under the eyes and protrusion of intraorbital fat pads, which may be seen as early as the second decade of life. A word of caution here is that when botulinum toxin A is used to treat periorbital lines, including infraorbital wrinkles, pan-weakening of the orbicularis oculi muscle may cause exacerbation of the intraorbital fat pad protrusion, enhancing the appearance of eye bags. There are two ways to prevent this aesthetically unacceptable outcome. First, limit the dose of toxin used in the periorbital region. Second, if periorbital volume loss is obvious (which may also enhance the lines in this area), reinforcement of the orbicularis muscle by injecting fillers in the sub orbicularis oculi fat pad (SOOF) first,

followed by a conservative treatment with botulinum toxin will allow a complete periorbital rejuvenation and a youthful appearance.

33.4 Nasal Tip Elevation with Botulinum Toxin

The nose, like every other part of the face, is not spared by the process of aging. Age-related changes are most prominent in the lower third of the nose, of which loss of nasal tip support is the most prominent feature (Figure 33.9). Ideally, the tip under rotation and under projection in an aging nose is corrected surgically by inserting a columellar strut to lengthen the conjoined medial crura of the nasal cartilage [12]. This lengthening, however, can be mimicked nonsurgically through botulinum toxin injection, albeit for a temporary period.

Depressor septi is a muscle that originates in the nasal spine of the maxilla and inserts into the medial crura of the lateral nasal cartilages. Its contraction pulls the nasal tip down during animation (smiling). In an aging nose, with an under-rotated tip, this downward pull of the depressor septi muscle further exaggerates the appearance of a ptotic nasal tip. A small dose of botulinum toxin A (2–4 U) causes chemodenervation of this muscle, elevates the nasal tip at rest and during smiling resulting in a temporary yet effective profile correction [13].

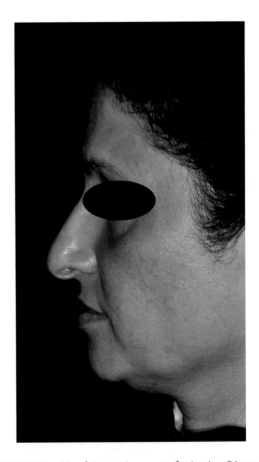

FIGURE 33.9   Nasal tip ptosis as part of aging in a 54-year-old Indian woman. The lower third of the nose, specifically the tip of the nose, shows a downward rotation due to the action of an overactive depressor septi muscle consequent to the loss of structural support with aging. This is amenable to treatment with botulinum toxin.

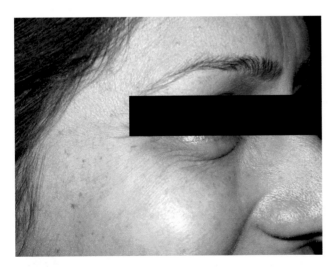

FIGURE 33.8   Minimal lateral canthal lines on a full smile in a 52-year-old Indian woman. Lack of photodamage and a thicker dermis in Indians reduce the appearance of facial rhytides compared to age-matched Caucasians.

This judicious use of a small amount of toxin is even more relevant in Indians, who tend to have a prominent nose with flared ala that sits on a retruded maxilla providing minimal structural support [13]. This, when coupled with bony resorption that happens with aging, causes over-contraction of the depressor septi muscle contributing further to the ptosis of the nasal tip. The use of botulinum toxin alone or in combination with fillers (to provide structural support) offers an effective nonsurgical treatment option for nasal tip elevation in an aging nose.

33.5 Botulinum Toxin Treatment for Perioral Lines

Photoaging is the prime contributor to extrinsic aging, manifesting as fine lines and wrinkles as a result of UV-induced degradation of collagen fibers and an increase in elastosis within the dermis [11]. This is most commonly seen in periorbital and perioral areas in Caucasians. These lines are not of major concern in ethnic skin types due to the protective role of melanin against the harmful effects of ultraviolet radiation [14]. Therefore, botulinum toxin is rarely used in the perioral area in Asians as compared to Caucasians.

33.6 Botulinum Toxin A Treatment of Masseter

The oval facial shape remains the universal standard for beauty and is the desired facial shape across ethnicities [15]. Asians, in particular, desire narrow, heart-shaped faces [13]. Indians specifically prefer a slimmer look in addition to an oval face. This is because Indians, per anthropometric measurements, have a shorter lower facial third and increased bigonial width giving them a rounded facial shape and a heavy lower face [4]. As such, a slimmer face is the desired aesthetic feature. This can be achieved by injecting botulinum toxin A into the masseter muscle to reduce the bulk of the muscle, thereby reducing the width of the lower face (Figure 33.10). The bulk of the masseter muscle may contribute to the wider lower face in Indians even without overt masseter hypertrophy. As such, the dose of botulinum toxin A required is usually lower than what is traditionally used in Asians with hypertrophic masseters [16].

Indians also tend to have heavier lower faces due to the presence of excess jowl fat [17]. In such cases, if the masseter muscle is treated overenthusiastically with high toxin doses, it may result in exaggeration of the jowls due to the lack of muscular support laterally, giving a more sagged appearance a few weeks post-treatment [4].

33.7 Botulinum Toxin A for Parotid Gland

As an adjunct to the injection of the masseter, botulinum toxin A may be injected into the parotid gland to enhance the slimming effect on the face and to make the angle of the mandible more apparent to give the jawline a shaper look [18].

A prominent parotid gland can be seen as a diffuse swelling behind the posterior border of the mandible (Figure 33.11) on each side, giving a "bull neck" appearance. This may sometimes become more apparent after the masseter muscle bulk has been reduced with botulinum toxin A injections. A dose similar to that used for masseter injections is usually needed. Twenty to forty units of onabotulinum toxin A is injected into the swelling (lower part of the parotid gland) lateral to the

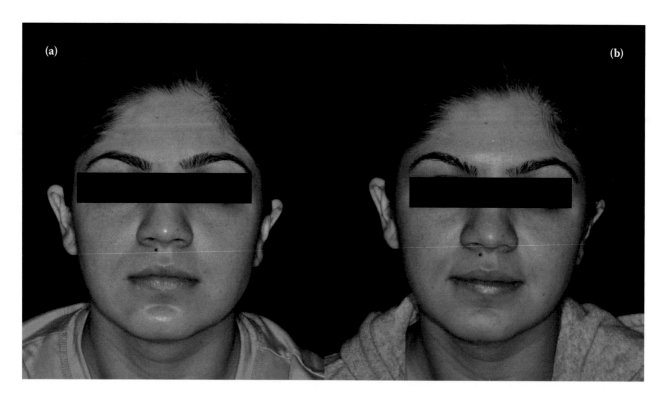

FIGURE 33.10 Facial slimming with botulinum toxin A injection of the masseter. A 29-year-old Indian woman with a wide lower face despite any obvious masseter hypertrophy (a) treated with 40 U of onabotulinum toxin A injection to achieve a slimming effect on the face (b).

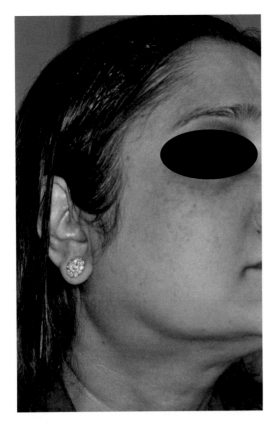

FIGURE 33.11 Parotid swelling in the infra-auricular area posterior to the angle of the mandible. The swelling, if present, may become more apparent after treatment of the masseter with botulinum toxin. This can then be injected additionally to amplify the slimming effect on the face.

angle of the mandible as three to four injection points 1 cm apart after pinching the swelling between the thumb and index finger. Caution must be taken not to inject too deep to avoid diffusion of the toxin into the underlying sternocleidomastoid muscle. The parotid injection can be done at the same time as masseter treatment or a few weeks after the masseter has been injected to better visualize the swelling or parotid hypertrophy. It takes four to six weeks for the treatment to show effect. No adverse effects like dry mouth [20], weakness of the neck muscles or nerve injury have been observed by the author. A definite slimming of the face is noted (Figure 33.12), and the effect typically lasts for four to five months, at which point the treatment with botulinum toxin A may be repeated. A wider lower face in Asians and Indians, as compared to Caucasians, makes toxin use for facial slimming a popular procedure.

33.8 Botulinum Toxin for Chin (Mentalis)

The chin is one anatomical area most commonly treated with botulinum toxin in Indians. It is also the indication where a combination of toxin and dermal filler are used synergistically to achieve an aesthetically superior result. This has a very sound anatomical basis pertinent to the Asian or Indian face. Anthropometric data has shown that Indians have a shorter vertical facial height compared to Caucasians [19]. This is attributed to a retruded mandible and a short chin (Figure 33.13). An obvious consequence of this structural framework is an overactive mentalis due to lack of bony support, rendering toxin injection in this muscle a suitable choice. Anatomically, the mentalis muscle has its origin on the mentum (bone) with multiple fibrous dermal insertions giving the chin a *peau d'orange* appearance on animation. Bone resorption and loss of subcutaneous fat with aging causes overactivity

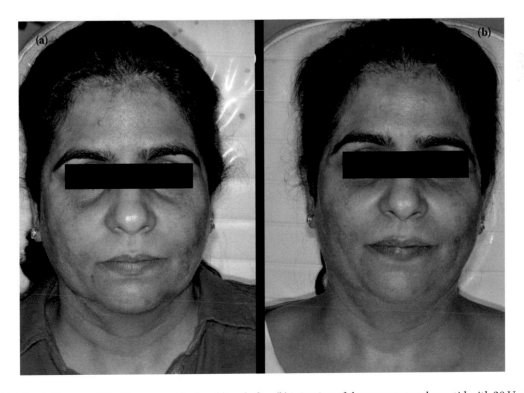

FIGURE 33.12 A 49-year-old Indian woman before (a) and after (b) injection of the masseter and parotid with 20 U of onabotulinum toxin A per side to reduce the width of the lower face for facial slimming.

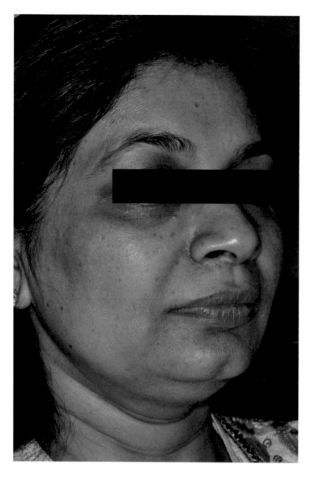

FIGURE 33.13 Quintessential lower face of an Indian woman, with a short chin, decreased vertical facial height, retruded mandible, and submental fullness.

of the mentalis muscle due to lack of underlying support, causing upward rotation of the chin, protrusion of the lower lip, and pebbly appearance of the overlying skin even at rest (Figures 33.14 and 33.15). Isolated treatment with botulinum toxin A to relax the mentalis muscle adequately serves the purpose of reducing chin dimpling in younger individuals. The dose of toxin needed for treating the mentalis is typically higher in Asians and Indians compared to Caucasians [3].

However, toxin treatment alone may not be effective when treating the chin in older age groups. One, more toxin may be needed to relax the overactive mentalis even at rest. Two, the effect of the toxin may not last as long as anticipated [3]. To overcome this, dermal fillers can be used in combination with toxins for better aesthetic outcomes. Combining the use of toxin and dermal fillers offers several advantages. First, the placement of fillers on the bone or subcutaneous fat provides structural support to the mentalis muscle. Second, when placed within the muscular layer, the filler serves as a mechanical block, thereby reducing the activity of an overactive mentalis. Utilizing the principle of myomodulation [21], dermal fillers act synergistically with botulinum toxin to reduce the overcontraction of the mentalis to give a more efficacious and longer-lasting effect. An added advantage of this combination treatment is the improvement in facial shape. By preventing the upward rotation of the chin by placing the filler in the labiomental fold and with the placement of filler on the menton, there is an increase in the

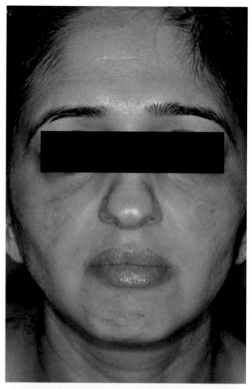

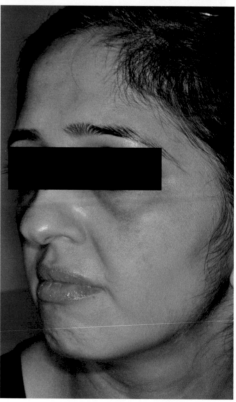

FIGURE 33.14/FIGURE 33.15 Upward rotation of the chin, protrusion of the lower lip, and dimpling of the skin overlying the chin even at rest. A retruded mandible and a short chin provide no underlying structural support to the mentalis muscle causing it to be overactive, which gives a *peau d'orange* appearance to the chin, making it right for the use of botulinum toxin either alone or in combination with fillers.

height of the lower third of the face, making the face look more oval and less round [22], which is the desired aesthetic outcome of an Indian face.

Then comes the question if botulinum toxin and dermal fillers should be injected at the same time or in different sessions. If both toxin and fillers are injected in the same session, the filler should be injected first as it may require some degree of molding, and if the toxin is already placed in the muscle, then massaging the filler may cause the toxin to spread into neighboring muscles, such as the depressor anguli oris or the depressor labii inferioris, increasing the incidence of adverse events such as asymmetrical smile. If fillers and toxin are injected on separate occasions, then the toxin should be injected first to relax the mentalis muscle so that when the dermal filler is placed on the chin subsequently, it should not get displaced by the otherwise overactive muscle fibers [23].

33.9 Botulinum Toxin Treatment for the Neck and Jawline

Botulinum toxin A has been primarily used in the neck for the treatment of platysmal bands responsible for a "turkey neck" appearance. These bands are more prominent in Caucasians with photodamaged skin, making the use of the toxin a popular treatment for neck rejuvenation. With a lack of photodamage and a thicker dermis in ethnic skin types [8], sagging rather than wrinkling is a more prominent feature of an aging neck. Indians, in addition, tend to have excess jowl and submental fat that masks the appearance of platysmal bands. Consequently, botulinum toxin treatment does not offer much advantage when used for treating the platysmal bands in an aging neck in Asians and Indians. Nonetheless, injection of the platysma with botulinum toxin can be used for one other purpose—a better definition of the jawline. Platysma is a paired muscle with a broad expanse over the neck up to the mandible. The anterior portion of the platysma depresses the mandible, while the posterior part is a depressor of the corner of the mouth. As the muscle pulls down with age, it aggravates jowl formation causing loss of jawline definition. The use of botulinum toxin A for jawline redefinition is now well understood after Levy described the "Nefertiti lift" [26], which involves the injection of the toxin into the lateral platysmal band and superficial injections along the mandible to reduce the downward pull of the platysma releasing the skin and making it more amenable to the elevator muscles. Although the technique remains quintessentially the same, there is one modification needed while treating heavier lower faces like that of Indians. The presence of excess jowl fat in this area should be accounted for by injecting the toxin slightly deeper along the mandible to target the underlying muscle as compared to the superficial (intradermal) injections described in the original technique.

33.10 Side Effects of Botulinum Toxin Treatment

The side effects of toxin treatment, such as pain, erythema, and edema at the site of injection, are common among all ethnicities. Similarly, adverse events related to injection technique like brow ptosis, eyelid ptosis, spocking of brows, asymmetrical smile, and weakening of neck muscles are dependant upon the expertise of the injector and uninfluenced by the color of the skin. Nonetheless, there are a few adverse events pertinent to ethnic skin.

1. Ecchymosis combined with post-inflammatory hyperpigmentation (ECPH) has been reported in Asians [25]. Although rare, this phenomenon is unique to skin of color. Inflammation triggered by the injury of needle pricks or by bruising post-injection stimulates melanocytes to release excessive melanosomes causing post-inflammatory hyperpigmentation at the site of injection or bruise. ECPH may persist for weeks or months if left untreated and can be a cause of considerable distress to the patient.

2. The incidence of brow ptosis varies greatly and is largely dependent on the injector rather than the toxin itself. Although there is no data in the literature to show that the incidence of brow ptosis is higher in Asians, it is more likely to be observed in Asians with pre-existing heavy upper eyelids [26], leaving less room for error with toxin injections.

3. Chin hypoplasia and mentalis hypertrophy, commonly seen in Asians, are frequently treated with botulinum toxin. Overzealous toxin treatment in this area to address the chin dimpling can result in the inability to evert the lower lip. This can lead to alteration in speech and the inability to close the mouth. Providing structural support with fillers as an adjunct to the toxin can reduce the incidence of this adverse event.

33.11 Conclusion

Injection of botulinum toxin A is a safe, effective, and popular approach to efface facial rhytides that develop as part of aging, both intrinsic and extrinsic. Ethnic skin is thicker, and there is less photodamage requiring lower doses of botulinum toxin. Combination treatment with resurfacing laser for static lines is often not required in darker skin types. Instead, treatment with fillers for myomodulation and structural support is the most common adjunct to treatment in ethnic skin types. Keeping ethnic considerations in mind, be they anthropometric or structural, will allow injectors to achieve superior aesthetic outcomes and better patient satisfaction with botulinum toxin treatments.

33.12 The Future of Botulinum Toxin

For decades, millions of botulinum toxin treatments to treat facial expression lines have been performed across the globe. It still remains the most efficient way to address fine lines and wrinkles resulting from repetitive muscle action on the face. A recent report [27] based on a global survey to understand facial aesthetic priorities across varied geographical regions suggested that crow's feet lines and forehead lines were the greatest aesthetic concern expressed by the surveyed respondents. However, the same survey also cited that "fear of injections" or "procedure-related pain" were among the major concerns expressed by the same group of respondents. In keeping with this information, a topical or non-injectable delivery system for the administration of botulinum toxin would be a befitting future for this "golden molecule" in the field of aesthetics for times to come.

33.13 Botulinum Toxin in Times of the Pandemic

In 2020, the world as we know it changed in more ways than one. Everything from travel to social life to businesses came to a standstill. The economies of countries and individuals alike suffered. The mood was somber, and the morale was down. As with every other field, the aesthetic industry took a hit. However, humans as a race stood the test of time, and their resilience overtook all adversities. As the world reopened its doors to the "new normal," there was a paradigm shift in the way we as human beings worked and socialized. The era of work from home and Zoom parties had begun. Computer screens and video conferencing became our new best friends during the pandemic. What ensued was an interesting and intriguing phenomenon.

Conventionally, we have always looked at ourselves in the mirror, that is, a two-dimensional view. Although the advent of selfies introduced our minds to see ourselves in a three-dimensional format, making us more aware of our appearance, something was still amiss. There was still a disconnect in the way we saw ourselves as opposed to how we were perceived by others. This is because, be it the mirror or photographs, we still didn't view ourselves in animation like others saw us. This missing piece in the puzzle was brought to light during the pandemic through computer screens when everything from conferences to meetings to socializing became virtual. While interacting with our peers in the virtual world, we started to see ourselves in animation for prolonged periods for the very first time! In one study, 25% of people reported that they spent more time looking at themselves than their colleagues during video conferencing [28]. This brought to attention the frown lines, the forehead lines, the dimpling of the chin, and many such expression lines that one didn't think needed to be addressed previously. As botulinum toxin is the gold standard for treating such dynamic facial expression lines that become obvious during animation, the demand for toxin treatments has risen exponentially across the globe. Whether this novel trend is here to stay, time will tell.

Frequently Asked Questions

1. Q: *How long can a vial of botulinum toxin A (Botox) be used after it has been reconstituted?*

   A: The efficacy of botulinum toxin A (Botox) is not reduced after it is reconstituted for up to four weeks if it is stored in the refrigerator at 4°C. However, multiple withdrawals from the same vial over an extended period can cause bacterial contamination, raising concerns regarding sterility and hence safety [29].

2. Q: *Should the area injected with botulinum toxin A be massaged post-injection?*

   A: Massaging or aggressive pressure post-injection should be avoided to prevent diffusion of the product beyond the target muscles, increasing the incidence of adverse events.

3. Q: *Can botulinum toxin A be used for the treatment of static lines?*

   A: Contrary to the traditional view that botulinum toxin A should only be used to treat dynamic facial rhytides, there is enough data to support that static lines can also be treated with botulinum toxin A either alone or in combination with dermal fillers. When used alone, a standardized dose of the toxin should be administered at regular intervals to note the efface-ment of static lines after repeated treatments. When used in combination with dermal fillers, not only is the effect on static lines immediate, the duration of the

toxin and the filler effect is likely to last longer than either modality alone [30].

4. Q: *Would repeated treatments with botulinum toxin A in the same individual get less effective with time, or would a higher dose of the toxin be required to achieve the same effect?*

   A: Long-term continuous treatments with botulinum toxin A are associated with high patient satisfaction. Response to toxin treatment is reproducible across mul-tiple treatment cycles without any reduction in efficacy. Based on the author's experience, the effect of the toxin may even last longer if the dose of toxin administered is kept constant. This can be explained by the possibil-ity of muscle atrophy with repetitive toxin treatments at regular intervals.

5. Q: *Can botulinum toxin and dermal fillers be used in the same anatomical area at the same time?*

   A: Botulinum toxin and dermal fillers can be used as a combination treatment on the same location in the same session. However, when done so, dermal fillers should be injected first so that when the filler is molded or mas-saged post-injection, any toxin, if injected prior to the filler, should not get dispersed into neighboring muscle groups, causing untoward side effects.

References

1. PLASTIC SURGERY STATISTICS REPORT 2020. n.d.
2. Choudhury S, Baker MR, Chatterjee S, Kumar H. Botulinum Toxin: An Update on Pharmacology and Newer Products in Development. Toxins (Basel). 2021 Jan 14;13(1):58
3. Wu WTL, Liew S, Chan HH, Ho WWS, Supapannachart N, Lee HK, et al. Consensus on Current Injectable Treatment Strategies in the Asian Face. Aesthetic Plastic Surgery 2016;40:202–14. https://doi.org/10.1007/s00266-016-0608-y.
4. Kapoor KM, Chatrath V, Anand C, Shetty R, Chhabra C, Singh K, et al. Consensus recommendations for treatment strategies in Indians using botulinum toxin and hyaluronic acid fillers. Plastic and Reconstructive Surgery - Global Open 2017;5. https://doi.org/10.1097/GOX.0000000000001574.
5. Sundaram H, Signorini M, Liew S, Trindade De Almeida AR, Wu Y, Vieira Braz A, et al. Global Aesthetics Consensus: Botulinum Toxin Type A - Evidence-Based Review, Emerging Concepts, and Consensus Recommendations for Aesthetic Use, Including Updates on Complications. Plastic and Reconstructive Surgery 2016;137:518e–29e. https://doi.org/10.1097/01.prs.0000475758.63709.23.
6. Yalçınkaya E, Cingi C, Söken H, Ulusoy S, Muluk NB. Aesthetic anal-ysis of the ideal eyebrow shape and position. European Archives of Oto-Rhino-Laryngology 2016;273:305–10. https://doi.org/10.1007/s00405-014-3356-0
7. Cotofana S, Freytag DL, Frank K, Sattler S, Landau M, Pavicic T, et al. The Bidirectional Movement of the Frontalis Muscle: Introducing the Line of Convergence and Its Potential Clinical Relevance. Plastic and Reconstructive Surgery 2020;145:1155–62. https://doi.org/10.1097/PRS.0000000000006756.
8. Rawlings A v. Ethnic skin types: are there differences in skin struc-ture and function? International Journal of Cosmetic Science. 2006 Apr;28(2):79–93..
9. Vashi NA, Buainain Castro Maymone M de, Kundu R v. Aging Differences in Ethnic Skin. J Clin Aesthet Dermatol. 2016 Jan;9(1):31–8.
10. Yakimov BP, Shirshin EA, Schleusener J, Allenova AS, Fadeev V v., Darvin ME. Melanin distribution from the dermal–epidermal junction to the stratum corneum: non-invasive in vivo assessment by fluorescence and Raman microspectroscopy. Scientific Reports 2020;10. https://doi.org/10.1038/s41598-020-71220-6.
11. Taylor SC. Skin of color: Biology, structure, function, and implica-tions for dermatologic disease. Journal of the American Academy of Dermatology 2002;46. https://doi.org/10.1067/mjd.2002.120790.
12. Quatela VC, Pearson JM. Management of the aging nose. Facial Plastic Surgery 2009;25:215–21. https://doi.org/10.1055/s-0029-1242032.

13. Liew S, Wu WTL, Chan HH, Ho WWS, Kim HJ, Goodman GJ, et al. Consensus on Changing Trends, Attitudes, and Concepts of Asian Beauty. Aesthetic Plastic Surgery 2016;40:193–201. https://doi.org/10.1007/s00266-015-0562-0.

14. Liew S. Ethnic and gender considerations in the use of facial injectables: Asian patients. Plastic and Reconstructive Surgery 2015;136:22S-27S. https://doi.org/10.1097/PRS.0000000000001728.

15. Goodman GJ. The oval female facial shape-A study in beauty. Dermatologic Surgery 2015;41:1375–83. https://doi.org/10.1097/DSS.0000000000000571.

16. Cheng J, Hsu SH, McGee JS. Botulinum toxin injections for masseter reduction in east asians. Dermatologic Surgery 2019;45:566–72. https://doi.org/10.1097/DSS.0000000000001859.

17. Shome D, Vadera S, Khare S, Ram MS, Ayyar A, Kapoor R, et al. Aging and the Indian Face. Plastic and Reconstructive Surgery - Global Open 2020;8:e2580. https://doi.org/10.1097/gox.0000000000002580.

18. Wu WTL. Botox Facial Slimming/Facial Sculpting: The Role of Botulinum Toxin-A in the Treatment of Hypertrophic Masseteric Muscle and Parotid Enlargement to Narrow the Lower Facial Width. Facial Plastic Surgery Clinics of North America 2010;18:133–40. https://doi.org/10.1016/j.fsc.2009.11.014.

19. Sundaram H, Huang PH, Hsu NJ, Huh CH, Wu WTL, Wu Y, et al. Aesthetic applications of botulinum toxin A in Asians: An international, multidisciplinary, pan-Asian consensus. Plastic and Reconstructive Surgery - Global Open 2016;4. https://doi.org/10.1097/GOX.0000000000000507.

20. Kalra S, Bagga DK, Agrawal P. Evaluation of various anthropometric proportions in Indian beautiful faces: A photographic study. APOS Trends in Orthodontics 2015;5:190–6. https://doi.org/10.4103/2321-1407.163418.

21. de Maio M. Myomodulation with Injectable Fillers: An Innovative Approach to Addressing Facial Muscle Movement. Aesthetic Plastic Surgery 2018;42:798–814. https://doi.org/10.1007/s00266-018-1116-z.

22. Rho NK, Chang YY, Chao YYY, Furuyama N, Huang PYC, Kerscher M, et al. Consensus recommendations for optimal augmentation of the asian face with hyaluronic acid and calcium hydroxylapatite fillers. Plastic and Reconstructive Surgery 2015;136:940–56. https://doi.org/10.1097/PRS.0000000000001706.

23. Molina B, David M, Jain R, Amselem M, Ruiz-Rodriguez R, Ma MY, et al. Patient Satisfaction and Efficacy of Full-Facial Rejuvenation Using a Combination of Botulinum Toxin Type A and Hyaluronic Acid Filler. Dermatologic Surgery : Official Publication for American Society for Dermatologic Surgery [et Al] 2015;41:S325–32. https://doi.org/10.1097/DSS.0000000000000548.

24. Levy PM. The "Nefertiti lift": A new technique for specific re-contouring of the jawline. Journal of Cosmetic and Laser Therapy 2007;9:249–52. https://doi.org/10.1080/14764170701545657.

25. Zhao Y, Yu J, Liu S, Zhou J, Wang J, Wang Z, et al. Ecchymosis combined with postinflammatory hyperpigmentation associated with acupuncture therapy: An observational study of 167 subjects. Medicine (United States) 2020;99. https://doi.org/10.1097/MD.0000000000018721.

26. Park DD. Aging Asian Upper Blepharoplasty and Brow. Seminars in Plastic Surgery 2015;29:188–200. https://doi.org/10.1055/s-0035-1556853.

27. Jamie Ballard. A quarter of the people on your work zoom call are watching themselves. 2021.

28. Fabi S, Alexiades M, Chatrath V, Colucci l et al. Facial aesthetic priorities and concerns: a physician and patient perception global survey. (Manuscript under review for publication.)

29. Park MY, Ahn KY. Effect of the refrigerator storage time on the potency of Botox for human extensor digitorum brevis muscle paralysis. Journal of Clinical Neurology (Korea) 2013;9:157–64. https://doi.org/10.3988/jcn.2013.9.3.157.

30. Coleman KR, Carruthers J. Combination therapy with BOTOX and fillers: the new rejuvnation paradigm. Dermatol Ther. 2006 May-Jun;19(3):177–88.

CHAPTER 34: INJECTABLES
Fillers—Intrinsic Aspects and Special Precautions
Sanjeev Nelogi and Meenaz Khoja

34.1 Introduction

People have been in quest for beauty and attractiveness, especially in the current era. There is no specific definition of beauty or attractiveness; it depends on the individual, although symmetry and proportions are significantly important when defining beauty. As a result, the art of beautification involves a well-contoured jawline that gives a perception of beauty and youth. The rejuvenation and beautification is becoming more common and injectable fillers can help in reshaping the jawline improving symmetry and proportion hence enhancing beauty and attractiveness.[1] People with a youthful appearance are termed as being more attractive than those appearing older. Studies indicate that there is heterogeneity based on the type of skin origin of both normal and pathological skin. External factors and intrinsic differences are central elements in determining skin types. Ethnic skin types are diverse in human populations and reveal a multifactorial adaptation through evolution that results in different cutaneous physiology. Differences in pigmentation, signs of aging, and stratum corneum function reflect the versatility of epidermal functions among ethnic skin. The stratum corneum differs in ethnic skin and is usually greater in darkly pigmented skin.[2]

Skin aging is a complex event that is influenced by extrinsic and intrinsic factors and varies depending on the age of onset, severity, or other specific concerns among ethnic populations. The ethnic group is a leading population seeking cosmetic procedures, thus it is important to understand the structural and functional differences of the skin and the aging process of different skin types.

34.2 Structural and Functional Differences of Ethnic Skin

Darkly pigmented skin has larger, numerous melanosomes with more melanin and is singly dispersed throughout the epidermis compared to lightly pigmented skin. The high levels of melanin content in darkly pigmented skin provide photoprotection, thus reducing the severity of photoaging in darker skin. Also, the structural differences in the dermis and epidermis can influence variations in aging. The stratum corneum in darkly pigmented skin has more layers that are compactly arranged compared to lightly pigmented skin. Moreover, the fibroblasts are numerously larger and more frequently binucleated or multinucleated in darker skin compared to lighter skin. Thus the darker skin has greater compact collagen bundles that are arranged more parallel to the dermis. The increased fibroblast activity usually contributes to a lower incidence of facial rhytides; however, it increases the risk of keloids in ethnic skin.[3]

34.3 Skin Aging Assessment in Ethnic Skin

Aging is bound to happen. It is a complex process characterized by the appearance of wrinkles, sunspots, uneven skin color, or sagging skin, all influenced by both intrinsic and extrinsic factors. On the other hand, the processes vary depending on ethnic origin due to underlying structural and functional differences. The differences reflect biological, environmental, and genetic influences, as well as other multidimensional factors, including physical, psychological, and social changes that are also influenced by cultural and social standards. The human desire to have a homogeneous skin color and texture and have the skin firm and without wrinkles has fueled the need for cosmetic treatments and surgical procedures, such as the use of dermal fillers and hyaluronic acid. The treatments improve wrinkles, sagging eyelids, and loss of volume.

Intrinsic aging is associated with the genetic background of an individual that occurs over time. It is characterized by smooth and unblemished skin with fine wrinkles, fat atrophy and soft tissue redistribution, and bone remodeling. On the other hand, extrinsic aging is associated with environmental exposures, health, and lifestyle of an individual, for example, exposure to the sun, tobacco use, diet, and exercise.[4]

There are several assessments for skin aging that dermatologists use to improve the quality of life of the aging population—for instance, three-dimensional camera, dermoscopy, and sample analysis of color, a measure of elasticity.[5] According to research conducted by Boston Medical Center,[6] the older population is expected to increase by the year 2030. As a result, their skin will age biologically as well as from being exposed to environmental factors such as sunlight that cause skin damage. All skin types show signs of aging due to exposure to ultraviolet rays from the sun leading to skin discoloration and loss of elasticity. However, each person has a unique experience with how the skin changes with advance with age. Meaning that the effects of skin aging are based on ethnicity[6] and are more pronounced in ethnic skin. For African Americans, facial wrinkles and fine lines appear later than in Caucasians, and in some cases, the wrinkles and fine lines may not appear until late in the fifth or sixth decade. On the other hand, white women showed more signs of moderate to severe facial aging than Asian and Hispanic women beginning in the fourth decade.[3] Nevertheless, hyperpigmentation and uneven skin tone are major concerns for people of color compared to lighter skin types. Lighter skin types report wrinkles and fine lines frequently. The ethnic skin is prone to develop benign facial neoplasms, textural irregularities, more so, intrinsic structural changes.

The need for cosmetic procedures for ethnic skin is to achieve maximal results and to reduce epidermal and dermal injury with minimal cases of post-inflammatory pigment alteration and scarring.[3]

34.4 Indications

Due to increasing patient diversity in clinical practice, there is a need to encompass patient age, ethnicity, and sex for effective facial rejuvenation and facial harmonization. Skin aging is a major concern associated with reduced epidermal and dermal thickness and reduced water content in the stratum corneum that results in dry-looking skin. There is decreased collagen content due to the inability of the dermal fibroblasts to synthesize collagen fibers and denatured elastic fibers and lose elasticity. Hyaluronic acid also decreases year after year. The procedures are also indicated for wrinkles and loose and

DOI: 10.1201/9780429243769-34

dropping skin.[7] Clinicians have achieved better outcomes and patient satisfaction through injectable dermal fillers. The hyaluronic acid fillers achieve results that are long-lasting and more satisfying in the treatment of volume loss. Volume restoration is a critical part of facial rejuvenation, and it replaces and augments soft tissue in the deflated malar zygomatic regions. The effects are visible after treatment and include a glowing, hydrated appearance of the skin around the injected regions.[8]

The aim is to create beautiful works of art and enhance natural facial beauty. The most common indications include the reshaping of the forehead, glabella, eyebrows, tear troughs, cheekbones, nose, nasolabial folds, upper and lower lips, marionette lines, jaws, and chin.

34.5 Patient Workup/Counseling

Consultation should include a physician who evaluates and provide information about the benefits that injectable dermal fillers may bring to the patient. At this point, the patient should understand that it does not involve a surgical procedure and that fillers promote a mild volumetric augmentation of the eyebrows. Therefore, the patient should be evaluated for eyebrow position and mobility, eyelid function, and the excess of skin and eye bags. The physician can begin a pre-treatment plan that includes photographic documentation and a clear explanation of the final result.[9]

34.6 Pre-Procedure Care

Pain is the most fearful experience during injections or cosmetic procedures, and topical anesthetics, infiltration, and nerve blocking have been utilized to make the procedure more tolerable.[9] For the majority of injectable dermal fillers, the procedure is undertaken with insufficient topical or without anesthesia for various reasons. Preoperative evaluation involves the selection of anesthetic procedures to be used moreover, the need for pain relief after treatment. In most cases, simple

procedures do not require the use of adjunctive agents except for very anxious patients. However, a physical examination should be performed before the use of any medication in addition to medical history. Preexisting conditions such as hypertension and heart disease can influence the use of anesthetics in combination with epinephrine. Blood thinners should be discontinued ten days before treatment to lessen the possibility of bleeding or bruising. Alcohol should also be avoided, and the procedure should not be performed if there are open sores in the treatment area. To avoid infections, if a patient has had an infection (such as a cold, virus, or flu), undergone a surgical procedure, received any immunizations, or gotten tattoos, all in the past 30 days; has taken immunosuppressives medication; or has contraindications, such as pregnancy, breastfeeding, allergies to any component of the dermal fillers, or open sores in areas to be treated, these should be taken into consideration before initiating treatment.[10] Pre-procedure care also involves understanding how the skin ages and knowing the fillers and techniques.

34.7 Procedure

Injectable hyaluronic fillers are mainly used in photoaging wrinkles, nasolabial folds, lip rhytides, volume enhancement, cheek and chin augmentation, and the treatment of tear lines. However, hyaluronic acid is more suitable for deep folds and volume augmentation. Preparations with smaller molecules show good effects on superficial wrinkles. The patient undergoes a pre-treatment assessment and pre-treatment photographs, after which the correct product is selected. A gel with greater viscosity offers a better ability to resist shear and can better exert a deformational force on the surrounding tissue to correct the deformity. On the other hand, if an injection is more superficial, it increases the risk of visibility.

The procedure is carried out in an outpatient clinic setting. The patient sits in an upright position for gravitational wrinkles to be visible, with the head supported on a headrest to prevent

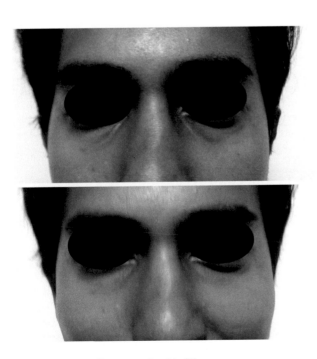

FIGURE 34.1 Tear trough with fillers.

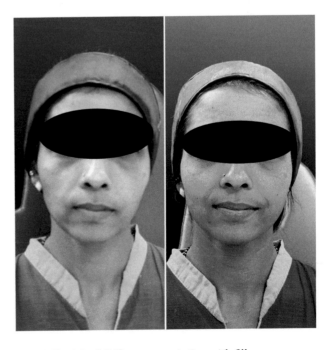

FIGURE 34.2 Midface augmentation with fillers.

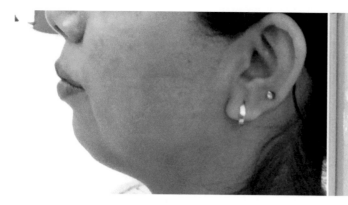
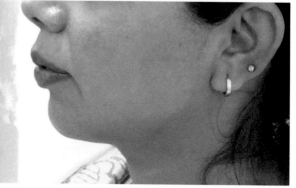

FIGURE 34.3   Chin augmentation with fillers.

sudden movements. Anesthesia is applied in the form of a topical anesthetic; alternatively, field blocks or nerve blocks are required, especially for lip procedures, which can otherwise be painful.

A 27–30 gauge needle is used to inject the agent into the middle to deep dermis. On the lips, it is injected intramuscularly rather than intradermally. Administration of hyaluronic acid with larger molecules requires larger gauge needles. The material is wasted if it is injected subcutaneously since its bioavailability is very short for the reason that it is quickly enzymatically degraded, making the effect limited.[11]

34.8 Post-Procedure Care for Ethnic Skin

Ethnic skin has a unique pattern that can successfully be augmented with minimal adverse outcomes. The patient should not apply anything on the skin, such as cleansers, moisturizers, or makeup, until the day after treatment. The injected area should not be massaged, touched, or manipulated, and any exercise should be avoided on the day of treatment. Dental work should be avoided for 30 days after filler injections. It is advisable that the patient avoids sleeping on the sides and the stomach but sleeps on the back using pillows to create stability. Sleep with the head elevated to decrease swelling, and take acetaminophen to reduce discomfort.[10]

34.9 Side Effects and Their Management

Dermal fillers are associated with risks that can have short-duration or long-duration complications due to the expanded indications and the number of treatments performed. However, the side effects are mild and transient, although more serious adverse events can occur, leaving the patient with long-term or permanent functional and aesthetic deficits. Some side effects can occur immediately after the treatment, while others have a delayed onset. Side effects include bruising, itching, infections, erythema, edema, pain or tenderness, formation of acne papules, abscess, hypersensitivity, non-fluctuant nodules, lumps, irregular contour, skin discoloration, redness, or local tissue necrosis[12] Bruising is treated by the use of cold compresses after the procedure and vitamin K cream. Patients are also advised to avoid all blood-thinning medications one week prior to the procedure and avoid direct sunlight and exercises as long as bruising continues. Edema can resolve spontaneously after a few hours or days; however, swelling and itching are short-lived and responsive to antihistamines. Alternatively,

oral prednisolone is the main treatment. Steroids are used for erythema, but their long-term use should be avoided. Studies indicate that ethnic skin tends to develop hyperpigmentation following trauma. In such a case, dermal fillers can cause post-inflammatory hyperpigmentation, especially in individuals with Fitzpatrick skin types IV–VI. A bleaching agent is used as a first-line treatment for the management of hyperpigmentation. Sometimes hyaluronic acid fillers can be inappropriately implanted into the superficial dermis or epidermis, resulting in a bluish hue caused by the scattering of light by suspending particles (Tyndall effect). The dyspigmentation is treated by nicking the skin using a small-gauge needle or surgical scalpel (gauge 30 and #11 blade, respectively). Infections are treated with appropriate antimicrobials. If nodules appear after treatment with hyaluronic acid, they are treated with hyaluronidase. Different injectable dermal fillers have different properties and side effects. Therefore, the physician should be experienced in selecting and using suitable products since most side effects are avoidable with appropriate planning and technique.[12]

34.10 Clinical Pearls in Treating Ethnic Skin or Skin of Color

It is important to note that the treatment of skin can manifest differently in specific populations. The population-based differences exist that can optimize treatment. The skin of color is a little bit different, an attribute that affects the presentation and management of various cutaneous diseases. Ethnic skin is not specific to a racial group, and post-inflammatory hyperpigmentation can be similar among populations of distinct population backgrounds.[13]

34.11 Special Precautions Do's and Don'ts

Dermal fillers are significant in dermatology for aging skin and have been approved for wrinkle management. Do's and don'ts include the following:

- Do schedule treatment when minor swelling or bruising cannot affect social life.
- Do lessen the likelihood of bleeding or bruising by discontinuing the use of blood thinner products, such as aspirin, ibuprofen, naproxen, fish oil, St. John's wort, flax, vitamin E, vitamin D, garlic, ginkgo biloba, and ginseng.
- Do not take alcohol before and after treatment.
- Do notify the physician about any history of cold sores.

- Do sleep elevated on the back post-treatment.
- Don't apply anything on the skin until a day after treatment.
- Don't massage, touch, or manipulate the treatment area.
- Don't take heavy exercises a day after treatment.
- Don't sleep on the side or stomach within 24 hours after treatment.

34.12 Precautions during COVID-19 Times for Dermal Fillers, Especially in India

The coronavirus pandemic has affected human life significantly. Since the first case was reported, there have been various interventions put in place to curb the pandemic. Countries, including India, were put on lockdown with the suspension of all non-essential services, including aesthetic practices. Nevertheless, with the introduction of the vaccines, things are gradually returning to normalcy despite fear of infectious disease, leaving the question of whether the aesthetic field is prepared to continue with the practices without fear of spreading infections. To cope with the pandemic, clinical facilities have been reorganized to increase the capacity for intensive or sub-intensive care units. Some departments have been closed or readapted to only focus on emergencies such as non-deferrable dermatological visits.[14]

The government advocates for the use of telemedicine in clinical practice to diagnose, treat, and prevent diseases, including research and evaluation for continued education in healthcare. Due to the pandemic, emphasis should be put on scheduling clinic visits in advance, and prior appointments should be compulsory. Patients scheduled should not be accompanied, while walk-in patients are not allowed without an appointment. There was an increased number of patients with unusual dermatological conditions, especially initially among children and later in adults. Studies showed a possible correlation between COVID-19 and dermatological eruptions, such as skin rashes mainly seen during viral infections.[14] During the unprecedented changes, there was a need for social distancing; therefore, tele-dermatology was made possible to ensure patients are taken care of remotely. Also, it is high time to organize and implement telemedicine services in dermatology to manage patients with skin problems from the safety of their homes. On the other hand, the facilities should ensure well-spaced appointments. All clinical facilities should adhere to decontamination protocols, such as disinfection and sterilization, before treatment, to ensure the safety of both the staff and patients visiting the clinic. Surfaces can be disinfected with 1% sodium hypochlorite or 70% ethanol to reduce infectivity.[15] The outbreak harmed dermatological services offered since it reduces the time spent between a dermatologist and a patient, which can increase the risk of missed observations. Therefore, it is important to take precautions for safe injections. Life in India is about to return to normal, and people have begun venturing out and finding ways to improve their looks. As a result, aesthetic services will see an increase in demand hence safety is paramount.

34.13 CK$_2$ Point in Indian Men beyond 40 Years and Bony Resorption

Aging can lead to osteoporosis, a common chronic metabolic bone disease. Osteoporosis is characterized by increased bone fragility. Bone resorption involves the dissolution of bone minerals and degradation of bone matrix.[16] Malar eminence enhancement is quite a challenge, particularly when using nonsurgical interventions, since the majority of available fillers do not meet the demand for structural support or longevity correction. CK$_2$ is the most prominent part of the zygomatico-maxillary complex.

Cheek augmentation should be well planned in the context of the entire face and not just the area overlying the malar eminence. In particular, it should precede any treatment of the nasolabial folds and the suborbital rim.[18] Studies in anthropology show differences in craniofacial features and body characteristics among different populations. The difference in facial morphology is due to differential growth that helps us to distinguish individuals. They are controlled by a number of factors, such as genetics, climate, or environment, where we live. According to a study conducted in India, North Indian males and females have higher facial height and upper facial height. South Indians have more facial width compared to north Indians in both sexes.[19] Similarly, cheekbones vary from culture to culture. India is a large country with a diverse population. Low cheekbones can make a face sag, especially around the lateral portion of the eyes, thus causing premature aging.[20, 21]

Confounding factors measure the association that occurs between the primary exposure of interest and other factors, such as the association between aging and environmental factors. Patient factors that contribute to early aging or wrinkled skin include smoking, dehydration, vigorous exercise, late nights, partying, and runners. In addition, other factors that influence the outcomes of injectable dermal fillers include the quality and quantity of the product and doctors' factors such as skills or experience.

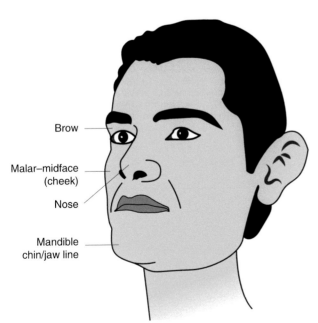

Brow

Malar–midface (cheek)

Nose

Mandible chin/jaw line

FIGURE 34.4 An illustration of the major promontories of mass and volume, the nose, malar-midface, and mandible jawline. (From Terino, 2018.)

34.14 Conclusion

Specific manifestations, such as nasojugular creases, tired upper eyelids, saggy, tired, and angry eyebrows, sadness in the under-eye area, eyebrow hooding, tense forehead, part and kiss-tense-hyperactive mentalis, corneas that turn downward, and tensed perioral areas can be treated with injectable dermal fillers. Hyaluronic acid stimulates collagen and offers a complementary treatment for volume loss. It is evident that volume deficit results from the loss and repositioning of the malar fat pad, as well as minor bone remodeling leading to facial aging. Fillers improve appearance by enhancing fullness and reducing fine lines and wrinkles. Patient satisfaction is used to measure success as people are immersed in looking great and realizing that a youthful look is the best thing to wear. Regardless of age or ethnic background, people share a common interest in beauty. Volume restoration is significant for facial rejuvenation. It replaces or augments soft tissue, especially in the deflated malar, zygomatic regions, brows, and infraorbital hollows. Hyaluronic acid is beneficial in facial rejuvenation, and the effects are visible immediately after treatment, with a glowing and hydrated appearance of the skin over the injected areas. Patients can return to their daily activities even on the same day, and adverse events are rare.

Frequently Asked Questions

1. *Q: What happens after injectable dermal filler treatment?*
   A: The outcome depends on the type of filler the dermatologist will use, what part of the skin is to be treated, and the medical history.
2. *Q: Can I go back to normal activities after a filler?*
   A: Yes, the majority of the patients can return to normal activities after the treatment.
3. *Q: Are there complications?*
   A: Yes, although not to all patients. Be sure to consult with an experienced dermatologist to avoid complications.
4. *Q: Are the side effects manageable?*
   A: Yes, the majority of side effects are easily managed.
5. *Q: How soon can I get the results?*
   A: It depends on the filler; nevertheless, they produce immediate results or close to immediate results.

References

1. Braz, A., & Eduardo, C. C. (2020). Reshaping the lower face using injectable fillers. *Indian Journal of Plastic Surgery*, 53(02):207–218. https://doi.org/10.1055/s-0040-1716185.
2. Girardeau-Hubert S, Deneuville C, Pageon H, Abed K, Tacheau C, Cavusoglu N, et al. Reconstructed skin models revealed unexpected differences in epidermal African and Caucasian skin. *Scientific Reports*. 2019; 9(1).
3. Alexis FA, Obioha OJ. Ethnicity and aging skin. *Journal of Drugs in Dermatology*. 2017; 16(6): 77–80.
4. Vashi AN, Castro, M, Kundu VR. Aging differences in ethnic skin. *Journal of Clinical Aesthetic Dermatology*. 2016; 9(1): 31–38.
5. Buranasirin P, Pongpirul K, Meephansan J. Development of a global subjective skin aging assessment score from the perspective of dermatologists. *BMC Research Notes*. 2019; 12(1).
6. The effects of skin aging vary depending on ethnicity, review finds [Internet]. *Eurelalert*. 2021 [cited 26 July 2019]. Available from: www.eurekalert.org/news-releases/505162.
7. Efficacy and safety of skin care product in aging facial skin—full text view—clinicaltrials.gov [Internet]. *Clinicaltrials.gov*. 2018 [cited 28 August 2021]. Available from: https://clinicaltrials.gov/ct2/show/NCT04015063.
8. Carruthers J, Carruthers A, Tezel A, Kraemer J, Craik L, Volumizing with a 20-mg/mL Smooth, highly cohesive, viscous hyaluronic acid filler and its role in facial rejuvenation therapy. *American Society for Dermatologic Surgery*. 2010; 36: 1886–1892. DOI: 10.1111/j.1524-4725.2010.01778.x.
9. Mario M, Rzany B. Injectable fillers in aesthetic medicine [Internet]. 2006 [cited 28 August 2021]. Available from: www.anme.com.mx/libros/Injectable%20Fillers%20in%20Aesthetic%20Medicine.pdf.
10. Dermatology F. Pre and post-care instructions for dermal filler [Internet]. *Fargoderm*. 2020 [cited 28 August 2021]. Available from: www.fargoderm.com/wp-content/uploads/2020/01/Dermal-Filler-Treatment-Instructions-1.pdf.
11. John H, Price R. Perspectives in the selection of hyaluronic acid leers for facial wrinkles and aging skin [Internet]. *Research Gate*. 2009 [cited 28 August 2021]. Available from: www.researchgate.net/publication/40029468_Perspectives_in_the_selection_of_hyaluronic_acid_fillers_for_facial_wrin.
12. Pavicic T, Funt D. Dermal fillers in aesthetics: An overview of adverse events and treatment approaches. *Clinical, Cosmetic and Investigational Dermatology*. 2013; 6:295–316.
13. Torres V, Herane M, Costa A, Martin J, Troielli P. Refining the ideas of "ethnic" skin. *Anais Brasileiros de Dermatologia*. 2017; 92(2):221–225.
14. Conforti C, Lallas A, Argenziano G, Dianzani C, Di Meo N, Giuffrida R et al. Impact of the COVID-19 Pandemic on dermatology practice worldwide: Results of a survey promoted by the international dermoscopy society (IDS). *Dermatology Practical & Conceptual*. 2021; 11(1).
15. Sethi N, Singh S, Kaur J, Raghukumar S, Ramchandani C, Dharmana S, et al. Consensus guidelines on opening up of aesthetic practices in India during the COVID-19 Era. 2021. http://doi.org/10.2147/CCID.S267528.
16. Maes C, Kroneneberg. Bone resorption: Osteoclast action and proteolytic enzymes. *Science Direct*. 2016. Available from: www.sciencedirect.com/topics/agricultural-and-biological-sciences/bone-resorption.
17. Nguyen. CK2.3 Promots bone formation and inhibits osteoclastogenesis through activation of ERK MAPK signaling pathway. 2020. Available from: file:///C:/Users/user/AppData/Local/Temp/Nguyen_udel_0060D_14309.pdf.
18. Terino E. Three-dimensional alloplastic midface volumization [Internet]. *Ento Key*. 2018 [cited 4 September 2021]. Available from: https://entokey.com/three-dimensional-alloplastic-midface-volumization/#.
19. LC P. Facial indices of North and South Indian adults: Reliability in stature estimation and sexual dimorphism. *Journal of Clinical and Diagnostic Research* [Internet]. 2013; 7(8):1540–1542. Available from: www.ncbi.nlm.nih.gov/pmc/articles/PMC3782890/.
20. Shah A. *Indian cheeks and chins | Dr. Anil Shah* [Internet]. Facial Plastic Surgery | Chicago, IL; 2016 [cited 4 September 2021]. Available from: www.shahfacialplastics.com/articles/plasticpediuropaan-cheeks-chins.
21. Rawlings A. Ethnic skin types: Are there differences in skin structure and function? 1. *International Journal of Cosmetic Science*. 2006; 28(2):79–93.

CHAPTER 35A: EMERGING TECHNIQUES
Platelet-Rich Plasma Therapy

Nina Madnani and Kaleem Khan

35A.1 Introduction

The ongoing quest for anti-aging has led to regenerative medicine as the next exciting discovery. Interventions for anti-aging were initially aimed at repairing and reversing damaged tissue. Now that the aging process is better understood, the aim is to make structurally and functionally new tissue!

Platelets (thrombocytes) play a crucial role in wound healing, and platelet-rich plasma concentrate has been adapted for tissue regeneration. The first documented evidence came in 1974 by Ross et al., who proposed that platelet-derived growth factor (PDGF) helped in arterial smooth muscle proliferation in vitro.[1]

Platelets are non-nucleated components of whole blood, derived from bone marrow precursors, the megakaryocytes. Platelets contain alpha-granules and dense granules, which are storage vesicles for various cytokines and stimulatory proteins, all of which play a role in wound healing.[2]

- Alpha granules contain seven fundamental growth factors: platelet-derived growth factors (PDGF), transforming growth factor (TGF-β), vascular endothelial growth factor (VEGF), epidermal growth factor (EGF), fibroblast growth factor (FGF), connective tissue growth factor (CTGF), and insulin-like growth factor (IGF-1).
- The dense granules contain bioactive agents, including histamine, dopamine, serotonin, adenosine, and calcium.

Activation of platelets causes the granules to fuse with the cell membrane and discharge the pre-formed growth factors at the site of activation, a process known as degranulation. This secretion of growth factors begins as early as within ten minutes of activation, and more than 95% of the stored growth factors are secreted within one hour.[3]

Platelet-rich plasma (PRP) contains an increased concentration of these growth factors and also numerous cell adhesion molecules, including fibrin, fibronectin, thrombospondin, and vitronectin.

Red blood cells (RBCs) form the major cellular component (94%) of whole blood. Platelets are only 6%, and white blood cells make up barely 1%. The whole purpose of creating PRP is to reverse the RBC-to-platelet ratio to achieve 95% platelets and 5% of RBCs. In 2001, Marx proposed a platelet concentration of 1 million/mcl (10 lakhs/mcl) as the defining criteria for PRP.[3] This was later confirmed by Giusti et al., who showed that maximum stimulation of endothelial cell proliferation occurs at a platelet concentration of 1.5 million/mcl.[4] It is generally accepted that for a PRP preparation to be effective, the achieved concentration of platelets should be four to eight times the baseline for the individual.

35A.2 Indications

PRP, because of its regenerative potential, has gained popularity in all fields of medicine, including dentistry for periodontal regeneration, bone grafting, and bone regeneration, cosmetic and plastic surgery including fat grafting, tendinopathies in sports medicine, corneal ulcers in ophthalmology, hepatocyte recovery, soft tissue ulcers and skeletal muscle injury and many others.

In aesthetic dermatology, it has been conclusively proven that activated PRP stimulates dermal fibroblast proliferation.[5]

TABLE 35A.1: List of Essential Growth Factors Released from Platelets and Their Biological Actions

Platelet Growth Factor	Growth Factor Source	Biological Actions
Platelet-derived growth factor (PDGF) (α, β)	Platelets, osteoblasts, endothelial cells, macrophages, monocytes, smooth muscle cells	Mitogenic for mesenchymal cells and osteoblasts; stimulates chemotaxis and mitogenesis in fibroblast/gial/smooth muscle cells; regulates collagenase secretion and collagen synthesis
Transforming growth factor (TGF) (α, β)	Platelets, extracellular matrix of bone, cartilage matrix, activated tH1 cells, natural killer cells, macrophages/monocytes, neutrophils	Stimulates undifferentiated mesenchymal cell proliferation; regulates endothelial/fibroblastic/osteoblastic mitogenesis; regulates mitogenic effects of growth factors; stimulates endothelial chemotaxis and angiogenesis
Vascular endothelial growth factor (VEGF)	Platelets, endothelial cells	Increases angiogenesis and vessel permeability; stimulates mitogenesis for endothelial cells
Epidermal growth factor (EGF)	Platelets, macrophages, monocytes	Stimulates endothelial chemotaxis/angiogenesis; regulates collagenase secretion; stimulates epithelial/mesenchymal mitogenesis
Fibroblast growth factor (FGF)	Platelets, macrophages, mesenchymal cells, chondrocytes, osteoblasts	Promotes growth and differentiation of chondrocytes and osteoblasts; mitogenic for mesenchymal cells, chondrocytes, and osteoblasts
Connective tissue growth factor (CTGF)	Platelets through endocytosis from extracellular environment in bone marrow	Promotes angiogenesis, cartilage regeneration, fibrosis, and platelet adhesion
Insulin-like growth factor (IGF-1)	Plasma, epithelial cells, endothelial cells, fibroblasts, smooth muscle cells, osteoblasts, bone matrix	Chemotaxis for fibroblasts; stimulates protein synthesis; enhances bone formation by proliferation and differentiation of osteoblasts

DOI: 10.1201/9780429243769-35

This has prompted the use of PRP for collagen remodeling in the following indications:[6, 7]

- Photodamaged and aged skin
- Skin rejuvenation
- Atrophic acne scars
- Delayed or non-healing ulcers of varied etiology
- Scar management
- Striae distensae

Li et al. provided significant evidence about the specific role of PRP in promoting hair growth.[8] Since then, it has been used for the following:

- Androgenetic alopecia in men and women
- As an adjunct to hair transplant
- Telogen effluvium
- Alopecia areata

35A.3 Patient Workup/Counseling

PRP makes use of autologous serum, so there is a high rate of acceptance among patients toward PRP. Among the many variables which affect the outcome of PRP (discussed in the following section), an important factor is the platelet count of the patient. So a baseline hemogram is essential. It is also imperative to rule out any bleeding disorders before considering this therapy.

35A.4 Pre-Procedure Care

PRP involves handling hematological products, so strict asepsis must be maintained, and protocol for handling body fluids must be followed. Depending on the indication and the method of delivery, PRP is either injected or applied to the treatment site. The latter must be sterile to avoid contamination and cross-infection.

35A.5 Procedure

Preparation of PRP involves the basic steps of blood collection followed by separating the platelets using differential centrifugation. (Figure 35A.1) The prepared PRP may or may not be activated before being used for the proposed indication.

Each step is briefly discussed here:

- *Withdraw of blood*: Peripheral venous blood is drawn in vacutainer tubes with minimal handling because the coagulation cascade (intrinsic/contact pathway) begins upon contact of blood with glass or an external surface.[9]
- *Anticoagulant*: The use of an anticoagulant prevents this coagulation cascade from progressing and prevents consequent platelet activation. Various anticoagulant agents have been used, including heparin sodium, sodium citrate, ACD-A (acid citrate dextrose solution-A), and EDTA (ethylenediaminetetraacetic acid). Each anticoagulant maintains the structural integrity of platelets for various durations and their subsequent spontaneous activation, thus resulting in a different quality of PRP.[10] ACD-A is considered the best for the purpose of PRP preparation.[11]
- The amount of blood collected varies between 10 ml and 30 mL, depending on the protocol followed and the kit used. The collected blood is mixed thoroughly with the anticoagulant and then centrifuged.
- *Differential centrifugation*: the centrifugation process is broadly grouped into single-spin or double-spin method. (Figure 35A.2) Commercially available kits promote the single-spin method for ease of use and reduced preparation time. However, the double-spin method allows for a greater concentration of platelets (>5 times) in the final PRP.[12] The variables in this step include the speed and the duration of the spin. The speed of centrifugation should be calculated in terms of g (gravitational force) rather than rpm (revolutions per minute). The g is calculated by the formula: $g = (1.118 \times 10^{-5})\,R\,S^2$, where r is the radius of the rotor of the centrifuge machine and s is the speed in rpm.

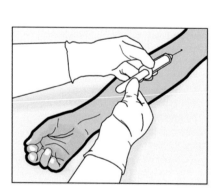
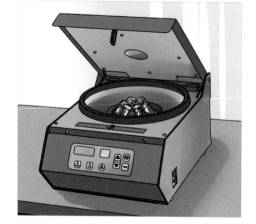
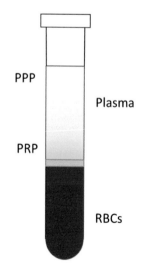

Step 1: Draw Blood
Step 2: Centrifuge
Platelet Rich Plasma

PPP
Plasma

PRP

RBCs

FIGURE 35A.1 Process of PRP therapy.

Abbreviations: PRF: platelet-rich fibrin; PRP: platelet-rich plasma; separator gel.

In the single-spin method, the collected blood is centrifuged at a fixed speed for a fixed duration (as decided by the manufacturer). The RBCs (red blood cells) are dense and settle at the bottom of the tube. A buffy coat (mixture of white blood cells and some platelets) forms a thin layer between the RBCs below and the plasma above. (Figure 35A.3a)) The separated plasma contains a gradient of platelet concentration. The lower third where the concentration is the highest constitutes PRP. The upper third contains a low concentration of platelets and forms PPP (platelet-poor plasma). Some commercial kits contain a separator gel. This gel traps the RBCs and granulocytes below it, while the less dense elements like monocytes and platelets float above the gel. Thus, a physical barrier is created to allow for easier and better separation of PRP. (Figure 35A.3b)

In the two-step method, the initial spin (soft spin) is used to separate the blood components while the second spin (hard spin) helps in the formation of a platelet pellet—a very high concentration of platelets—at the bottom of the tube. The pellet is then reconstituted with the plasma to prepare the final PRP solution.

- Another important variable to be considered for PRP preparation is the temperature at which the blood is processed. A lower-than-ambient temperature (21–24 degrees) retards platelet activation and is ideal. But this requires a specialized refrigerated centrifuge which may not be available to all.[11]

- *Activation*: The final PRP can then be activated by adding calcium gluconate, 10% calcium chloride ($CaCl_2$), 10% autologous thrombin, or a combination of both. They cause a progressive release of growth factors from the PRP over 24 hours and promote clot formation. Interestingly, Cavallo et al. showed that platelets get activated spontaneously upon exposure to dermal collagen (type 1) and that PRP does not require an external agent for activation.[13]

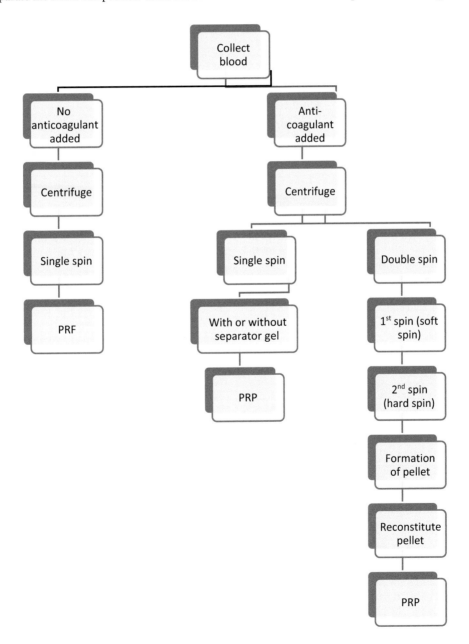

FIGURE 35A.2 Different steps in preparation of PRP.

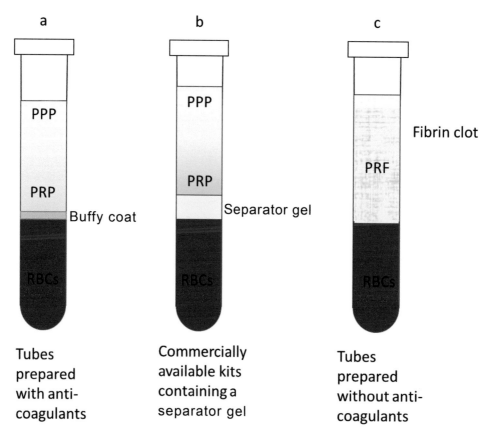

FIGURE 35A.3 Platelet-rich fibrin.

Abbreviations: PRF: platelet-rich fibrin; PRP: platelet-rich plasma; separator gel.

- The PRP thus prepared must be used immediately. The aim is to deliver the PRP in the dermal layer or the hair bulge (depending on the indication). This may be achieved in numerous ways:
  - Inject using a needle.
  - Use a derma roller (microneedle device) to create channels in the skin.
  - Use an ablative laser to remove the stratum corneum and allow for greater penetration into the dermis.

Platelet-Rich Fibrin (PRF)

PRF is a platelet concentrate therapy, like PRP. The process is extremely simple and involves collecting venous blood in a glass test tube, without any anticoagulant. This blood is immediately centrifuged at 3,000 rpm for ten minutes. The intrinsic clotting pathway gets activated and results in the formation of PRF in the middle of the tube. (Figure 35A.3c) It has a jellylike consistency, and unlike PRP, it cannot be injected. It can be spread into a membrane or used as a plug iuropaous dental procedures to cover non-healing wounds and bone grafts.[14, 15]

Various attempts have been made to classify PRP for the purpose of uniformity in the formulation process and for comparing the outcomes following PRP use. Ehrenfest *et al.* (2009) proposed a classification based on the concentration of platelets and leucocytes and the presence or absence of fibrin in the final PRP.[16] He described four categories as P-PRP (high-platelet, poor-leukocyte concentration a low-fibrin preparation), L-PRP (high-platelet, leucocyte-rich preparation with a low-fibrin concentration), P-PRF (high-platelet, leucocyte-poor preparation set in a thick fibrin mesh), and L-PRF (high-platelet, leucocyte-rich preparation set in a thick fibrin mesh).

Mishra et al. (2012) proposed a different classification system based on the presence or absence of leukocytes, whether an activating agent was used and the platelet concentration coefficient compared with the whole-blood baseline.[17]

Recently, Magalon et al. (2016) proposed yet another classification of PRP called DEPA, which is based on four components: dose of injected platelets, efficiency of the production, purity of PRP obtained, and activation process used.[18]

Irrespective of the classification, for PRP therapy to be effective, the consensus is to repeat the procedure monthly for the first three months. Subsequent sessions may be spaced three months apart or six months apart for the next one year to maintain the beneficial effect of the treatment.[19]

35A.6 Post-Procedure Care

Post-procedure care includes maintaining asepsis and the use of a barrier cream. Topical antibiotics may be essential, as would cold compresses, to reduce swelling and hematoma formation.

35A.7 Contraindications

There are a few contraindications for PRP therapy, and those would include patients who are anemic and those with low platelet count or platelet dysfunction syndromes. Patients on anticoagulant therapy or those with liver disease must be evaluated and treated with caution. Active infection at the site of PRP therapy is a relative contraindication, and therapy can be initiated once the infection is clear.

35A.8 Side Effects and Their Management

PRP usage is a safe procedure, and most adverse events are related to the delivery method. When injecting intradermally or subdermally, there may be transient pain and discomfort. Swelling and bruising can be expected, but hematoma formation, although uncommon, can occur. When injecting deeper into the subcutaneous plane or on the supra-periosteal area, dull ache, and soreness may continue for a couple of days. Post-inflammatory pigmentation, scar formation, and calcification have been reported, albeit rarely.

Most complications can be easily managed with rest and cold compresses. Topical antibiotics prevent the chance of contamination and secondary infection. Oral analgesics may be used in patients with severe discomfort.

35A.9 Clinical Pearls in Treating Ethnic Skin

PRP therapy is independent of skin phototype and can be used in all patients safely. When used for skin of color, the risk of post-inflammatory hyperpigmentation is possible. When combined with other procedures like fractional ablative lasers, wound healing and skin recovery are faster with better outcomes than either modality used independently.[20–22]

35A.10 Special Precautions

The commercially available kits make PRP preparation simpler but may not be cost-effective. Also, each preparation may provide for a different concentration of platelets in the final PRP. So it is best to check the specifications of each company.

Manual preparation of PRP yields good results if proper guidelines are followed. Each laboratory must formulate its own protocol depending on the common indications catered to. The protocol must also take into account the centrifuge machine and its settings, as they can play a crucial role in the final platelet concentration of the PRP.

Frequently Asked Questions

1. *Q: How quickly does PRP work?*
   A: Most patients will see improvement within two months of therapy, and improvement may continue for up to six months post-procedure.
2. *Q: Is PRP painful?*
   A: Most patients tolerate the procedure well. In a few, using topical anesthetic cream makes the procedure comfortable. Post-procedure soreness may last for 24 hours.
3. *Q: Who is a good candidate for PRP?*
   A: Age is not limiting the criteria for PRP. If a patient can benefit from PRP and is in good health, he/she is a good candidate for PRP.
4. *Q: Can it be combined with other treatments?*
   A: When combined with other interventions, PRP has a synergistic effect and improves the outcome of the procedure.
5. *Q: Is PRP safe?*

A: Since it uses autologous serum, there is no risk of contamination or introducing a foreign body into the system. When maintaining strict asepsis, the procedure is very safe.
6. *Q: Is PRP effective?*
   A: There is enough clinical evidence to strongly suggest the beneficial effects of PRP in skin rejuvenation and hair regrowth.

References

1. Ross R, Glomset J, Kariya B, Harker L. A platelet-dependent serum factor that stimulates the proliferation of arterial smooth muscle cells in vitro. *Proc Natl Acad Sci USA*. 1974 Apr;71(4):1207–1210.
2. Sunitha Raja V, Munirathnam Naidu E. Platelet-rich fibrin: Evolution of a second-generation platelet concentrate. *Indian J Dent Res*. 2008 Jan–Mar;19(1):42–46.
3. Marx RE. Platelet-rich plasma (PRP): What is PRP and what is not PRP? *Implant Dent*. 2001;10(4):225–228.
4. Giusti I, Rughetti A, D'Ascenzo S, Millimaggi D, Pavan A, Dell'Orso L, et al. Identification of an optimal concentration of platelet gel for promoting angiogenesis in human endothelial cells. *Transfusion*. 2009;49:771–778.
5. Kim DH, Je YJ, Kim CD, Lee YH, Seo YJ, Lee JH, Lee Y. Can platelet-rich plasma be used for skin rejuvenation? Evaluation of effects of platelet-rich plasma on human dermal fibroblast. *Ann Dermatol*. 2011 Nov;23(4):424–431.
6. Arshdeep, Kumaran M S. Platelet-rich plasma in dermatology: Boon or a bane? *Indian J Dermatol Venereol Leprol*. 2014;80:5–14.
7. Leo MS, Kumar AS, Kirit R, Konathan R, Sivamani RK. Systematic review of the use of platelet-rich plasma in aesthetic dermatology. *J Cosmet Dermatol*. 2015 Dec;14(4):315–323.
8. Li ZJ, Choi HI, Choi DK, Sohn KC, Im M, Seo YJ, et al. Autologous platelet-rich plasma: A potential therapeutic tool for promoting hair growth. *Dermatol Surg*. 2012;38:1040–1046.
9. Smith SA, Travers RJ, Morrissey JH. How it all starts: Initiation of the clotting cascade. *Crit Rev Biochem Mol Biol*. 2015;50(4):326–336.
10. Zhang N, Wang K, Li Z, Luo T. Comparative study of different anticoagulants and coagulants in the evaluation of clinical application of platelet-rich plasma (PRP) standardization. *Cell Tissue Bank*. 2019 Mar;20(1):61–75.
11. Dhurat R, Sukesh M. Principles and methods of preparation of platelet-rich plasma: A review and author's perspective. *J Cutan Aesthet Surg*. 2014 Oct–Dec;7(4):189–197.
12. Mautner K, Malanga GA, Smith J, Shiple B, Ibrahim V, Sampson S, Bowen JE. A call for a standard classification system for future biologic research: The rationale for new PRP nomenclature. *PM R*. 2015 Apr;7(4 Suppl):S53–S59.
13. Cavallo C, Roffi A, Grigolo B, Mariani E, Pratelli L, Merli G, et al. Platelet-rich plasma: The choice of activation method affects the release of bioactive molecules. *Biomed Res Int*. 2016;2016:6591717.
14. Dohan DM, Choukroun J, Diss A, Dohan SL, Dohan AJ, et al. Platelet-rich fibrin (PRF): A second-generation platelet concentrate. Part I: Technological concepts and evolution. *Oral Surg Oral Med Oral Pathol Oral Radiol Endod*. 2006 Mar;101(3):e37–e44.
15. Agrawal M, Agrawal V. Platelet rich fibrin and its applications in dentistry—A review article. *Natl J Med Dent Res*. 2014;2:51–58.
16. Dohan Ehrenfest DM, Rasmusson L, Albrektsson T. Classification of platelet concentrates: From pure platelet-rich plasma (P-PRP) to leucocyte- and platelet-rich fibrin (L-PRF). *Trends Biotechnol*. 2009 Mar;27(3):158–167.
17. Mishra A, Harmon K, Woodall J, Vieira A. Sports medicine applications of platelet rich plasma. *Curr Pharm Biotechnol*. 2012 Jun;13(7):1185–1195.
18. Magalon J, Chateau AL, Bertrand B, Louis ML, Silvestre A, Giraudo L, et al. DEPA classification: A proposal for standardising PRP use and a retrospective application of available devices. *BMJ Open Sport Exerc Med*. 2016 Feb 4;2(1):e000060.
19. Stevens J, Khetarpal S. Platelet-rich plasma for androgenetic alopecia: A review of the literature and proposed treatment protocol. *Int J Womens Dermatol*. 2018 Sep 21;5(1):46–51.
20. Makki M, Younes AEKH, Fathy A, Abd ElDayem OY, Morsy H. Efficacy of platelet-rich plasma plus fractional carbon dioxide laser in treating posttraumatic scars. *Dermatol Ther*. 2019 Jul 25:e13031.
21. Alser OH, Goutos I. The evidence behind the use of platelet-rich plasma (PRP) in scar management: A literature review. *Scars Burn Heal*. 2018 Nov 18;4:2059513118808773.
22. Faghihi G, Keyvan S, Asilian A, Nouraei S, Behfar S, Nilforoushzadeh MA. Efficacy of autologous platelet-rich plasma combined with fractional ablative carbon dioxide resurfacing laser in treatment of facial atrophic acne scars: A split-face randomized clinical trial. *Indian J Dermatol Venereol Leprol*. 2016;82:162–168.

CHAPTER 35B: NON-FDA SKIN-LIGHTENING PROCEDURES

Nina Madnani

In the last decade, the quest for skin lightening has exploded beyond the realm of creams and lotions and has barged into the procedural world of dermatology aesthetics. The eternal hope of a "quick fix."

Though well-established clinical studies have shown benefits on pigment lightening, with procedures like chemical peels, microdermabrasion, lasers (Q-sw Nd:YAG/fractional CO_2/Er:YAG/pulsed dye) or light systems (IPL), none of the above are specifically FDA approved for the skin-lightening indication. They have also not been labeled as non-FDA approved.

A single procedure recently gaining popularity has specifically been labeled as non-FDA approved by the authorities (e.g., FDA in the United States and FDA in the Philippines) in view of reports coming in on its side effects, some life-threatening. This refers to parenteral glutathione (GSH) injections, which are recently being administered by various clinics for "fairness" and "glow."

Asian populations across the world are thronging to clinics for this "magic injection." IV glutathione injections are solely approved for addressing the adverse effects of chemo drugs. Sae Yong Hong et al., in their publication, demonstrated that GSH was useful in dealing with acute ROS injury (parquet poisoning). They measured the metabolites cysteine and methionine and inferred that the required dose for effective treatment needed to be at least 50 mg/kg body weight every 427.4 minutes.

Glutathione, an SH-containing compound, is present in all living cells. It is involved in several important biological steps, especially for its antioxidant effect. It is also hypothesized to compete with tyrosinase-binding sites and hence affect melanogenesis. When taken orally, it gets rapidly metabolized within ten minutes in the GI tract. It comes under the category of nutraceuticals.

Very few reports in the scientific literature with small numbers of participants have shown evidence of some skin lightening among patients taking oral glutathione for four weeks. There are none reported for parenteral glutathione for skin lightening. The dose generally used for skin lightening in various clinics and medispas range from 600 to 2,400 per dose twice a week, although the exact dosage recommended or duration has no scientific guidelines laid down.

The adverse effects reported have ranged from very serious ones, such as angioedema, Steven-Johnson's syndrome, toxic epidermal necrolysis, and septic shock, to less life-threatening ones, such as urticaria and rashes. A report of batches of glutathione injections causing endotoxin poisoning was reported by Johnstone et al. These vials were used at a complementary medicine center.

In view of these adverse effects, the Philippine FDA issued an advisory against its use and labeled it as a non-FDA-approved drug for indications other than in chemo patients in 2011. Similarly, the US FDA on consumer forums stated that they had not approved any drug for skin lightening, and injectable glutathione is under the drug category and cannot be administered without prescriptions. Also, in an interesting editorial in the *BMJ* 2016, the authors voiced concern that since glutathione switches the eumelanin to the phaeomelanin pathway, there could be chances of developing cancers in the future.

Until large double-blind placebo-controlled studies are done on the use of IV glutathione for a cosmetic indication like "fairness," dermatologists and aestheticians who administer it are walking a very narrow path, almost like playing Russian roulette. No court of law can save them from a legal suit slapped for a severe drug reaction when administering a drug that is not-FDA approved for an aesthetic indication with no scientific backing.

Recommended Reading

1. Sae Yong Hong et al. Pharmacokinetics of glutathione and its metabolites in normal subjects. *J Korean Med Sci*. 2005; 20:721–726.
2. T. Johnstone, E. Quinn, S. Tobin, R. Davis, Z. Najjar, B. Battye, L. Gupta. Seven cases of probable endotoxin poisoning related to contaminated glutathione infusions. *Epidemiol Infect*. 2018 May; 146(7): 931–934.
3. FDA Philippines Advisory DOH-FDA No 2011–004 dated 12 May 2011.
4. US FDA Consumer forum: Injectable Skin Lightening and Skin Bleaching Products May Be Unsafe.
5. OE Dadzie. Unethical skin bleaching with glutathione. *BMJ*. 2016; 354:1486.
6. www.fda.gov.ph › wp-content › uploads › 2019/07.

DOI: 10.1201/9780429243769-36

CHAPTER 35C: NON-SURGICAL THREAD LIFTS

Nina Madnani and Kaleem Khan

35C.1 Introduction

Polydioxanone (PDO) threads have been in use for several years with cardiac surgeons and have been adopted in aesthetics for various indications. Their ease of use and decent results in selected patients have made them a good option for patients averse to plastic surgery and who are comfortable with mini-invasive options. Also, their versatility in lifting and rejuvenating skin makes them useful in sequential combination treatments with fillers, neurotoxins, dermo-cosmeceutics, and so on.

The use of threads for tissue suspension is not new. Dr. Sulamanidze described the use of non-absorbable barbed threads in the late 1990s, and he named it Aptos (anti-ptosis).[1] The expertise required, long downtime, and high rate of complications made this procedure unappealing. However, better understanding of the aging process, availability of newer materials, limited tissue interaction of these materials, and refining thread implantation techniques have led to the resurgence of the use of threads for rejuvenation and non-surgical face lifts.

35C.2 Indications

1. Improving skin texture, including pore tightening and brightening[2]
2. Improving the nasolabial folds, marionette lines, and neck lines[3, 4]
3. Jawline definition[5]
4. Forehead tightening[6]
5. Nose reshaping[7]
6. Eyebrow lift
7. Reduce submental fat

35C.3 Types of Threads

1. *PDO threads* for aesthetic indications were introduced in 2003. As a suture material, PDO offers distinct advantages over vicryl, in having a less inflammatory response and better absorbability.[8] The majority of monofilament and spiral threads available today are PDO threads. Many cog threads are now available as PDO threads too.
2. *Poly-L-lactic acid (PLLA)* threads became popular when the US FDA approved their use for aesthetic indications in 2006. They are biocompatible, synthetic polymers that degrade slowly and promote the gradual deposition of collagen over months.

TABLE 35C.1: Various Parameters Used When Describing Threads

Parameter	Variation	
Number of threads	Single	Multiple
Orientation	Straight	Twisted, spiral
Presence of projections	Smooth	Cog/barb
Direction of projections	Unidirectional	Bidirectional
Type of needle	Blunt-tipped	Sharp-tipped
Material	PDO	PLLA/PLC

3. *Polycaprolactone (PCL) threads* have been used only recently for aesthetic purposes. They are a biodegradable synthetic polyester, which has the advantage of an even slower rate of disintegration than PLLA.
4. *Poly(lactic-co-glycolic acid) (PLGA/PLG) threads* are biodegradable co-polymers composed of two monomers, glycolic acid, and lactic acid. The ratio of these two monomers decides the characteristics of PLGA. It has been used for drug delivery but has now been incorporated in threads due to its collagen stimulatory property. Specifically, the cones in Silhouette Soft threads are composed of PLGA.
5. *Aptos threads* were first introduced as polypropylene threads with barbs in 1998.[9] These are non-absorbable biocompatible thermoplastic polymers that had to be placed through a small incision in the temporal region. Subsequent iterations include threads made of a combination of polypropylene, PLLA, PLG, and PCL.

Threads are available in various configurations depending on their characteristics (Table 35C.1).

35C.4 Mechanisms of Action

Understanding the tissue reaction provides better insight into a mechanism of action and the outcome of threads.

PDO threads:[10, 11] Once the thread is placed in the required plane, a foreign body reaction ensues, which attracts polymorphs and eosinophils. Granulation tissue starts forming around the thread, followed by neo-vascularisation. Myofibroblasts typically appear within 12 weeks, whereas fibroblast proliferation continues up to 24 weeks. New collagen is laid. This persists beyond 48 weeks and provides a scaffolding for the overlying skin, improving skin sag and elasticity. Another reaction is the breakdown of fat cells adjacent to the thread, thought to be due to the inflammatory response.

The inserted thread retains its shape for up to 12 weeks, after which it starts degrading. By 24 weeks, it is fragmented and completely absorbed by 48 weeks.

Poly-L-lactic acid (PLLA) threads:[12] Upon insertion, an immediate but mild inflammatory response is seen. Initially consisting of neutrophils, the infiltrate changes to predominantly lymphocytes, macrophages, and foreign body cells in three weeks. The infiltrate encapsulates the thread, and there is fibroplasia. By 12 weeks, the inflammatory response starts reducing, and the fibroblasts start laying down collagen fibers. By 24 weeks, the number of macrophages and fibroblasts is significantly less, but collagen production continues to increase. This neocollagenesis continues beyond 24 months and is seen along the entire tract of PLLA thread insertion.

Threads made of PLLA are broken down slowly by the lactic acid metabolic pathway, where at the end of 12 weeks, only 32% of the thread is degraded. By 24 weeks, only 58% of the threads are degraded, but new collagen formation is well underway by then.

DOI: 10.1201/9780429243769-37

35C.5 Patient Workup/Counseling

Pre-procedure patient counseling is of utmost importance. Reasonable expectations need to be set in accordance to the intended procedure.

The outcome of the procedure, whether it is skin rejuvenation or tightening or lifting of sagging skin, must be defined and would depend upon the type and number of threads used. The total number of threads to be used during the procedure must be discussed with the patient for anticipated patient outcome and financial reasons.

Patients must be informed about post-procedure downtime which may be up to three weeks.

Clinical photographs of the patient in five standard positions must be taken to document any pre-existing asymmetry.

35C.6 Pre-Procedure Care

As a foreign material is going to be introduced into the tissues, utmost sterility must be maintained to prevent infections, as these threads remain in the skin for several weeks before being absorbed. This is especially true if the entry or exit points are within the hairline. Tying up the hair in small bunches reduces the need to cut/trim the hair. When using longer threads, it is best to cover the entire field with a sterile plastic sheet/drape to avoid contamination. Having an assistant to handle the needles and threads helps to keep the procedure streamlined and decreases the risk of complications.

For simple PDO threads, topical anesthesia with EMLA cream under occlusion for 30 minutes seems sufficient to make the procedure comfortable. The area to be treated must be cleaned and sterilized with betadine or chlorhexidine. The entire field of procedure must be covered with a sterile drape to prevent accidental contamination.

Since barbed threads or more advanced ones are placed deeper, topical anesthesia is not sufficient. The entry and exit points need to be anesthetized with 2% lidocaine: adrenaline (1:80,000). Anesthesia along the line of insertion is not required if the depth of placement is correct.

35C.7 Procedure

Hands-on training is recommended before embarking solo for this procedure. The operator must be familiar with certain terms relevant to the procedure:

Entry point: This is the point from where the thread is inserted into the skin.
Exit point: This is the point from where the thread emerges under the skin after traveling along a defined path. This is of significance when using threads with projection.
Vector: The direction along which thread must be placed so that the force is redistributed and the sagging tissue is lifted. This is the most important parameter, and a good understanding of the vectors is essential for proper placement and successful lifting and rejuvenation.
Depth: The level at which the threads must be placed for maximum efficacy. This is usually in the subdermal or subcutaneous region.

A brief protocol is provided here:

1. Plan the types and numbers of threads to be used.
2. After cleansing, apply topical anesthesia for 45 minutes with/without occlusion as needed or infiltrate topical xylocaine: adrenaline at the entry and exit points.
3. Sterilize the area.
4. Mark the vectors.

For monofilament PDO threads, some suggested vectors are shown in (Figure 35C.1). Once the vector(s) is decided, insert the threads parallel to the surface of the skin in a wave-like fashion,

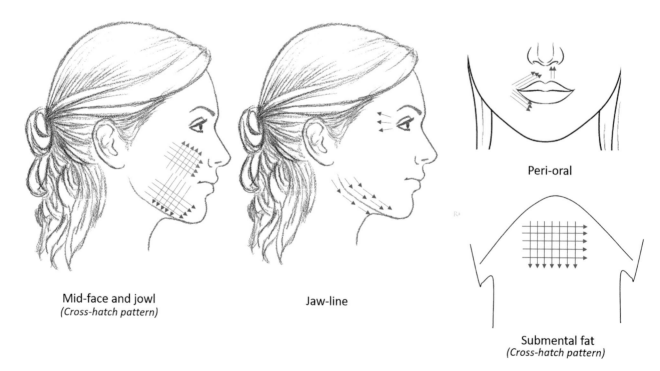

Mid-face and jowl
(Cross-hatch pattern)

Jaw-line

Peri-oral

Submental fat
(Cross-hatch pattern)

FIGURE 35C.1   Some common vectors used with monofilament threads for various areas of the face.

making sure the needle does not breach the epidermis. These threads are usually placed parallel to each other or cross/hatched. Once the thread is inserted up to the full length of the needle or even beyond the fixing sponge, the needle must be twisted a couple of times and then pulled out. Threads projecting out of the skin must be trimmed to just below the level of the skin.

For barbed threads, one must remain in the subcutaneous fat above the superficial muscular aponeurotic system (SMAS). Blunt cannulas are safer to use in this plane, and needles must be used with caution (Figure 35C.2). shows a few configurations for the entry points and their vectors. Some threads come with needles on both ends. These threads have a single entry point and two exit points. The vector may be linear, at an angle, or in a U configuration (Figure 35C.3). The threads emerge at the exit point and need to be trimmed at the appropriate depth. One must tug gently at the exiting thread and cut it while pressing down on the skin. This causes the thread to retract into the skin at the subcutaneous level. On pulling the thread, the physician can see the amount of lift. It is best not to pull with a lot of force, as doing so will cause puckering of the skin. The barbs on the thread must be fixed in place by pressing on the overlying skin. A distinct snapping sound can be heard, which corresponds to the projections attaching to the skin and thus confirming the placement of the thread.

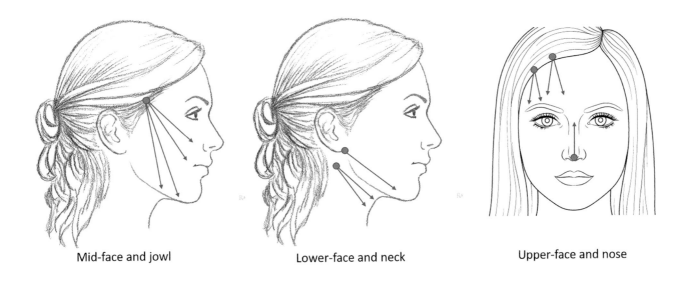

Mid-face and jowl   Lower-face and neck   Upper-face and nose

● Entry point

FIGURE 35C.2   Some recommended vectors for use with cog threads to achieve the lifting of tissue.

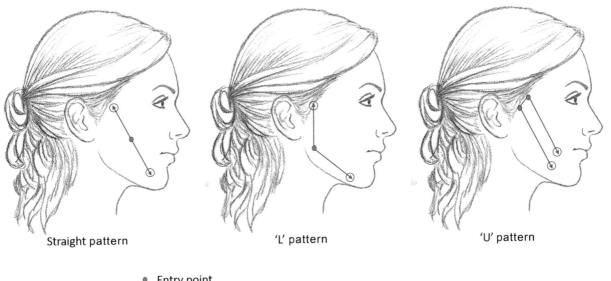

Straight pattern   'L' pattern   'U' pattern

● Entry point
⊙ Exit point

FIGURE 35C.3   Suggested vectors when using cog threads with needles on both ends.

35C.8 Post-Procedure Care

Immediate application of ice/cold compress is recommended to allay the discomfort and swelling from tissue manipulation. Topical antibacterial creams like mupirocin need to be applied and continued for up to five to seven days. Paracetamol can be used for pain relief. Anti-inflammatory agents like ibuprofen should be avoided.

Patients must be instructed to avoid facial massage for up to two weeks, and all dental procedures should be deferred for up to four weeks. Makeup is to be avoided for one week.

35C.9 Contraindications

Patients with unrealistic expectations are best avoided. Those with keloidal tendencies or with connective tissue diseases like SLE or scleroderma must be deferred. Avoid this procedure in patients with any bleeding disorders or those currently taking anticoagulants.

Patients with active infections, like herpes, impetigo, folliculitis, tinea, acne, or any skin disease, on the procedure area are a relative contraindication. They must be treated for the same and can be taken for the procedure once clear. Patients with a history of recurrent herpes labialis need acyclovir prophylaxis.

35C.10 Side Effects and Their Management

The common complications encountered with threads and their management are discussed in Table 35C.2.[2, 13–17] Most complications can be attributed to inadequate planning and poor technique but the quality of the thread matters too.[18]

35C.11 Clinical Pearls in Treating Ethnic Skin/Skin of Color

Ethnic skin is thicker and more seborrhoeic than Caucasian skin. It is more forgiving to bruising and is associated with less downtime compared to Caucasian skin but may require more a number of threads to achieve better lifting.

Post-inflammatory dyspigmentation and keloid formation are more common.

35C.11.1 Combination Treatments

Threads are designed to stimulate collagen formation. Platelet-rich plasma (PRP) therapy also helps in tissue repair and neocollagenesis. The two procedures can be combined in the same session to give better results.[19]

Neuromodulators can be used in conjunction with threads. However, it is best to use the neuromodulators two weeks prior to using threads.

Threads help to achieve lift with little volumizing. When combined with fillers, 3D restructuring of the face is possible. Fillers must be done at least four weeks before implanting the threads.

Frequently Asked Questions

1. *Q: Are threads safe?*
   A: Absorbable threads, when used correctly, are safe and effective.
2. *Q: Is there any difference between threads?*
   A: The main difference between threads is the material they are made of and their longevity.
3. *Q: Do they achieve the lifting of sagging tissue?*

TABLE 35C.2: **Common Side Effects Seen with Threads and Their Management**

Complication	Cause	Management
Bleeding, bruising, hematoma	• Sharp needles, fine gauge cannula • Blood vessels at the point of entry/exit, especially in the temple area • Bruising due to damage to the superficial dermal plexus of blood vessels	• Evaluating the entry and exit points by visualization and palpation esp in the temporal area • Immediate withdrawal of needle/cannula followed by pressure
Infection	• Non-sterile field of operation • Hair entanglement at the entry/exit sites	• Maintain strict asepsis • Cleaning the site with antiseptic solution/betadine and using sterile sheets to cover the entire field of operation
Skin puckering/dimple formation	• Incorrect dept of insertion • Thread being cut at the improper depth at the exit site. • Incorrect insertion technique when using U pattern vectors	• Maintain uniform depth of insertion • At the exit, cut close to the skin after pulling gently on the thread • Use subcision to align the threads in the same plane
Thread protrusion	• May be noted immediately after the procedure • Bump after a few weeks, which becomes more evident on making exaggerated facial movement	• Tugging on the thread and cutting the excess part away • Bump may be incised, and the thread size reduced by excision
Thread breakage/ thread migration	• Due to overzealous tightening • If bidirectional cog threads are cut in the middle	• Do not over-tighten to achieve more lift • Creating a lattice or mesh pattern helps to keep the threads in place
Asymmetry	• Improper placement • Excessive pull on the threads • Unequal number of threads used	• Planning the procedure • Marking the vectors correctly at the start of the procedure • Improving the technique
Facial nerve paralysis/ facial paraesthesia	• Diffusion of the local anesthetic into the deeper layers	• Wears off after a few hours

A: Bidirectional PLLA cog threads have an excellent lifting capacity, and the results may last for up to a couple of years.

4. *Q: Can they replace facelift surgery?*
A: Threads have their own limitations, but with the right candidate and the correct choice of threads, the need for surgery can be deferred.

5. *Q: Who is an ideal candidate for a thread lift?*
A: Patients with mild ptosis and good skin elasticity. Thread lift could achieve ideal rejuvenation and recontouring results.

6. *Q: Can they be combined with other procedures?*
A: Threads work best when combined with other procedures, including neurotoxins, fillers, and PRP.

7. *Q: How long does the effect last?*
A: Rejuvenation usually lasts for up to six months, and depending on the number of cog threads used, the lifting effect lasts up to nine months to a year.

8. *Q: When would I need to repeat the procedure?*
A: The need to repeat the procedure would depend upon the speed of intrinsic and extrinsic aging.

References

1. Sulamanidze MA, Shiffman MA, Paikidze TG, Sulamanidze GM, Gavasheli LG. Facial lifting with APTOS threads. *Int J Cosmetic Surg Aesthetic Dermatol.* 2001;3:275–281.
2. Lee H, Yoon K, Lee M. Outcome of facial rejuvenation with polydioxanone thread for Asians. *J Cosmet Laser Ther.* 2018;20(3):189–192.
3. Arora G, Arora S. Neck rejuvenation with thread lift. *J Cutan Aesthet Surg.* 2019;12(3):196–200.
4. Kim J, Kim HS, Seo JM, Nam KA, Chung KY. Evaluation of a novel thread-lift for the improvement of nasolabial folds and cheek laxity. *J Eur Acad Dermatol Venereol.* 2017;31(3):e136–e179.
5. Karimi K, Reivitis A. Lifting the lower face with an absorbable polydioxanone (PDO) thread. *J Drugs Dermatol.* 2017;16(9):932–934.
6. Ko HJ, Choi JY, Moon HJ, et al. Multi-polydioxanone (PDO) scaffold for forehead wrinkle correction: A pilot study. *J Cosmet Laser Ther.* 2016;18(7):405–408.
7. Lee HY, Yang HJ. Rhinoplasty with barbed threads. *Plast Reconstr Surg Glob Open.* 2018;6(11):e1967.
8. Laufer N, Merino M, Trietsch HG, DeCherney AH. Macroscopic and histologic tissue reaction to polydioxanone, a new, synthetic, monofilament microsuture. *J Reprod Med.* 1984;29(5):307–310.
9. Sulamanidze M, Sulamanidze G. Facial lifting with Aptos methods. *J Cutan Aesthet Surg.* 2008;1(1):7–11.
10. Yoon JH, Kim SS, Oh SM, Kim BC, Jung W. Tissue changes over time after polydioxanone thread insertion: An animal study with pigs. *J Cosmet Dermatol.* 2019;18(3):885–891.
11. Kim J, Zheng Z, Kim H, Nam KA, Chung KY. Investigation on the cutaneous change induced by face-lifting monodirectional barbed polydioxanone thread. *Dermatol Surg.* 2017;43(1):74–80.
12. Fitzgerald R, Bass LM, Goldberg DJ, Graivier MH, Lorenc ZP. Physiochemical characteristics of poly-L-lactic acid (PLLA). *Aesthet Surg J.* 2018;38(suppl_1):S13–S17.
13. Suh DH, Jang HW, Lee SJ, Lee WS, Ryu HJ. Outcomes of polydioxanone knotless thread lifting for facial rejuvenation. *Dermatol Surg.* 2015;41(6):720–725.
14. Ahn SK, Choi HJ. Complication after PDO threads lift. *J Craniofac Surg.* 2019;30(5):e467–e469.
15. Sarigul Guduk S, Karaca N. Safety and complications of absorbable threads made of poly-L-lactic acid and poly lactide/glycolide: Experience with 148 consecutive patients. *J Cosmet Dermatol.* 2018;17(6):1189–1193.
16. Ali YH. Two years' outcome of thread lifting with absorbable barbed PDO threads: Innovative score for objective and subjective assessment. *J Cosmet Laser Ther.* 2018;20(1):41–49.
17. Makhecha M, Singh T, Yadav T, Atawane M. Cutaneous pseudolymphoma secondary to facial thread lift procedure. *Indian Dermatol Online J.* 2019;10(3):322–324.
18. Aitzetmueller MM, Centeno Cerdas C, Nessbach P, et al. Polydioxanone threads for facial rejuvenation: Analysis of quality variation in the market. *Plast Reconstr Surg.* 2019;144(6):1002e–1009e.
19. Ali YH. Two years' outcome of thread lifting with absorbable barbed PDO threads: Innovative score for objective and subjective assessment. *J Cosmet Laser Ther.* 2018;20(1):41–49.

CHAPTER 36: HOME-USE DEVICES
An Overview and Regulatory Aspects

Godfrey Town and Christine Dierickx

36.1 Introduction

Media exposure of light-based technologies and medical and scientific validation that lasers and intense pulsed light devices produce measurable results in hair removal, acne and psoriasis reduction, and skin rejuvenation has led to the introduction of miniaturized, low-cost devices for home use by the consumer (home-use devices, or HUDs). Several leading brands are now entering this expanding market sector but are these low-cost systems credible, and how do they compare with professional treatments? A number of review articles have been published since 2011 reflecting upon the growing consumer use of HUDs and their potential role as "companion products" to professional treatments [1–7].

As the cost of technology has come down, there has been an expansion in North America and most European countries in the use of intense pulsed light devices by non-medically qualified therapist operators outside of the medical clinic and in spas and salons. Given the huge consumer demand for cosmetic hair removal, it is perhaps unsurprising that companies are eager to offer new technology products to the general public for personal use.

Facial cleansing devices dominate the consumer skin care appliances market (Clarisonic) with a range of both professional and at-home devices. However, cleansing devices are not considered in this chapter, where the focus is on light-based therapies.

36.2 Hair Reduction

Home-use light-based treatments by consumers have been documented as far back as 2003, and recent years have seen the launch, through the high street and online, of a number of HUDs for hair removal and skin rejuvenation [8]. These include major consumer brands for hair removal, such as SpectraGenics Tria Hair Removal Laser 4X, Philips SatinLux, iPulse Smooth Skin Bare, Braun Glow, and Remington iLight Pro. Manufacturers of home-use hair removal devices have been granted FDA clearance in the United States for over-the-counter sale to consumers (e.g., SpectraGenics Tria and Home Skinovations Silk'n) (Figure 36.1).

36.2.1 Mode of Action

The concept of low fluence laser and intense pulsed light to produce significant hair growth delay is not a new hypothesis. Manstein *et al.* first proposed this at the Annual Meeting of the American Society for Lasers in Medicine and Surgery (ASLMS) in 2001 [9]. The theory of extended hair growth delay in clinical and *in vitro* studies was again presented at the ASLMS meeting in 2008 [10] and again in 2014 [11]. Other researchers have also reported on the efficacy of using low fluence for successful hair reduction using professional alexandrite [12] and diode lasers [13].

Roosen *et al.* (2008) found in an *in vitro* study that one low-fluence IPL treatment caused mild trauma to the hair shaft, interrupting the hair cycle and inducing temporary hair loss

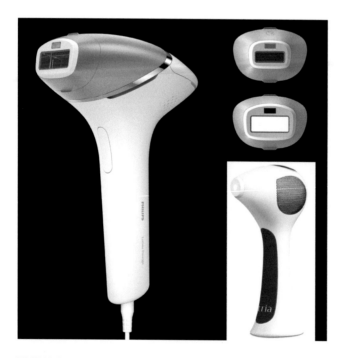
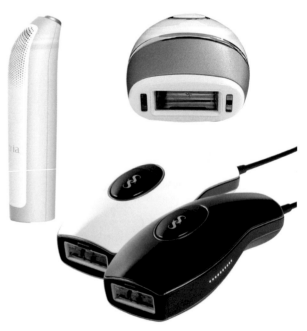

FIGURE 36.1 Popular IPL and laser home-use hair reduction devices.

DOI: 10.1201/9780429243769-38

(A) **(B)**

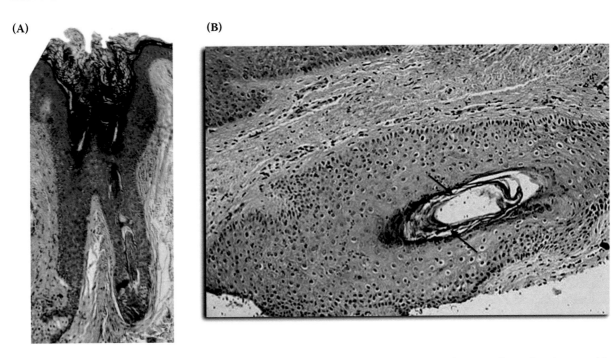

FIGURE 36.2A Hair follicle biopsy taken 15–20 minutes after treatment, stained with hematoxylin and eosin, magnification 10×, showing disintegration with retraction of the intraluminal hair shaft and plugging of keratin (longitudinal section). The epidermis presents with no damage, and slight coagulation is seen in the upper part of the hair structure.

FIGURE 36.2B Hair follicle showing infundibular dilatation and plugging of keratin with mild trauma of the intraluminal hair shaft. Notice disruption (separation) of the trichilemmal keratinization and a few inflammatory cells in the dermis.

[14]. A preliminary histology study with the iPulse home-use IPL by Trelles (2014) confirms that in several phototype II subjects, primary thermal effects were evident in the hair shaft due to thermal absorption, including an immediate inflammatory infiltration reaction of the perifolliculum, together with changes in hair architecture and detachment from the skin [15] (Figure 36.2a, b).

A recent review by Town *et al.* (2019) proposed mechanistic differences in light delivery regimes and the resulting divergences in the mode of action between high-fluence professional devices and low-fluence home-use appliances. This review concluded that *in vivo* studies demonstrated that low fluence home-use hair removal devices could result in high hair reduction efficacy after a short treatment regimen, while prolonged and less frequent (once in six weeks) maintenance treatment over a year can lead to high and sustained hair reduction even one year after cessation of treatment [16] (Figure 36.3).

However, further histological studies involving dynamic observation of the hair follicle (i.e., terminal vs. vellus) over the whole cycle of treatment with these HUDs are needed to confirm the proposed mode of action of low fluences in combination with treatment and maintenance regimes and the extent of hair damage.

36.2.2 Clinical Efficacy and Safety

To date, the majority of published clinical studies have focused on hair reduction using low fluence, home-use laser, and intense pulsed light devices confirming meaningful hair reduction figures and relatively few side effects but still inferior to some professionally delivered treatments.

While all of these studies were medically supervised rather than performed at home, it is clear that permanent hair

reduction results are achievable [17]. However, a recent systematic review of published trials of light-based HUDs for hair removal found only seven prospective studies, of which only one was controlled, and none were randomized [18]. The data so far indicate that the devices tested provided short-term efficacy, but further studies will be required to confirm and extend the results and to establish the incidence of adverse events in selected cohorts of patients. Longer-term surveillance studies will then be required to demonstrate the safety profile of HUDs in real-world use.

Safety is a major consideration for the consumer, and the literature indicates that ocular safety systems incorporated by reputable manufacturers position home-use lasers as class I (i.e., eye-safe) laser devices. To date, several safety studies have appeared in international, peer-reviewed journals examining measurement and safety issues [19–23].

36.2.3 Side Effects and Adverse Incidents

The most probable adverse effect of visible and infrared light is skin burns, which might include blistering and possibly scarring, as seen in several reported cases following professional laser, IPL, and radiofrequency (RF) hair reduction and skin rejuvenation treatments. Notwithstanding that other side effects, such as triggering of skin infections, photoallergic and photo-toxic reactions, leucotrichia (temporary hair bleaching), hair growth induction, and photosensitive drug interaction, might arise with HUDs, these are likely to be considerably less common than with professional treatments owing to the built-in limitations on treatable phototypes, skin color sensors, conservative energy settings, small aperture size, comparatively low pulse energy, and so on, inherent in HUDs. Side effects are most likely to occur

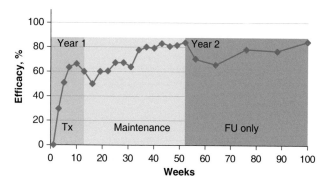

FIGURE 36.3 Progression of hair reduction recorded in a study using a commercially available IPL consumer appliance (IPL, 6.5 J/cm², 1.8 ms) in simulated home use. Treatment was administered by a test leader on a lower leg of N=90 female study participants (Fitzpatrick skin phototype I–III). Four initial biweekly treatments were followed by periodic treatment sessions at six-week intervals for a full year. Follow-up observation sessions without treatment were held for another year. Manual hair counting was performed at all sessions. (From Nuijs T, Bartula L, Reiter S, van den Broek L. Long-term hair reduction with a home-use IPL device. Laser Surg Med 2014;46(S25):22–23; Nuijs T, Evers L, Roosen G, et al. Clinical and in-vitro investigation of low-fluence photoepilation with an IPLsystem. Lasers Surg Med 2008;40:S20.)

through intentional misuse by a consumer through repeated application on the same skin area.

While it has been suggested anecdotally that paradoxical hair growth might be attributed to low fluences used in home-use appliances, there have been no published studies or case reports on the incidence of hair growth induction by home-use laser or intense pulsed light devices. A review of the literature by Town and Bjerring in 2016 provided a scientific explanation of why there is no simple correlation between low-level laser therapy at 655 nm used on the scalp in patients with androgenic alopecia and the suggestion that stray or scattered radiation might stimulate dormant hair follicles [24].

Although some adverse event cases that might arise following incorrect or inappropriate use of HUDs may require medical care, most of them will heal without treatment over time. Permanent side effects may consist of scarring and hyper-/hypopigmentation. Although this risk of skin damage seems tolerable, eye injury due to the non-functioning of safeguards or due to misuse of the equipment is a serious concern. Although millions of units have already been sold [25–28], apparently there are only a few reports available about incidents of any type in the home use area, the most notable of which was the withdrawal from the market by Neutrogena of its LED therapy mask over fears of ocular damage in a small subset of users. This should not prevent those who are concerned from collecting data and evaluating the true risks.

36.3 Skin Rejuvenation

One of the most frequent signs of aging is the appearance of fine lines and wrinkles. Regardless of when wrinkles are first seen, they are often an undesirable indicator of age, especially for people who are seeking ways to look and feel their best. Energy-based skin rejuvenation is a process of reversing the effects of aging by reducing wrinkles, pigmentation, vascular dyschromia, and minor scars following acne vulgaris. By using controlled, invisible thermal "wounds" to the skin, fresh new cells and structural components are created to replace damaged aged skin cells and matrix.

Radiofrequency (RF) and massage devices dominate the consumer anti-aging sector (e.g., Tripollar Stop, Trinity NuFACE, Clarisonic Smart Profile Uplift), with laser devices and microdermabrasion taking a smaller but rapidly expanding role (e.g., Tria Age-Defying Laser, Silk'n FaceTite, Nira Skin, MZ Skin). Consumer-use light-emitting diode (LED) arrays, LED masks, and hand-held applicators for anti-aging treatments are also gaining in popularity (e.g., Omnilux Contour, Lustre Skin Renew, iDermalight, Iderma Masque, Talika Genius Light LED Mask, NuFACE Trinity Wrinkle Reducer) (Figure 36.4).

These consumer-use masks are based on larger LED arrays originally designed for professional use in assisting wound healing after invasive ablative laser resurfacing procedures. Several larger arrays are also now sold for home use (e.g., Aesthetic Technology Dermalux Flex MD, Trophy Rejuvalite MD, and Celluma PRO) with flexible options for treating other body areas (Figure 36.5).

36.3.1 Mode of Action—Thermally Based Technology

Brit and Marcus (2017) reviewed available literature from 2011 to 2016 *for professional use* and found that there are three broad categories of thermally based technologies used for facial rejuvenation: lasers, light therapy, and other non-laser-based thermal tightening devices such as radiofrequency (RF) and intense focused ultrasonography (IFUS). Laser light therapy has continued to diversify with the use of ablative and nonablative resurfacing technologies, fractionated lasers, and their combined use [29].

The first at-home wrinkle treatments were released by professional laser developers (SpectraGenics Tria Skin Rejuvenating Laser, PaloVia Skin Renewing Laser, and Solta Philips RéAura). These early devices used mid-infrared laser diode wavelengths (1,410 nm, 1,435 nm, and 1,440 nm, respectively) with scanner fractional delivery of sub-ablative fluences to create microthermal zones (MTZ) of dermal injury below the epidermis, which produce sub-millimeter diameter columns of thermal damage, ejected as microscopic epidermal necrotic debris (MENDs) without ablating the epidermis. The Iluminage non-scanning laser diode also uses the 1,440 nm wavelength with a 60 ms pulse duration, maximum peak power of 10 W per pulse, and is manufactured to medical device safety and performance standards.

A typical protocol involved daily treatments for up to 30 days, followed by biweekly maintenance treatments. Like professional nonablative treatments, skin dyschromia is expelled in the MENDS, and neocollagenesis has been shown in the treated tissue. Although poorly understood, Dams *et al.* concluded that short-pulsed heat shocks, together with upregulation of gene expression, show that it is possible to stimulate human dermal fibroblasts to produce more collagen [30]. However, in clinical trials, the side effect profile of these mid-infrared laser devices included erythema in most subjects and skin dryness, roughness, bronzing, flaking,

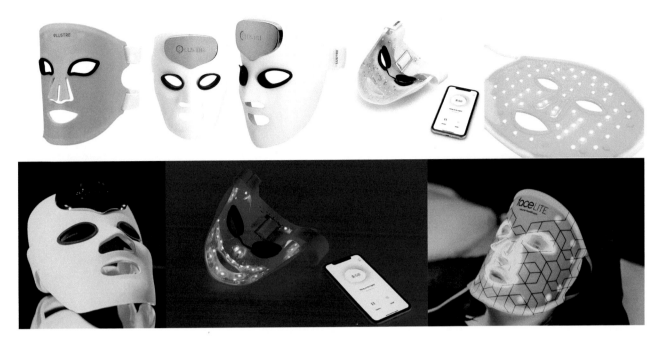

FIGURE 36.4 Examples of popular home-use LED skin rejuvenation masks, including both flat flexible masks and mouldable masks shaped to the contours of the face. Some masks now come with mobile phone- and tablet-compatible software to monitor treatment progress.

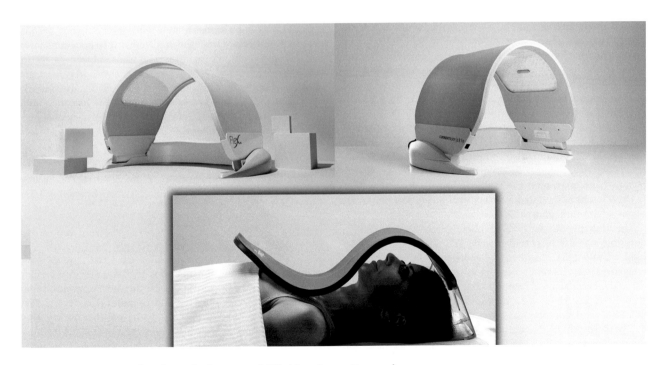

FIGURE 36.5 Examples of popular home-use LED skin rejuvenation masks.

edema, and itching, which made these treatments generally unattractive to consumers, and two of these devices have since been withdrawn from the market [31]. Only the Tria Age-Defying Laser and Nira Skin laser remain on sale (Figures 36.6 and 36.7).

Further developments in miniaturized laser diodes based upon mass-market core technology have resulted in lower consumer prices and fewer side effects, with the added benefit of internet connectivity. The Dermal Photonics Nira Skincare Laser uses 1,440 nm infrared diode non-scanning technology and a very low side-effect profile.

36.3.2 Mode of Action—Non-Thermal Technology

LEDs are complex semiconductors that convert electrical current into incoherent narrow-spectrum light. They have been around since the 1960s but were limited to very simplistic

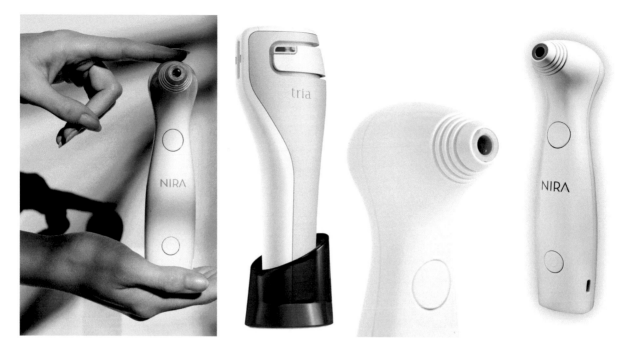

FIGURE 36.6   Examples of two popular home-use laser skin rejuvenation devices.

applications as they could only produce red, green, and yellow but not white light. In 1993, Nichia Chemical of Japan started producing blue LEDs, which permitted the combination of blue, red, and green to produce white light. Initial work on non-thermal light therapy in humans was conducted by the National Aeronautics and Space Administration (NASA) to seek solutions to deficient levels of wound healing experienced by astronauts in zero-gravity space conditions and Navy SEALs in submarines under high atmospheric pressure. NASA investigated the use of LED therapy in wound healing and obtained positive results [32, 33]. Originally referred to as *low-level laser therapy* (LLLT) but now also accepted to be referred to as *low-level light therapy*, LED-LLLT delivers non-coherent, highly narrow band quasi-monochromatic light with more than 95% of the photons at the rated wavelength allowing precise targeting of skin chromophores [34].

The therapeutic use, called photobiomodulation (PBM), describes the use of specific visible and near-infrared (NIR) light wavelengths absorbed by endogenous chromophores, triggering non-thermal, non-cytotoxic biological reactions through photochemical responses but more recently published studies suggest the involvement of opsin photoreceptors [35, 36]. PBM works predominantly on a protein in the mitochondria oxidative chain (cytochrome c oxidase) to increase adenosine triphosphate (ATP) and reduce oxidative stress. A cascade of mitochondrial and intracellular downstream effects leads to improved tissue repair and reduced inflammation.

Karu *et al.* (2005) showed that LED therapy, a nonthermal noninvasive treatment, can trigger natural intracellular photobiochemical reactions [37–39].

According to Ohshiro and Calderhead (1988 and 1991), the level of biological activity achieved by incident photons on tissue depends on the strength of the stimulus, where low-photon intensities excite the cell, moderate ones sustain the cell, strong intensities will damage the cell through the generation of a photothermal reaction, retarding cellular activities, and very strong ones will kill the cell [40, 41].

36.3.3 Clinical Efficacy and Safety

Home-use, thermally mediated, nonablative fractional laser technology is comparatively new, and several major brands have been withdrawn from the market owing to poor consumer acceptance of levels of discomfort and transient side effects. In a study by Leyden *et al.*, 10% of 100 subjects withdrew from the study because of post-treatment erythema, edema, discomfort, or viral meningitis during treatment [42]. There has, therefore, been very little published clinical data on the efficacy of home-use cosmetic laser treatments.

36.3.4 Side Effects and Adverse Incidents

There have been no published or anecdotal reports of any injuries sustained to the skin through the application of LED technology.

36.4 Hair Growth Stimulation

Alopecia is a common disorder that touches more than half of the world's population, with the most common type, *androgenic alopecia*, affecting 50% of males over 40 and 75% of females over 65 years [43]. Conventional therapy involves either medication such as finasteride and minoxidil for long periods or hair transplant surgery. *Alopecia areata*, an autoimmune inflammatory condition, is also typically treated with topical and systemic medication or contact sensitizers, psoralen plus blue UVA light, or narrowband UVB (phototherapy).

The first over-the-counter products for male pattern hair loss were FDA-cleared for sale in the United States in 2007 and 2011 to treat *androgenetic alopecia* and promote hair growth in males who have Norwood Hamilton Classifications of IIa to V patterns of hair loss and to treat *androgenetic alopecia* and promote hair growth in females who have Ludwig (Savin) scale I-4, II-1, or II-2, or frontal alopecia, both with phototypes I to IV. Early home-use models were in a brush/comb design, while

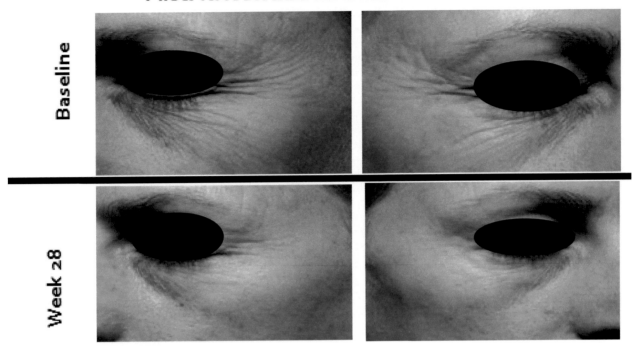

FIGURE 36.7 Examples of the efficacy of a home-use nonablative fractional laser device for wrinkle treatment, from baseline to week 28, showing complete resolution of side effects and maintenance of wrinkle improvements throughout the follow-up phase. (From: This image was published in *J Acad Dermatol*. 2012; 67(5): Figure 4, page no. 980 by Leyden J, Stephens TJ, Herdon JH. Copyright Elsevier (2012).)

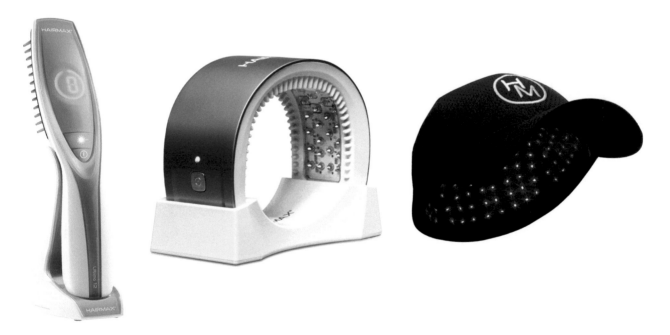

FIGURE 36.8 Examples of popular home-use hair stimulation devices.

later LED and laser diode devices adopted headband and helmet formats emitting continuous wave (cw) and pulsed red or near-infrared light, predominantly 650–660 nm. LaserComb (Hairmax, Boca Raton, FLA, USA), the early market leader, now has a total of seven FDA clearances to market hair growth devices (Figure 36.8).

36.4.1 Mode of Action

It is postulated that light phototherapy initiates and prolongs the anagen hair growth phase, increases the rate of proliferation in active anagen follicles, and prevents early catagen transition; however, the exact mechanism of action is unclear [44]. However, Mignon *et al.* (2016) described important drawbacks in existing knowledge and inconsistencies in optical parameters chosen for photobiomodulation (PBM) in hair growth stimulation. Mignon *et al.* compared the wide variation in radiant energy densities recommended by manufacturers of hair growth HUDs and concluded there was a lack of consistency in experimental and translational approaches in photobiomodulation studies both *in vitro* and *in vivo* citing treatment methods, experimental conditions, and inconsistency in the clear transition between *in vitro* and *in vivo* studies [45].

In a subsequent commentary on Mignon's work, Keene (2016) identified the reduced cost and increased speed of the US FDA's 510K clearances to market for medical devices compared with the FDA pre-market approval (PMA) process as having an impact on PBM device development, including choice of power output and wavelength. Keene argues that the 510K process of demonstrating "substantial equivalence" and safety to an existing product is much cheaper, simpler, and quicker than the PMA process to achieve market commercialization. This may explain the delay in seeing novel devices with optimal wavelengths and more effective power being developed [46, 47].

36.4.2 Clinical Efficacy and Safety

Mignon *et al.* reported in 2016 that more than 20 light-based devices based on PBM had been safety-cleared to market by the FDA for the management of hair regrowth with efficacy reported to be similar to that of existing FDA-cleared drugs for hair growth (i.e., minoxidil and finasteride) and inherently free from potential side effects [48].

36.4.3 Side Effects and Adverse Incidents

In the LaserComb study treating *androgenic alopecia*, only mild paraesthesia (burning or prickling sensation) and urticaria were observed in four cases (total of eight cases).

36.5 Medical Use of Huds

Numerous blue light LED, hand-held acne-clearing appliances can be purchased online or may be recommended by a dermatologist for supplementary home care (e.g., Ambicare Lustre Pure Light, Quasar MD, Tria Positively Clear, Foreo Espada) (Figure 36.9).

36.5.1 Mode of Action

There is an abundance of published literature covering dermatological applications of phototherapy using visible and near-infrared light. Numerous clinical studies support the efficacy of blue light (narrowband UVB) therapies across a range of conditions, such as jaundice, acne, psoriasis vulgaris, and eczema. Such treatments rely on photobiological interactions between visible light, in particular 400–495 nm blue light and target tissues, but the underlying mechanism of any therapeutic approach is not fully understood. As described earlier in this chapter, the most feasible theories are based upon the photostimulation of terminal molecules in the mitochondrial electron transport chain (cytochrome C oxidase) with two immediate consequences: an increase in adenosine triphosphate (ATP) concentration and elevation of reactive oxygen species (ROS), which can enhance the cellular functions of both epidermal and dermal cells through specific mitogen-activated protein kinase (MAPK) signaling pathways. As high- and low-dose blue light suppress dendritic cell activation (like UV irradiation), the effects of blue light on keratinocytes and immune cells may explain the reduced inflammation and diminished epidermal thickness of lesional psoriatic skin after treatment [48].

Dermatologists most often employ photodynamic therapy (PDT) in the treatment of cancerous skin cells (including superficial basal cell carcinoma, actinic keratosis, and

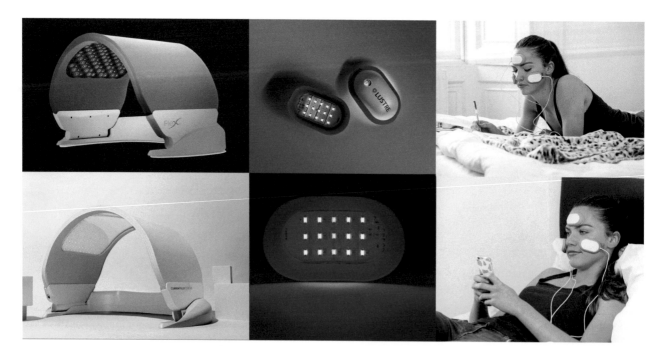

FIGURE 36.9 Examples of home-use acne care devices, including rigid LED arrays, powered face masks, and rechargeable wearable devices.

Bowen's disease) and have noted concomitant improvements in skin quality [49]. The combination of light and a photoactive 5-aminolevulinic acid (ALA) or its derivative methylaminolevulinic acid (MAL) has now become the accepted treatment for these dermatological conditions [50].

Reactive oxygen species (ROS) produced by absorption of light in bacterial porphyrins are also formed in the presence of certain wavelengths of light in the UV ("Soret band" 415 nm peak) and visible spectrum ("Q-band" 508–635 nm) alone. This is the primary mode of action hypothesized in the use of HUDs for maintenance therapy in the treatment of mild to moderate acne vulgaris. A bactericidal effect has been proposed by several authors [51, 52].

36.5.2 Clinical Efficacy and Safety

The majority of published clinical studies that demonstrate the efficacy of LEDs and laser diodes used professional devices or consumer devices in simulated home-care studies.

36.5.3 Side Effects and Adverse Incidents

Many of the HUDs are fitted with skin contact switches to prevent light emission into free space when not in full skin contact and/or temperature sensors that switch off the device if a pre-set skin temperature is exceeded (typically 41°C). Although side effects of phototherapy for these conditions are known to include erythema, hyperpigmentation, edema, pruritus, pain, purpura, transient petechiae, and others, reported side effects for consumer-use LEDs are reported as mild and transient. At the same time, the safety of skin irradiation with blue light remains a topic of some controversy.

36.6 Standards

For optical radiation hazard, home-use IPL devices should comply with several international standards, including IEC 60601-2-57,[1] which focuses on radiation aspects and related markings but hardly provides any product-specific safety requirements; IEC 60335-2-113,[2] which provides such specific requirements for household appliances with light sources for cosmetic and beauty care but does not apply to equipment with medical purposes; and IEC 60601-2-83,[3] which addresses all safety requirements for home light therapy equipment and has taken over relevant requirements from IEC 60335-2-113 and IEC 60601-2-83.

Manufacturers should also rely upon IEC 60825-1:2014,[4] IEC TR 60825-14,[5] and the International Committee on Non-Ionizing Radiation Protection (ICNIRP) Guidelines on Limits of Exposure to Broad-band Incoherent Optical Radiation family of standards.[6] At least one home-use hair removal IPL has been tested under these international standards [53].

36.6.1 Embedded Lasers—Class 1C

Home-use laser products have "accessible emission limits" from embedded lasers that would result ordinarily in laser hazard classifications of Class 3R, 3B, or 4, but because of interlocks and design features, cannot emit hazardous radiation when the product is not in contact with the skin. With no "free" emission, control measures in current standards do not make much sense. Therefore, the Electrotechnical Committee for Standardization (CENELEC) has defined a new laser category, Class 1C, in its latest revisions to IEC standard 60825-1:2014, "Safety of Laser Products—Part 1: Equipment Classification and Requirements," which may be applied to laser products

that are being marketed for skin treatments in the home. The most recent IEC 60825-1 ed3.0: 2014-05 "parent" standard, while specifying the requirements for a Class 1C laser, clearly states that if an applicable IEC ("vertical") standard specifying engineering controls to prevent emission into the surrounding space or to the eye does not exist, then classification to laser Class 1C is not permitted. Typical Class 1C laser products would embrace those intended for home-use hair removal, skin wrinkle reduction, and acne reduction.

Meanwhile, the IEC has also published the vertical standard IEC 60335-2-113:2016, "Household and Similar Electrical Appliances—Safety—Part 2–113: Particular requirements for Cosmetic and Beauty Therapy Appliances Incorporating Lasers and Intense Light Sources," where their operation relies upon contact with the skin. This standard incorporates the new laser classification wording contained in IEC 60825–1 ed.3.0: 2014 and provides the necessary design features, engineering controls, interlocks, skin pigment detection, and suitable user instructions to ensure safe use by a consumer [54].

The invention of the laser Class 1C and acceptance of the definition of Class 1C in the new IEC 60825-1 ed3.0: 2014 opens the market for new products being offered by manufacturers of cosmetic light-based appliances. This makes sense since the laser appliances, otherwise classified as laser Class 3B or 4, would be regarded as being very hazardous to the eyes (which they are not when interlocked) and hence are subject to strong regulation of their usage. In similar cases, such as UV-emitting devices, national regulation comes into play in some countries. However, lasers and IPL sources discharging in the visible and infrared spectrum present no risk of cancer as compared with malignancy-provoking UV sources [55].

36.7 Regulatory Aspects

36.7.1 General

Since their introduction, manufacturers of HUDs have relied upon existing international standards and national regulations covering household electrical appliances to achieve safety compliance [56]. In the absence of specific national regulations, in the European Union this would typically include compliance with the General Product Safety Directive, Electromagnetic Compatibility legislation, and international standards covering household and similar electrical appliances, such as the IEC 60335 family of standards. In order to obtain FDA marketing clearance for over-the-counter sale of HUDs in the United States, some consumer device manufacturers have sought to comply with existing laser and lamp standards as far as they could be reasonably applied. These have included the current IEC "parent" standard for lasers, 60825-1 and the IEC 60601 family of standards, which were largely formulated for professional medical, dental, diagnostic, and cosmetic electrical equipment.

The European Medical Device Regulation (MDR), published in March 2017 and scheduled for full implementation by May 2020 but delayed by the COVID-19 pandemic to March 2021, seeks to capture all equipment emitting high-intensity electromagnetic radiation (e.g., infrared, visible light, and ultraviolet) intended for use on the human body, including coherent and non-coherent sources, monochromatic, and broad spectrum, such as lasers and IPL equipment, for skin resurfacing, tattoo or hair removal, or other skin treatments. This includes those groups of products without an intended medical purpose [57]. As these products are not covered by Harmonised Standards, the MDR contains a provision for an alternative to Harmonised Standards—namely, Common Specifications (CS). The challenge for the European regulator and its expert groups is to develop suitable Common Specifications that can be used by manufacturers of these appliances before full implementation of the MDR. Manufacturers of HUDs will need a new quality management system and involve notified bodies, and further product evaluation (e.g., post-market clinical follow-up studies [PMCF]) will comply with safety and performance (efficacy) requirements for medical products.

Until 2012, evidence-based guidelines on light-based, home-use hair removal devices did not exist for this new product category. No national, European, or international guidelines had been established for the treatment of unwanted body and facial hair. Based on the available literature, an independent group of experts developed "Guidelines on the Safety of Light-Based Home-Use Hair Removal Devices from the European Society for Laser Dermatology," which is recognized in the EU [58].

36.7.2 Regulations outside the European Union and the United States

International efforts continue to develop consistency in regulatory frameworks, and in the EU and the United States, regulatory controls usually include a three-tiered approach:

- Pre-market assessment, assuring quality and safety for sale
- In-market monitoring of advertising, claims, and labeling
- Post-market surveillance to check adverse events and ensure continuing safety in use

While Australia and New Zealand treat home-use light-based devices in a similar way to other household electrical appliances as in the EU, no clear pattern is seen in most other world markets.

Japanese and Chinese manufacturers produce significant numbers of home-use lasers and intense light devices, which are both exported and actively sold in the domestic market. However, the regulatory position of such devices in Japan and China is at best ambiguous, with strong opinions expressed by professional interest groups about who should use light-based devices, such as lasers, but are not backed by any visible statutory framework or guidelines from government ministries. Despite many anecdotal reports of adverse events in the media and at national medical conferences, between 1999 and 2003, there were only seven complaints to the Consumers' Centre of the Tokyo Metropolitan Government about home-use laser hair removal devices.

36.8 Where Does This Leave the Professional Practitioner and the Client?

First, experts in the field need to recognize that HUDs are already here and growing in number and popularity. Some devices are ineffective, and some may not be safe. They must be informed about the devices themselves and be ready to "pick up the pieces" when home-use treatments go wrong. Opportunities should be explored to use proven HUDs alongside our own professional treatments (e.g., for ongoing homecare top-up treatments as part of a total professional treatment regimen).

Second, light-based HUDs are not suitable for all skin types (usually excluding phototypes V–VI), and most FDA clearances do not so far allow use on the face and neck. These HUDs also require significantly more treatments than is commonplace in the clinic environment where higher fluences, larger spot sizes, and faster repetition rates permit a speedier and more efficient treatment with the reassurance of professional counseling and support.

Third, many consumers will be uncertain about issues of safety, suitability for use with underlying medical conditions (e.g., diabetes, epilepsy, hormonal conditions), and contraindicated medication.

Last, many home-device users will still require professional treatments for difficult body areas and conditions not treatable at home, such as intimate body areas, backs, pilonidal sinus, pseudofolliculitis barbae, polycystic ovaries, acne, and benign pigmented and vascular lesions.

As experts in this field, we must maintain our professional position and be ready to offer paid-for consultation support to cosmetic clients seeking help in resolving any issues related to self-treatments or offering in-salon treatments where HUDs are unsuitable.

As the beauty industry has seen with previous examples of home-use products, home waxing kits and home electrolysis have had no impact on professional services. Another example is the recent popularising of at-home teeth-whitening among consumers, which has driven the demand for professional treatments in almost every dental practice in the UK. With the recent increased publicity for home-use laser and IPL devices and the consequential raising of consumer understanding and awareness, it is reasonable to suppose that the same may already be true of driving demand for professional hair removal and skin rejuvenation treatments.

36.9 Conclusion

The HUD category is a new and fast emerging market worth many millions of dollars annually. The emergence of HUDs reflects the needs of an aging, wealthy, and wellness-oriented population. These new miniaturized products and appliances entering the market employing powerful and complex technology do, however, raise some health concerns. Safety standardization and national regulation, however, seem to be somewhat behind the market development.

Manufacturers are strongly motivated to provide safe products in order to make products available to as wide a consumer base as possible and to avoid negative press coverage and expensive litigation.

Notes

1 IEC 60601-2-57:2011, Medical electrical equipment – Part 2–57: Particular requirements for the basic safety and essential performance of non-laser light source equipment intended for therapeutic, diagnostic, monitoring and cosmetic/aesthetic use.
2 IEC 60335-2-113:2016, Household and similar electrical appliances – Safety – Part 2–113: Particular requirements for cosmetic and beauty care appliances incorporating lasers and intense light sources.
3 IEC 60601-2-83: 2019, Medical electrical equipment—Part 2–83: Particular requirements for the basic safety and essential performance of home light therapy equipment.
4 IEC 60825-1:2014, Safety of laser products – Part 1: Equipment classification and requirements.
5 IEC TR 60825-14:2004, Safety of laser products – Part 14: A user's guide.
6 IEC 62471:2006, Photobiological safety of lamps and lamp systems.

References

[1]. Hodson DS. "Current and future trends in home laser devices," *Semin Cutan Med Surg.* 2008; 27:292–300.

[2]. Brown AS. "At-home laser and light-based devices,". *Curr Probl Dermatol.* 2011; 42:160–165.

[3]. Metelitsa AI, Green JB. "Home-use laser and light devices for the skin: An update," *Semin Cutan Med Surg.* 2011; 30(3):144–147. [PubMed: 21925367].

[4]. Keller EC. "Home-use devices in aesthetic dermatology," *Semin Cutan Med Surg.* 2014; 33:198–204.

[5]. Hession MT, Markova A, Graber EM. "A review of hand-held, home-use cosmetic laser and light devices," *Dermatol Surg.* 2015; 41:307–320.

[6]. Greaves A.J. "The effects of narrow bands of visible light upon some skin disorders: A review," *Int J Cosmet Sci.* 2016; 38:325–345. doi: 10.1111/ics.12305.

[7]. Juhasz MLW, Levin MK, Marmur ES. "A review of available laser and intense light source home devices: A dermatologist's perspective," *J Cosmet. Dermatol.* 2017; 16:438–443.

[8]. Rohrer TE, Chatrath V, Yamauchi P, et al. "Can patients treat themselves with small a novel light based hair removal system?" *Laser Surg Med.* 2003; 33:25–29.

[9]. Manstein D, Pourshagh M, Anderson R. "Effects of fluence and pulse duration for flashlamp exposure on hair follicles," *Presented at the 21st Annual ASLMS Meeting.* New Orleans, 2001. *Lasers Surg Med.* 2001; 28:S13:46.

[10]. Nuijs T, Evers L, Roosen G, Westgate G, Bjerring P, van Kemenade P, Roersma M, "Clinical and in-vitro investigation of low-fluence photoepilation with an IPL system," Abstract 117 *Lasers Surg Med.* 2008; 40:S20.

[11]. Nuijs T, Bartula L, Reiter S, van den Broek L. "Long-term hair reduction with a home-use IPL device," Abstract 68 *Laser Surg Med.* 2014; 46:S25:22–23. doi: 10.1002/lsm.22229.

[12]. Drosner M, Stangl S, Hertenberger B, et al. "Low dose epilation by alexandrite laser: A dose response study," *Med Laser Appl.* 2001; 16:293–298.

[13]. Braun M. "Permanent laser hair removal with low fluence high repetition rate versus high fluence low repetition rate 810 nm diode laser—a split leg comparison study," *JDD.* 11/2009; 8(11 Suppl):s14–s17.

[14]. Roosen G, Westgate G, Philpott M, Berretty P, Nuijs T, Bjerring P. "Temporary hair removal by low fluence photoepilation: Histological study on biopsies and cultured human hair follicles," *Lasers Surg Med.* 2008; 40: 520–528.

[15]. Trelles M, Ash C, Town G. "Clinical and microscopic evaluation of long-term epilation effects of the iPulse personal home-use intense pulsed light (IPL) device," *J Eur Acad Dermatol Venereol.* 2014; 28(2): 160–168.

[16]. Town G, Uzunbajakava N, Nuijs A, van Vlimmeren M, Botchkareva N, Ash C, Dierickx C. "Light-based home-use devices for hair removal: Why do they work and how effective they are?" *Lasers Sur Med.* 2018 Accepted for publication 2018 Jan 3. doi: 10.1002/lsm.23061. [Epub ahead of print].

[17]. Hodson DS. "Current and future trends in home laser devices," *Semin Cutan Med Surg.* 2008; 27:292–300.

[18]. Thaysen-Petersen D, Bjerring P, Dierickx C, Nash JF, Town G, Haedersdal M. "A systematic review of light-based home-use devices for hair removal and considerations on human safety," *J Eur Acad Dermatol Venereol.* 2012; 26(5):545–553. doi: 10.1111/j.1468-3083.2011.04353.x. Epub. 2011 Nov 30.

[19]. Town GA, Ash C, Eadie E, Moseley H. "Measuring key parameters of intense pulsed light (IPL) devices," *J Cosmet Laser Ther.* 2007; 9:3:148–160.

[20]. Thomas G, Ash C, Hugtenburg R, Kiernan M, Town G, Clement M. "Investigation and development of a measurement technique for the spatial energy distribution of home-use intense pulsed light (IPL) systems," *J Med Eng Technol.* 2011; 35:3–4:191–196.

[21]. Town G, Ash C. "Do home-use hair removal lasers & intense light devices deliver what they promise?" *J Cosmet Surg Med.* 2010; 5:3:48–55.

[22]. Town G, Ash C. "Measurement of home use laser and intense pulsed light systems for hair removal: Preliminary report," *J Cosmet Laser Ther.* 2009; 11:157–168.

[23]. Town G, Ash C. "Are home-use intense pulsed light (IPL) devices safe?" *Lasers Med Sci.* 2010; 25:773–780.

[24]. Town G, Bjerring P. "Is paradoxical hair growth caused by low-level radiant exposure by home-use laser and intense pulsed light devices?" *J Cosmet Laser Ther.* 2016; 18:6:355–362.

[25]. Schmitt L, Resai K, Karsai S. "Are IPL home devices really foolproof?" Letters to the Editor. *JEADV.* 2016; 30:857–858.

[26]. Thaysen-Petersen D, Erlendson AM, Nash JF, et al. "Ultraviolet radiation after exposure to a low-fluence IPL home-use device: A randomized clinical trial," *Lasers Med Sci.* 2015; 30:2171–2177. doi: 10.1007/s10103-015-1796-4.

[27]. Thaysen-Petersen, D., Lin, J. Y., Nash, J., Beerwerth, F., Wulf, H. C., Philipsen, P. A. & Haedersdal, M. "The role of natural and UV-induced skin pigmentation on low-fluence IPL-induced side effects: A randomized controlled trial," *Lasers Surg Med.* 2014; 46:104–111.

[28]. Friedman DP, Mishra V, Buckley S. "Keloidal scarring from the at-home use of intense pulsed light for tattoo removal," *Lett Commun Dermatol Surg.* 2017; 43:8 1113–1114.

[29]. Brit CJ, Marcus B. "Energy-based facial rejuvenation: Advances in diagnosis and treatment," *Lasers Med Sci.* 2017; 19:1:64–71. doi: 10.1001/jamafacial.2016.1435.

[30]. Dams SD, Liefde-van Best M.de, Nuijs AM, Oomens CWJ, Baaijens FPT. "Pulsed heat shocks enhance procollagen type I and procollagen type II expression in human dermal fibroblasts," *Skin Res Technol.* 2010; 16:354–364.

[31]. Leyden J, Stephens TJ, Herndon JH. "Multicenter clinical trial of a home-use non-ablative fractional laser device for wrinkle reduction," *J Am Acad Dermatol.* 2012; 67:(5):975–984.

[32]. Whelan HT, Houle JM, Donohue DL, Bajic DM, Schmidt MH, Reichert KW et al., "Medical applications of space light emitting diode technology—Po¨ space station and beyond," *Space Technol Appl Int Forum.* 1999; 458:3–15.

[33]. Whelan HT, Houle JM, Whelan NT, Donohue DL, Cwiklinski J, Schmidt MH et al. "The NASA light-emitting diode medical program—Po¨ progress in space flight and terrestrial applications," *Space Technol Appl Int Forum.* 2000; 504:37–43.

[34]. Calderhead GR, Vasily DB. "Low level light therapy with light-emitting diodes for the aging face," *Clin Plastic Surg.* 2016; 43:541–550.

[35]. Haltaufderhyde K, Ozdeslik R N, Wicks N L, Najera J A, Oancea E. "Opsin expression in human epidermal skin," *Photochem Photobiol.* 2015; 91:117–123.

[36]. Kim H J, Son E D, Jung J Y, Choi H, Lee T R, Shin D W. "Violet light down-regulates the expression of specific differentiation markers through Rhodopsin in normal human epidermal keratinocytes," *PLoS One.* 2013; 8:e73678.

[37]. Karu TI, Kolyakov SF, "Exact action spectra for cellular responses relevant to phototherapy," *Photomed Laser Surg.* 2005; 23:355–361.

[38]. Karu TI, Pyatibrat LV, Afanasyeva NI. "Cellular effects of low power laser therapy can be mediated by nitric oxide," *Lasers Surg Med.* 2005; 36:307–314.

[39]. Karu TI, Pyatibrat LV, Kolyakov SF, Afanasyeva NI. "Absorption measurements of a cell monolayer relevant to phototherapy: Reduction of cytochrome c oxidase under near IR radiation," *J Photochem Photobiol B.* 2005; 81:98–106.

[40]. Ohshiro T, Calderhead RG. *Low level laser therapy: A practical introduction.* Chichester, UK: John Wiley & Sons, Limited; 1968.

[41]. Ohshiro T. *Low reactive-level laser therapy: Practical application,* Chichester, UK: John Wiley & Sons, Limited; 1991.

[42]. Leyden J, Stephens TJ, Herdon JH. Multicenter clinical trial of a home-use nonablative fractional laser device for wrinkle reduction. *J Acad Dermatol.* 2012; 67(5):975–984.

[43]. Otberg N, Finner AM, Shapiro J. Androgenetic alopecia, *Endocrinol Metab Clin North Am.* 2007; 36(2):379–398. doi: 10.1016/j.ecl.2007.03.004.

[44]. Wikramanayake TC et al. "Effects of the Lexington LaserComb on hair regrowth in the C3H/HeJ mouse model of alopecia areata," *Lasers Med Sci.* 2012; 27:431–436. doi: 10.1007/s10103-011-0953-7.

[45]. Mignon C, Botchkareva NV, Uzunbajakava NE, Tobin DJ. "Photobiomodulation devices for hair regrowth and wound healing: A therapy full of promise but a literature full of confusion," *Exper Dermatol.* 2016; 25(10):745–749. doi: 10.1111/exd.13035.

[46]. Fargan K, Frei D, Fiorella D, McDougal C, Myers P, Hirsch J, Mocco J, "The FDA approval process for medical devices: An inherently flawed system or valuable pathway for innovation?" *J. NeuroInterv Surg.* 2013; 5(4):269–275. doi: 10.1136/neurintsurg-2012-010400. Epub. 2012 Jul 4.

[47]. Keane SA. "Illuminating current pitfalls in optimal photobiomodulation device development and assessment for treating hair loss," *Exp Dermatol.* 2016; 25(10):758–759. doi: 10.1111/exd.13142.

[48]. Fisher MR, Abel M, Lopez Kostka S, et al. "Blue light irradiation suppresses dendritic cells activation *in vitro*," *Exp Dermatol.* 2013; 22:558–560. doi: 10.1111/exd.12193.

[49]. Le Pillouer-Prost L, Cartier H. "Photodynamic rejuvenation: A review," *Dermatol Surg.* 2016; 42(1):21–30. doi: 10.1097/DSS.0000000000000528.

[50]. Philipp-Dormston WG, Sanclemente G, Torezan L, Tretti Clementoni M, Le Pillouer-Prost A, Szeimies RM, Bjerring P. "Daylight photodynamic therapy with MAL cream for large-scale photodamaged skin based on the concept o' 'actinic field dama'e': Recommendations of an international expert group," *Eur Acad Dermatol Venerol.* 2016; 30(1): 8–15. doi: 10.1111/jdv.13327. Epub. 2015 Nov 9.

[51]. Kjeldstad B, Johnsson A. "An action spectrum for blue and near Ultraviolet inactivation of propionibacterium acnes; With emphasis on a possible porphyrin," *Photochem. Photobiol.* 1986 43, 67–70.

[52]. Dai T, Gupta A, Murray CK, et al. "Blue light for infectious diseases: Propionibacterium acnes, Helicobacter pylori, and beyond?" *Drug Resist Updat.* 2015; 15:223–236. doi: 10.1016/j.drup.2012.07.001. Epub. 2012 Jul 28.

[53]. Eadie E, Miller P, Goodman T, Moseley H. "Assessment of the optical radiation hazard from a home-use intense pulsed light (IPL) source," *Laser Surg Med.* 2009; 40:520–528.

[54]. IEC 60335–2–113:2016, "Household and similar electrical appliances—safety—part 2–113: Particular requirements for cosmetic and beauty therapy appliances incorporating lasers and intense light sources," Available at: https://webstore.iec.ch/publication/24535.

[55]. Ash C, Town G, Whittall R, Tooze L, Phillips J. "Lasers and intense pulsed light (IPL) association with cancerous lesions," *Lasers Med Sci.* 2017 Nov; 32(8):1927–1933.

[56]. Town G, Gorisch W. *International progress in standards and regulation for light-based home-use devices* (Paper No: 104). Orlando, FL: Proceedings of the ILSC, 2013 Mar 18–21.

[57]. Regulation (EU) 2017/745 of the European Parliament and of the Council of 5 April 2017 on medical devices, amending Directive 2001/83/EC, Regulation (EC) No 178/2002 and Regulation (EC) No 1223/2009 and repealing Council Directives 90/385/EEC and 93/42/EEC, Article 2: Definitions (1) <http://eur-lex.europa.eu/legal-content/EN/TXT/?uri=CELEX:32017R0745>.

[58]. Town G, Ash C, Dierickx C, Fritz K, Bjerring P, Haedersdal M. "Guidelines on the safety of light-based home-use hair removal devices from the European Society for Laser Dermatology (ESLD)," *J Eur Acad Dermatol Venereol.* 2012; 26(7):799–811. doi: 10.1111/j.1468-3083.2011.04406.x. Epub. 2012 Jan 3.

Part VI

CHAPTER 37: DIGITAL MARKETING AND SOCIAL MEDIA BRANDING

Wendy Lewis

Dermatologists acquire a wealth of knowledge and experience during their extensive training on how to manage the care of patients. However, what is rarely taught in medical school or residency is how to venture out into the real world with this expertise to actually practice dermatology and make a living. Of course, this is not specific to dermatology; rather, it is common among most medical specialties.

If you manage your own practice or run a small group practice, you will undoubtedly need to carve out some time to run your business, oversee the finances, hire staff, invest in the right technology, and plan the marketing to drive patients in the door. This will take quite a lot of time away from being able to take good care of patients. Regrettably, not all dermatologists are cut out to manage the business side of their practice, nor do they have the proper training to be successful at it. In fact, for many dermatologists I know, managing the nitty-gritty details of managing their practices is the last thing they really want to do.

In many ways, dermatologists have some distinct advantages over other specialists. The skin is the human body's largest organ;[1] thus, most people will be in need of medical attention at some point in their lives, leaving a massive group of potential patients to pull from. Organizations like the American Academy of Dermatology (AAD.org) and the European Academy of Dermatology and Venereology (EADV.org) are now offering informative programs to assist their members in learning about business matters.[2]

What has changed over the past five to ten years are the sweeping effects of digital marketing and social media on both the cosmetic and the general practice of dermatology. In fact, the growth of digital health and advice offered online have changed what consumers want, and dermatologists have shifted to keep up.[3] Patients are becoming more eager to take their healthcare into their own hands as more digital health platforms and apps are giving them the power to monitor many aspects of their skin health.

37.1 Dermatology Trends on Social Media

Today's dermatology residents are savvier about business and marketing than previous generations. This is partly due to the advent of digital marketing and the meteoric rise of social media in a relatively short period of time. It is also a necessity born out of the intense competition young dermatologists just out of residency face from well-established dermatology groups, plastic surgeons, and other medical specialties, as well as physician extenders and medspas offering many of the same or similar treatments.

It is abundantly clear that social media is where information is most widely shared and disseminated today. Instagram was launched in 2010, and 10,000 people downloaded it in the first few hours. Ten million joined in the following year. As of this printing, Instagram, which was bought by Facebook/Meta in 2012, has over 1.3 billion users.[4] If you want to get your message across to the general public and your own patients, the three social media channels are considered to be a must to be active on: Facebook, Instagram, and YouTube. However, this depends to a large extent on your geographic market and the demographic of patients you most want to attract. For example, TikTok has gained enormous traction since its inception in 2016 and most recently surpassed one billion users.[5] Although this app created in China initially became popular with younger millennials, it has blossomed to attract the attention of all age groups of consumers as well as a wide range of dermatologists.

The explosion of social media channels has created valuable opportunities for both aesthetic and medical dermatologists. Patients are flocking to social channels to get educated about their skin conditions, in particular acne, as well as a wide range of other concerns, including hair loss, pigmentation, rosacea, melasma, scarring, skin laxity, telangiectasia, and vascularity.

Searching on Instagram by hashtag revealed some of the key cosmetic issues that patients may be seeking out dermatologists for by the number of posts found in descending order.[6] The hashtags #dermatology and #dermatologist also ranked in the millions of posts:

#acne	10,661,998
#lipfiller	3,828,288
#hairloss	2,818,241
#melasma	2,235,926
#pigmentation	1,599,310
#rosacea	701,483
#darkspots	465,619
#dermatology	2,996,172
#dermatologist	1,556,314

More cosmetic procedures generate even higher levels of interest on many channels, such as #lipfiller as an example. Instagram is flooded with lip filler injections posted by patients and providers, and these tend to get very good engagement.

DOI: 10.1201/9780429243769-39

37.2 More Dermatologists Turn to Social Media to Communicate with Patients

It is understandable that more dermatologists would flock to the most popular social media channels to open a dialogue with consumers and potential patients. In addition, many dermatologists are quite frustrated with the high levels of misinformation found on social channels about skin issues and treatments, some of which may even be harmful. Although their primary goal may be to re-educate the public, this also presents an ideal way for dermatologists to join the conversation and elevate their own platforms.

Once upon a time, dermatologists who finished their training may have opened a solo practice, and in a relatively short period of time, patients would find them and their practice grew based on demand and referrals. This is not a feasible strategy today in many or most markets.

For example, I reside in New York City on the Upper East Side near many world-class cosmetic dermatologists. The results of a Google search for "Dermatologist near me" revealed "About 1,110,000,000 results (0.58 seconds)." This does not take into consideration the additional count of other practitioners who offer dermatologic procedures in my neighborhood. My search for "BOTOX near me" resulted in "About 153,000,000 results (0.63 seconds)." Try this exercise from your own practice to see how vast the competition is. It may be enlightening.

If you are still on the fence about whether or not to get active on social media, consider that a high percentage of your current patients, as well as the new patients you would like to bring into your practice, are definitely active. Therefore, if you are not present on at least the most relevant social media channels in your market, you may be restricting your visibility to key target audiences who are seeking out the treatments you specialize in.

37.3 Increasing Your Brand Awareness

To be successful at growing your practice and expanding your patient reach, consider how you can distinguish yourself from your top competitors. Focus on special areas of expertise, published articles, extensive training, speaking engagements, your media presence, research work, and anything else that will resonate with the patients you want to attract. Boosting your presence on social media is a reasonably cost-effective way to promote yourself early on in your career.

While you may have a personal Facebook or LinkedIn account as an individual, you will want to also create business

TABLE 37.1: Consumer-Facing Social Channels for Dermatologists

- Facebook
- Instagram
- YouTube
- TikTok
- WhatsApp
- Twitter
- Snapchat
- Pinterest
- WeChat

* Note these channels may not be popular or available in all markets.

accounts for your practice across multiple platforms, even if you are not ready to be active on them. Personal and business accounts should be maintained separately on all channels for safety and privacy.

Consider creating active accounts on any other channels that your target audience of patients spends time on. For example, TikTok started out attracting younger users, from teens to millennials. However, over time, most social channels will expand and become popular for older demographics. Therefore, even if you are currently treating a mature population who are keen to have age-reversing procedures such as dermal fillers, botulinum toxin, laser therapies, and body sculpting, they may be on TikTok now or in the near future. Thus, it is wise to reserve your practice name early on for channels that have the potential to be important for your practice down the road. If you don't reserve your name, you may find that another company or competitor has taken your practice name or brand, and you will be unable to get it back.

Casting a wider net across social channels can be effective in attracting more patients to your practice. Plan a strategy to leverage social media to accomplish the goals you have for your practice in the long term. You may be most eager to stay visible to your current patients, attract new patients, gain the attention of influencers and media, network with colleagues and partners, do more research studies, or some or all of these. Each of your goals may necessitate a slightly different strategy which can be more time-consuming. Start by focusing on one or two of your main goals and expand from there over time.

Many successful dermatology practices have now implemented a vigorous digital marketing and social media plan that includes an updated website featuring content on every service offered in detail, a web marketing plan designed to convert web traffic to leads to actual patients, an email platform to automate e-blasts directly to their patient base at specific intervals, plus a social media calendar to include boosting specific posts, promoting the most important posts, as well as taking advantage of many of the other tools available to get more eyes on their content.

37.4 Five Core Benefits of Social Media Marketing for Dermatologists

1. Increase opportunities to attract new patients
2. Increase brand awareness to build confidence in patients
3. Grow patient loyalty and encourage referrals
4. Improve patient retention by staying visible and relevant
5. Enhance per-patient revenue with additional treatments and services

37.5 Best Practices for Creating Compelling Content

The extensive rise of social media has changed the way patients want to interact with practitioners of all specialties, in particular cosmetic dermatologists. A sensible content strategy may include leveraging the most valuable channels to stay connected with your loyal patients, implementing an advertising strategy to reach a new patient base, plus ongoing efforts to raise awareness by utilizing the assets that appeal most to these unique audiences. To learn which content is performing best, check the analytics on each platform. If a specific type or format is working well, you will learn what your audience is most interested in and can go from there.

It is important to note that users of each channel want to absorb content in a specific way. Facebook offers the opportunity to write a lot of content and add videos, photos, memes, GIFs, emojis, and more. Many channels allow several forms of content to be posted in different ways. YouTube and TikTok, however, are all video-only. The format and tone of your content should also match the standards of the users on the channel. Spend some time on the channels of interest to you to see what kinds of content are getting good engagement for guidelines.

Instagram offers several opportunities to express your personality quite effectively. The Reels format is similar to TikTok, Instagram Live is a video platform where you can speak live to your audience, and the Stories format is used for short-form videos or still images with stickers and other special effects. Fortunately, most of the content you create for one channel can be repurposed for other channels by making a few changes in format tone and images.

Creating content that revolves around your most popular services, unique treatments, practice philosophy, special expertise and training, and superior outcomes can help to drive traffic to your practice website, where patients can schedule an appointment. Be sure to add contact information and utilize any live links that are available on each platform so users can take the next step to reach out to your practice directly. For example, Instagram allows only one live link, but you can change it as often as you want to direct followers as needed.

Video has evolved as a vital component of a successful digital marketing strategy. It is an invaluable asset in all forms of marketing today, from your practice website to the TikTok channel. People have developed very short attention spans over time, most especially younger generations. This accounts in part for the appeal of TikTok that started by limiting users to posting up to 15-second videos. Now users can string video clips together on most social channels. In general, short videos that get to the key points you want to make quickly tend to perform best.

During the pandemic and beyond, many dermatology practices started offering virtual consultations and follow-up visits. This trend is here to stay in all facets of healthcare and medicine. The concept of telemedicine in the form of virtual visits has gained popularity with patients and many doctors, as well as a time-saving and cost-effective measure. If you do offer virtual visits, it would be valuable to include this on all of your digital marketing channels, including your website, to attract patients who may be unable to travel or cannot break away from work or children to come in.

37.6 Monitoring Your Online Reputation

Reputation management has emerged as a critical success factor for all medical professionals, especially dermatologists,

who often tend to see many patients in a day of office hours. It is imperative to build and protect your online reputation because negative reviews can deter patients from coming to see you. Today, even patients who are referred by word of mouth will check out your reviews before scheduling an appointment. If your practice ranks lower than four out of five stars, you may be at risk.

Maintaining a solid reputation management strategy can turn negative reviews around by encouraging your real patients to leave reviews that are positive and honest. This process should never be done by coercion or any underhanded methods like payoffs or free treatments. Rather, simply letting your happy and loyal patients know that positive reviews are important to your practice in a subtle way can be effective. Posting your best reviews on social media channels and on your website may encourage other patients to leave a great review for you too.

This is also true of mishaps in social media management. A staff member or agency should be enlisted to monitor your social channels 24/7 to delete any abusive or inappropriate posts, respond to complaints or negative comments in a speedy fashion, and answer questions from fans and followers. Your social media presence offers a glimpse into your practice and brand, including who you are as a physician and how you care for your patients. Every detail counts.

37.7 Conclusion

Social channels are always in a state of flux, and algorithms, rules, and restrictions may change frequently with no advance notice. This can be very frustrating to busy dermatologists, and it is difficult to stay up-to-date without external assistance.

Despite all of the challenges, the value of social media for dermatologists, both medical and cosmetic specialists, is indisputable. You would be well-served to consider this vital marketing strategy for your practice in whatever way makes sense for your goals, staffing, bandwidth, and how much time you can set aside to be active. The less time you have to spend on social media, the more you may need to delegate these tasks to key staff members or consider an external marketing company to help manage the logistics for you.

References

1. https://pubmed.ncbi.nlm.nih.gov/21087182/.
2. www.aad.org/member/career/epm.
3. www.businessinsider.com/social-media-digital-health-dermatologists-compete-startups-2021-9.
4. www.abc.net.au/triplej/programs/hack/a-brief-history-of-the-first-10-years-of-instagram/12731664.
5. www.businessofapps.com/data/tik-tok-statistics/.
6. Instagram search as of 20 December 2021.

CHAPTER 38: NEWER COSMECEUTICALS

Zoe Diana Draelos

38.1 Introduction

Cosmeceuticals remain a scientifically undefined category for everyone except for the consumer. Consumers expect cosmeceuticals to deliver more skin benefits than a simple moisturizer, but many consumers purchase based on claims and are sadly disappointed. This drives a multi-billion dollar market driven by hope, dreams, and new product introductions. Advances in the availability of biologically derived skin-relevant materials have brought much new technology to the cosmeceutical category. This chapter will examine some of these novel ingredients added to moisturizers to provide skin benefits.

38.2 Peptide-Containing Cosmeceuticals

The ability to easily synthesize peptides has launched biologically modeled ingredients into the cosmeceutical marketplace. Since peptides, which are the building blocks of proteins, are felt to be safe, peptides can easily be added to moisturizers. Cosmeceutical peptides have been developed by fragmenting skin proteins hoping to induce some positive biological response. Thus, peptides may function as cellular messengers purported to induce receptor modulation, activate enzyme release, or regulate the production of proteins. Currently, marketed cosmeceutical peptides belong to the following functional families: carrier peptides, signal peptides, and neurotransmitter peptides.[1]

38.2.1 Carrier Peptides

The first cosmeceutical peptides to enter the marketplace were carrier peptides, so named because they are intended to attach to an active ingredient and facilitate the transport of the ingredient to the intended active skin site.[2] The first commercialized carrier peptide GHK-Cu was designed to deliver copper into wounds. It was used for ulcers and other open wounds to promote healing in high-risk patients, such as those with venous insufficiency and diabetes, based on the in vitro observation of increased dermal keratinocyte proliferation. Copper is a trace element important for wound healing, so it was theorized that increasing the copper concentration in a wound would promote wound closure.[3] The peptide was named GHK, indicating the order and presence of the following amino acids: glycine, histidyl, and lysine. This amino acid group was isolated from human plasma and synthetically replicated. GHK-Cu was commercialized as the active ingredient in a cosmeceutical designed to minimize the appearance of fine lines and wrinkles.

38.2.2 Signal Peptides

The most widely used peptide group in cosmeceuticals is signal peptides, which are designed in vitro to increase collagen, elastin, fibronectin, proteoglycan, and glycosaminoglycan production.[4] Pal-KTTKS, known as palmitoyl pentapeptide, is an example of a commercialized signal peptide composed of the amino acids lysine, threonine, threonine, lysine, and serine. This signal peptide is a fragment of procollagen I. In vitro, this peptide stimulated the production of collagen I, III, and IV.[5] Signal peptides are used in very low concentrations, such as four parts per million, whereby the "signal" initiates a cascading effect. It is theorized the procollagen fragments will downregulate collagenase production, thereby increasing dermal collagen synthesis; however, the exact mechanism of action is unknown.

38.2.3 Neurotransmitter Peptides

The final category of peptides is classified as neurotransmitter peptides functioning by inhibiting the release of acetylcholine at the neuromuscular junction. These peptides attempt to mimic the cutaneous effects of botulinum toxin, which selectively modulates the 25,000 Dalton synaptosome-associated proteins, known as SNAP-25. The most commonly used neurotransmitter peptide is acetyl hexapeptide-3, which mimics the N-terminal end of the SNAP-25 protein that inhibits the SNARE (soluble N-ethyl-maleimide-sensitive factor attachment protein receptor) complex formation.[6] Acetyl hexapeptide-3 inhibits vesicle docking through the prevention of the SNARE complex formation, inducing muscle relaxation. However, this is challenging in vivo since the prevention of the SNARE complex formation requires the ability to reach the neuromuscular junction molecularly intact with sufficient concentration to maintain the duration of effect.

38.3 Platelet-Rich Plasma Cosmeceuticals

Platelet-rich plasma (PRP) is a novel concept that has come to dermatology from orthopedic and dental surgery.[7–9] Platelets are composed of a cytoskeleton and intracellular structures such as glycogen, lysosomes, and two granules, the dense granule and the alpha granule. The dense granule contains adenosine diphosphate (ADP), adenosine triphosphate (ATP), serotonin, and calcium, while the alpha granule contains clotting factors, growth factors, and proteins.[10] PRP is defined as 1,000,000 platelets per microliter, as compared to the normal human blood platelet count of

DOI: 10.1201/9780429243769-40

150,000–350,000/microliter, in a small volume of plasma with a full complement of clotting factors.

The efficacy of PRP can be attributed to the[7] growth factors in the biological material: platelet-derived growth factors (PDGFaa, PDGFbb, PDGFab), transforming growth factors (TGF-b1, TGFb2), vascular endothelial growth factor (VEGF), and epithelial growth factor (EGF).[11, 12] PRP may have a role in facial rejuvenation cosmeceuticals for its ability to upregulate cellular mitogenesis and angiogenesis; however, PRP is typically used via injection and not topically.[13] It is prepared from freshly drawn blood from the patient with an added anticoagulant followed by centrifugation.[14] The first spin, known as the hard spin, separates the red blood cells from the plasma containing the platelets, white blood cells, and clotting factors. Three layers result from the hard spin: an upper layer containing platelets and white blood cells, a middle layer (known as the buffy coat) containing white blood cells, and a bottom layer containing red blood cells. The red-blood-cell layer is removed and discarded.

The second spin, known as the soft spin, separates the platelet-rich plasma in the bottom of the tube from the platelet-poor plasma (PPP) in the top of the tube by removing more red blood cells.[15] Proper preparation and centrifuge technique are critical to obtaining high-quality active PRP. PRP works through the degranulation of the alpha granules in platelets, which contain the growth factors. When the platelet becomes activated, the granules fuse to the cell membrane activating the secretory growth factors, which bind to the transmembrane receptors of target cells, such as mesenchymal stem cells, fibroblasts, endothelial cells, and epidermal cells.[16] This binding activates intracellular signal proteins that express a gene sequence directing cellular proliferation, collagen synthesis, extracellular matrix formation, and numerous other pathways to promote healing and repair processes.[17]

Injection of PRP is typically carried out immediately after preparation; however, topical uses for PRP are now being popularized. PRP can be added to a stabilizing moisturizing vehicle to deliver benefits topically to the skin with or without penetration enhancement. The PRP cosmeceutical must be refrigerated at 4°C to maintain PRP stability, and the vehicle must be carefully constructed not to destroy the platelets. This means a special selection of preservatives and incorporation of nutrient sources for the platelets.

Topical PRP is part of the new wave of personalized cosmeceuticals gaining popularity where biological materials from the patient are used to develop active moisturizers only for personal use. Since the cosmeceutical contains autologous blood products, no one other than the biological donor can use it. It is also necessary to have a knowledgeable physician properly prepare the PRP and put it into formulation. Typically, one bottle of customized PRP will be stable for around[3] months refrigerated, requiring quarterly preparation.

38.4 Prebiotic, Probiotic, and Postbiotic Cosmeceuticals

Another area of active innovation is the development of cosmeceuticals designed to maintain or modify the skin microbiome. Actually, all cosmeceuticals interact with the skin microbiome in one dimension or another. The skin is covered with over 100 species of bacteria with one million microorganisms per square centimeter: Actinobacteria (51.8%), Firmicutes (24.4%), Proteobacteria (16.5%), Bacteriodetes (6.3%), fungi (*Malassezia* species), and mites (*Demodex* species).[18] The composition of the

skin microbiome varies based on the body area affected by apocrine, eccrine, and sebaceous gland secretions.[19] Microbiome-based cosmeceuticals attempt to improve skin health by "improving" or "normalizing" the skin bacterial colonization.

There are three types of microbiome-based cosmeceuticals: prebiotics, probiotics, and postbiotics. Each of them will be discussed. Prebiotics are substances that promote the growth of beneficial organisms and inhibit harmful organisms on the skin surface. Oral prebiotic substances include the nondigestible carbohydrates found in fibrous foods, such as legumes, whole wheat, garlic, onions, oats, and berries. These foods contain fructo-oligosaccharides and galacto-oligoaccharides providing nutrition for beneficial bacteria. These sugars can be applied topically to provide nutrition for beneficial bacteria. Most prebiotic skin care products are based on sugars or plant oils. This is not a new concept. Many currently marketed skin care products contain sugars, such as glucose, which can be used as a natural thickening agent. Plant oils are also commonly incorporated into current cosmeceuticals, such as sesame, olive, hemp, and grapeseed oils. These oils have been used as occlusive moisturizers for many years, but now these ingredients are being repurposed as the basis for prebiotic cosmeceuticals.

The second type of microbiome-based cosmeceuticals is probiotics. Probiotics cosmeceuticals contain live bacteria, usually dairy propionic bacteria organisms, designed to repopulate the skin. However, it is not easy to modify the skin microbiome. For a probiotic cosmeceutical to be effective, the bacteria must adhere to the skin, must be capable of transient colonization, must exhibit resistance toward potential pathogens, and must produce antimicrobial substances.[20] In vitro studies have demonstrated a 4–16% propionic bacteria adhesion rate to the stratum corneum in some preparations.[21]

It is very difficult to formulate probiotic skin care products because preservatives will destroy the bacteria, which is what preservatives are designed to kill. True probiotic cosmeceuticals must be refrigerated and will only remain stable for about two weeks. Most consumers are not willing to invest this type of time and money in cosmeceuticals; thus, many probiotic skin preparations contain ultrasound-inactivated bacterial extracts from propionic acid bacteria (PAB) since dead bacteria can exist in unrefrigerated, preservative-containing cosmeceuticals.[22]

Probiotic cosmeceuticals may also contain fermented bacterial ingredients, not necessarily live bacteria. The theory is that the topical bacterial extracts may provide a protective shield through competitive inhibition of binding sites preventing colonization by pathogenic bacteria.[23, 24] This concept is known as bacterial interference. Staph epidermis, a nonpathogenic bacteria, has been demonstrated to inhibit the growth of p. acnes, the causative bacteria for acne.[25] Much research is currently ongoing to develop cosmeceuticals capable of modifying the facial microbiome based on bacterial interference.

Finally, postbiotic cosmeceuticals contain non-viable bacterial products or metabolic by-products from probiotic bacteria. Postbiotics are produced during the fermentation process. Examples of postbiotics include enzymes, peptides, peptidoglycan-derived muropeptides, polysaccharides, cell surface proteins, and organic acids. The use of postbiotics is not new in skin care. Bacterial fermentation products include glycerol and lactic acid, both of which have been used in therapeutic moisturizers in dermatology for many years.

The microbiome is becoming a very important concept in cosmeceutical formulation. It appears that microbial biodiversity is key to healthy skin. Microbiome-based cosmeceuticals include sugar and oil prebiotics to promote bacterial growth, bacterial lysate probiotics to change the microbiome, and postbiotics containing bacterial fermentation by-products.

38.5 Conclusion

Cosmeceuticals are developing sophisticated technologies based on the current scientific literature, yet they must remain within the unregulated cosmetic space taking care not to enter the highly regulated pharmaceutical space. Thus, claims are carefully constructed to only describe appearance benefits and not physiological benefits. The commercialization of peptides designed to modify cellular behavior will continue to expand as more fragments of skin structures are developed. Topical PRP is just in its infancy but heralds the development of the personalized cosmeceutical market. Finally, microbiome-modifying products can produce important physiological changes without ever entering the body. Developing topical product technology will continue to provide more sophisticated cosmeceuticals in the future.

Frequently Asked Questions

1. Q: *When is the best time to apply lip balm?*
   A: The best time to apply lip balm is at night when the lips are at rest. Lip balm places an oily or waxy film over the lips stopping transepidermal water loss from the transitional mucosa. Patients who mouth breathe at night tend to have extra dry lips, and a nighttime lip balm is definitely recommended.

2. Q: *What can be done easily for under-eye bags?*
   A: There are many factors contributing to undereye bags, including extracellular fluid. During sleep at night, this fluid distributes evenly to all tissues; however, during the day gravity draws fluid to the feet. In the morning, the under-eye tissue may be puffier due to edema in the skin under the eye. During the day, while standing, this extracellular fluid will be drawn by gravity to the feet. Sleeping with the head elevated on several pillows is the quickest way to minimize under-eye edema, termed under-eye bags by consumers.

3. Q: *How does charcoal face wash work?*
   A: A new fad in facial cleansing is ground charcoal. Charcoal can be added to facial cleansers to work as an exfoliant since the particles are slightly rough and can be rubbed over the face to induce desquamation and improve skin smoothness. Ground nut pits can also be used for the same purpose. Some charcoal products claim to aid in oil control; however, the charcoal does not remain on the skin surface long enough to absorb much oil.

4. Q: *Does clinical strength antiperspirant work better than regular antiperspirant?*
   A: Clinical strength antiperspirants do work better than regular antiperspirants, but for one very good reason. They are applied twice a day, once in the morning and once before going to bed. Clinical strength products do contain an increased amount of antiperspirant ingredients, but the most important aspect is the evening application. Most people do not sweat as much at night, so the antiperspirant remains in the armpit longer and is not washed away by sweat. Twice daily application of antiperspirants is necessary for optimal performance.

5. Q: *How can you fix hair split ends?*
   A: Unfortunately, hair split ends cannot be fixed, only temporarily mended. Split ends occur when the hair cuticle is missing. The protective cuticle is lost with repeated hair trauma, such as shampooing, brushing, combing, and so on. Once the cuticle is lost, the next layer, known as the cortex, is traumatized, exposing the weak medulla. The medulla then splits and causes the appearance at the end of the hair shaft, known as split ends. Split ends can be temporarily mended by sticking the pieces of the medulla back together. Conditioners can effect this change, making the hair ends less frizzy; however, the conditioner is removed with shampooing, at which time it must be reapplied.

References

1. Litner K. Peptides, amino acids and proteins in skin care? *Cosmet Toilet.* 2007;122:26–34.
2. Gruchlik A, Jurzak M, Chodurek E, Dzierzewicz Z. Effect of Gly-Gly-His, Gly-His-Lys and their copper complexes on TNF-alpha-dependent IL-6 secretion in normal human dermal fibroblasts. *Acta Pol Pharm.* 2012;69(6):1303–1306.
3. Maquart FX, Pickart L, Laurent M, et al. Stimulation of collagen synthesis in fibroblast cultures by the tripepetide-copper complex glycyl-L-histidyl-L-Cu²⁺. *FEBS Lett.* 1988;238:343–345.
4. Zhang L, Falla TJ. Cosmeceuticals and peptides. *Clin Dermatol.* 2009;27(5):485–489.
5. Katayama K, Armendariz-Borunda J, Raghow R, et al. A pentapeptide from type I procollagen promotes extracellular matrix production. *J Biol Chem.* 1993;268:9941–9944.
6. Blanes-Mira C, Cemente J, Jodas G, et al. A synthetic hexapeptide (Argireline) with antiwrinkle activity. *Int J Cosmet Sci.* 2002;24:303–310.
7. Sommeling CE, Heyneman A, Hoeksema H, Verbelen J, Stillaert FB, Monstrey S. The use of platelet-rich plasma in plastic surgery: A systematic review. *J Plast Reconstr Aesthet Surg.* 2013;66:301–311.
8. Carter MJ, Fylling CP, Parnell LKS. Use of platelet rich plasma gel on wound healing: A systematic review and meta-analysis. *Eplasty.* 2011;11:e38.
9. Li ZJ, Choi HI, Choi DK, Sohn KC, Im M, Seo YJ, Lee YH, et al. Autologous platelet-rich plasma: A potential therapeutic tool for promoting hair growth. *Dermatol Surg.* 2012;38:1040–1046.
10. Everts PA, Knape JT, Weibrich G, Schönberger JP, Hoffmann, J, Overdevest EP, Box, HA, van Zundert A. Platelet-rich plasma and platelet gel: A review. *J Extra Corpor Technol.* 2006;38(3):174–187.
11. Eppley BL, Pietzak WS, Blanton M. Platelet rich plasma: A review of biology and applications in plastic surgery. *Plast Reconstr Surg.* 2006;118:147e–159e.
12. Marx RE. Platelet-rich plasma (PRP): What is PRP and what is not PRP? *Implant Dentistry.* 2001;10:225–228.
13. Sclafani AP, Azzi J. Platelet preparations for use in facial rejuvenation and wound healing: A critical review of current literature. *Aesthec Plast Surg.* 2015;39:495–505.
14. Dhurat R, Sukesh M. Principles and methods of preparation of platelet-rich plasma: A review and authors perspective. *J Cutan Aesthet Surg.* 2014;7(4):189–197.
15. Boswell SG, Cole BJ, Sundman EA, Karas V, Fortier LA. Platelet-rich plasma: A milieu of bioactive factors. *Arthroscopy.* 2012;28:429–439.
16. Sclafani AP, McCormick SA. Induction of dermal collagenesis, angiogenesis, and adipogenesis in human skin by injection of platelet-rich fibrin matrix. *Arch Facial Plast Surg.* 2012;14:132–136.
17. Eppley BL, Pietrzak WS, Blanton M. Platelet-rich plasma: A review of biology and applications in plastic surgery. *Plast Reconstr Surg.* 2006;118:147e.
18. Grice EA, Kong HH, et al. Topographical and temporal diversity of the human skin microbiome. *Science.* 2009;324(29):1190–1192.
19. Kong HH, Segre JA. Skin microbiome: Looking back to move forward. *JID.* 2012;132:933–939.
20. Zeeuwen P, Boekhorst J. et al. Microbiome dynamics of human epidermis following skin barrier disruption. *Genome Biology.* 2012;13:R101.
21. Seite S, Zelenkova H, Martin R. Clinical efficacy of emollients in atopic dermatitis patients. *Clin Cosmet Investig Dermatol.* 2017;10:25–33.
22. Ouwehad AC, Batsman A, Salminen S. Probiotics for the skin. *Lett Appl Microbiol.* 2003;36:327–331.
23. Gueniche A, Bastien P, Ovigne. Bifidobacterium longum lysate. *Exp Dermatol.* 2010;19(8).
24. Brook I. Bacterial interference. *Crit Rev Microbiol.* 1999;25:155–172.
25. Wang Y, Kuo S, Shu M, et al. Staph epi in the human skin microbiome mediates fermentation to inhibit the growth of P. acnes. *Appl Micro Biotechnol.* 2014;98(1):411–424.

CHAPTER 39: NEW DEVICES FOR TREATING DARKER SKIN TYPES

Paula Celeste Rubiano Mojica and Michael H. Gold

39.1 Introduction

One of the purposes of aesthetic treatment might be described as facial rejuvenation encompassing patient age, ethnicity, and sex, which yields the more accurate objective of facial harmonization—through correction of acquired (usually age-related) disharmonies, together with modification of congenital characteristics.

A recent survey in Australia showed that 85% of dermatologists do not feel confident in treating cosmetic issues in ethnic men; they would have liked more teaching in that field.[1]

Ethnic mixing, because of intermarriage, adds to the multiplicity of facial morphotypes. These considerations inform qualitative and quantitative differences in treatment.[2]

Variations in incidence and presentation of photoaging among ethnic groups are attributable in part to physical differences, for example, variations in fibroblast size and structure, and in part to differences in lifestyle.[2]

In the same way, understanding cultural differences and preferences among ethnic patients are as important as technical proficiency in procedures.

39.2 Ethnic Population

In this chapter, we will focus on treating darker skin types, which might reflect one of many phototypes seen in ethnic populations.

Ethnic populations are considered to be Africans, Caribbean people, Asians, Pacific Islanders, Latin Americans, Native Americans, Hispanics, Indians, and Middle Easterners.

There are some biological and pathophysiological differences between ethnic and fair skin that affect cosmetic treatment needs. The following are some general characteristics, but we emphasize that every patient is different, and the treatment should be individualized:

1. Patients of color have a thicker and more compact dermis and stratum corneum with more cornified layers than light-skinned patients.[1]
2. Due to increased melanin, patients with darker skin have inherent protection against extrinsic factors of aging, such as damage from ultraviolet light. Therefore, photoaging appears decades later compared with those with lighter skin tones. This photodamage is typically manifested as pigmentary aberrations such as lentigines, macules, melasma, and rhytides.[1]
3. Facial aging in these populations is due to volume loss from deeper muscular layers than from dermal layers.[1]
4. Perioral and periorbital lines may not occur as early in patients of color, but there is a tendency toward mid- and lower-face aging, including the formation of nasolabial folds and sagging of the jowl.[1]
5. Hair structure: Black individuals have flat elliptical-shaped hair shafts with curved hair follicles and fewer elastic fibers anchoring hair follicles to the dermis.[1]

Besides biological differences, there are also cultural aspects that differentiate cosmetic concerns, habits, and goals. We would like to encourage the development of culturally/gender-sensitive approaches to beauty, including advanced techniques.

39.3 Laser Tissue Interactions

Laser principles are important when treating darkly pigmented skin due to the increased melanin content within the epidermis, which will interfere with the absorption of laser energy intended for another target, which may lead to hyperpigmentation of the treated area.[3]

The darker skin of ethnic patients is more prone to dyschromia and scarring, which are common in cosmetics consultations.

It is critical to have a thorough medical history, where we must ask for isotretinoin regimen consumption before initiation of any laser surgical corrective procedure. Also, we should ask about any personal or family history of hereditary hemolytic diseases that may affect any postoperative healing, in addition to a history of scarring and keloidal tendency

In the pre-procedure consultation, it is very important to discuss the patient's expectations, post-operative period, and outcomes to be realistic for what we are planning to do.[3]

39.4 Anti-Aging Treatments

Energy-based devices such as those that harness energy from laser/lights and radiofrequency in combination with fillers, neurotoxins, and topical cosmeceuticals can reduce the appearance of wrinkles, pore size, and laxity and replete any areas of volume loss.

39.5 Lasers

Most laser therapy has been focused on Caucasian patients. However, nowadays, the face of aesthetics is more representative of the ethnic diversity of the population.

It is anticipated that by the year 2056, more than 50% of the US population will be of non-European descent, which brings a large number of ethnic patients with cosmetic concerns; thus, it is imperative for the dermatologist to recognize the unique needs of darker skin, risks, and benefits of cutaneous laser procedures.[3]

Lasers are the first line of therapy for the reduction of fine lines and wrinkling, textural abnormalities, and pore size. They have excellent safety profiles and, for most procedures, short downtimes.

For instance, the nonablative fractional laser resurfacing procedures can be used successfully in these types of patients due to the fact melanin is not at risk of targeted destruction. Candidates for this treatment include those with mild/moderate photodamage acne scarring and striae.[1]

An ideal treatment regimen typically includes a series of four to six treatments with low densities allowing for adequate recovery between sessions. Moreover, pre-treatment and post-treatment with hydroquinone or another skin-lightening medication are useful for preventing secondary or post-inflammatory hyperpigmentation. Also, there must be caution for patients with melasma or keloid scars.[1]

Kono and colleagues also demonstrated the safety and efficacy of a nonablative fractional 1550 nm laser in patients of color, noting that patient satisfaction was higher when their

DOI: 10.1201/9780429243769-41

skin was treated with high fluences than with high densities. Pore size reduction was also noticed in another study using the fractionated nonablative 1440 nm laser in 20 patients (skin types I–VI).[1, 3]

39.6 Radiofrequency

These devices transmit thermal energy to the dermal layers and can stimulate wound-healing mechanisms promoting collagen production and remodeling, which leads to skin rejuvenation.

The monopolar Thermage (Solta, Hayward, CA, USA) system has been shown to be effective in improving periorbital and jowl laxity in patients of darker skin types.[1]

The newest technologies have developed fractional microneedle radiofrequency in dark-skinned patients (three treatments, four-week intervals), showing improvement in periorbital wrinkling and high satisfaction.[1]

39.7 Microfocused Ultrasound

Mostly used for skin laxity, it delivers ultrasound energy to the reticular dermis and, by producing microcoagulation zones, stimulates denaturation, collagen remodeling, and skin rejuvenation without influencing the epidermal layer of the skin.[1]

The interesting feature for dark-skinned types is that this energy is not selectively absorbed by chromophores; therefore, it is safe for darker complexions that have excess laxity.

39.8 Toxins and Fillers

According to the Global Aesthetic Consensus (2), clinical data supports the safety and efficacy of botulinum toxin type A and hyaluronic acid fillers in persons of color. The general principles of individualized analysis and correction apply to every patient.

Men and women of all races may have brow furrows, glabellar creases, and crow´s feet.

Neurotoxins can give a more relaxed and youthful appearance.

It has been seen that in men, the treatment with neurotoxins should preserve a lower position of the brows and a flatter arch for a more male-looking end result.[1]

Botulinum toxin A is the most common neurotoxin used for the relaxation of glabellar frown lines and off-label for the relaxation of the upper and lower hyperkinetic muscles in patients of color. The response rate to botulinum toxin type A for aesthetic applications is very high. In cases of apparent nonresponses or partial responses to any toxin formulation, practitioners should first consider causes such as inappropriate patient selection, dosing, or placement of injection sites.[1]

A recent prospective study of onabotulinum toxin A raised the possibility of a biomechanical restoration, demonstrating increased skin pliability and elastic recoil after injection of the lateral orbital, forehead, and glabellar regions of 40 women.[2]

People with darker skin also present age-related muscle and volume loss, which can be fixed with volume repletion.

Ethnic skin has a reduced rate of collagen degradation. Therefore, fewer treatments may be needed to achieve volume restoration. The most common fillers used include hyaluronic acid (Juvederm; Allergan, Parsippany, NJ, USA), poly-L-lactic acid (Galderma, Fort Worth, TX, USA), and calcium hydroxylapatite (Radiesse; Merz Aesthetics, Raleigh, NC, USA).[1]

Deep volumizing fillers typically have a higher elasticity (G′), which confers firmness and resistance to applied forcés and a higher viscosity to give resistance to spread. For instance, the deep volumizer Vycross (Voluma) has a higher elasticity than the midlevel Vycross (Volift), which has a higher elasticity than the superficial volumizer (Volbella).[2]

Likewise, science-based selection of filler products and injection techniques allows a more evidence-based approach toward safety and efficacy. Treatment outcomes can be predicted by a product's scientific design in the context of its target tissue and the techniques that are used to implant it.

Histopathologic and ultrasonographic studies directly correlate a filler's viscosity and cohesivity to its pattern of spread and tissue integration after in vivo, intradermal implantation.[2]

Finally, there are some considerations to remember, such as minimizing the use of multiple puncture techniques due to more risk of hyperpigmentation, and keep in mind that the greatest benefits are obtained if patients return for treatment when the previous results start to diminish rather than after they disappear completely.

39.9 Skin Tone and Pigmentation Disorders

Pigmentation disorders are one of the most common complaints of dark-skinned patients; some in which laser therapy has been applied include melasma and post-inflammatory hyperpigmentation.

Melasma affects all ethnic groups but is more prevalent in fair-complected African American and Hispanic women living in tropical climates where the sun exposure is higher.[3]

The prevalence of melasma in men has been estimated to approximately 20%, and it is generally recognized to be more common in individuals with Fitzpatrick skin types IV–VI.[1]

Melasma and hyperpigmentation treatments include topical medications, chemical peels, lasers, and light but also involve an integrated regimen, in which we should encourage sun avoidance and the daily use of broad-spectrum ultraviolet A and B sunscreens with factor 30 or greater as one of the pillars of treatment.

It is important to counsel patients and communicate in the best way possible that photoprotection underscores all treatment modalities for disorders of pigmentation, and without photoprotection, minimal benefit will be seen with any other therapeutic option.

In addition, some patients may have both melasma and post-inflammatory hyperpigmentation (PIH), which makes it a really challenging treatment.

In regard to topical formulations, these do little to alleviate pigment centered in the dermal layer of skin, and prolonged use of topical hydroquinone may cause paradoxical hyperpigmentation due to exogenous ochronosis, and irritation secondary to topical retinoids may induce skin irritation, increasing the risk of PIH.[3]

The increased baseline pigment of the epidermis and larger melanosomes more widely distributed throughout epidermal keratinocytes confer a greater risk of dyschromia following laser procedures using wavelengths that have melanin as a chromophore.

However, energy-based devices are a good option for darker skin tones, and caution needs to prevent hypopigmentation and post-inflammatory hyperpigmentation. Here we present some of the most commonly used in daily practice:

1. Nd:YAG 1064 nm laser can penetrate and target deep dermal melanin while sparing the normal epidermal melanin.[1]
2. Picosecond lasers destroy melanocytes via high-pressure photoacoustic effect, decreasing thermal damage on surrounding structures.[1]
3. Fractionated microneedle radiofrequency creates microablation in the deep dermis and can improve texture, tone, and color in all skin types. There is little risk of hyperpigmentation because melanin is not the target.[1]

On the other hand, a prospective randomized study comparing tranexamic acid microinjections to microneedling followed by topical tranexamic acid application in 60 patients (Fitzpatrick skin types IV–V) with moderate to severe melasma showed that the combination of microneedling with tranexamic acid was superior in improving the Melasma Area Severity Index score with no adverse effects reported.[1]

As we noted, lasers that selectively target and destroy epidermal pigment should be efficacious in the treatment of dyschromias.

The wavelengths of the 510 nm pigmented lesion dye laser, 511 nm copper vapor laser, 514 nm argon laser, 694 nm ruby laser, and 755 nm alexandrite laser fall within the peak absorption spectrum of melanin, making them appropriate therapeutic options for the treatment of a range of epidermal and vascular lesions, including melasma and post-inflammatory hyperpigmentation; however, this little data were not conducted in ethnic patients populations.[3]

In order to bypass epidermal pigment, several studies have attempted pre-treating with an ablative laser to remove the epidermis, thereby decreasing intervening epidermal pigment between a Q-switched (QS) laser and dermal pigment. A combination of intense pulsed light (IPL) followed by a QS 1064 nm Nd:YAG fractionated laser also had a significant lightening effect in patients with type III–IV skin with no PIH noted.[4]

It has been hypothesized that the success of the treatment relied on the large action spectrum of the two lasers, with IPL covering epidermal pigment and dermal pigment covered by the QS Nd:YAG

Post-inflammatory hyperpigmentaton is likely to be resolved if the causative factor is eliminated, whereas melasma often needs ongoing or intermittent therapy. Topical hydroquinone or kojic acid preparations alone or in combination with chemical peels remain the treatment of choice, yet it has been seen that a combination of laser treatment does appear to be a viable option in patients with melasma unresponsive to topical therapy alone.

Optimizing laser parameters, such as increasing pulse durations, longer wavelengths, and attached cooling devices, minimize the risk of adverse events. Nonetheless, treatment of darkly pigmented patients continues to be associated with an increased risk of post-inflammatory hyperpigmentation (PIH) and prolonged erythema.

39.10 Acne and Other Scarring

Acne is a very common dermatoses in patients with darker skin, often accompanied by post-inflammatory hyperpigmentation and scarring, followed by increased fibroblast in the dermis, which might influence hypertrophic scarring following injury and more risk of keloid formation.[3]

With that said, it is prudent to initiate aggressive treatment in ethnic skin to avoid dyschromia and scarring, both of which can have a significant psychologic effect on the patient. Scars may or may not be dyschromic.

Note: Scars may or may not be dyschromic.

It is crucial to convey the goal of scar revision to the patient, which is to obtain a more aesthetically pleasing scar with improvement rather than perfection.

Without adequate treatment, the scarring and pigmentary changes may persist indefinitely despite the clearance of the acne itself. It is common to have different types of scarring at the same time. Thus, severe acne and acne scarring may be better treated with multiple modalities able to target the underlying lesions most effectively.

Dermabrasion is a procedure with diminished popularity since the mid-1990s and requires more technical skill but offers potentially fewer risks when treating patients with dark skin.

Ablative resurfacing lasers (CO_2, erbium [Er]) produce heat that is deposited into the dermis. The heat causes the collagen contraction necessary for the tightening effect desired when using these lasers to resurface for the improvement of rhytides.[3]

For the available nonablative laser-resurfacing technologies, such as the Nd:YAG 1320 nm, 1450 nm diode, and 1540 nm Er:YAG glass lasers, the laser beam penetrates through the epidermis without disruption to act on dermal collagen to induce remodeling. Studies show promising results and the potential to avoid the complications often seen with darker skin.[3]

Traumatic and postsurgical hypertrophic scars have been successfully treated with the 585 nm pulsed dye laser. Tumor thickness found in keloids limits the effectiveness of this therapy. Pigmented epidermis imposes additional limitations on the effective absorption of light energy by the target tissue because the epidermis absorbs and reflects the laser light energy.[3]

By using a combination of both ALA-PDT (5-aminolaevulinic acid-photodynamic therapy) treatment with an ablative fractional Er:YAG 2,940 nm laser in 40 patients with skin types III–IV, Yin et al. showed complete resolution of all active acne lesions after four to five monthly sessions and no new scars.[4]

ALA is applied to the face after extractions and exfoliation with a vibrating microdermabrasion system (Vibraderm, Grand Prairie, Texas) are performed. It is then degreased with acetone wash.

In a study using microfocused ultrasound (MFU-V) with the use of 1.5-mm- and 1-mm-depth probes, sebaceous glands are targeted for coagulation while bypassing the basal layer. Data from this pilot trial suggest that MFU-V could prove to be a promising novel treatment option to improve acne clearance in those with moderate to severe inflammatory acne.[4]

With the use of 1.5-mm and 1-mm depth probes, sebaceous glands are targeted for coagulation while bypassing the basal layer. Data from this pilot trial suggest that MFU-V could prove to be a promising novel treatment option to improve acne clearance in those with moderate to severe inflammatory acne.

Radiofrequency (RF) treatment devices use one or two electrodes to heat the dermis and cause collagen contraction and skin tightening. Thermal damage also recruits fibroblasts to the areas of injury, which increase collagen synthesis. When RF devices are combined with nonablative lasers, atrophic acne scars have been shown to improve by 60–72%.[4]

Additionally, high-intensity bipolar RF (Inni, Lutronic Inc., Burlington, Massachusetts) targets the dermis in a highly focused manner by varying the depth of the microneedles on the device. This technique bypasses the epidermis and directly heats the dermis to maximize remodeling beneath acne scars. This protective epidermal effect is particularly beneficial in pigmented skin while maintaining efficacy deeper in the tissue.[4]

There is also a treatment with the conditioned medium of adipose-derived stem cells (ADSCs) with the aim that the healing of laser-damaged skin would be accelerated. Following two passes of fractional CO_2 laser, there was a significant improvement.[4]

39.11 Facial Photodamage and Rejuvenation

Because of the photoprotective nature of melanin in patients with darker skin, crow's feet, lipstick lines, and fine perioral and periorbital lines seen as early as age 20 in the Caucasian patient tend to occur much later, if at all, in patients with darker skin.

Patients with darker skin, particularly African Americans, tend to manifest signs of aging in the deeper muscular layers of the face, with sagging of the malar fat pads toward the nasolabial folds.

A combination of ADSC and fractional CO_2 laser has shown efficacy for rejuvenation.[4]

It has been hypothesized that microscopic holes in the skin make drug delivery significantly enhanced; therefore, the growth factors in the ADSC medium should be able to more efficiently recruit dermal fibroblasts and increase dermal collagen.

Moreover, histological analysis showed increased dermal collagen density and more ordered collagen than the facial side treated with laser alone.

For the noninvasive treatment of wrinkles, a combination of optical energy with RF or heat energy is thought to work synergistically with each other. Twenty-three patients were treated for facial and neck wrinkles with up to three sessions of a combination diode laser and RF system (Polaris, Syneron Medical Ltd, Yokneam, Israel), after which 30% experienced at least a 50% improvement and 66% noted at least a 25% improvement, with no reports of pigmentary change. Importantly, patients had skin phototypes ranging from II to IV, though there were no notable differences in efficacy based on skin type.[4]

39.12 Benign Cutaneous Tumors

Laser-resurfacing procedures are effective treatments to smooth benign cutaneous tumors such as syringomas, dermatosis papulosa nigra, and acne keloidalis nuchae, all of which are more prevalent in ethnic groups.

Many treatment modalities, such as dermabrasion, electrodesiccation, and scissor excision, have been tried with success. Recently, CO_2 lasers alone and in combination with trichloroacetic acid have shown good results.[3]

Long-term follow-up is necessary to determine the efficacy of treatment. Because of the depth of the lesion, a complete removal is unlikely without an increased risk of scarring.

It is important for the patient to understand the goal of the procedure, which is to flatten, smooth, or improve the appearance of the lesion and not completely remove it.

Regarding papulosis nigra, although no treatment is needed, they are often of cosmetic concern and are easily removed through scissor excision, electrodesiccation, and laser ablation. When using an ablative laser such as the CO_2, Er:YAG laser, or 532 diode, one must be careful to use a spot size that does not exceed the diameter of the lesion to minimize the risk of collateral thermal damage and hyperpigmentation of the surrounding skin.[3]

39.13 Hair Disorders

39.13.1 Acne Keloidalis Nuchae

This is a chronic condition where we might find firm alopecic keloidal plaques in the posterior region of the scalp.

The commonly used treatment is based on topical steroids, systemic agents (antibiotics, retinoids), surgery, and lasers/light devices, such as Nd:YAG. In the same way, a CO_2 laser in cutting mode is used to excise the tumor below the level of the hair follicles to deep subcutaneous tissue, and the wound is left to heal by second intention.[1]

We want to emphasize changes in hair care practices in our patients for better results, such as reducing anything that creates friction and aggravates papules.

39.13.2 Hypertrichosis

Hypertrichosis has been defined as excessive hair growth anywhere on the body in either males or females, for which hair removal devices have been a topic of interest among aesthetics.[5]

First hair removal technologies (mid-'90s) caused hyperpigmentation, blistering, and scarring in darker-skinned patients.[3]

For the melanin within the hair shaft and follicle to be selectively targeted and destroyed, laser energy should be transmitted unimpeded through the skin toward its target.

On the basis of studies performed by Dr. Brooke, longer pulse durations of 40 ms using the long-pulsed alexandrite laser (Cynosure, Chelmsford, MA) were found to be safer in dark skin and were able to destroy the hair follicle while protecting epidermal melanin; this is possible through thermokinetic selectivity. Current laser hair-removal devices incorporate longer pulse durations and a variety of cooling devices, all of which may allow the safe treatment of dark skin.[3]

With these modifications, laser hair removal is now a successful treatment for hypertrichosis and pseudofolliculitis barbae.

39.14 Conclusion

In this chapter, we have explored energy-based devices, toxins and fillers, and conditons associated with darker skin types. By understanding how best to approach these patients, treating darker skin types can be successfully accomplished.

Bibliographic References

1. Henry M. Cosmetic concerns among ethnic men. *Dermatol Clin.* 2018 Jan;36(1):11–16.
2. Sundaram H, Liew S, Signorini M, Vieira Braz A, Fagien S, Swift A, De Boulle KL, Raspaldo H, Trindade de Almeida AR, Monheit G. Global aesthetics consensus group. Global aesthetics consensus: Hyaluronic acid fillers and botulinum toxin type a-recommendations for combined treatment and optimizing outcomes in diverse patient populations. *Plast Reconstr Surg.* 2016 May;137(5):1410–1423.
3. Jackson BA. Lasers in ethnic skin: A review. *J Am Acad Dermatol.* 2003 Jun;48(6 Suppl):S134–S138.
4. Guss L, Bolton JG, Fabi SG. Combination therapy in skin of color including injectables, laser, and light devices. *Semin Cutan Med Surg.* 2016 Dec;35(4):211–217.
5. Saleh D, Yarrarapu SNS, Cook C. Hypertrichosis. In: *StatPearls* [Internet]. Treasure Island, FL: StatPearls Publishing; 2021 Jan 5.

Part VIII

CHAPTER 40: POST-COVID-19
Where Are We Headed?

Mukta Sachdev

The COVID-19 pandemic has touched each of our lives in some way or another—be it losses—personal, financial, self-realization, and just gratitude to have made it through the past two years in good health.

With the world being thrust at the mercy of a tiny organism over the past couple of years, there are many lessons that the pandemic has taught us.

It has been testing times for both practitioners and patients.

Needs, desires, and patient expectations have changed due to varying reasons, and patient interactions from safety standpoints have been difficult, to say the least, over recent times.

Dermatology—aesthetic dermatology, in particular—is a field that involves a rather close contact with patients. Therefore, at the outset, the priority is to keep both the patient and physician as safe as possible. Notwithstanding, this is something that, as physicians, we have been able to relate to considering the colossal changes that had to be made with patient approach during this pandemic. Eventually, though, as we have witnessed, this involves simply not compromising on precautionary measures, regardless of circumstances.

General measures of wearing masks, keeping the designated workspace and equipment clean, and sanitizing are recommended as per specific guidelines, which may vary from country to country.

Patients with suspected symptoms, however mild, must be evaluated first before proceeding with any skin treatment. The uncertainty with regard to how long the pandemic may last, with the emergence of new variants and waves making their presence felt every few months, confirms that we have to remain vigilant and careful.

Hence, having a structured protocol for all procedures, consultations, and processes based on one's practice is of the essence.

Moving forward, we must remember that we are all still vulnerable with ongoing resurgences and variants resurfacing globally. However, there will always be a certain amount of risk, and minimizing them is key. The lessons learned now should serve as a reminder of what must be followed in the event that we are faced with a similar situation sometime in the future.

Newer treatments and procedures are now suddenly all emerging, and everyone is now motivated to move forward and revive their practice.

There has been an unprecedented interest in the use of skin care cosmeceuticals, lasers and injectables like toxins and fillers are gaining unprecedented popularity, with increased enthusiasm.

One is noticing less fear and concern among patients for these procedures. It is imperative that correct patient selection for all treatments is maintained, as unrealistic expectations and body dysmorphic disorder are still high in cosmetic and aesthetic dermatology patients.

Newer terminologies such as 'proageing', 'immune fitness', 'inflammaging', skin and gut microbiome are all now concepts to introduce a body equilibrium and enhance longevity and quality of life.

Newer triggers like the exposome including blue light and pollution awareness are now part of our daily skin protection professional advice.

The future trend is a proactive approach and a new attitude towards 'ageing beautifully'.

DOI: 10.1201/9780429243769-42

INDEX

Note: Numbers in **bold** indicate a table. Numbers in *italics* indicate a figure.